Cardiac Catheterization

Concepts, Techniques, and Applications

Cardiac Catheterization

Concepts, Techniques, and Applications

Edited by

Barry F. Uretsky, M.D.
H. H. Weinert Professor of Medicine
Director, Cardiac Catheterization Laboratory
University of Texas Medical Branch at Galveston
Galveston, Texas

**Blackwell
Science**

Blackwell Science
Editorial offices:
Commerce Place, 350 Main Street,
  Malden, Massachusetts 02148, USA
Osney Mead, Oxford OX2 0EI, England
25 John Street, London WC1N 2BL, England
23 Ainslie Place, Edinburgh EH3 6AJ, Scotland
54 University Street, Carlton, Victoria 3053,
  Australia

Other Editorial offices:
Arnette Blackwell SA, 224 Boulevard Saint
  Germain, 75007 Paris, France
Blackwell Wissenschafts-Verlag GmbH
  Kurfürstendamm 57, 10707 Berlin, Germany
  Zehetnergasse 6, A-1140 Vienna, Austria

Distributors:

USA
  Blackwell Science, Inc.
  Commerce Place
  350 Main Street
  Malden, Massachusetts 02148
  (Telephone orders: 800-215-1000 or
  617-388-8250; fax orders: 617-388-8270)

Canada
  Copp Clark, Ltd.
  2775 Matheson Blvd. East
  Mississauga, Ontario
  Canada, L4W 4F7
  (Telephone orders: 800-263-4374 or
  905-238-6074)

Australia
  Blackwell Science Pty, Ltd.
  54 University Street
  Carlton, Victoria 3053
  (Telephone orders: 03-9347-0300;
  fax orders: 03-9349-3016)

Outside North America and Australia
  Blackwell Science, Ltd.
  c/o Marston Book Services, Ltd.
  P.O. Box 269

Abingdon
Oxon OX14 4YN
England
(Telephone orders: 44-01235-465500;
fax orders: 44-01235-465555)

The Blackwell Science logo is a trade mark
  of Blackwell Science, Ltd., registered at the
  United Kingdom Trade Marks Registry

Acquisitions: Chris Davis
Development: Kathleen Broderick
Production: Colophon
Manufacturing: Lisa Flanagan
Typeset by G&S Typesetters, Inc.
Printed and bound by Maple Vail
© 1997 by Blackwell Science, Inc.
Printed in the United States of America
97 98 99 00 5 4 3 2 1

All rights reserved. No part of this book may be
  reproduced in any form or by any electronic
  or mechanical means, including information
  storage and retrieval systems, without
  permission in writing from the publisher,
  except by a reviewer who may quote brief
  passages in a review.

**Library of Congress
Cataloging-in-Publication Data**
Cardiac catheterization : concepts, techniques,
  and applications /edited by Barry F. Uretsky.
      p.   cm.
    Includes bibliographical references and
    index.
    ISBN 0-86542-406-3 (alk. paper)
    1. Cardiac catheterization.   I. Uretsky,
    Barry F. [DNLM: 1. Heart Catheterization.
    WG 141.5.C2 C2673 1997]
  RC683.5.C25C384   1997
  616.1′2—DC20
  DNLM/DLC
  for Library of Congress   96-32624
                                                   CIP

To Sybil

CONTENTS

Part II
APPLICATIONS OF CARDIAC CATHETERIZATION IN SPECIFIC DISEASE STATES

Part III
NEWER CATHETER DIAGNOSTIC MODALITIES

Part IV
THERAPEUTIC INTERVENTIONS

CONTRIBUTORS

Richard G. Bach, M.D.
Associate Professor of Internal
  Medicine and Associate Director,
  Coronary Care Unit
St. Louis University Health
  Sciences Center
St. Louis, Missouri

Kenneth Baughman, M.D.
Professor of Medicine
Chief of Cardiology
Johns Hopkins School of Medicine
Baltimore, Maryland

Lee Beerman, M.D.
Professor of Pediatrics
Division of Pediatric Cardiology
Children's Hospital of Pittsburgh
Pittsburgh, Pennsylvania

John D. Carroll, M.D.
Professor, Department
  of Medicine
Director, Interventional
  Cardiology and Cardiac
  Catheterization
Division of Cardiology
University of Colorado Health
  Sciences Center
Denver, Colorado

Andrew P. Chodos, M.D.
Assistant Professor of Medicine
Evans Memorial Department of
  Clinical Research
Department of Medicine
Section of Cardiology
Boston University Medical Center
Boston, Massachusetts

Anthony C. DeFranco, M.D.
Department of Cardiology
The Cleveland Clinic Foundation
Cleveland, Ohio

Bart G. Denys, M.D.
Director, Thibodaux Division
Cardiovascular Institute of the
  South
Thibodaux, Louisiana

David P. Faxon, M.D.
Professor of Medicine
Chief, Division of Cardiology
University of Southern California
  School of Medicine
Los Angeles, California

Michael A. Fifer, M.D.
Associate Professor of Medicine
Director, Coronary Care Unit
Massachusetts General Hospital
Boston, Massachusetts

James A. Goldstein, M.D.
Director, Coronary Care Unit
William Beaumont Hospital
Royal Oak, Michigan

Alan J. Greenfield, M.D.
Professor of Radiology
Tufts University School of
    Medicine
Chief, Cardiovascular and
    Interventional Radiology
New England Medical Center
    Hospital
Boston, Massachusetts

Neil J. Halin, D.O.
Instructor of Radiology
Tufts University School of
    Medicine and
Assistant Radiologist
    Cardiovascular;
    Interventional Radiology
New England Medical Center
    Hospital
Boston, Massachusetts

Howard C. Herrmann, M.D.
Associate Professor of Medicine
Director, Interventional
    Cardiology
University of Pennsylvania Medical
    Center
Philadelphia, Pennsylvania

Alice K. Jacobs, M.D.
Associate Professor of Medicine
Director, Cardiac Catheterization
    Laboratory and Interventional
    Cardiology
Boston University School of
    Medicine
Boston, Massachusetts

Edward K. Kasper, M.D.
Assistant Professor of Medicine
Division of Cardiology
Johns Hopkins School of Medicine
Baltimore, Maryland

Stephen Keim, M.D.
Director, Cardiac
    Electrophysiology Laboratory
Watson Clinic
Lakeland, Florida

Carey D. Kimmelstiel, M.D.
Assistant Professor of Medicine
Associate Director, Adult Cardiac
    Catheterization Laboratory
Tufts University School of
    Medicine and New England
    Medical Center Hospital
Boston, Massachusetts

Marvin A. Konstam, M.D.
Professor of Medicine and
    Radiology
Chief of Cardiology
Departments of Medicine and
    Radiology
Tufts School of Medicine and New
    England Medical Center
Boston, Massachusetts

Peter A. McCullough, M.D.,
    M.P.H.
Chief Clinical Fellow
Division of Cardiology
William Beaumont Hospital
Royal Oak, Michigan

Srinivas Murali, M.D.
Associate Professor of Medicine
Director, Heart Failure/
    Transplantation Section
Division of Cardiology
University of Pittsburgh Medical
    Center
Pittsburgh, Pennsylvania

Jan B. Namyslowski, M.D.
Instructor of Radiology
Department of Radiology
Assistant Radiologist, Cardiovascular and Interventional Radiology
Tufts School of Medicine and New England Medical Center
Boston, Massachusetts

Ira S. Nash, M.D.
Assistant Professor of Medicine
Associate Director, Cardiovascular Institute
The Mount Sinai Medical Center
New York, New York

Steven E. Nissen, M.D.
Vice Chairman
Department of Cardiology
Director, Clinical Cardiology
Director, Coronary Intensive Care Unit
The Cleveland Clinic Foundation
Cleveland, Ohio

Igor F. Palacios, M.D.
Associate Professor of Medicine
Harvard Medical School
Director of Interventional Cardiology
Director of Cardiac Catheterization Laboratories
Massachusetts General Hospital
Boston, Massachusetts

Richard D. Patten, M.D.
Instructor of Radiology
Tufts University School of Medicine
Assistant Radiologist
Cardiovascular and Interventional Radiology
New England Medical Center Hospital
Boston, Massachusetts

Michael Ragosta, M.D., F.A.C.C.
Assistant Professor of Medicine
Cardiovascular Division
University of Virginia Health Sciences Center
Charlottesville, Virginia

Robert D. Rifkin, M.D.
Associate Professor of Medicine
Tufts University School of Medicine
Director, Echocardiography Laboratory
Division of Cardiology
Baystate Medical Center
Springfield, Massachusetts

Marc J. Schweiger, M.D.
Director, Cardiac Catheterization Laboratories
Baystate Medical Center
Springfield, Massachusetts

Chris C. Shaw, Ph.D.
Associate Professor
Department of Radiology
University of Pittsburgh
Pittsburgh, Pennsylvania

E. Murat Tuzcu, M.D.
Department of Cardiology
The Cleveland Clinic Foundation
Cleveland, Ohio

Barry F. Uretsky, M.D.
H. H. Weinert Professor of Medicine
Director, Cardiac Catheterization Laboratory
University of Texas Medical Branch at Galveston
Galveston, Texas

Ronald E. Vlietstra, M.D., Ch.B.,
F.A.C.C.
Clinical Professor of Medicine
University of South Florida
Tampa, Florida and
Clinical Professor of Medicine
University of Florida College of
Medicine
Gainesville, Florida
Cardiologist
Watson Clinic
Lakeland, Florida

Andrew A. Ziskind, M.D.
Associate Professor of Medicine
Director, University of Maryland
Cardiac Network
University of Maryland
Baltimore, Maryland

PREFACE

Cardiologists with a good memory may recall the mystique surrounding cardiac catheterization twenty years ago. At that time it was made clear during training that not everyone was cut out to be an invasive cardiologist. Today catheterization is considered an essential element in a clinical cardiology training program. This book has been written to provide the first level of knowledge in this area. Its approach is primarily practical: to provide the concepts, techniques, and overview of pathologic states studied in the catheterization laboratory. To accomplish this goal, an outstanding group of clinical teachers (all of whom are respected investigators and clinicians) was assembled. They were given the following instruction: Share with the reader that information which you consider essential for a trainee to be considered a competent graduate of your program. Their combined efforts have resulted in a strong basic text on invasive cardiology. We hope that the reader concurs.

The text is divided into four major sections: (1) concepts underlying and diagnostic techniques utilized in the catheterization laboratory, (2) clinical application of these concepts and techniques in various pathologic states, (3) newer intracoronary diagnostic modalities, and (4) therapeutic procedures. By design we have not included chapters on interventional procedures such as balloon angioplasty, nor have we included information on invasive evaluation of arrhythmias. It is our feeling that these areas have grown to such an extent that a cursory discussion in this text would be unsatisfactory to the would-be interventionist and unnecessary to the non-interventional invasivist. We would emphasize, however, that the contents of this book should be considered background material for those who embark on the aforementioned subspecialities.

The reader may wonder why we have included chapters on the intracoronary diagnostic modalities of ultrasound, angioscopy, and angiometry. The answer is that any or all of these techniques may become part of the invasive cardiologist's diagnostic tool kit. Should their use expand beyond therapeutic interventional procedures, so will the group of cardiologists performing them. At the very least, these chapters will provide the reader with the concepts, techniques, and applications of these tools as utilized today. The fourth section describes therapeutic procedures with which all catheterizing physicians should be familiar.

All of the authors are expert practitioners as well as teachers in their respective fields. They were encouraged to present their material as if it were a "chalk talk." They were requested to end the chapter with a group of selected readings. This approach worked fairly well in the early chapters (e.g., Chapter 1, "Pressure, Flow, and Resistance"). In the chapters on specific pathophysiologic states, it became apparent that citations of individual studies in the text might facilitate the reader in exploring the subject further. We left it to the authors as to whether citations have or have not been placed in the chapter body.

To minimize duplication, we have attempted to concentrate each subject in one chapter and refer the reader to it where mentioned elsewhere. There are some small areas that do not totally conform to this approach (e.g., indications for low versus high osmolar contrast media). We have maintained discussions in two chapters because of differences in emphasis or conclusions by the authors despite attempts by the editor to smooth out these differences. Such differences of opinion are probably inevitable in a multi-author book. Where appropriate, such as in the example of angiographic dye, we have left both discussions in place because they are instructive in illuminating current controversies within clinical practice.

From a personal viewpoint, this project has been an enjoyable one. It has afforded me the opportunity to work with an outstanding group of people. Not unexpectedly, I have learned from all of them. This project has also provided me the opportunity to reread texts and articles and review them from an instructional perspective. I am particularly sentimental toward Grossman's first edition of *Cardiac Catheterization,* published in 1974. I read this book many times during fellowship and have continued to refer to it in both teaching and practice situations over the past 17 years. Even at the time of its publication, the book was considered short (and comprehensive). The result was a book with a high "informational specific gravity." At this time we demur (as did Dr. Grossman in his first edition) in stating that our text is "complete." It is likely that no text can be unequivocally considered complete in covering as broad a topic as cardiac catheterization. We have tried vigorously to produce a central core of knowledge that the reader can use to accrete further layers of knowledge over time. We hope that the reader enjoys this task as much as the editor has in putting this book together.

The authors collectively express their appreciation and gratitude to those individuals who helped in the preparation of their chapters and to those individuals who provided the supportive environment to succeed. I would especially like to express my thanks and appreciation to Mrs. Rhonda Oliver, who helped in the organization of the project at its inception in Pittsburgh and carried it through to its conclusion in Galveston. I also express my appreciation to Ms. Darla Webb and Ms. Avis Morgan, who provided invaluable secretarial support and to Mr. Lee Rose and Ms. Joann Aaron for creating the superb illustrations necessary to complete this project at Galveston.

Barry F. Uretsky, M.D.
Galveston, Texas

Notice
The indications and dosages of all drugs in this book have been recommended in the medical literature and conform to the practices of the general medical community. The medications described do not necessarily have specific approval by the Food and Drug Administration for use in the diseases and dosages for which they are recommended. The package insert for each drug should be consulted for use and dosage as approved by the FDA. Because standards for usage change, it is advisable to keep abreast of revised recommendations, particularly those concerning new drugs.

I

CONCEPTS AND TECHNIQUES

1

PRESSURE, FLOW, AND RESISTANCE

Ira S. Nash
Michael A. Fifer

O UR UNDERSTANDING OF cardiovascular pathophysiology, as well as our assessment of the state of health of a particular individual, rests on the accurate determination of key indices of cardiovascular performance. This chapter is devoted to the theory and practice of measuring (1) the pressure of blood in various locations in the circulation and (2) the flow of blood through the circulation, allowing for calculation of (3) the resistance offered to that flow. For each of these measures, particular attention will be paid to techniques required to obtain consistently reliable clinical data in the cardiac catheterization laboratory.

Pressure

Theoretical Background

Pressure is defined as force per unit area. It is a measure of how vigorously a fluid presses against the wall of the vessel containing it. Pressure may be expressed in metric units as dynes per cm^2, but is more familiarly expressed in units of millimeters of mercury (mm Hg).* A pressure that does not change appreciably over time, like that in a balloon or bicycle tire, is said to be static. A pressure that varies from one moment to another, and whose fluctuations are of interest, like that in the left ventricle, is a dynamic pressure, and the fluctuations themselves are termed *pressure waves.*

Dynamic pressures place greater demands on the devices used to measure and record them than do static pressures. A simple tire pressure gauge is adequate to measure the static pressure in a bicycle tire. It cannot, however, respond rapidly to changes in pressure; it must be reset and reapplied to make another measurement. In contrast, capturing the changes in pressure over time (reproducing the form of a pressure wave) is the essence of physiologic recording systems; a single "snapshot" of the pressure at a given instant is of no clinical value.

Fourier Analysis

Before considering the elements of a system needed to capture, display, and record dynamic pressures, we must examine the nature of pressure waves more closely. A pressure wave, no matter how complex its shape, may be described mathematically as the sum of sine waves of successively higher frequencies (Fig 1-1). This is the Fourier principle; use of this powerful concept is called Fourier analysis. In the case of repetitive waveforms (as are observed in the cardiovascular system), where the basic pattern of pressure occurs over and over again, the frequency with which the basic pattern repeats is termed the *fundamental frequency.* In this example, the fundamental frequency is the heart rate. Frequency is measured in units of repetitions or "cycles" per second, or Hertz (Hz). A pressure wave from a patient with a heart rate of 60 beats per minute has a fundamental frequency of 60 cycles per minute or 1 cycle per second or 1 Hz. The higher frequencies, which, when added to the wave at the

---

*The conversion between dynes per cm^2 and mm Hg can be derived if one calculates the pressure exerted by a column of mercury 10 mm high, with a base of one square cm:

$$\text{Force} = \text{Force}$$
$$(\text{Pressure})(\text{Area}) = (\text{Mass})(\text{Acceleration})$$
$$(\text{Pressure})(\text{Area}) = (\text{Density})(\text{Volume})(\text{Acceleration})$$
$$(10 \text{ mm Hg})(1 \text{ cm}^2) = (13.6 \text{ g/cm}^3)(1 \text{ cm}^3)(9.8 \text{ m/sec}^2)$$
$$10 \text{ mm Hg} = (133.3 \text{ g-m/sec}^2)(100\text{cm/m})(1/\text{cm}^2)$$
$$\text{mm Hg} = (1333 \text{ g-cm/sec}^2)(1/\text{cm}^2)$$
$$\text{mm Hg} = 1333 \text{ dynes/cm}^2$$

where 13.6 g/cm^3 is the density of mercury and 9.8 m/sec^2 is the acceleration due to gravity.

Figure 1-1 The lower panel shows three sine waves of increasing frequency and decreasing amplitude. Harmonic 1 is equivalent to the fundamental frequency. The upper panel demonstrates increasing proximity of the sum of the sine waves to the straight diagonal line with the addition of higher harmonics. The Fourier principle states that any curve can be built up in this way through the addition of sine waves of increasing frequency. (*Adapted from Nichols WW, O'Rourke MF, eds. McDonald's blood flow in arteries. 3rd ed. Philadelphia: Lea & Febiger, 1990:272.*)

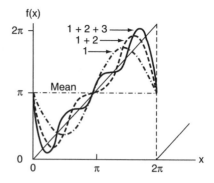

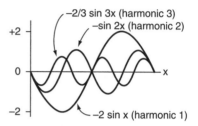

fundamental frequency, recreate the detailed pressure waveform, are called higher *harmonics.** These higher harmonics occur at frequencies that are multiples of the fundamental frequency. In the previous example, in which the fundamental frequency was 1 Hz, the second harmonic would have a frequency of 2 Hz, the third 3 Hz, and so on.

Because a complex pressure waveform can be considered as a sum of simpler sine waves, the task of accurately reproducing a complex pressure wave is equivalent to reproducing a pressure wave at the fundamental frequency and a sufficient number of the higher harmonics to define the details of the wave contour. Just as a dynamic pressure is more difficult to measure than a static one, higher frequency harmonics are more difficult to measure than lower frequency harmonics. This is because, by definition, higher frequency harmonics require the measuring system to adjust more rapidly to the fluctuations in pressure. In general, a recording system able to capture up to the tenth harmonic produces a waveform of sufficiently high fidelity for all clinical applications. The actual frequency of these higher harmonics (or the *frequency content* of the pressure wave) depends on the fundamental frequency. For example, at a heart

---

*This is a familiar concept in music, in which the tone of a note corresponds to a its fundamental frequency. The sounds of different musical instruments are distinguishable from each other because each instrument contributes a unique set of higher harmonics to the fundamental frequency. Thus, the "same" note can be played on a clarinet or a violin, but the ear can identify which instrument was used.

rate (fundamental frequency) of 60 beats per minute (1 Hz), the tenth harmonic has a frequency of 10 Hz; at a heart rate of 90 beats per minute or 1.5 Hz, the tenth harmonic has a frequency of 15 Hz. Therefore, a recording system capable of capturing 10 harmonics and producing a high fidelity record at low heart rates may not be able to do so at high heart rates.

Frequency Response

What, then, determines the capability of a measuring and recording system to reproduce these pressure waves? Pressure measuring devices depend on the physical movement or deformation of a flexible element or membrane in response to changes in pressure. This movement is then detected and, in general, amplified before it is displayed and recorded. For example, in the case of the tire pressure gauge, an indicator stick extends out of the gauge a distance proportional to the tire pressure, which it displays along a graduated scale.

In systems designed to measure *dynamic* pressure, there must be some self-restoring capacity to the flexible element, so that after it moves or bends in response to a change in pressure, it can reset automatically and respond to the next fluctuation. Like a spring-loaded supermarket scale, which must respond promptly to adding or removing weight and automatically come back to registering zero when the load is removed, an idealized pressure sensor should respond rapidly and proportionally to changes in pressure and come back to its baseline position when the pressure wave has passed. Any physical system characterized by movement in response to an applied stimulus and a tendency to restore itself back to its original condition, if stimulated, tends to oscillate. This behavior can be described by considering two parameters: the natural frequency and the damping coefficient.

The *natural* or *"resonant" frequency* (ω_0) is the characteristic frequency of these oscillations and is dependent only on the physical characteristics of the system, not the nature of the stimulus. For example, a violin string, if plucked, does not simply return to its original position, but vibrates, oscillating back and forth around its original position. This oscillation defines a particular tone (it will occur at a given frequency) regardless of how hard the string is plucked.*
A violin string vibrates at higher frequency if the tension on the string is increased, thereby increasing the force necessary to displace it. Likewise, pressure sensors that have stiffer sensing elements have higher resonant frequencies than systems built around less rigid sensors.

The *damping coefficient* (β) is a dimensionless ratio that describes what happens to these oscillations over time. In physical systems, in which friction always

---

*Plucking the violin string harder, by pulling it farther away from its rest position before letting go, changes the loudness of the tone, which is a function of the amplitude of the oscillations, but not its frequency.

impedes movement, oscillations decrease in amplitude over time. The plucked violin string does not vibrate forever; a child on a playground swing slows to a stop without an occasional push. The rapidity with which the oscillation diminishes is described by the damping coefficient. In underdamped systems ($\beta<1$), the amplitude of oscillations diminishes exponentially over time. In overdamped systems ($\beta>1$), there is so much frictional opposition to movement that there are no true oscillations (or overshoots of the equilibrium position) in response to a perturbation. Rather, the system returns relatively slowly to its original position. Plucking an overdamped violin string (imagine a string suspended in a viscous fluid like honey) would result in the string slowly returning to its original position without ever passing it. When β equals 1, the system is critically damped. A critically damped system also does not oscillate. Rather, it returns to equilibrium in a fashion similar to an overdamped system, but does so as fast as possible without overshooting the starting point.

We are now in a position to examine more closely how the characteristics of pressure waves interact with the nature of physical recording systems. The ability of a recording system to reproduce pressure waves to which it is exposed depends on β, as well as how the frequency content of the wave compares with ω_0. This complex interaction is best shown graphically in the form of a Bode plot (Fig 1-2). The x-axis is frequency relative to ω_0, and the y-axis is the ratio of the magnitude of the output signal (the "recording") to the input signal (the pressure wave). As can be seen, for all frequencies well below ω_0, the ratio of output/input is 1 regardless of the damping coefficient. This means that a low-frequency sine wave could be reproduced exactly by such a system. It also implies that the very low frequency components of a more complex wave would also be reproduced with high fidelity. The frequency response of the system is said to be "flat" in this range. In underdamped systems, as the frequency of the input signal increases, or, equivalently, as one considers the fate of higher frequency components of a complex wave, it is apparent that the input gets progressively amplified (output/input > 1) as ω_0 is approached. The selective amplification of input frequencies at or near ω_0 is termed *resonance*. Input frequencies much above ω_0 are attenuated by the measuring system (output/input < 1). Input waves of different frequencies are also transmitted with different time or phase delays.

These phenomena have important implications. Because different component frequencies of the same complex pressure wave are amplified and delayed nonuniformly, the output wave is distorted. This problem is exaggerated when the frequency content of the pressure wave is high (e.g., at high heart rates), the natural frequency of the recording system is low, or the damping coefficient is much less than 1. Conversely, systems that offer high natural frequencies capture many more of the higher harmonics without systematic distortion and thereby produce recordings of much greater fidelity.

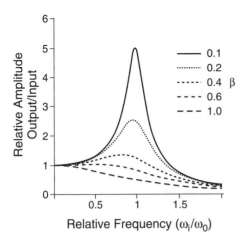

Figure 1-2 Bode plot demonstrating resonance amplification of input frequencies near the resonant frequency, ω_0 and attenuation of input frequencies above ω_0, plotted for various values of β. Note that when β equals 0.6, the frequency response is "flat" out to the highest relative frequency.

Practical Considerations

Transducers

It is not a simple matter to design practical pressure recording systems that optimize natural frequency and damping. The systems in daily use in catheterization laboratories represent effective trade-offs among frequency response, damping, cost, and durability. At the center of the recording system is the pressure transducer or manometer. In general terms, a transducer is any device that converts energy from one form to another. For example, a photovoltaic cell, which converts light to electricity, is a transducer. The pressure transducer transforms mechanical energy into an electrical signal. This is done through the use of an electrical strain gauge.

Within the strain gauge, a thin but relatively rigid metal foil, called the transducer membrane, moves or bends slightly in response to the pressure wave. The membrane is physically connected to an electrical circuit, and its movement compresses or stretches thin wires that have a known voltage applied to them. Because the resistance of a wire changes in direct proportion to how much it is stretched, the current passing through the circuit corresponds to the degree to which the wires attached to the membrane have been stretched. This, in turn, is directly proportional to the displacement of the transducer membrane, which is proportional to the pressure applied against the membrane. In this way, an electrical signal directly proportional to pressure is produced.

It is critically important that the response of such a strain gauge transducer be *linear* over the range of pressures that might be anticipated. That is, if the pressure, for example, increases by 25%, so must the electrical output. This proportionality depends on the linear change in resistance in wires under tension, which holds true only for small amounts of stretch. It follows then that the linearity of the strain gauge depends on allowing only small movements of the transducer membrane in response to pressure. This action, in turn, demands small displacement transducers with stiff sensory elements.

Stiff transducer membranes are desirable not only for optimizing amplitude linearity, but because they have higher natural frequencies as well. Why not, then, make transducer membranes as rigid as possible? The reason is that, as we have seen, the electrical signal from the transducer is proportional to the actual movement of the membrane. The more rigid the membrane, the less it moves. The less it moves, the lower the output. If a signal becomes too faint, it may be lost in the electrical "noise" of the circuit. Therefore, the greater the transducer *sensitivity*, or the ability to detect small fluctuations in pressure, the lower its natural frequency. Because it is desirable to have all of the attributes of linearity, high frequency response, high sensitivity, and good signal-noise ratio, a practical transducer design must strike a balance among all of these characteristics.

Pressure Recording Systems

The strain gauge transducer is not the only element of the pressure measuring and recording system; rather, it defines the transition between physical pressure waves transmitted to the transducer and the analog electronic representations of those waves. The pressure wave is conveyed to the transducer through a column of fluid contained in a catheter and, in most laboratories, an interposed length of "pressure tubing." It is the oscillatory tendency of this *combination* of fluid column and transducer membrane that determines ω_0 and β for the pressure measurement system.

The natural frequency of the system can be maximized by taking steps that facilitate the movement of very small volumes of fluid back and forth in the catheter in response to pressure waves.* These steps include minimizing the combined length of the catheter and the pressure tubing to minimize the volume (and mass) of fluid that must be moved. Using tubing and catheters with as large a diameter as possible also maximizes the natural frequency of the system, because the same volume displacement at the level of the transducer can be achieved with a smaller longitudinal movement of fluid.

The catheter and tubing should also be as stiff as possible. That is, the catheter and tubing should resist expansion radially in response to transient increases in pressure. The combined distensibility of the transducer membrane

---

*It is important to distinguish the movement of very small volumes of fluid necessary to deform the transducer membrane from frank fluid flow through the catheter. The former is a consequence of the transient pressure wave traveling through a closed system constituted by the column of fluid and the transducer. The latter, which is not under consideration here, is bulk flow, which occurs as a consequence of pressure differences from one end of a catheter to another.

and the catheter and tubing connected to it can be expressed quantitatively as the *capacitance* of the system, defined as $\Delta V/\Delta P$, or the change in volume divided by the change in pressure. A system of low capacitance has a higher natural frequency than one of higher capacitance.

A potential source of higher than desirable capacitance is the presence of air bubbles, which are readily compressible. The expansion and contraction of air bubbles in response to pressure waves act to lower the natural frequency of the entire recording system, just as an excessively elastic catheter or flaccid transducer membrane would. Several investigators have reported significant gains in the frequency response of catheter transducer recording systems through the use of techniques that remove air bubbles that are too small to see. These techniques include the use of detergent agents to reduce the ability of bubbles to cling to the inner surfaces of catheters, the use of boiled saline to reduce the content of microbubbles, and the use of carbon dioxide flushes to rid the fluid path of undissolved gasses.

Strict adherence to the principle of reducing system capacitance maximizes the natural frequency of the recording system. Because friction plays a role in all physical systems, however, the overall ability of the system to reproduce pressure waves with high fidelity also depends on the damping coefficient. The damping coefficient not only helps describe the resonance behavior of the system, but also governs the actual (observed) *damped* natural frequency (ω_D), rather than the ideal, undamped natural frequency (ω_0), according to the formula

$$\omega_D = \omega_0 \sqrt{1 - \beta^2}$$

Thus, minimizing damping allows the system to operate as closely as possible to the theoretical maximum natural frequency. As Figure 1-2 demonstrates, however, very low damping also causes increased resonance amplification at relatively lower frequencies. Attempts to increase the damping coefficient in an effort to minimize resonance amplification results in diminishing the natural frequency.

It is therefore necessary to strike a balance between keeping the damping coefficient low, to operate near the theoretical maximum of resonant frequency, and keeping the damping coefficient high, so that most of the physiologically relevant frequencies are not significantly amplified or attenuated by the fluid-transducer system. In practical terms, most fluid-filled catheter systems are highly underdamped. A damping coefficient of approximately 0.6 to 0.7 is considered ideal. In this range, there is minimal resonance amplification of frequencies relatively near the natural frequency, and the observed (damped) natural frequency is close enough to the ideal (undamped) that a well-designed system will be able to capture the physiologically relevant information with an acceptable amount of resonance distortion. Put another way, a damping co-efficient in this range maximizes the flat portion of the system's frequency response.

Because damping is a measure of the internal frictional losses in the system, it can be increased by design changes that make it more difficult for fluid in the catheter to quickly move back and forth in response to rapid changes in pressure. Filling the catheter and pressure tubing with a fluid that is more viscous than saline, such as x-ray contrast material, is a common technique. Other commonly employed techniques to "reduce resonance," such as the use of smaller diameter catheters or the introduction of a small air bubble, *appear* to have a similar effect as well. It is important to recognize, however, that these latter maneuvers do not work only by increasing the damping coefficient. Rather, they simultaneously lower the natural frequency of the system enough that the higher frequency components of the pressure wave are attenuated rather than amplified. It is to be expected, then, that such techniques lead to the loss of physiologically relevant information in the pressure signal. It is much more desirable to have a more underdamped system with a high enough natural frequency that the high frequency components of the pressure wave still fall in the range of minimal resonance amplification. Only in this way can all of the high-frequency detail in the pressure wave be captured (Fig 1-3).

Once a catheter transducer system has been designed and assembled according to the principles outlined here, it is important to actually measure the damping coefficient and the natural frequency to determine whether they meet performance standards. Conceptually, the most straightforward way to test the system is to measure how well it reproduces input pressure waves of known amplitude and frequency. This can be done by placing the tip of the catheter into a test chamber that has a pressure signal generator. Signal generators are able to produce sine wave pressure signals of varying frequency. By gradually increasing the frequency of the input signal and recording the system output, it can be directly determined which frequencies are transmitted without distortion, which are amplified, and which are attenuated.

An alternative method that does not require a signal generator is the *pop test*, in which the response of the system to an abrupt change in pressure is analyzed. The name comes from a popular method of causing an abrupt change in pressure through the "popping" of an inflated rubber membrane (or surgical glove) above a fluid-filled syringe to which the test catheter is attached. Using a sphygmomanometer bulb, the fluid-filled syringe is pressurized and, with the recorder running, the rubber membrane is burst. To avoid a transient increase in pressure, the membrane can be ruptured by the application of a flame (or match) rather than by stabbing it with a blade or needle. The response of the system to the sudden fall in pressure in the syringe includes some "transients," or fluctuations, around the lower equilibrium pressure before the

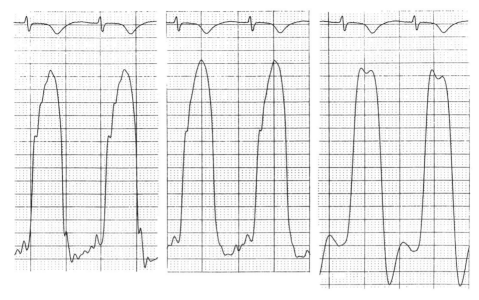

Figure 1-3   Three left ventricular pressure tracings taken from the same patient within minutes of each other. The first panel was recorded with the fluid-filled catheter filled with saline. Note the resonance phenomena, most apparent during mid diastole and the systolic upstroke. The second panel, recorded with relatively viscous x-ray contrast material in the catheter, demonstrates less resonance, characteristic of a higher β. The third panel shows the effects of a small air bubble in the catheter. In this case, ω_0 is markedly diminished, and resonance occurs at a much lower frequency. Note the loss of definition of the shape of the left ventricular pressure waveform because of attenuation of higher frequency components.

pressure settles out at a new constant value. The damping coefficient is calculated by taking the ratio of the magnitude of successive peaks, and applying the formula

$$\beta = \sqrt{\frac{\ln^2 (x_{n+1} / x_n)}{\pi^2 + \ln^2 (x_{n+1} / x_n)}}$$

where ln is the natural logarithm (logarithm base e) and x_{n+1} and x_n are the magnitudes of the overshoot in the pressure recording on successive oscillations (Fig 1-4). The actual or damped natural frequency of the recording system can be determined directly as the inverse of the period between successive peaks. The undamped natural frequency can then be calculated.

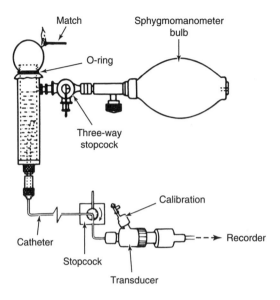

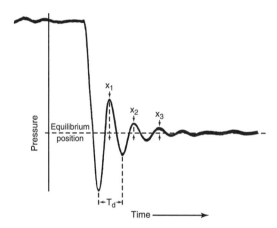

Figure 1-4 The upper panel is a schematic diagram of the apparatus needed for a "pop test." The syringe, into which the catheter is inserted, is pressurized with the sphygmomanometer bulb. The pressure is released instantaneously by holding a lighted match to the rubber membrane atop the syringe. The transient pressure response is plotted in the lower panel and demonstrates resonant oscillations around the equilibrium position from which the resonant frequency and damping coefficient can be calculated. (*Adapted from Nichols WW, O'Rourke MF,* eds. McDonald's blood flow in arteries. 3rd ed. Philadelphia: Lea & Febiger, 1990:148.)

Pressure System Components

We now turn to a discussion of the actual systems in use in cardiac catheterization laboratories, and how they can be optimized to obtain accurate physiologic information. If we trace the path of the pressure wave from the patient to the paper on which the tracing is recorded, the first element to be considered is the *catheter*. The characteristics of the catheter that have an impact on its ability to transmit pressure signals are largely governed by clinical considerations. For example, although it is desirable to have short catheters to obtain accurate pressure signals, catheter length is dictated by the necessity to reach various cardiac chambers from the standard sites of arterial or venous access in the groin or arm. Likewise, the diameter of the catheter is often chosen to be as small as possible to minimize vascular trauma and only large enough to allow for an adequate rate of infusion of x-ray contrast and to provide enough structural integrity to manipulate the catheter and prevent twisting and breakage. Trade-offs are also made in the selection of catheter material to provide enough flexibility to assure the safe passage of the catheter through the circulation while minimizing catheter capacitance.

The catheter is connected to a *manifold* containing several stopcocks, allowing the operator to manipulate the catheter, flush the catheter with saline, inject radio-opaque contrast material, or measure pressure without the need to disconnect and reconnect the catheter to separate lines. The manifold can be connected to the pressure transducer in either of two ways. Some laboratories use disposable pressure transducers, which are mounted directly on the manifold. This has the advantage of minimizing the length of the fluid column. More commonly, the manifold is connected to "off-table" transducers via a length of flexible, nondistensible pressure tubing. This system allows the reuse of transducers, but exacts a penalty in the form of a longer fluid column, which may diminish the natural frequency of the system. Regardless of how the transducer is mounted relative to the manifold, it must be balanced, leveled, and calibrated to function properly.

Balancing an electrical strain gauge transducer refers to the process whereby the electrical circuit to which the transducer membrane is attached is adjusted so that the voltage across the circuit registers zero (or baseline) when the pressure to which it is exposed is the zero reference pressure. Such adjustments are made at the level of the electronic amplifier to which the transducer is connected, rather than by physically modifying the transducer itself.

Because the pressure signal is being transmitted to the transducer through a column of fluid and the fluid column has mass, if the transducer is too low, some of the weight of that fluid is sensed by the transducer and a positive or added pressure results. If the transducer is too high, the fluid has a tendency to drain away from the transducer. This is reflected in a negative or diminished pressure. To minimize these effects, the zero reference is taken to be atmospheric pressure at the level of the mid-chest, with the patient supine.

In the case of off-table transducers, *leveling*, or adjusting the height of the transducers so that the transducer membrane is at mid-chest, can be done by measuring the anterior-posterior diameter of the patient's chest, using a graduated caliper designed for this purpose. Placing the transducers at half of the measured value above the level of the catheterization table assures their placement at mid-chest. Alternatively, the same location can be closely approximated by utilizing a carpenter's level placed against the patient at the mid-chest level and adjusting the height of the transducers directly.

In laboratories where the transducers are mounted directly on the stopcock manifold, the level of the transducer cannot be fixed. In this configuration, the reference pressure is established through the use of a "zero line," which is a fluid-filled length of pressure tubing that runs from the transducer to another manifold, open to atmospheric pressure, mounted at the mid-chest level off the sterile field. The height of this second manifold is established through the use of the graduated calipers or carpenter's level, as discussed.

Balancing and leveling the transducer assure that the baseline for subsequent measurements is zero, so that there is no "offset" in the recordings. *Calibrating* the transducer assures that "gain" in the transducer is properly adjusted, so that a particular voltage output can be reliably interpreted as representing a particular physical pressure. This is done by presenting the transducer with a known pressure (relative to atmospheric) and adjusting the transducer output accordingly. This pressure reference can be a mercury manometer (the absolute standard), inflated to a known pressure, such as 100 mm Hg. Some laboratories rely on nonmercury manometer calibration reference standards, but it is important that these devices themselves be calibrated against a mercury standard on a regular basis. Once a known pressure signal is applied, the output of the transducer is adjusted so that it registers the appropriate value on the paper or screen display. Once the calibration to a given pressure is performed, it is important to rebalance the transducer against zero. If adjustments of the zero are needed, then it should be recalibrated against the positive standard. Several iterations of progressively smaller adjustments may be required to assure a stable zero baseline and proper calibration.

The linearity of the system can and should be checked after it is properly calibrated. Graduated, known pressures can be applied and the output examined. If, for example, the system is properly zeroed and calibrated against a reference pressure of 100 mm Hg, then an input reference pressure of 50 mm Hg should produce an output signal of half the magnitude. If the system fails to behave in this way, the transducer should be replaced.

The main functions of the electronic equipment that connects the transducers to the visual displays are to amplify and filter the incoming signal. *Amplification* is the increase in amplitude of a signal and is required because the voltage produced by the transducer is quite small. In theory, this amplification is no different from a home stereo system that increases on the relatively small voltage coming from the stylus of a phonograph record before the signal can be used to "drive" the speakers and produce sounds. Like home stereo systems, modern catheterization laboratory recording systems are increasingly built around digital instead of analog signals.*

Filtering refers to the selective rejection, in this case by electronic means, of certain frequencies in the input signal. Because the input signal to the amplifier is not the actual pressure wave but rather the electronic representation of that wave coming from the transducer, it contains "noise" resulting from unavoidable imperfections in the transducer as well as from interference from other electronic signals, such as standard 60-Hz AC power. An analog electrical filter is constructed using the same theoretical framework discussed previously in the context of the frequency response of catheter manometer systems. Namely, an electrical circuit is designed that itself has a chosen frequency response. Passage of the transducer signal through such a circuit results in attenuation of frequencies significantly above a given value, so that the circuit acts as a low pass filter.

In digital systems, filtering is achieved, in part, through control of the rate at which the incoming signal is sampled to generate the sequence of numbers that represents it. For example, at a "sampling frequency" of 100 Hz, the transducer signal is transformed into a sequence of numbers that represents the voltage in that signal at successive moments in time, each separated by 1/100 second, or 10 msec. It can be shown that sampling a signal in this way does not capture any information that has a frequency of greater than one half the sampling frequency. Put another way, to reproduce a signal with a frequency content of N Hz requires a sampling frequency of 2N Hz. One can take advantage of this by setting the sampling frequency in the digital filter high enough to capture the anticipated frequency content of physiologic waveforms but low enough to "reject" high-frequency noise.

We have now traced the path of the pressure wave through the catheter and explored how it interacts with the catheter, tubing, and transducer to emerge as an electrical signal. This electrical signal, in turn, is then processed to yield a filtered and amplified signal that may be displayed in a number of different ways. The most familiar form of display is a cathode-ray tube (CRT), or "television" screen. In older, analog systems, the amplified transducer voltage is used to direct a focused beam of electrons onto a phosphorescent screen. The variable voltage controls the excursion of the beam up and down while the beam is

---

*Analog signals are so named because the electrical voltage varies continuously in a fashion analogous to the fluctuations of some physical measurement, in this case, pressure. In digital systems, the signal is converted to a sequence of numbers that correspond to the values of the input variable at closely spaced intervals of time.

"swept" across the screen from left to right at a constant rate. The net result is the visual reproduction of the pressure waveform in a bright line trace on a dark background. The scale of the display can be selected from a few standard options (which is equivalent to amplifying the signal further by a known amount) so that the vertical extent of the screen can represent, for example, 40 mm Hg, 100 mm Hg, 200 mm Hg, or 400 mm Hg.

More modern monitor displays bear more resemblance to the display monitors of computers than they do to analog oscilloscopes. As with a computer, a digital image is reproduced by specifying what should appear at each point on the monitor screen.* This allows for much greater control over the presentation of the image. Rather than just showing a glowing green trace against a dark background, these monitors can present several waveforms using a range of colors. They can also maintain an image on the screen, rather than have it fade gradually as the tracer beam moves along. This allows for a bright, sharp screenful of data that can be overwritten continuously by new information. The use of digital techniques also allows for the display of mixed data on the same screen, so that pressure tracings, text, alarms, timers, and fluoroscopic images can all be presented simultaneously.

The simplest way to create permanent records of pressure waveforms is to generate a paper copy. Analog *printers* are required to do this function. Like the electronic amplifiers and display monitors, analog printers are being replaced by digital equipment. In an analog printer, also called a strip chart recorder, a printing element moves up and down a continuous paper strip in response to a variable voltage input that is proportional to the pressure of clinical interest. The actual printing element in an analog strip chart recorder can be an inked pen or a heated pointer that creates a dark line when it is applied to heat-sensitive or "thermal" paper. The advantage of the pen-based recorder is that inexpensive, conventional paper rolls can be used, rather than relatively expensive thermal paper. Pen-based recorders, however, tend to be messy and more difficult to maintain than thermal printers.

More modern, digital printers work according to the same principles that govern the operation of computer laser printers and fax machines. The printer is "told" what the value of the pressure waveform is at each point in time and applies a tiny dot of ink to the paper at the appropriate location. By having the ability to apply very small dots (modern laser printers achieve more than 600 dots per inch), the spatial resolution of the tracing is improved, and the waveform appears much sharper on the page than it would have had it been inscribed by a pen or thermal printing element. In addition to sharper lines, dig-

---

*Although the image on a computer monitor, like the oscilloscope, is ultimately produced by an electron beam hitting a phosphorescent screen, the beam is rapidly swept across the screen in a regular scanning pattern, "hitting" every point on it many times per second.

ital printers also offer the advantage of being capable of printing annotations on the paper along with the pressure waveforms. For example, pressure reference lines of constant value can be printed, along with their labels (10 mm Hg, 20 mm Hg, etc.), as well as waveform labels and user-generated comments identifying a concurrent clinical event ("inspiration," "Valsalva," etc.). Finally, such printers have few moving parts, which makes maintenance easier, and can use inexpensive paper that can be "Z-folded" for easy storage.

Digital representation of pressure waveforms offers the opportunity to replace paper recordings as the primary form of data archiving. With waveforms transformed into sequences of numbers, the numbers themselves, rather than the "pictures" they represent, can be stored. *Digital storage* is inexpensive and also allows for direct computer-based analysis of pressure waveforms, such as the calculation of valvular gradients. In addition, digital storage provides the capability to reproduce the pressure waveforms "from memory" without any degradation in the quality of the tracing. It then becomes possible, for example, to include pressure tracings in the clinical procedure record, to transmit those waveforms to distant facilities via computer networks, and to examine them simultaneously at multiple workstations scattered throughout a hospital.

Sources of Error

Potential sources of error in pressure measurement may be grouped into three broad categories: errors made in setting up systems, the changes in system characteristics over time, and effects incurred by the movement of catheters.

Errors in system set-up are the most straightforward to consider. The interposition of extra lengths of tubing and stopcocks should be avoided. Extra tubing decreases the natural frequency of the system. Stopcocks are problematic because they can harbor small air bubbles, which may be very difficult to detect and purge. In addition, the abrupt change in diameter of the fluid column brought about by passage through a stopcock degrades the transmission of the pressure wave by setting up wave reflections. The transducer itself must also be incorporated into the recording system with close attention to flushing out all air bubbles. In addition, failure to properly balance, level, and calibrate the transducer leads to spurious results. Specifically, if the transducer (or zero reference) is mounted higher than the mid-chest level, the pressure recorded will be artifactually low; if mounted too low, the pressure will appear high.

A potential source of a decline in system performance during a catheterization procedure is transducer drift. *Drift* refers to a slow change in transducer output in response to a constant input. This means that apparent differences in pressure collected at two points in time may be falsely attributed to a change in clinical information rather than to system error. Further, if a comparison between two simultaneous pressures is being performed, as would be the case in the evaluation of stenotic valvular lesions, disparities in the rate or extent of drift in the two transducers may lead to spurious conclusions about the relationship of those pressures. For these reasons, it is important to periodically check the zero of the transducers in use.

Another source of diminished system performance during a catheterization is the the deposition of fibrin on the inner surface of the catheter. Even a small layer of material can lower the effective internal diameter of the catheter, causing a decline in the natural frequency. Finally, the risk of introduction of air bubbles into the system must be guarded against throughout the procedure. Although proper flushing of the catheter prevents the routine changing of catheters from introducing bubbles into the recording system (and the patient), bubbles may still be introduced into "closed" systems if the associated sources of saline flush and radiocontrast are themselves not completely bubble-free.

The third source of error in pressure measurements from fluid-filled catheter manometer systems is *catheter movement artifact*. Because the heart is in constant motion, any catheter in the heart or central circulation is likely to move as well. As a consequence of its mass, the fluid in the catheter has inertia. That is, the fluid in the catheter resists the motion of the catheter and the two elements do not move in perfect step with one another, which leads to relative motion of the fluid in the catheter.* This phenomenon causes a positive pressure wave when the catheter is accelerated toward its tip and a negative pressure wave when it is accelerated toward its hub.

Catheter impact artifact occurs when a fluid-filled catheter hits up against something, such as the wall of the ventricle or a leaflet of a heart valve. In this case, the impact causes the catheter to vibrate, or "ring" in a fashion analogous to the ringing of a struck wine glass or plucked violin string. It is a pure resonance phenomenon and generates oscillations in the pressure recording at the damped natural frequency of the system.

End-hole pressure artifact is caused by the orientation of the catheter in relation to the flow of blood. The transmission of pressure waves in the circulation is accompanied by a large, pulsatile flow of blood, which has both potential energy reflected in its pressure and kinetic energy associated with its movement. As the blood interacts with a catheter, some of the kinetic energy is dissipated as some of the fluid "stops" at the open end of the catheter. This causes a local increase in pressure, which results in apparently higher pressures being recorded from end-hole catheters that point "upstream" instead of "downstream." The absolute magnitude of this effect is dependent on the velocity of blood flow, but is small enough to be safely ignored in clinical practice.

Close attention to the quality of the pressure waveforms and the magnitude of the measured pressures is an essential part of the quality control needed to

---

*More precisely, the fluid resists the acceleration, or change in motion, of the catheter.

assure accurate tracings. Loss of fine detail in a pressure waveform should alert the physician to search for air bubbles; check the connections among the catheter, stopcocks, manifold, and transducer; and flush the catheter and pressure tubing. An unexpectedly high or low pressure should prompt a rebalancing of the transducer and reassessment of the height of the transducers or zero reference line. Any comparison among pressures, either at the same location at two points in time (e.g., after administration of a drug or as part of an experimental protocol) or at different locations simultaneously, should be preceded by confirmation of the zero reference. Transducers should be calibrated on a daily basis (for reusable, off-table ones) or prior to each case (for disposable ones).

Micromanometer Catheters

With proper attention to the aforementioned considerations, fluid-filled catheter manometer systems are reliable for obtaining the pressure waveforms needed for clinical decision making. There are, however, situations that require a higher standard of waveform fidelity than can be achieved easily with these systems. In a wide variety of research applications, the distortions caused by resonance, subtle changes in system performance over time, and catheter movement are unacceptable. In these settings, fluid-filled catheter manometer systems have generally been supplanted by micromanometer catheters (Fig 1-5).

As the name implies, micromanometer catheters contain very small pressure transducers that are mounted on the catheters themselves. The transducers are connected to the amplifiers and recording devices through wires that run the length of the catheter. By virtue of their small size and inherent stiffness, these transducers have very high resonant frequencies. In addition, the pressure is converted into an electrical signal inside the circulation, eliminating distortion due to the column of fluid in the catheter and tubing. The superb frequency response comes at the cost of a markedly diminished sensitivity, so that the electrical signal produced by these devices is very small and requires

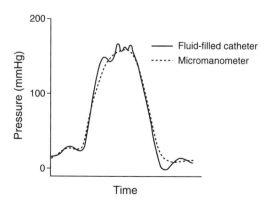

Figure 1-5 Simultaneous tracings of left ventricular pressure obtained from a micromanometer catheter and a fluid-filled catheter attached to an off-table strain gauge transducer. Note the presence of resonance artifact in the tracing from the fluid-filled catheter.

specially designed amplifiers. In addition, micromanometer catheters are considerably more expensive than standard catheter manometer systems and are relatively fragile.

Flow

Cardiac Output

Pressure is a reflection of a fluid's potential energy, indicating how "hard" it presses against the vessel or chamber containing it. By contrast, *flow* is a reflection of a fluid's kinetic energy, or the energy associated with its bulk movement. The total amount of blood flowing through the cardiovascular system per unit time is the cardiac output, usually expressed in units of liters per minute. Although the right ventricle and left ventricle do not match their output precisely on each beat, continuity of the circulation obviously demands that, in the absence of a shunt, the average "right-sided" and "left-sided" outputs are equal to each other. Because most of the variation in beat-to-beat output is a consequence of variable filling caused by respiratory changes in intrathoracic pressure, averaging in this instance incorporates measurements spanning at least one full respiratory cycle.

For most clinical applications, the cardiac output is not as useful as the *cardiac index,* which takes into account the subject's body size, as reflected by the body surface area (BSA), expressed in units of square meters (m^2):

$$\text{Cardiac index (CI)} = \text{Cardiac Output (CO)}/\text{BSA}$$

Cardiac index is expressed in units of liters/min/m^2. To determine BSA, most laboratories rely on the empiric formula derived by Dubois and Dubois in 1916:

$$\text{BSA} = .007184 \; W^{0.425} \; H^{0.725}$$

where W is the weight in kg and H is the height in cm. A graphic application of this formula is provided by a nomogram (Fig 1-6). The cardiac index at rest is normally at least 2.5 liters/min/m^2 in adults and is higher in adolescents and children.

Determination of Cardiac Output

We will review four methods for determining the cardiac output. Three of these, the Fick oxygen method, the indicator dilution method, and the thermodilution method, are based on the Fick principle, first articulated by Adolphus Fick in 1870, which states that the rate of delivery to or withdrawal from

BSA

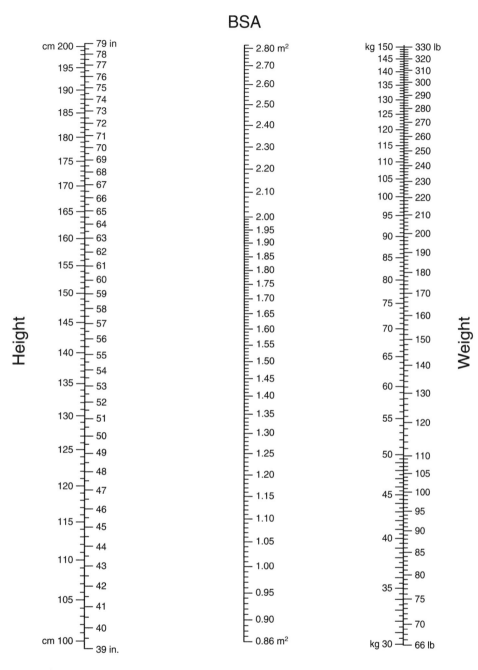

Figure 1-6 Nomogram for the calculation of BSA based on height and weight. To use, find the patient's height and weight on their respective scales and connect the points with a straight line. The point at which the line intersects the middle scale indicates the BSA. *Adapted from Grossman W, Baim DS*, eds. Cardiac catheterization, angiography, and interventions. 4th ed. Philadelphia: Lea & Febiger, 1991.

the circulation of a substance is equal to the product of the blood flow and the difference in concentration across the point of delivery or withdrawal:

Rate of delivery or withdrawal = (Blood flow)(Concentration difference)

Fick Oxygen Method

The Fick principle indicates that the rate of oxygen consumption is equal to the difference in oxygen content between arterial and venous blood multiplied by the total flow of blood through the circulation, or the cardiac output. To see why this is the case, consider the total amount of oxygen presented to the body for consumption per unit time. This is equal to the amount of blood presented per unit time (the cardiac output) times the oxygen content of that blood, in units of volume of O_2/volume of blood, or

Available O_2 per unit time = (CO)(Systemic arterial O_2 content)

Clearly, not all of the oxygen presented to working tissues is actually taken up and used in active metabolism. Much is "left over" and remains in mixed venous blood, which is then re-oxygenated when it passes through the lungs. The unused oxygen remaining in venous blood (returning to the lungs per unit time) is

Residual O_2 per unit time = (CO)(Venous O_2 content)

The rate of actual oxygen utilization is the difference between the available oxygen and the residual oxygen

O_2 utilization = (CO)(Arterial O_2 content) − (CO)(Venous O_2 content)
             = (CO)(Arterial O_2 content − venous O_2 content)

At steady state, the rate of oxygen utilization by the tissues is equal to the rate of oxygen consumption by the subject. The rate of oxygen utilization cannot be measured directly, but the rate of oxygen consumption via the lungs can be. Substitution of consumption for utilization yields

O_2 consumption = (CO)(Arterial O_2 content − venous O_2 content)

Rearranging this equation yields

$$CO = \frac{O_2 \text{ consumption}}{(\text{Arterial } O_2 \text{ content} - \text{venous } O_2 \text{ content})}$$

Thus, by measuring the oxygen consumption and the oxygen content of arterial and venous blood, one can derive the cardiac output.

Oxygen consumption can be measured by either of two techniques. The first depends on the use of a machine expressly designed for this purpose (Deltatrac Metabolic Monitor, SensorMedics Corporation, Yorba Linda, CA; Fig 1-7). It consists of a loosely fitting hood, which is placed over the patient's head. The hood is attached to a hose, which gently pulls in ambient air through the hood, where it mixes with the patient's expired air. From the flow rate of the mixed air in the hose (which is controlled by the machine), the concentration of oxygen in the flow (directly measured), the concentration of oxygen in ambient air (a constant), and the respiratory quotient (the relationship between oxygen consumption and carbon dioxide production—assumed to be constant), the machine calculates oxygen consumption.

Alternatively, a timed collection of expired air can be made by clamping the patient's nose and having him breathe through a mouthpiece connected to a valve that allows in ambient air and directs all expired air to a *Douglas bag*. The concentration of oxygen in the bag, along with the volume of expired gas, the respiratory quotient, ambient temperature, and atmospheric pressure can be used to calculate the oxygen consumed during the time of the collection. Dividing the total amount of oxygen consumed by the duration of the

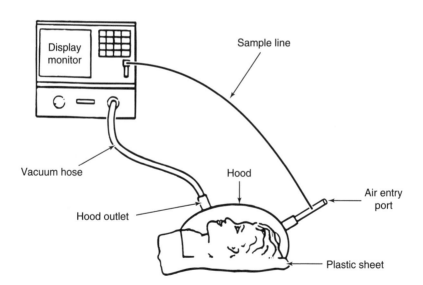

Figure 1-7 Schematic drawing of a device for measuring oxygen consumption. Ambient air is drawn through the hood and sampled as it enters and exits. The hood is made air-tight through the use of a plastic sheet, which can be folded under the patient's pillow.

collection yields a rate of oxygen consumption. Both the bag collection and the direct measurement of oxygen consumption require that the patient breathe in a relaxed and steady fashion to reflect the true oxygen consumption at rest. The normal rate of oxygen consumption for adults at rest is 75 to 175 ml $O_2/min/m^2$.

Once the oxygen consumption is known, measurement of the *oxygen content* in samples of arterial and mixed venous blood allows calculation of the cardiac output. Samples of blood should be obtained at the same time as the determination of oxygen consumption. Arterial samples may be obtained from any arterial location, such as the radial or femoral artery or the central aorta (or, for that matter, the left ventricle). The venous sample should be drawn from the pulmonary artery to assure adequate mixing of venous blood through the right side of the heart. For both locations, it is important to withdraw enough blood to clear the catheter so the sample reflects the oxygen content of blood at the catheter tip. It is also good practice to draw two samples from each location and average the results and to avoid air bubbles in the samples with which oxygen can equilibrate. The oxygen content of each sample of blood can be determined directly, or can be calculated from the equation

$$O_2 \text{ content of blood} = (O_2 \text{ carrying capacity}) (\text{Percent } O_2 \text{ saturation}).$$

The oxygen carrying capacity is the maximal amount of oxygen that can be bound by hemoglobin (Hgb) in a particular sample:

$$O_2 \text{ carrying capacity} = (\text{Hgb concentration}) \ (\text{Hgb } O_2 \text{ binding constant})$$

The hemoglobin binding constant is 1.36 ml O_2/g hemoglobin. If carrying capacity is expressed in units of ml $O_2/$liter blood, and hemoglobin concentration in the standard units of grams per deciliter, then a factor of 10 is required to rectify the units:

$$O_2 \text{ carrying capacity} = (\text{Hgb concentration}) (1.36) (10)$$

This equation is an approximation in that it does not account for the small amount of oxygen that is dissolved in blood but not bound by hemoglobin. *Oximeters* are used to provide direct and rapid determination of the percent hemoglobin saturation.

As an example, suppose a patient weighing 80 kg and standing 180 cm is found to have an oxygen consumption of 250 ml O_2/min at rest. Her arterial blood samples, drawn at the time the oxygen consumption was measured, had saturations of 96% and 98%, while her pulmonary artery (mixed venous) samples both had a saturation of 74%. Her hemoglobin concentration is

14 g/dL. What is her cardiac output? What is her cardiac index? Applying the provided equations,

$$O_2 \text{ carrying capacity} = (14 \text{ g Hgb/dL})(1.36 \text{ ml } O_2/\text{g Hgb})(10 \text{ dL/liter})$$
$$= 190.4 \text{ ml } O_2/\text{liter}$$
$$\text{Arterial } O_2 \text{ content} = (190.4 \text{ ml } O_2/\text{liter})(0.97) = 184.7 \text{ ml } O_2/\text{liter}$$
$$\text{Venous } O_2 \text{ content} = (190.4 \text{ ml } O_2/\text{liter})(0.74) = 140.9 \text{ ml } O_2/\text{liter}$$
$$CO = \frac{250 \text{ ml } O_2/\text{min}}{(184.7 - 140.9) \text{ ml } O_2/\text{liter}}$$

$$= 5.7 \text{ liters/min}$$
$$BSA = 2.0 \text{ m}^2 \text{ (by nomogram)}$$
$$CI = 2.9 \text{ liters/min/m}^2$$

Error in the determination of the cardiac output by the Fick method can be introduced at any step in the collection of the data utilized in the calculation. The measured oxygen consumption can be spurious if the respiratory quotient, most often assumed to be equal to 1, is significantly lower. This results in a lower volume of expired air than inspired air, which means that the oxygen concentration in a Douglas bag is artifactually high, or that the oxygen consumption and, by extension, the cardiac output are artifactually low. Douglas bag determinations also can fall prey to mistimed or incomplete collections (leaks) and must be carefully corrected to account for temperature and barometric pressure effects. The continuous oxygen consumption measuring devices must be carefully calibrated and allowed to "warm up." Because of wide interpatient variability in oxygen consumption, the oxygen consumption must be measured; the use of an "assumed" oxygen consumption is not recommended. The determination of oxygen content also requires careful calibration of the oximeter and is limited by the assumptions about oxygen binding to hemoglobin discussed previously.

Indicator Dilution Method

This technique is also based on the Fick principle. Consider the fate of a substance, or indicator, that is injected as a rapid bolus. Assuming that there is no destruction of the indicator, all of it will pass a point in the circulation downstream to the injection site. If we could detect the presence of the indicator in the downstream flow, we could apply the same concept used in the Fick output determination. Namely, the total amount of a substance carried by a flowing stream is equal to the concentration of that substance in the stream multiplied by the flow rate, or

Total amount of indicator detected per unit time = (Flow) (Concentration)

Rearranging this equation yields

Total amount of indicator detected = (Flow) (Concentration) (Time)

The total amount of indicator detected is equal to the amount injected. The flow is equal to the cardiac output, so that

Amount of indicator injected = (CO) (Concentration) (Time)

In considering what happens to an injected bolus of indicator, it is clear that the downstream concentration of indicator is not constant. Prior to the injection, it is zero; it remains zero until the blood carrying it flows from the injection site to the detection site. The concentration then rises rapidly, as the bolus—now "spread out" because of the mixing of indicator and blood—passes the detection site, and then declines as the remnants of the indicator bolus trail off (Fig 1-8). When concentration is not constant over time, the product of concentration and time must be replaced by the *integral* of concentration over time (which is the area under the concentration curve):

$$\text{Amount of indicator injected} = (\text{CO}) \int_0^\infty C(t)\,dt$$

where $C(t)$ is the instantaneous concentration of the indicator at the downstream detection site. Rearranging this equation yields

$$\text{CO} = \frac{\text{Amount of indicator}}{\displaystyle\int_0^\infty C(t)\,dt}$$

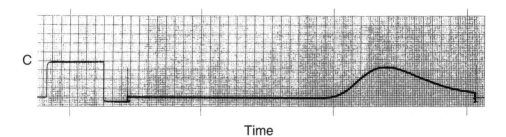

Time

Figure 1-8   Indicator-dilution curve, preceded by a calibration signal. Note the rise and gentle decline in indicator concentration over time. The area under this curve is inversely proportional to the cardiac output.

In practice, this method is used with one of two different indicators. The older indicator is *indocyanine green ("green dye")*. A known amount of indicator is injected as a rapid bolus into the central venous circulation, the right side of the heart, the pulmonary artery, or the left ventricle. Blood is sampled continuously at an arterial site by withdrawing it at a constant rate through a calibrated densitometer, which then plots the concentration of dye as a function of time, also called an indicator dilution curve.

Thermodilution Technique

More commonly, the indicator dilution method is applied by injecting cold saline as the indicator and plotting the dip in blood temperature downstream from the injection site. This technique, known as the thermodilution method, has the advantages of not requiring the withdrawal of blood and using a universally available indicator (iced saline). Pulmonary artery catheters incorporating a separate lumen for injecting saline, which terminates proximal to the end of the catheter, as well as a thermistor (temperature sensor) near the end of the catheter, are generally used for this purpose. If the end of the catheter is placed in the pulmonary artery, the injectate "port" is in the right side of the heart. Injecting a known volume of iced saline (usually 10 ml) allows a dedicated "cardiac output computer" to plot the indicator dilution curve for "cold." For either indicator, the area under the dilution curve is theoretically equal to the integral in the denominator of the preceding equation. In practice, the shape of the curve deviates from the mathematic ideal, and computer-based or manual corrections are used to calculate the value of the integral. Correction factors, or warming constants, are also utilized to account for the warming of the injected saline by the blood surrounding the catheter before the saline enters the circulation. Once the value of the integral is calculated, the cardiac output is derived.

A potential source of error in indicator dilution techniques is the injection of less than the full amount of indicator. This can occur if the indocyanine has partially decomposed prior to use or if the saline, in a thermodilution system, has warmed; in both cases, the actual amount of indicator is diminished and the cardiac output will be overestimated. Detectors and automated computers must be properly calibrated. Thermodilution, because of the usual location of the injectate port in the right atrium, is unreliable in the presence of significant tricuspid regurgitation, which has the effect of warming the injected bolus with blood from the right ventricle which is not part of the forward stream.

Angiographic Output

Finally, one can determine the cardiac output as the product of the stroke volume (the volume of blood ejected by the heart on each beat) and the heart rate. Stroke volume can be measured by contrast ventriculography, as long as a length calibration standard is utilized. A length standard, filmed with the x-ray source and image intensifier in the same relative position used for filming the ventriculogram, allows one to derive absolute volumes from the end-diastolic and end-systolic frames of the cineangiogram. The difference in volume between the two is the stroke volume. The cardiac output measured this way is called the angiographic output. Because this technique requires cineangiography and a contrast injection, it is not practical for serial determinations. Beat-to-beat variation in stroke volume, as occurs because of ectopy or the variable cardiac cycle length of atrial fibrillation, makes this technique inappropriate in those settings. In the presence of mitral or aortic regurgitation, the angiographic output is greater than the true "forward" cardiac output (a phenomenon that is the basis for determination of regurgitant fraction).

Resistance

Pressure is the motive force responsible for the flow of blood through the circulation. The opposition to that flow, which resides in the vasculature, is termed the *vascular resistance.* By definition (and in analogy to Ohm's Law),

$$\text{Pressure} = (\text{Flow})(\text{Resistance})$$

More precisely, *pressure* is not an absolute measure, but is the difference in pressure between two points (the pressure "drop").

It is also important to note that this simple equation relating pressure, flow, and resistance does not take account of the fluctuations in each of these measures as a function of time. It is strictly true only in (the nonexistent) steady state in which pressure and flow are constant (nonpulsatile). If we allow pressure and flow to vary with time, then the opposition to that flow is more properly termed *vascular impedance.* Nevertheless, the bulk of the vascular impedance is provided by the vascular resistance, and the latter, because of the simplicity of its calculation, is widely used clinically.

The circulation consists of two circuits: the pulmonary blood flow from the right ventricle to the left atrium and the systemic blood flow from the left ventricle to the right atrium. The resistances of these circuits, termed the *pulmonary vascular resistance (PVR)* and the *systemic vascular resistance (SVR),* respectively, are

$$PVR = \frac{\text{Mean pulmonary arterial pressure} - \text{mean left atrial pressure}}{\text{Cardiac output}}$$

and

$$SVR = \frac{\text{Mean systemic arterial pressure} - \text{mean right atrial pressure}}{\text{Cardiac output}}$$

The mean pulmonary capillary wedge pressure is commonly substituted for mean left atrial pressure in the determination of the PVR.

These resistances can be expressed in two different units. If pressure is expressed in millimeters of mercury and cardiac output in liters per minute, their quotient is resistance in so-called *hybrid resistance units* or *Wood units*. If pressure is converted to dynes per square centimeter (see section on pressure) and flow to cubic centimeters per second, resistance can be expressed as absolute resistance units, which are equal to dynes-sec/cm^5. Wood units are easily converted to *absolute resistance units* by multiplying by 80.

Because vascular resistance is dependent on the cardiac output, some authors advocate *indexing* the resistance to account for variation in cardiac output based on body size. This can be done by substituting the cardiac index for the cardiac output in the preceding equations. Note that this is equivalent to *multiplying* the resistance by the BSA. Although this has appeal on theoretical grounds, it is not often done. Normal values for systemic vascular resistance range from 500 to 1500 dynes-sec/cm^5, and for pulmonary vascular resistance, from 20 to 150 dynes-sec/cm^5.

SELECTED READING

Nichols WW, O'Rourke MF, eds. McDonald's blood flow in arteries, 3rd ed. Philadelphia: Lea & Febiger, 1990.

2

RADIOGRAPHIC PRINCIPLES

Chris C. Shaw

Radiographic Principles and Equipment

DESPITE ADVANCES IN new imaging techniques like computed tomography (CT), ultrasonic (US) imaging, and magnetic resonance imaging (MRI), contrast angiography remains the gold standard in imaging cardiac chambers and coronary arteries. In this chapter, we briefly describe and discuss the principles and equipment of contrast angiography as used in cardiac imaging. Quality control and radiation safety also are addressed.

Radiographic Principles

Like visible light or microwaves, x-rays are a special form of electromagnetic radiation that have wavelengths between 1.2×10^{-5} to 4.1×10^{-14} cm. This wavelength range corresponds to a photon energy of 10 to 3×10^{10} eV. With this range of wavelengths or energies, the x-ray photons can partially penetrate many objects. Thus, since the discovery of x-rays, they have been widely used to probe and study internal structures of various objects, including the human body.

Radiographic techniques used in cardiac angiography are part of a large category of x-ray imaging techniques referred to as *projection radiography*. In projection radiography, x-rays from a stationary point source are collimated to form a divergent x-ray beam that is used to penetrate and probe the internal structures of the patient's body (Fig 2-1). Some of the x-rays pass through the body without interaction, while others are absorbed or scattered. These absorption and scatter phenomena together are referred to as the *x-ray attenuation*. The factor by which x-rays are attenuated depends on the energy of x-ray photons and the thickness and composition of the patient's body along the specific x-ray path. As a result, the intensity of transmitted x-rays varies spatially with the patient's anatomic structures. Typically, the x-ray intensity is attenuated by a factor ranging from 2 to 3 in the lung area to more than 20 in the mediastinum and abdomen. Although the intensity variation of the transmitted x-rays contains useful information, it can not be viewed directly by the eye, and an x-ray detector system must be used to convert the transmitted x-ray pattern into either a film image to be viewed on a viewing box or with a film projector or a video signal to be displayed on a cathode ray tube (CRT) monitor. The two most widely used detector systems are the screen-film combination and image-intensifier (II)-based imaging systems.

With the screen-film systems, a phosphor screen is used to convert x-rays into visible light, which exposes a film that is placed in close contact with the screen in a light-tight cassette. X-ray imaging systems designed for screen-film combinations are often referred to as "radiographic" imaging systems because large exposures are often used to obtain high-quality images, which are typically acquired one at a time. Such systems are widely used for imaging stationary anatomic structures like extremities, abdomen, breast, and so on, or for tasks that do not require dynamic changes to be studied. However, there are also film

Figure 2-1   Attenuation and scattering of x-rays and formation of an x-ray image.

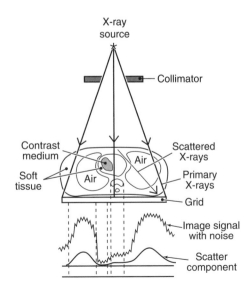

changer systems that can transport the exposed film to a "receiving cassette," retrieve a fresh film from the "supply cassette," and move it behind a fixed screen for new exposure. Such systems can achieve an image rate of up to 2 to 6 per second with formats as large as 14″×14″.

An x-ray II converts x-rays into a minified and intensified optical image that can be viewed indirectly through a lens-mirror system or most often recorded with television or film cameras. The II-based imaging systems are mainly designed for monitoring or studying moving structures (e.g., patient positioning, monitoring catheter placement, cardiac imaging, etc.). When the II is used for positioning, monitoring, or other less critical tasks, the x-rays are often turned on continuously at a reduced exposure level to allow real-time image acquisition and display for long periods. This mode of operation is referred to as "fluoroscopy," which has been existent since shortly after the x-rays were discovered by Roentgen in 1895. However, modern II-based imaging systems also have provisions for "serial radiographic" imaging. This is often achieved by coupling a cut film or cine film camera to the output of an II and using shorter but high-exposure x-ray pulses. In digital angiography, a high-quality TV camera is used in conjunction with digital image acquisition, display, and storage equipment to perform the tasks of serial radiographic imaging.

Cardiac Angiography

Cardiac chambers and vessels, when filled with blood, provide little inherent image contrast for diagnostic purposes. Thus, radiopaque contrast agent must be injected to enhance the vessels or chambers being studied. This technique in general is referred to as *angiography*. The angiography procedures used for cardiac imaging are referred to as cardiac angiography or angiocardiography. They resemble other angiography procedures for examining noncardiac vessels. Cardiac angiography, however, has some stringent requirements. The primary targets in cardiac angiography—heart chambers or coronary arteries—are constantly moving in a pulsating fashion. To minimize image blurring due to cardiac motion, short x-ray exposures must be used to "freeze" the motion so that reasonably sharp images of cardiac chambers or vessels can be obtained. Furthermore, to study blood flow or cardiac function, a rapid image sequence covering several heart beats is necessary. To achieve reasonable temporal resolution, a minimum framing rate of 15 frames per second (fps) or higher is required, with rates as high as 60 fps used for pediatric cardiac angiography.

The block diagram for a typical angiography imaging system used in a cardiac catheterization laboratory is shown in Figure 2-2. It consists of the x-ray tube, collimator, antiscatter grid, II, video camera, and cine film camera. These components are generally mounted on a C-arm or similar mounting system. An x-ray generator with control panel is located nearby to provide high-voltage and filament current for the x-ray tube. A video recorder and CRT monitor are used

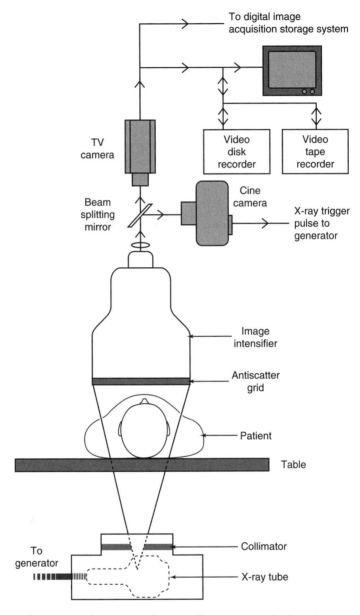

Figure 2-2   Schematic drawing for a cardiac angiography imaging system.

to record and display images during both fluoroscopy and cine film studies. A cine film processor and projector are required to develop and display, respectively, the exposed cine film. A digital image acquisition, storage, and processing system is needed for digital angiography. In this section, we discuss the processes and equipment related to x-ray generation and detection.

Other equipment is discussed separately in the subsequent sections dealing with the three major techniques: cinefluorography, fluoroscopy, and digital angiography.

Image Characteristics

Image quality is characterized by four major characteristics: brightness, contrast, sharpness, and noise. Images, be they electronic signals displayed on a CRT monitor or films displayed on a viewing box, must have sufficient brightness to allow the eyes to function optimally to perform the diagnostic tasks. *Image contrast* refers to how well the image details or objects of interest are rendered as various degrees of brightness. When the rendered brightness difference among these image details or objects decreases, it would become more difficult to visualize them. Image sharpness, also known as the spatial resolution, refers to how well image details are preserved without blending with each other. In the extreme case, image details may not be resolved if they are rendered in an excessively blurry fashion. Image noise, on the other hand, measures how much the image signals fluctuate. For the objects of interest to be detected, the contrast level should be several times greater than the noise level. Another rule is that the smaller the objects, the more contrast it requires to detect them. Lowering the noise level (by using higher exposures and high-quality imaging equipment) also helps visualize smaller objects.

In cardiac angiography, image contrast depends on many factors, including the iodine concentration, thickness of vessels or chambers, and tube voltage. Contrast materials with higher iodine concentrations, faster injection rate, and proximity to the injection site tend to increase the iodine concentration and therefore the contrast of the opacified vessels or chambers.

Image noise, on the other hand, depends mainly on x-ray exposure level at the input of the II. When an x-ray photon enters the input phosphor of the II, it may either be absorbed as part of the image signal or pass through without interaction. This stochastic nature of x-ray absorption causes the resulting image signal to fluctuate both in the spatial domain (from one location to another) and in the time domain (from one frame to another), thus producing image noise. Lower peak kilovoltage (kVp) or tube current (mA) or larger patient habitus tends to produce fewer x-ray photons at the input of the II and therefore results in more statistical fluctuation and noisier images. Noise levels in heavily attenuated regions are higher than those in lightly attenuated regions.

The primary transmission ratio (discussed later) of the antiscatter grid and the quantum detection efficiency (discussed later) of the II also affect the noise level of the images. However, these are generally fixed factors for any specific imaging system. Film graininess, electronic noise, or other noises introduced in imaging equipment also contributes to image noise, but any properly designed and operated medical x-ray imaging system should produce images with noise contributed mostly by x-rays.

In fluoroscopy and digital angiography, the image contrast can be electronically or digitally enhanced or reduced. It should be realized, however, that such manipulation also increases the noise level in the images. Therefore, there is no fundamental improvement of the image contrast relative to noise. The value of electronic or digital contrast and brightness control is to present the images to human observers with proper image brightness and contrast level for optimal visualization of image details.

X-ray Generation

Diagnostic x-rays are generated inside an x-ray tube powered by an x-ray generator. The x-rays emitted from the x-ray tube are filtered and collimated to form an x-ray beam that can be used to produce quality x-ray images while minimizing patient exposure.

X-ray Generator

The main function of an x-ray generator is to convert commercially available 3-phase AC power (440–480 volts) to nearly DC voltage at 60 to 100 kV for accelerating the electrons in the x-ray tube. The generator consists of a step-up transformer to produce alternating high voltage. It also consists of a step-down transformer and circuitry to provide a low-voltage current to heat the cathode (filament) and generate electrons for acceleration. For cooling and insulation, the transformers are placed in a large tank and submerged in oil. Also contained in the tank is rectifier circuitry, which converts alternating high voltage into DC voltage for accelerating the electrons. A modern angiography facility should use generators capable of producing so-called 12-pulse (per 1/60 sec) voltage output that has only minimal fluctuations at a frequency of 720 per second. Some new generators, often referred to as high-frequency x-ray generators, employ voltage inversion and switching technology to produce nearly constant voltage output. The use of 12-pulse or constant-voltage generators is essential in cardiac angiography because it allows x-ray pulses as short as 1 msec to be made with consistent exposure output.

X-ray Tube

As shown in Figure 2-3, an x-ray tube is essentially a large vacuum tube consisting of the cathode, focusing cup, and anode. The tube housing contains lead shielding, which blocks x-rays emitting in all directions except through a small window. It is filled with oil to prevent arcing from high voltage and to help dissipate heat from the anode. The cathode is a fine filament coil made of tung-

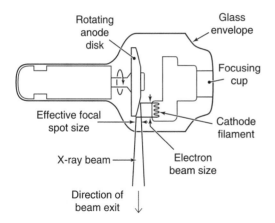

Rotating anode disk

Glass envelope

Focusing cup

Effective focal spot size

Cathode filament

X-ray beam

Electron beam size

Direction of beam exit

Figure 2-3   Schematic drawing of an x-ray tube.

sten alloy, which is heated by low-voltage current to emit thermal electrons. The electrons are accelerated toward the anode by a high voltage current applied between the cathode and anode. A focusing cup behind the filament shapes the electric field around the filament and causes the electron beam to converge at a small area on the anode, referred to as the *focal spot,* where x-rays are produced.

X-rays are generated when high-energy electrons bombard nuclei in the target material. To increase the efficiency of x-ray generation, the target is usually made of elements with large atomic numbers, such as tungsten or rhenium-tungsten alloy. The majority of x-rays are generated through the bremsstrahlung ("braking radiation") process in which the electrons are deaccelerated by the nuclei of target material and emit a continuous spectrum of x-rays. These x-rays have energies ranging from zero to the maximum energy of accelerated electrons, as determined by the kVp. However, more x-rays are generated with lower energy. As the result, the x-ray intensity decreases linearly with the photon energy until it decreases to almost zero at the maximum photon energy.

A significant but minor fraction of x-rays are generated as characteristic x-rays, which are emitted when inner shell electrons in the target atoms are freed and replaced with free or outer shell electrons. Unlike the bremsstrahlung x-rays, the characteristic x-rays are emitted with specific energies that are equal to the differences between the energy levels of the freed and replacing electrons. X-ray production through electron bombarding is inefficient. Only about 1% of the energy is converted into x-rays. The rest of the energy is dissipated in the target as heat. This heat must be dissipated from the focal spot to the entire anode, from the anode to the tube housing, and from the housing to the atmosphere.

For more efficient cooling and heat-loading capacity, most tubes use rotating anodes constructed of a tungsten-rhenium alloy bonded to a molybdenum disk. With the cathode pointing at an off-center location near the edge, the target surface of the anode is beveled away from the cathode (see Fig 2-2). The angle of the bevel (with respect to the axis of the disk or direction of the electron beam) is referred to as the anode or target angle, ranging from 7 to 12 degrees for most angiographic tubes. During exposure, the electron beam focuses on and hits a fixed small area on the tilted surface. Because the anode is rotating at a high speed (typically from 3000 to as high as 10,800 rpm), the electron beam actually traverses and hits a much larger area in the shape of an arch on the target surface, the length of which depends on the exposure time. This helps spread the heat over the entire anode.

Focal Spot Size

The generated x-rays exit through a low-attenuation window in the tube in a direction perpendicular to the electron beam. Because the target surface is tilted toward the cathode at a small angle (7–12 degrees) with respect to this direction, the effective x-ray focal spot, as viewed along the x-ray beam, appears to be smaller than the actual spot on the target where electrons are focused and x-rays are generated. This allows the electron beam to be focused at a long and narrow rectangular area on the target while producing a smaller, more square-like x-ray focal spot. This helps spread the heat generated during x-ray production over a larger target area. Most tubes employ two filaments to allow the focal spot size to be changed between two different values to accommodate different imaging conditions. Typical small focal spots used in cardiac angiography are 0.5 to 0.6 mm in size, and typical large focal spots are 0.9 to 1.1 mm in size.

X-ray Techniques

The intensity of x-ray tube output is determined by two factors: the kVp, and mA. The mA measures how many electrons are accelerated to hit the target per unit time. Therefore, it is directly proportional to the intensity of the x-rays generated. In fluoroscopy, the x-rays are continuously turned on and the rate of x-ray exposure generated is proportional to the mA used. In cine film or digital angiography studies, the x-rays are pulsed and the amount of x-ray exposure generated for each image is proportional to both the mA and the exposure time. Due to the need to minimize motion blurring, it is generally more desirable to use short exposures at high mA.

The intensity of the x-rays generated is approximately proportional to the third power of the kVp used. It increases with the kVp at a faster rate because both the number of photons produced and average beam energy increase with the increasing kVp. X-ray photons with higher energies are also more penetrating than those with lower energies. Thus, high kVp x-rays are often used to achieve higher x-ray tube output and to reduce x-ray attenuation so that the intensity of transmitted x-rays at the input of the x-ray detector (II) can be maintained for consistent image quality. However, high kVp x-ray beams also tend to produce lower image contrast because x-ray attenuation by the patient's body and contrast material generally decreases at a slower rate as the photon energy increases. In contrast, low kVp x-ray beams are less penetrating but produce higher image contrast. A further consideration is related to the x-ray absorption properties of the iodinated contrast material used to enhance the visualization of cardiac vessels or chambers in cardiac angiography. Because the K shell electrons in iodine atoms have a binding energy of 33.2 keV, they absorb x-rays most efficiently when the photon energy is slightly above 33.2 keV. This energy is referred to as the K-edge energy. Thus, to optimize the iodine contrast, it is best to use x-rays generated with a kVp between 60 and 70 and keep the average x-ray beam energy slightly above 33.2 keV. The kVp used in cardiac angiography ranges from 60 to 90 kVp, depending on the patient's habitus. In general, lower kVp should not be used because iodine contrast would be significantly decreased when the average beam energy goes below the iodine K-edge energy.

Power Rating

The product of the kVp and the mA is the power delivered to the x-ray focal spot by the accelerated electrons hitting the x-ray target. The power rating for an x-ray tube is the maximum power that can be delivered without damaging the focal spot itself. Obviously, larger focal spots have higher power ratings. Therefore, for tubes with two or more focal spots, ratings for each different spot size should be given. Tubes used in cardiac angiography should have a minimum of 35 to 40 kilowatts (1 kW = 1 kV × 1000 mA). The power ratings of modern angiography tubes are significantly improved by using a rotating anode with a beveled target surface.

Heat Loading and Dissipation

The product of the mA and exposure time is often referred to as the mAs. Together with the kVp and the x-ray source to detector distance, it determines the exposure for each image during cine film or digital angiography studies. The anode heat-loading capacity is specified in terms of heat units (HUs). The number of HU for a single exposure generated with a 3-phase generator is determined by multiplying the kVp with the mAs and 1.35. This number can be multiplied by the number of images to determine the total number of HUs for an image sequence obtained in a cine film and digital angiography study. Similarly, numbers of HUs from all cine film and digital angiography studies can also be summed to determined the total number of HUs for the entire patient examination procedure. Typical x-ray tubes used in cardiac angiography have an anode heat-loading capacity of 400,000 HU or higher. For procedures involving more frequent high-dose pulsed x-ray imaging or high-dose fluoroscopic studies (i.e., PTCA), a tube with a capacity of at least 800,000 HU should be used. When heated to maximum capacity, the anode should cool down to 50% of its maximum capacity in 4 minutes or less, so that subsequent procedures can be performed with minimum delay.

Heat accumulated in the anode needs to be dissipated into the tube housing, mainly through thermal radiation emission. The housing may be cooled by fan or by air or water circulation. Typical x-ray tubes used in cardiac angiography have a housing heat capacity of at least 1.5 million HU and require less than 30 minutes to cool down from 100% loading to 50% loading. For more demanding usage, tubes with a heat capacity of at least 2 million HU and a 50% cooling time of 10 minutes or shorter should be used.

X-ray Collimation and Filtration

X-rays generated inside the x-ray tube exit through a minimally attenuative window. However, they need to be further collimated to define the x-ray beam to accurately match the image field defined by the detector. Both circular and rectangular formats are used by the components of an II-based imaging system. Specifically, the II, used as the primary x-ray detector, has a circular input screen, whereas the TV and cine film cameras use rectangular or square image formats. For this reason, x-ray tubes used in angiography are typically fitted with both circular and rectangular adjustable collimators. With these two collimators, the x-ray field should be reduced to cover just the active part of the II input. An additional collimator is also added near the exit window of the x-ray tube to further reduce the off-focus x-rays. Accurate x-ray collimation minimizes scattered and off-focus x-rays and is crucial for optimizing the image quality and for reducing patient and staff exposures.

X-rays coming directly from the x-ray tube contain low-energy x-rays that will be totally absorbed by the patient. These low x-rays do not contribute to image signals but significantly increase radiation exposure to the patient. The use of aluminum or copper filters of appropriate thicknesses are required to attenuate the low-energy x-rays to minimize the radiation risk to the patient without degrading the image quality. Another type of filter used in cardiac angiography are the shaped bolus filters that are often used (placed on the tube side) to decrease the incident x-ray intensity in the lung region surrounding the heart. This helps decrease the exposure range and avoid the blooming or signal saturation effects associated with the TV camera.

X-ray Detection

The II is the sole detector used in cardiac angiography. It is a versatile x-ray detector ideal for high-speed x-ray imaging, as required by cardiac angiography. Coupled to a TV camera, cine film camera, and digital image acquisition system, the II can be used for fluoroscopy, cine film, and digital angiography studies. In this section, we describe and discuss how an II converts the x-rays into optical images. The use of antiscatter grids for scatter removal is also addressed. The cine film camera, TV camera, and digital image acquisition and storage systems are discussed in subsequent sections addressing the three imaging techniques used in cardiac angiography: cinefluorography, fluoroscopy, and digital angiography.

Image Intensifier

Figure 2-4 shows a schematic drawing of an II. A modern x-ray II consists of the input screen, focusing electrodes, accelerating anode, and output phosphor, enclosed in an evacuated cylindrical glass container. The input screen consists of a thick layer of cesium iodide (CsI) crystals followed by a thin deposition of photocathode layer. The CsI crystal layer absorbs about half of the input x-rays and converts them into visible light by fluorescence. The photocathode layer converts the fluorescent light into photoelectrons whose density is proportional to the light intensity. These electrons are then accelerated and focused at the output screen (type P20 or ZnCdS), which converts the accelerated electrons into fluorescent light. Thus, the intensity variation of the transmitted x-rays, which contains information on the patient's internal structure, is transformed into a smaller but much brighter image. The increased image brightness is achieved by both image intensification and image minification. In the first process, the photoelectrons are accelerated by a high voltage (about 30 keV) before they reach the output phosphor. Therefore, each electron hits the phosphor with a large amount of energy and produces a large number of visible photons, which is much higher (by a factor of about 10^4) than the number of photons required to generate the photoelectron in the photocathode layer.[3–5] In the second process, the photoelectrons are converged into a phosphor screen much smaller than the input screen (e.g., 0.5-1.0″ compared with 4.5-12.0″), thus the density of electrons reaching the output screen is much higher than the density of the electrons emitted from the photocathode layer.

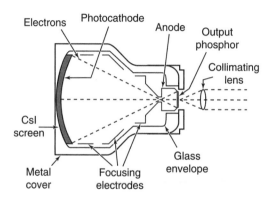

Figure 2-4   Schematic drawing of an x-ray image intensifier.

Conversion Factor

The gain of brightness of an II is often characterized by the conversion factor, defined as the amount of light emitted from the output phosphor per unit exposure of the x-rays striking the input phosphor during fluoroscopy. The conversion factor is usually expressed in units of candelas per square meter per milliroentgen per second ($cd/m^2/mR/sec$). Obviously, high conversion factor is an important feature to look for when selecting an II. The conversion factors are determined by many factors, including the quantum detection efficiency of the input screen and the ratio of the input field of view (FOV) to the size of the output screen. For a 6- or 7-inch mode of a typical II, the conversion factor ranges from 75 to 100 $cd/m^2/mR/sec$. It decreases significantly for 4.5- or 5.0-inch modes due to reduced minification gain. Some newer IIs are of high quantum detection efficiency design. They have thicker input phosphor (330 instead of 200 μm) and therefore absorb more x-rays (about 60% vs. 40%). They have higher conversion factors when compared with older IIs of comparable size.

Spatial Resolution

Another important characteristic is the spatial resolution, which sets a limit on how sharp fluoroscopic or cine film images look. The spatial resolution of an II is mainly determined by the thickness of the input phosphor and to a lesser extent by the accuracy of electronic focusing. Toward the edge of the input screen, the projected phosphor thickness becomes greater and the focusing becomes less optimal. Thus, the spatial resolution is significantly degraded toward the edge of an II. Typical IIs have a spatial resolution of 4 to 5 lps/mm at the center. The resolution at the edge could be lower by as much as 10%.

Contrast Ratio

The image intensifier is subject to the effects of "veiling glare," a result of a combination of x-ray scatter in the II tube housing, stray electrons, and light scatter in the output window. Like scattered radiation, veiling glare results in a significant loss of image contrast. The standard method to measure this contrast loss is to measure the light output with and without a 1/4-inch-thick lead disk, with an area equal to one tenth of the active area of the input phosphor, positioned at the center of the field. The contrast ratio is then computed as the ratio of the brightness without the beam stop to that with the beam stop. The contrast ratio has been significantly improved with the use of a metal input window and specially coated output window. A modern II for cardiac angiography should have a contrast ratio of 12:1 or higher. The II contributes to the image noise mainly through the input phosphor structure. However, this noise, which is generally of lower level, should normally be masked by the quantum noise that originates from the fluctuations in x-ray detection and by the structures to be imaged.

Optical Distribution

The output of the IIs is often fitted with a collimator lens with an f/stop of 1.2 or smaller. This lens turns the output image into a parallel beam for optical distribution and coupling to various cameras. Through the use of beam splitters and mirrors, a combination of as many as three different cameras can be optically coupled to the output of the II. In a cardiac catheterization laboratory, the II is typically fitted with a TV camera for fluoroscopy and a cine film camera for cinefluorography studies. A high-quality TV or charge-coupled device (CCD) camera is sometimes added for digital angiography or high-quality fluoroscopy.

Electronic Magnification

Most IIs have provisions to vary the FOV to a smaller size. This process, sometimes referred to as "electronic magnification," is achieved by varying the voltages on the focusing electrodes to focus the electrons in a magnifying way. Thus, only electrons from a selected central part of the input screen reach the output screen. The diameters of the different FOVs available with an II are referred to as the mode of operation. Using smaller modes of an II allows an electronically magnified view at the expense of smaller FOV. With some larger IIs using smaller modes also helps improve the overall spatial resolution. This should be distinguished from "magnification radiography" in which the magnification is achieved "geometrically" by shifting the patient toward the x-ray tube, providing a physically larger x-ray image at the x-ray detector.

Geometric Magnification

Because of the divergence of x-rays from the focal spot, image magnification can also be achieved by varying the geometric relationship among the x-ray focal spot, patient, and x-ray detector (II). This magnification technique is referred to as "geometric magnification." In cardiac angiography, the x-ray tube and II are often mounted on a C-arm or U-arm, with a fixed distance between the tube and II. Thus, the patient-to-II distance dictates the geometric magnification achieved. The farther the patient from the II, the larger the geometric magnification. Geometric magnification is achieved at the expense of a smaller FOV. In addition, it requires a small x-ray focal spot to be used to reduce the blurring effect generated by the penumbra (projection of focal spot on II) of x-ray spot. Because of the availability of electronic magnification capability with the II and need to obtain full view of the heart, geometric magnification is seldom used in cardiac angiography. It should be realized, however, that based on the principle of geometric magnification, structures farther from the II may look slightly larger than those farther from the II.

Scattered Radiation

X-rays entering the patient's body may transmit through it without interacting with it (see Fig 2-1). They are referred to as the primary x-rays, which form the useful signal in the x-ray detector and the resulting images. Their intensity indicates how many x-rays have interacted with the body structures. However, x-rays interact with matter via several processes. For diagnostic x-rays, the two most important processes are the photoelectric effect and Compton scattering. With the latter effect, x-ray photons are simply deflected and part of their energy is taken away by electrons. These photons are referred to as scattered x-rays. Scattered x-rays could be scattered again, resulting in so-called multiple scatter. Because scattered x-rays are deflected at least once, they could transmit through the patient's body and be absorbed by the detector at various locations (see Fig 2-1). Therefore, they do not contribute to the image signal in a useful way. Instead, they degrade the image contrast and make it more difficult to visualize image details. The effect of scattered x-rays depends on the ratio of the scatter component to the primary component in the image signals, not on the absolute size of the scatter component. For instance, the scatter components are actually weaker in the mediastinum and abdomen when compared with those in the lung field. However, because primary signals in these regions are heavily attenuated, resulting in much higher scatter-to-primary ratios, the effects of x-ray scatter are most serious in these regions.

Antiscatter Grids

To reduce the relative strength of scatter component in image signals, an antiscatter grid is often attached to the front of the II. The grid consists of thin lead foils oriented in parallel or toward the x-ray source. They are separated by relatively x-ray–transparent material. Because scattered x-rays come from the irradiated part of the patient's body from all directions, they tend to be blocked unless they arrive in directions parallel with the foils. The primary x-rays, on the other hand, transmit with a much greater ratio, thus resulting in an overall reduction of scatter-to-primary ratios. When the lead foils in a grid are oriented in a parallel way, the grid is called unfocused. This type of grid tends to transmit more primary x-rays in regions closer to the center line. When the FOV is large compared with the source-to-detector distance, cutoff may occur in regions far from the center line. The focused design orients all foils toward the x-ray source and therefore transmits primary x-rays in the same way throughout the FOV.

However, they require careful alignment and operate only for a narrow range of the source-to-detector distances.

The antiscatter grids are characterized by the grid ratio and line density. The grid ratio refers to the ratio of the height of the grid strips to their separation distance. Grid ratios range from 5:1 to as high as 16:1. Grids with larger ratios reject x-ray scatter more efficiently. The line density, also referred to as the strip density, is the number of grid strips per inch or centimeter. The line density ranges from 60 to 110 lines per inch. High line density is important because the grid lines are less obvious and therefore do not interfere with image reading.

It should be remembered that the use of an antiscatter grid improves the image contrast at the expense of attenuating the information carrying primary x-rays or alternatively increased patient exposure (if exposure is increased to compensate for this attenuation). Selection of the grid used is a compromise between scatter rejection ability and transmission of primary x-rays. Most modern cardiac angiography systems use grids with a ratio of 10:1, a line density of 100 lines per inch, and a focal range of 34 to 40 inches. Grids with the more transmissive carbon-fiber interspace material should be used because they allow an exposure reduction of 10% to 25%, compared with aluminum. Lower ratio grids may be used for pediatric cardiac imaging and may not be necessary for studies of neonates because of the smaller scatter volume. In reality, most grids can not be easily removed from the housing of the II for interchange.

Cine Fluorography

Cine fluorography refers to the technique of using a cine film camera optically coupled to the II output to acquire high-quality x-ray images with a rapid sequence of short pulsed exposures. The cine film camera has its own lens, focused at infinity into the light beam from the II output (reflected by the beam splitter). Unlike the TV camera, which is limited in speed by the long target readout time (typically 33 msec or longer), a cine film camera can achieve very high speed. However, cameras used in cardioangiography are typically operated at from 30 to 60 fps. When the cine film study begins, a beam splitter swings into place, directing about 10%-20% of the light from the II output to the TV camera and the majority of the light to the cine film camera. During the study, a segment of fresh, unexposed cine film is retrieved from the supply spool and transported into the exposure position, the shutter opens and an x-ray pulse is fired, resulting in an exposure of the cine film frame. Following the exposure, the shutter is closed again and the exposed frame is transported into a receiving spool while a fresh new frame is retrieved from the supply spool and transported into the exposure position again. The cycle of cine filming starts over again. For 60-fps operation, this cycle must be completed within 16.7 milli-seconds. The film transportation time is generally minimized to allow an exposure time of as long as 10 milliseconds, although an exposure time of 5 milliseconds or shorter is more commonly used.

Cine Film Framing

Most cine film cameras used in cardiac angiography are the 35-mm type, using a 24-mm-wide and 18-mm-high frame area, the same as that used in the so-called half-frame 35-mm photography. There are various methods to magnify and match the circular II output image with the rectangular cine film format. These methods are referred to as the overframing methods. Usually, the II output image is magnified in such a way that its diameter is equal to the width (maximum horizontal overframing) or diagonal (total overframing) of the cine frame or somewhere in between (subtotal overframing). Depending on the overframing method used, a camera lens with the appropriate focal length should be selected for the magnification factor required. The film exposure may vary when a different overframing method is used. Thus, different overframing methods may require different settings in the lens aperture or exposure level, or both, for proper exposure of the film.

Automatic Exposure Control

The automatic exposure control (AEC) system is used to maintain the II output light level at a constant level and therefore achieves consistent film density from one frame to another and from one patient to another. A small prism is positioned between the beam splitter and the cine camera lens to deflect a small portion of the light beam onto a photocell, which converts the light into a voltage signal. This signal is compared with a reference voltage, which can be varied to set the overall level of film exposure. If the photocell signal is different from the reference voltage, x-ray techniques will be varied until the two signals are identical with each other. The x-ray kVp, current, and exposure time can be varied alone or in combination to vary the exposure (per frame) at the II input. However, the range of variation in mA and pulse width is rather limited, therefore, the kVp is typically varied when the mA and pulse width are increased to their maximum limits. The kVp and mA can also be varied in such a way that their product is kept fixed. Thus, the power delivered to the target is constant, while the kVp is varied to alter the average energy and therefore the penetrating ability of the x-ray beam. Notice that the camera aperture can also be changed to vary the film exposure. However, this adjustment is outside the AEC feedback system. It provides a method to alter the overall density of the exposed cine film.

Film Characteristics

Films used in x-ray imaging are characterized by measuring the characteristic curve, which is also called the H&D curve and defined as the plot of the measured film density against the log of relative exposures. The curve approaches a straight line in the middle density range while turning flat on both ends. Based on this curve, several parameters can be computed. The base plus fog density is the density measured on unexposed film. This density typically ranges from 0.06 to 0.20, depending on the film type, storage, and processing conditions. The film gamma, or gradient, is the slope of the straight portion of the curve. Its value is a direct indication for the contrast of the film. The speed of the film is indicated by the position of the characteristic curve along the log exposure axis. In comparing the speed of different films, the same set of exposures should be used. Both contrast and speed can be modified by changes in processing conditions such as the development time, temperature, and concentration of the developer.

One important film characteristic that cannot be measured from the characteristic curve is the film graininess. Film graininess refers to the size and contrast of mottle originated from the silver halide grains in the emulsion. Film graininess is not independent of film speed and contrast. For instance, film speed and contrast are often increased by using larger silver halide grains in the emulsion to allow easier activation by light. As the result, high-speed film tends to look grainier. Like film speed and contrast, variation in processing conditions also changes the film graininess.

Cine Film Selection

Cardiac angiography involves an anatomic region where the degree of x-ray attenuation varies dramatically, resulting in a large range of exposure to cine film. Therefore, it is preferred that films of modest contrast be used. Modern IIs generally provide bright output images. The intensity of these images can be modulated to accommodate films of various speeds. This can be achieved by using diaphragms of appropriate size to control the size of the collimated light beam from the II output or by varying the aperture in the cine camera lens, or both. Film graininess, on the other hand, bears close relationship to the image quality. Therefore, selection of the cine film should be based mainly on the contrast and graininess of the film rather than the speed.

Cine Film Processing

As mentioned in the previous section, film speed, contrast, and graininess are all affected by film processing. Processing with higher temperature or longer development time (often referred to as "push processing") may result in higher film density and contrast, but also produce grainier images. The film processing factors should be specifically optimized for each different type of film used. However, both processing factors and film quality should be monitored on a daily basis by technical staff associated with the catheterization laboratory to ensure stable and consistent film quality and to find processing or film problems in their early stages before they jeopardize patient examinations.

Cine Film Projector

The cine projection system is the image display component in the cine fluorography imaging chain. It plays just as important a role in determining the quality of the final visual image as other components. There are two types of projectors: the intermittent film advance and the rotating prism types. The intermittent film advance type of projectors operates in the same manner as the movie projector or the cine camera itself. With it, each cine frame is stationary for a brief period for projection. The film advances only intermittently from one frame to the next while the shutter closes. This design should provide the best resolution. However, it is also limited in projection speed to under 30 fps. With the rotating prism-type projectors, the cine film is moved continuously while being projected through a rotating polygon prism. A higher projection speed can be achieved with this type of projector.

Image brightness is essential to the visualization of details. It is important to achieve and maintain the screen brightness, without film projected, above 16-foot lambert. Selection and use of a high-intensity lamp and a projection screen with good reflectivity can help achieve this goal. This is particularly helpful when projecting films whose overall density is on the darker side. There should be provisions for proper darkening of the room. The viewing room should be maintained at a reasonably clean level to avoid dust accumulation on lenses, projecting screen, or film itself. Projector optics and projecting screen should be checked regularly for cleanliness and cleaned carefully if necessary.

Fluoroscopy

Modern fluoroscopy employs a TV camera optically coupled to the output of the II to provide real-time (30 fps) imaging capability. The camera converts the optical image from the output of the II into electronic video signals that are sent to a CRT monitor for display and to video recording devices for recording and playback. Fluoroscopy is used primarily for positioning and framing for cine studies and monitoring catheter and wire position. For these applications, image quality does not have to be extremely high, and low-dose operation is often used. In interventional procedures such as percutaneous transluminal coronary angioplasty (PTCA), high-quality fluoroscopy is required for visualizing smaller guide wires and lesions. This is generally achieved by using a high-quality TV camera and high-dose operation.

Although most fluoroscopy systems employ continuous x-rays, some newer systems provide the option of using pulsed x-rays. Some systems incorporate digital image acquisition and storage capability for higher image quality and more flexibility. Because the features and capabilities of the x-ray generator and tube are often specified for the more demanding cine film studies, they are generally more than suitable for fluoroscopic use.

Television Camera

The TV camera consists of the lens, image pick-up tube, and electronics for operating the tube and amplifying the signal output. The lens (with multiple components) of the TV camera is used to focus the image from the output of the II at the target in the TV pick-up tube. The TV target consists of a large matrix of small capacitors made of photoconductive material. Each capacitor, if charged first, can be discharged by light photons falling on it. Thus, the optical image focused on the target can produce a spatially varying charge pattern. A focused electron beam scans and recharges the target in a faster scanning fashion. Depending on the degree of discharge in the scanned region, a signal current proportional to the incident light exposure is generated by the recharging process. This signal current is amplified and read out as a voltage signal. Appropriate timing signals are then added to form a standard composite video signal for display or recording.

Conversion of the light exposure into an electronic signal may not be a linear process. Different target materials often result in different signal responses. The older camera tubes use an antimony trisulfide target and are designed to accommodate larger exposure range at the expense of contrast loss. Because of the need to use the same camera for digital angiography and high-quality fluoroscopy, most modern angiography systems employ the newer types of pick-up tubes, for example, Plumbicon (North American Philips Company, Inc., Shelton, Conn.) (using a lead monoxide target), which are designed to produce a nearly linear signal response and almost no contrast loss. These tubes often have better resolution and signal-to-noise ratio as well. The disadvantage of these tubes, however, is that they can be easily saturated with excessively bright light and therefore are less forgiving to overexposures. Careful framing and x-ray collimation are necessary to avoid overexposing the TV target, which can cause permanent damage to the target, in addition to producing saturated TV signals with washed-out details.

Another characteristic of TV pick-up tubes is the persistence or lagging in image readout. This refers to the effect of the scanning electron beam failing to fully recharge the charge and therefore leaving a discharge pattern that would be read out as a residual image shadow in subsequent image frames. This is particularly serious for the antimony trisulfide (vidicon) target (lasting for 100–200 msec) and for target areas that are exposed to intense light exposure and therefore heavily discharged. The image persistence or lagging is more obvious when bright spots are present during rapid panning movement, resulting in streaks in images. The modern pick-up tubes [e.g., Plumbicon, Primicons (North American Philips Company, Inc., Shelton, Conn.)] are typically designed to have reduced persistence (10% or less of signals carried over to the next frame or field).

There are two ways that the electron beam scans the TV target: interlaced or non-interlaced. The North American standard divides a TV image into 525 lines for scan. The electron beam must scan all lines and retraces to its initial position within one thirtieth of a second. The video signal generated during this cycle is called a frame. Therefore, there are 30 frames for each second. With an interlaced scan, each frame is divided into an odd field, consisting of all odd lines, and an even field, consisting of all even lines. A complete frame of image is acquired by scanning the odd lines first and then the even lines. The interlaced scan is used to reduce flickering without going to a higher scanning rate. Because scanning one field tends to partially erase the other field, the interlaced scan is often used with continuous x-rays to achieve more uniform signal readout. With the non-interlaced scan, also referred to as the progressive scan, all 525 lines are scanned in one pass. The non-interlaced scan is more demanding in camera design. For instance, to achieve flickerless display during fluoroscopy, the target must be scanned at 60 or more fps. The non-interlaced scan is often used when high-resolution images are required, or when pulsed x-rays are used, as in digital angiography or pulsed fluoroscopy studies.

In recent years, high-quality TV systems have become available for use in angiography. These systems generally provide a resolution of at least 1000 lines in both horizontal and vertical directions. However, their use should be limited to digital angiography or high-dose fluoroscopy. The x-ray noise present in low-dose fluoroscopic images prevents their spatial resolution capability from being useful in regular fluoroscopy. However, many manufacturers upscan 525-line fluoroscopic images to 1025-line for display to decrease the perception of TV scan lines and achieve a smoother look. This technique does not increase the intrinsic resolution of the fluoroscopic images.

Display of TV Images

Video signals from the TV camera are generally sent to one or more CRT monitors for display. Inside the CRT, a scanning electron beam is accelerated and focused at a fluorescent screen (type P4 phosphor) to generate visible images. The electron beam scans the screen in much the same way the electron beam scans the target inside a TV pick-up tube. Synchronization between the monitors and camera relies on the synch pulses encoded in the video signals. The video signal is applied to a control grid to modulate the intensity of the electron beam to produce various levels of luminance (in foot-lamberts) on the screen. The contrast of CRT images may be characterized by the dynamic range defined as the ratio of the maximum luminance (slightly before saturation) to the minimum luminance (corresponding to the black video level). It is important to choose monitors with good brightness (50 foot-lamberts or higher) and dynamic range (250:1 or better) to optimize the visualization of image details.[7] It is also important to position the monitor and to adjust the room light in such a way that glares from the CRT screen are minimized. It is important to adjust the monitor-to-viewer distance for about 4 times the diagonal screen size (frequently 7 to 21 inches). For monitors with higher resolutions (i.e., 1000- or 2000-line monitors), this distance should be reduced to below 2 times the diagonal screen size.

Automatic Brightness Control and Automatic Gain Control

Under fixed x-ray techniques, the brightness of fluoroscopic images varies when the FOV is altered during panning or change of the II mode. This variation makes it difficult or impossible to visualize image details. Therefore, an automatic brightness control (ABC) system is generally provided to vary the x-ray techniques to compensate for this brightness change. The ABC system used in fluoroscopy is similar to the AEC system used in cinefluorography. With the system, the light output from the II is monitored and used to generate a feedback signal that is compared with a reference signal to determine whether to increase or decrease the x-ray tube output. Three methods are used to vary the x-ray tube output: variable kVp and mA, variable kVp and fixed mA, or fixed kVp and variable mA. These three methods can be used alone or combined to vary the output of the x-ray tube and maintain the brightness of the fluoroscopic images. The ABC system can also help adjust the x-ray output to accommodate patients of different sizes. When the x-ray output exceeds the legal dose limit, the automatic gain control (AGC) kicks in to maintain the brightness of the fluoroscopic images electronically without further increasing the x-ray tube output. The AGC system is basically a video signal amplification circuitry with its output used as a feedback signal to control the gain. The AGC system is designed to maintain the peak or average video signal at a preset value, thus resulting in a more consistent image display. Some AGC systems also incorporate a variable camera aperture that can open up to pass more light to the TV target before the amplifier-based AGC system kicks in.

Video Recording

With the help of video recording, fluoroscopic images can be saved and replayed almost immediately. Two types of video recording devices are available: videotape recorder and videodisk recorder. Both recorders can be used to save live video images from a standard TV camera. Tape recorders have a larger storage capability but are less convenient in locating and replaying specific images. Videodisk recorders, on the other hand, are convenient in freeze-framing, locating, and replaying specific images, but store many fewer images. Therefore, videodisk recorders are often used as a temporary recording and replaying device when freeze-frame or slow-frame advancement is required.

Video recording devices vary in image quality. State-of-the-art videotape recorders continue to be broadcast-quality helical scan, 1-inch type C recorders. They have a bandwidth frequency of 10 or 20 MHz for use with 525-line or 1,023/1,049-line TV systems, respectively. The signal-to-noise ratio can reach about 180:1. The best of this type of technology can almost compete with cine film in quality. Recorders of lesser quality are also available in various formats, including 3/4-inch U-matic and super VHS. Some of these recorders incorporate limited digital image storage and processing capabilities to provide features like freeze-framing and digital magnification, although locating specific images remains slow and inconvenient. Videodisk recorders have evolved to be able to record 10 or more seconds at 30 fps with an image resolution of at least 500 lines in both vertical and horizontal directions. The videodisk recorder is an ideal loop recording device to be used in conjunction with a videotape recorder. With such an arrangement, the disk recorder provides the abilities for random image access, true instant replay (no rewinding required), freeze-framing, and single-frame forwarding and backing, while the tape recorder provides long-term recording of all image runs in a catheterization procedure.

Digital Angiography

Digital angiography was developed initially for subtraction angiography with intravenous or reduced contrast injections. As the technology for TV camera, digital image acquisition, storage, display, and processing techniques have advanced, digital angiography applications have spread to many other angiographic procedures. Although the image enhancement and processing capabilities of digital angiography are still important, the convenience and speed it has brought to angiographic procedures has become equally important.

Digital Representation of Images

A digital image is basically a two-dimensional matrix of digital numbers stored in memory chips and various magnetic, or optical digital storage devices, including floppy disks, hard disks, and tapes. No matter how digital images are actually acquired and stored, they can be conceptually reviewed as obtained from a real analog image by dividing the image into columns and rows of little square boxes, averaging and digitizing the image signals within each box. These boxes and their dimension are called the pixel size. The average image signal for each pixel is digitized to form the digital image signal, pixel value, or grey value. The numbers of the columns or rows, generally identical with each other in digital angiography, are used to describe the dimension or size of the digital images. The dimensions of the digital images are often but not always in power of 2. The pixel values are generally represented by an integer number ranging from zero to some power of 2. This practice greatly simplifies hardware and software designs for image storage, display, and processing. For example, images used in cardiac angiography are typically 512×512 or 1024×1024 in size and have a 8- to 10-bit data depth. In digital chest radiography, the images can be as large as 4096×5000 and the data depth as large as 12 bits.

Digital Image Acquisition

Figure 2-5 shows the block diagram for a typical digital angiography system. With digital angiography techniques, a high-quality TV camera is coupled to II output for both fluoroscopy and high-dose serial imaging. The electronic signal output of the TV camera is digitized into digital data by an analog-to-digital converter (ADC). The digital image data are then sent to a digital image acquisition system for image display, processing, and storage. Digital angiography allows instant image replay, image enhancement, and easy formation of subtraction images. Furthermore, digital image data can be processed and analyzed by computer. This is particularly useful in cardiac angiography in which quantitative analysis is an important part of the diagnostic procedure.

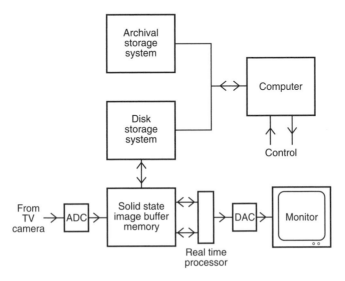

Figure 2-5 Block diagram for a typical digital image acquisition, storage, processing, and display system used in digital angiography.

The quality of a TV camera is often characterized by its spatial resolution capability and signal-to-noise ratio. Although many TV cameras are designed to produce 525-line video images, their spatial resolution capability may be further limited by the target used, by the scanning electron beam size, by the bandwidth frequency of the camera electronics, and by the use of interlaced scanning image readout. The TV camera used in digital angiography should have the provision for operation in non-interlaced scanning readout mode and have a resolution of at least 500 lines in both horizontal and vertical directions. It also should have linear signal response and high signal-to-noise ratio. For systems intended for coronary arteriography, the camera should be designed for 1000-line operation. This is considered as a necessary step for the digital angiography technique to approach the cine fluorography technique in spatial resolution quality.

Digital Image Storage

Although digital videotape recorders capable of recording 1000-line digital images at 30 fps exist, they are expensive and inconvenient for replaying. A more common arrangement is to use a high-speed hard disk storage system to record image data at the same rate as they are acquired. These images can be replayed instantly for clinical study and later archived at a slower data rate. Currently, there are disk systems that allow $1024 \times 1024 \times 8$-bit images to be stored at a rate of 30 fps and have sufficient capacity to hold images from several image runs. Such systems can be used in conjunction with a 1000-line TV system for high-resolution imaging applications such as coronary arteriography. Although systems with such capability are expensive now, their cost is likely to go down with advances in digital technology. Less capable systems can achieve a recording rate of up to 30 $512 \times 512 \times 8$-bit images or 7.5 $1024 \times 1024 \times 8$-bit images per second. Thus, either resolution or speed must be compromised for imaging coronary arteries. However, these systems should be adequate for imaging cardiac chambers or larger vessels. Both digital tape and writable optical disk storage technologies can be used for image archival storage. The tape devices have larger storage capacity and are generally available at lower cost. The writable optical disk system, while more expensive, offers reasonably large capacity (over 10 gigabytes on a single 14″ disk) and much faster and more convenient image retrieval.

Pulsed X-ray, High-Dose Applications

Digital angiography techniques can be used for fluoroscopy or high-quality pulsed x-ray imaging. When used for the latter, the TV camera is generally operated in the non-interlaced or progressive scan mode. The sequence of events during image acquisition are similar to those in a cine fluorography study. Prior to image acquisition, the TV camera aperture is stopped down to the proper f/stop value to accommodate the more intense light resulting from higher exposures. The TV target is first exposed to the pulsed x-rays and then read out with a non-interlaced electron beam scan. The readout signal is digitized instantaneously into digital data. Two image buffer memories are generally used so that one can be used to receive digitized image data while the other sends out the previous frame of image data to the disk storage system. One limitation of digital angiography is the excessive time required to read out the target. This limits the framing rate of most digital angiography systems to 30 fps or lower. While not as high as achieved by cine fluorography techniques, this rate is usable for many studies, in particular those of adult patients.

Digital Fluoroscopy

Traditionally, fluoroscopy is performed with continuous x-rays and the TV camera operated in the interlaced scanning mode. It is possible to operate the TV camera in the non-interlaced mode and use pulsed x-rays to perform so-called pulsed fluoroscopy. The advantage of pulsed fluoroscopy is that short x-ray exposures produce sharper images of moving objects such as cardiac chambers, pulsating vessels, or catheters. Pulsed fluoroscopy, however, requires the TV system to be operated in non-interlaced mode. This would cause flickering unless both the TV camera and monitor are operated at 60 fps. With a digital angiography system, the flickering problem can be handled easily by using its digital image memory buffers. The system can be programmed to use alternatively one of two image buffer memories to acquire a new image frame while using the other to display a previously acquired frame. This approach is more flexible because the images do not have to be displayed in the same way as they are acquired. Another advantage is the ability to reduce the x-ray pulsing rate while using image buffers to produce seemingly continuous image display. This allows reduction of patient/staff x-ray dose during some fluoroscopic studies in which changes or motion of the objects being imaged do not require 30 fps. This method allows the fluoroscopy radiation dose to be spread over fewer images, thus producing high-quality fluoroscopic images (at reduced fps).

Quality Control

The main objectives of a quality control program are to detect problems in their early phases and to avoid unsuccessful examinations due to equipment failure or poor image quality. Although unsuccessful or aborted examinations are obviously undesirable in all areas of radiologic imaging, it is particularly serious in cardiac angiographic studies for several reasons. Unlike most other radiographic examinations, cardiac angiographic studies involve risks from catheterization and injection of large amounts of contrast material. Catheterization procedures are relatively low throughput and expensive procedures. Furthermore, the total radiation dose received by the patient is enormous and among the highest in diagnostic radiology. Therefore, it is vital to have a vigorous quality control program for every cardiac catheterization laboratory.

A quality control program for a cardiac catheterization laboratory may be divided into three parts: (1) film processing, (2) daily test image quality and equipment function, and (3) annual test of image quality and radiation dose measurement. The first two parts of the tests are typically performed by technologists associated with the laboratory. The third part of the tests should be performed by a qualified physicist. Here, we discuss only the first two types of quality control.

Film Processing

Quality control of the film processor is generally carried out with the sensitometry technique using a device called the sensitometer. It consists of a stable calibrated light source filtered by a series of neutral filters to produce a set of gradually increasing light exposures. As a daily quality control procedure, a section of film is exposed by the sensitometer and then processed to produce an optical density step wedge. A densitometer is used to measure the optical density for selected density steps. Three parameters are measured and plotted each day to monitor the performance of the processor and detect any change: the base-plus-fog optical density, the optical density at the "speed step," and the contrast index.

The base-plus-fog density is measured to monitor the condition of the unexposed film. It is defined as the density in the unexposed area of the film. This density varies with the film type and may increase with the storage conditions. It can range from 0.06 for clear-base film to 0.31 for tinted-base films. Higher than normal base-plus-fog densities may indicate incorrect film type or improper film storage. The speed step is defined and identified as the step that produces a density value closest to 1, at which the film speed is often evaluated. The optical density at the speed step is measured daily to monitor fluctuations of film speed, which may be affected by the processing conditions. The contrast index is measured as the difference between the optical density at the speed step and that at the next higher step. This is used to monitor the film contrast, which also may be affected by the processing conditions. The developer temperature also can be measured and recorded to directly monitor the processing conditions. These parameters should be measured and plotted on a daily basis. When excessive fluctuations—for example, ± 0.1 or greater for speed and contrast and ± 0.03 or greater for fog—are observed, the processing conditions should be checked carefully.

Fluoroscopy Imaging Chain

The fluoroscopy imaging chain should be tested for image resolution and brightness on a daily basis before any patient study begins. A standard tool for testing the overall resolution power of the II-based imaging system is a copper mesh pattern consisting of eight different sections with various line densities. The pattern should be taped to the input of the II and imaged with the ABC system turned on. The images should be viewed to determine the system resolution limit as indicated by the line density of the finest resolvable mesh pattern. The value should match previously measured values and those specified by the manufacturer. An anthropomorphic chest phantom can be imaged to check the image brightness and functions of the ABC system. If the anthropomorphic chest phantom is not available, copper plates of several different thicknesses (up to 2.4 mm for adult patients and 0.9 mm for child patients) can be grouped together to simulate the variation of x-ray attenuation in the chest regions. Panning, change of the II mode, or x-ray collimation may be used to see if the ABC system is functioning properly in maintaining adequate image brightness and contrast under various imaging conditions.

Cinefluorography Imaging Chain

Similar tests should be performed on the cinefluorography imaging chain on a daily basis before any patient study begins. Cine film images of the copper mesh pattern (taped to the input of the II) should be acquired and displayed on a viewing box. The overall system resolution should be checked with a magnifier and compared with previously measured values or those specified by the manufacturer.

Proper film exposure and functions of the AEC system should be checked by imaging a copper plate simulating an average adult (2.4 mm thick) or child patient (0.9 mm). Easily reproduced geometry and x-ray collimation should be used. A short cine film run should be performed for all frequently used II modes. Film densities should be measured at the center on three or more randomly selected frames. These densities should not vary from each other by more than 0.2. They should be recorded on a daily basis together with the kVp, mA, exposure time, focal spot size, cine camera aperture size, and camera frame rate used. They should not deviate from the optimal values, set during installation, by more than 0.05. If the deviation exceeds 0.05, the sensitometry data should be checked to see if the quality of films or film processing are in control. If they are, a new camera aperture should be chosen until the deviation falls below 0.05. If the aperture needs to be changed frequently or the largest aperture has to be used, chances are that either the x-ray generator, tube, or AEC system is malfunctioning, and service personnel from the manufacturer should be called in for correction measures.

The quality of the cine film projector should be checked and monitored on a daily basis. This can be done by projecting a test film strip containing the Society of Motion Picture and Television Engineers (SMPTE) test pattern. The cine film projection should be able to resolve all resolution and contrast patterns with no or minimal jittering.

Radiation Safety

Radiation exposure levels to both the patient and personnel in typical catheterization examinations are among the highest in diagnostic x-ray imaging procedures. Diagnostic x-rays have sufficient energy to ionize molecules in body structures and generate free radicals, which could cause cancer in the exposed persons some years later. This risk is generally considered to increase with the exposure level. A large number of personnel are often present around the patient during typical catheterization procedures. The examinations may require long fluoroscopic time for positioning and catheter placement and several long image sequences at high exposure levels. Thus, it is essential for both the patient and personnel's protection that the personnel involved in catheterization procedures understand the danger of radiation exposures and how to protect from such exposures.

Radiation Units

Three radiation units are often used for x-ray–related measurements. The unit *roentgen* is a unit of exposure. It is defined as the amount of ionization created by x-rays in a unit volume of air. The word *rad* is the acronym for "radiation absorbed dose." Used as a unit, it is defined as the amount of energy deposited to a unit mass of absorbing material when the x-rays ionize the molecules (including energy transferred to the kinetic energy of the ions and electrons generated). The word *rem* is an acronym for "roentgen equivalent man." It is another unit of rad that takes the relative effects of the radiation into account. For diagnostic x-rays, 1 rem equals 1 rad. This is not the case for other types of ionizing radiations like charged particles. Newer literature on radiation safety uses the units *gray* and *sievert*, which are equivalent to 100 rad and 100 rem, respectively.

Monitoring Radiation Exposure

There are several devices often used to monitor radiation exposures in a work environment. Film badge dosimetry employs the density of exposed films as the measure of the radiation received by the person who wears the badge. Although relatively insensitive and sometimes inaccurate, it is an inexpensive and convenient method to monitor the accumulated exposures for each worker. It also has the advantage of providing a permanent record of the dose. Thermoluminescent dosimetry (TLD) employs special phosphor crystals that can be excited by radiation and releases the absorbed energy when heated. TLD is more sensitive and accurate than film. It also can be used for monitoring personnel exposures. A pocket dosimeter is a simplified ionization chamber that, together with a portable charger-reader, can easily be used to measure x-ray exposure on a study-by-study or daily basis. It is most useful for checking or daily monitoring of exposure levels at various locations in a catheterization laboratory.

Maximum Permissible Dose

The concept of maximum permissible dose (MPD) was established for protecting radiation workers by the National Council on Radiation Protection and Measurements (NCRP). The MPDs currently applicable to personnel involved with radiographic procedures in the United States are as follows:

- Whole body exposure: 5 rem/yr
- Lens of eye: 15 rem/yr
- All other areas (e.g., red bone marrow, breast, lung, gonads, skin, extremities): 50 rem/yr

The MPDs should be used as guidelines in designing radiation protection methods and in controlling personnel exposures.

Radiation Risk

There are two categories of risks from x-ray exposures. Radiation may induce mutations and cause genetic damages. This risk, however, is low if lead aprons are worn and if radiation exposure outside the aprons is kept below the MPD levels. Because most catheterization laboratory workers receive only a small fraction of the MPD, the genetic risk should be even lower. High-level x-ray exposures in the order of hundreds or thousands of rads can cause cancer. The great majority of medical radiation workers, however, currently receive an occupational dose of 0.1 rem per year, comparable to that from natural background radiation. Thus, the risk of inducing fatal cancers to these workers should be similar to that caused by natural background radiation. This risk has been estimated to be 10 in a million per year, approximately equivalent to the risks of riding in an automobile for 1000 miles, making three coast-to-coast round-trip commercial flights, or smoking 30 cigarettes. Although the risk appears to be insignificant, effort should be made to avoid unnecessary exposures to reduce the radiation worker's risk to a minimum level. Large exposures to the eyes have been known to induce cataracts. Such effects, however, seem to require a high threshold exposure, and no incidence has been observed at low-dose levels.

Patient Exposures

In posteroanterior projection, the patient is lying on the table while the x-ray tube is underneath the table. Therefore, table-top exposures are often used as a measure of the patient entrance exposure in radiation safety considerations. Table-top exposures during fluoroscopy and cine film studies have been measured on a large number of systems. Average table-top exposure for cine film studies is approximately 26 mR per frame in the 6- or 7-inch mode and 18 mR in the 9- or 10-inch mode. Multiplying the exposures per frame with the image rate in fps, the average table-top exposure rate is 40 R/min at 30 fps and 122 R/min at 60 fps. Measurements also show that lower kVps often lead to higher patient/staff exposure as well as heat loading.

Table-top exposure rate during fluoroscopy ranges from 2 to 4 R/min, depending primarily on the mode of II used. All fluoroscopic equipment manufactured after August 1976 must comply with the Center of Devices and Radiological Health (CDRH) standards. Generally, they should not be operated if the automatic brightness control results in an exposure rate in excess of 10 R/min, unless the images are being recorded or an optional high-output mode is activated. Exposures in the high-output mode can be as high as 20 to 30 R/min.

The total patient entrance exposure for a typical cardiac angiographic study, involving 10 minutes of fluoroscopy and 1 minute of cine film studies, ranges from 42 to 100 R at 30 fps and from 60 to 160 R at 60 fps. These exposures are equivalent to 100 to 250 chest films and 150 to 400 chest films, respectively. Thus, the cancer risk for cardiac angiographic studies is high compared with those estimated for other diagnostic x-ray studies. The risk is estimated to be between 20 to 50 chances in a million for 30 fps and 30 to 80 chances in a million for 60 fps. This is compared with 0.2 chance in a million for a chest film.

Factors Affecting Patient Exposures

In general, patient exposures increase or decrease with personnel exposures. They are affected by many factors, including the x-ray kVp, beam filtration, exposure time, x-ray collimation, source-to-skin distance, and use of antiscatter grids. Many of these factors also affect the image quality. Thus, selecting these factors often becomes a process of compromising between image quality and increased patient/staff exposure. Decreasing the x-ray kVp generally increases patient exposure and tube heat loading. However, it also increases the image contrast. Low-energy x-rays are mostly absorbed in the patient, resulting in higher dose level. Therefore, most radiation safety regulations require that additional filtration be added to absorb low-energy photons before they reach the patient. For 70- or higher kVp x-rays, the total filtration should be at least 2.5 mm of aluminum or equivalent. The filtration should be checked once a year, or more frequently, by qualified professionals, usually a medical or health physicist. To minimize the exposure time during fluoroscopy, the exposure must be terminated at the end of any 5-minute period, unless the timer is manually reset. This keeps the staff aware of the exposure time used.

Personnel Exposures

Exposures to the laboratory personnel are mainly caused by direct scatter from the irradiated part of the patient. Thus, exposures depend on many factors, including the x-ray techniques, patient size, x-ray collimation, projection angle, and approaches to catheter placement. A useful guideline is that personnel standing at 1 meter from the patient receive 0.001 of the patient exposure. Both fluoroscopic and cine film studies contribute to personnel exposures. Personnel exposures during fluoroscopy are typically 0.5 to 0.8 mR/min for an average adult male patient. Personnel exposures during cine film studies are a factor of 10 to 20 times higher, depending on the framing rate. They range from 5 to 7 mR/min at 30 fps and 10 to 12 mR/min at 60 fps.

To reduce personnel radiation exposures, the "x-ray on" time should be minimized and the distance between the workers and patient should be kept as great as possible. Shielding devices should be used between the workers and the patient. At a minimum, lead aprons should be worn to reduce the exposure to 5% of the unattenuated level. As an extension of the lead aprons, individual thyroid shields of 0.5-mm lead or equivalent should be worn to further reduce the workers' occupational radiation risk by a factor of about 2. Depending on the work load, exposures to unprotected eyes could approach or even exceed the legal limit of 15 rems per year. Wraparound leaded eyeglasses can be worn to keep the eye exposure well under the limit.

The intensity of scattered radiation increases with the area of irradiation. Therefore, proper collimation is essential for minimizing the scattered radiation and personnel exposures. The personnel exposures also depend on the projection used, which largely determines the relative positions of the workers, x-ray tube, and patient. Because backscatter from the tube side of the patient is much more intense than that from the detector side, additional shielding should be used to protect workers from backscatter.

Room Shielding

The walls, doors, floors, and ceiling in a cardiac catheterization laboratory must be shielded with lead lining to protect people in neighboring rooms from receiving too much radiation. For controlled areas, where access, occupancy, or working conditions are supervised for radiation protection, the shielding should be designed to reduce the exposure level to below 5 rems per year. A more conservative approach is to keep the exposure about 0.5 rem/yr in controlled areas, assuming there is a pregnant technologist present (0.5 rem/gestation period in the MPD to the fetus). Exposures in adjacent office areas should be kept down to 0.1 rem/yr.

SELECTED READINGS

1. Sprawls P. Jr. Physical principles of medical imaging. 2nd ed. Gaithersburg, MD: Aspen, 1993.
2. Moore RJ. Imaging principles of cardiac angiography. Rockville, MD: Aspen, 1990.
3. Mistretta CA, Crummy AB, Strother CM, Sackett JF. Digital subtraction arteriography: an application of computerized fluoroscopy. Chicago, London: Year Book Medical, 1982.
4. Mancini CBJ. Clinical applications of cardiac digital angiography. New York: Raven, 1988.
5. Wasserman AG, Ross AM. Cardiac application of digital angiography. Mount Kisco, NY: Futura, 1989.
6. Proceedings of the ACR/FDA Workshop on Fluoroscopy. Washington, DC, October 16–17, 1992.
7. Blume H, Roehrig H, Brown M, Ji TL. Comparison of the physical performance of high resolution CRT displays and the need for a display standard. Medical Imaging IV: Image capture and display. Society of Photographic Imaging and Electronics, 1990;1232:97–114.

3

THE CARDIAC CATHETERIZATION LABORATORY: SET-UP AND MANAGEMENT

David P. Faxon

The Cardiac Catheterization Laboratory

THE CARDIAC CATHETERIZATION laboratory has undergone enormous changes over the past 40 years. Not only have there been remarkable advances in x-ray systems with the development of C-arm systems and digital imaging, but the laboratory has become the setting for a growing number of therapeutic techniques, such as angioplasty and radiofrequency ablation, that were not even conceived of only a few years ago. With the increased complexity of the laboratory's function, having an adequately equipped, organized laboratory and a highly trained and skilled staff is even more important than it was in the past. This chapter discusses the elements necessary to run a cardiac catheterization laboratory in today's environment.

The Laboratory and Equipment

The cardiac catheterization laboratory is a designated area that is specifically designed and staffed for the performance of cardiac catheterization and interventional cardiology techniques.[1] It is usually not advisable for the laboratory to be shared with other hospital departments, such as vascular radiology, because the special requirements of the cardiac catheterization laboratory can be compromised and less functional in a shared setting. It is advantageous for the laboratory or laboratories to be closely located to the cardiology patient care areas, such as the coronary care unit, as well as in close proximity to operating and emergency rooms in order to facilitate optimal transfer of patients to and from the laboratory.

The catheterization laboratory should include procedure, control, equipment, and utility rooms.[2-3] An example of a cardiac catheterization laboratory is shown in Figure 3-1. The suggested sizes of these rooms are shown in Table 3-1. Procedures rooms should be large enough to accommodate the x-ray system and the x-ray table. Sufficient storage and space for catheters and other disposable equipment should exist. It should also have space for movable equipment that might be used during the procedure, for instance, the intra-aortic balloon console, respirator, crash cart, or other imaging devices such as intravascular ultrasound. An adjacent room also may serve as storage facility, as long as these pieces of equipment can be rapidly moved into the catheterization laboratory. If space is limited, consideration of the type and acuity of cases done in the facility should be considered. These space considerations are particularly important for freestanding or mobile catheterization laboratories, which will be discussed later. The minimal space requirements for a catheterization laboratory are approximately 400 square feet, with sufficient height to permit ceiling mounts for x-ray or ancillary equipment.

The specific design of the room can vary, depending on the preference of the operators. Many laboratories have the control room incorporated into the procedure room to save on overall space, as well as to have the person who will operate the physiologic recorder and x-ray systems nearer the patient during the procedure. Alternatively, the control room can be a separate room with a microphone, permitting the technologist to communicate easily with the laboratory during the procedure. In some settings, a control room is shared between two adjacent cardiac catheterization laboratories. The advantage of this approach is that the area can share personnel and also serve as a nonsterile observation area. These two common configurations are shown in Figure 3-2. Another alternative is to use one large laboratory that shares a single x-ray system between two areas in a room that can be easily partitioned. This so-called swing laboratory allows one patient to be prepared while another procedure is ongoing in the adjacent alcove. Once the procedure is finished, the partition is removed and the x-ray gantry is swung into the adjacent area to permit an imme-

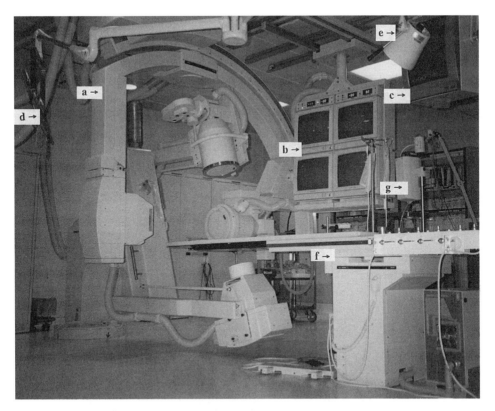

Figure 3-1 Interior of a typical cardiac catheterization laboratory. Major equipment includes the following: **(a)** C-arm x-ray gantry. This laboratory has a biplane configuration with a second C-arm also present. The x-ray tubes are below and to the left on the two C-arms. The image intensifiers are above and to the right; **(b)** monitors, which include one for fluoroscopy of each plane and one for digital imaging display; **(c)** monitor for physiologic signals, including ECG and pressures; **(d)** leaded glass shield to be placed between x-ray tube and operator to decrease radiation to operator; **(e)** high-intensity light source; **(f)** x-ray table; **(g)** power contrast injector.

diate procedure to take place there. The advantage of this design is that one large space can be utilized more efficiently. The disadvantage is that if the x-ray machine fails, a significant impact on laboratory operations occurs and thus, it is not ideal as the only x-ray facility for cardiac catheterization. This set-up is also not practical for biplane x-ray systems and would therefore be limited for interventional and pediatric use.

Other rooms that are necessary in the catheterization suite include a storage and equipment room and clean and dirty preparation rooms. Adequate storage space is frequently overlooked in the designing of cardiac catheterization laboratories. With the increasing demands on managing a rapidly changing inventory, it is important to have an adjacent storage area that is flexible

Table 3-1 Suggested Size of Rooms in
Cardiac Catheterization Laboratory

Use	Suggested area (ft/sq)
Procedure room	400
Soiled utility room	70
Staff dressing room	70
Darkroom and film processing	60
Patient preparation room	120
Recovery/observation room	120
Holding room	120
Reception/secretarial/transcription/ viewing/reporting room	70
Scrub facility	30
Film/record storage	60
Toilet facility	30
Patient dressing room	12
Janitorial space	20
Equipment storage	90
Pharmacy area	30
Blood gas area	20
Staff lounge	70
Conference room	120
Library	70
Office space (per office)	70

Source: Modified from American College of Cardiology/ American Heart Association Ad Hoc Task Force on Cardiac Catheterization. ACC/AHA guidelines for cardiac catheterization and cardiac catheterization laboratories. J Am Coll Cardiol 1991;18:1170.

in design, with movable shelves and closets that can accommodate hanging catheters. Storage within only the laboratory is too restrictive for the modern cardiac catheterization laboratory. The size of the storage room should be determined by the use the laboratory, the number of other catheterization laboratories in the area, and the efficiency and storage capacity of the central supply facilities. An equipment room next to the procedure room can house the x-ray generator and digital angiography equipment. Most manufacturers require this room to be specially climate controlled. In some laboratories, this equipment is placed in the procedure room or in the control room. This is not ideal, because proper climate control and protection from accidental damage are more difficult in this setting. The clean room should be large enough to allow sterile set-up of a number of tables for use in the laboratory during the day. The clean room also should not be used as a dirty room for table and equipment cleanup; a separate area is necessary for this function. In addition to these areas, it is important to have office space for the cardiac catheterization laboratory staff, the catheterization laboratory manager, and secretarial support staff. A breakroom,

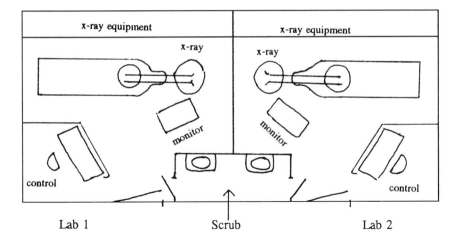

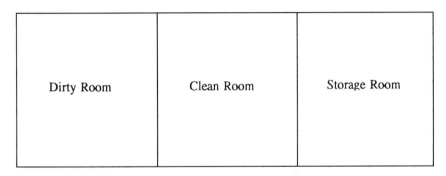

Figure 3-2 *(A)* Catheterization laboratory configuration with internal control room.

staff dressing room with shower, and small conference room are also desirable. A separate film reading room and storage area that is capable of storing at least 1 year's worth of cine films on-site is essential. This area is optimally located next to the cardiac catheterization laboratory, but it can be off-site if necessary. The reading area needs to be accessible to physicians and staff who are not in scrub clothes.

Finally, patient areas for outpatient cardiac catheterization, a waiting area for families, and a recovery area need to be in close proximity to the catheterization laboratory. While it is an attractive idea to share these areas with other patient care facilities, such as outpatient surgery, the coronary care unit, or stepdown areas, in a busy laboratory the patient turnover and staffing makes this arrangement logistically impractical.

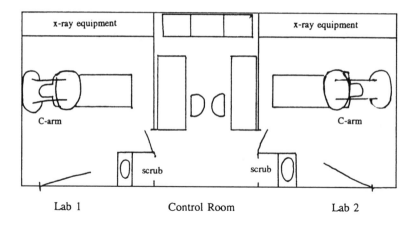

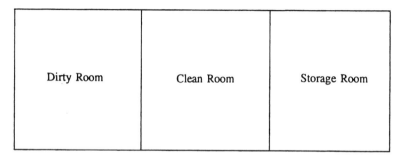

Figure 3-2   **(B)** Catheterization laboratory configuration with external control room.

Equipment Requirements

Continuous blood pressure and ECG monitoring is essential in the cardiac catheterization laboratory. In addition, most laboratories also include continuous arterial oxygen saturation. These monitoring functions are best done through the use of a centralized physiologic recording system, with ECG, BP, and/or oximetry connections directly under the catheterization table and wired into a central recording system. Likewise, pressure transducers should be mounted on a manifold on the x-ray table and connected directly into the base of the table. This permits optimal access to the patient, without excess wiring across the floor or from the ceiling.

One of the most neglected areas in the catheterization laboratory is proper physiologic recording of hemodynamic waveforms. The recording system should be capable of recording high-fidelity waveforms without excessive under- or overdamping. This requires attention to the transducer, the size and type of fluid-filled catheter system used, and the length and size of the conduit tubing from the transducer to the tip of the catheter. Many laboratories use strain-gauge pressure transducers that are mounted directly onto the end of the diagnostic catheters or with a very short tubing to reduce waveform distortion. Pressure channels should be calibrated by the technologist on a routine basis, as well as during the procedure to maintain a zero pressure reference level. When high-level fidelity tracings are necessary, catheters with micromanometers should be used, because fluid pressure wave distortions are not present. The physiologic monitor should be easily visible to the operators at the table, as well as to the technologist operating the physiologic recorder. This usually requires several monitors placed strategically about the room. The physiologic recorder should have a minimum of 5 input channels and, optimally, 6- to 12-channel recorders. A 12-channel recorder is necessary for electrophysiologic studies. Three pressure channels should be available for simultaneous recording and at least two ECG channels are usually needed. The physiologic recorder should be capable of a 12-lead ECG, or a separate ECG machine should be available for 12-lead ECG monitoring. The recorder should be capable of displaying all the hemodynamics simultaneously at variable speeds on the monitor and on paper, and it is useful to have the physiologic recorder display these in color to allow easy recognition of the location of the pressure recording. Most newer physiologic recorders use digital display and have computer capacity to process and accumulate data, as well as store pressure waveforms for later review. The physiologic recorder should also be capable of interfacing with other hemodynamic equipment, such as thermodilution cardiac output or dye dilution measurements, if necessary. The laboratory should also have facilities for arterial blood gas analysis or a reflectance oximeter to measure oxygen saturation. In addition, measurement of coagulation parameters, particularly activated clotting time (ACT), is essential for laboratories performing coronary angioplasty.

The radiographic equipment is critically important to provide the highest quality images and proper digital images for roadmapping during interventional procedures. The details of optimal radiographic equipment are provided in Chapter 2. In most laboratories, more than one x-ray monitor is necessary to provide separate digital images for roadmaps. If a biplane is utilized, four monitors are necessary. It is optimal to have this ceiling-mounted and movable, so that it can be adjusted depending on the location of the operator. The laboratory should be capable of doing procedures from the left as well as the right side of the patient. It is also advantageous to have the ability to replay the cine images from within the laboratory, either using a hand-held control or a table-mounted control, to review the procedure prior to its completion.

The laboratory should be equipped with adequate radiation protection, including a ceiling-mounted x-ray dense glass shield, that can be positioned between the operator and the x-ray tube. In addition, a movable x-ray dense glass partition also is helpful for protection of other personnel in the laboratory.

The power injector necessary to deliver adequate contrast for left ventricular angiography or aortography is also critically important. This may be mounted directly on the angiographic table, from the ceiling, or on the injector itself, which can be moved up to the patient when needed. A mobile injector permits removal to another laboratory if necessary; if space is a serious consideration, however, a table mounted injector may be a better option.

The laboratory should have a properly functioning defibrillator and a crash cart, which are mobile within the room and can be moved rapidly to the patient for immediate use during the procedure. The crash cart should include a defibrillator, equipment for intubation, and standard drugs for advanced life-support resuscitation. The crash cart and the function of the defibrillator should be checked routinely. A temporary pacemaker should be located either on the crash cart or somewhere conveniently placed in the laboratory for immediate use if necessary.

Cineangiographic Film and Processing

A separate cine film processing area, with proper ventilation, should be adjacent to the cardiac catheterization facility. This area should have a cine film processor that is capable of developing, fixing, washing, and drying the film, with a variable temperature control, development time, agitation, replenishment, filtration, and drying system. Several commonly available processors are optimally adapted for cineangiographic film. Proper maintenance of equipment with routine cleaning is also mandatory and should be done at least twice yearly by experienced service personnel. In addition, the processing area should have available a sensitometer to maintain routine quality control on cine film development. Most film companies provide support for instituting a standardized quality assurance program. A separate area for cine film viewing with a high-quality cineangiographic projector is necessary. In addition, a similar digital angiographic viewing area is important and should not be located solely within the procedure room. Optimally, the reading area should be next to the cardiac catheterization laboratory to allow easy transmission of images in the digital system to a proximate reading area for review and storage. The digital system should be such that image review can occur simultaneously with the acquisition of digital images during the procedure. An adjoining storage area for recent cineangiograms with a system that properly files and accounts for films is also important. Many laboratories store most of their cineangiograms off-site, and the duration of storage may vary from institution to institution, but in general should be at least 5 years. There are state requirements concerning the storage of x-ray film.

Safety

The cardiac catheterization laboratory should be monitored continuously by in-hospital electrical and radiation safety protection services.[4-7] Careful monitoring of radiation exposure for all staff and patients is mandatory. Standards for radiation exposure have been published previously. Personnel who are not directly involved in the procedure should stay behind leaded glass areas. Those who are involved should maintain a maximum distance from the x-ray source during angiography and fluoroscopy to minimize radiation exposure.

Electrical safety should be checked on a regular basis.[7] The catheterization laboratory should be placed on an emergency power line. This is particularly important, because most of the x-ray and digital imaging equipment involves computer software. Accidental power surges can significantly harm this equipment, and it should be protected by surge protectors and an adequate back-up system. Electrical safety officers should inspect the electrical safety of all the equipment used in the cardiac catheterization laboratory on a routine basis.

Staffing

Cardiac Catheterization Laboratory Director

The laboratory director is responsible for overseeing the overall operation of the cardiac catheterization laboratory. The Society for Cardiac Angiography and Interventions and the ACC-AHA Task Force on Cardiac Catheterization have provided guidelines for the appropriate qualifications of such individuals.[1,8] The physician director should be a board-certified specialist who is a recognized expert in cardiac catheterization, with at least 5 years of catheterization experience, performing at least 200 procedures a year. The director also should be thoroughly trained in radiation safety and imaging techniques. The director is responsible for setting up criteria for granting privileges, periodically reviewing performance, establishing and maintaining a quality assurance program, acting as a technical director, assuring the proper use of laboratory equipment, assisting the staff in scheduling of patient flow, overseeing the budget, and participating in evaluation and review of laboratory personnel. It is important that the director have the interpersonal skills to communicate and interface with laboratory personnel, clinicians, and hospital administration to ensure optimal patient care. The director should have sufficient dedicated time for catheterization laboratory administrative and oversight duties to optimally manage the facility. It is also advisable that an assistant director be designated to serve as a substitute in the director's absence.

Cardiac Catheterization Laboratory Administrator

The administrator should be responsible for the day-to-day operation of the cardiac catheterization laboratory and be directly responsible to the physician catheterization laboratory director.[9] This individual is most often the head nurse, nurse manager, or head technician. Because the cardiac catheterization laboratory is a complicated and unique facility, it is advisable that the administrator have at least 2 to 3 years experience in the catheterization laboratory before assuming the administrator position. Administrators should be responsible for directing the nonphysician personnel, maintenance of equipment, inventory control, darkroom operation, film quality control, supervision of staff training, and interaction with other hospital departments and services, such as specialized nursing units (CCU, SIU), central supply, radiology, and hospital administration.

Cardiac Catheterization Laboratory Personnel

The mix of nursing and nonnursing personnel varies from laboratory to laboratory. In most laboratory settings, however, there is a mixture of both nurses and cardiovascular technologists. In this setting, nurses should be familiar with the overall function of the laboratory and are directly responsible for nursing care for the patient prior to, during, and following the procedure. In addition, nursing personnel should be ready to respond rapidly and efficiently to an emergency. Most often, cardiac catheterization nurses have a background in critical care and are skilled in performing emergency procedures. Full knowledge of the operation of the catheterization laboratory is desirable, with a working knowledge of x-ray equipment and physiologic recording. In some laboratories, complete cross-training between nursing personnel and nonnursing personnel takes place to run the laboratory more efficiently.

The nonnursing personnel usually includes a cardiovascular technologist and a certified radiology technologist. The cardiovascular technologist is skilled in physiologic recording and the operation of the recorders, cardiac output machines, and blood gas oxygen saturation equipment. The monitoring technician should be trained to recognize cardiac arrhythmias, hemodynamic abnormalities, and in many laboratories also participate in the analysis and calculation of hemodynamic parameters. A certified radiology technician is mandated in most states and is responsible for operation of the cineangiographic equipment, film processing, and film quality control. In addition, the film x-ray technician should be knowledgeable about the operation of the catheterization laboratory and understand the role of the nurse and the cardiovascular technologist.

The catheterization laboratory staff should be adequately cross-trained, so that personnel can be rotated and available for 24-hour coverage. A training program for new personnel should be set up routinely in each laboratory, and if complete cross-training is desired, adequate training in pharmacology and drug administration is essential. An ongoing, continuing education program is imperative for the catheterization laboratory staff. This is best accomplished through weekly meetings, participation in cardiac catheterization laboratory conferences, and periodic seminars put on by professional organizations and industry. Certification in advanced cardiac life-support is desirable, while basic life-support training should be mandatory.

Physicians

Physicians participating in cardiac catheterization laboratories should be credentialed through a standardized process set up by the laboratory director and approved by the appropriate hospital credentialing committees.[1,10] Specific criteria for credentialing have been reported previously. It is generally accepted that physicians should be board eligible or board certified in cardiology, pediatric cardiology, or cardiovascular radiology and have received specialized, in-laboratory training for at least 1 year in a recognized and approved cardiovascular training program. The laboratory physician should be a fully accredited member of the hospital staff and have an anticipated caseload of approximately 150 cases per year (50–100 for pediatric laboratories). The exact number of cases should be determined at each laboratory. For all new physician personnel, a period of preceptorship or proctoring, with direct observation by a laboratory director, should be performed prior to granting full credentials. For physicians who have been away from the laboratory for at least 1 year, a longer period of preceptorship should be necessary.

Interventional cardiology procedures should be credentialed separately for PTCA, valvuloplasty, electrophysiological testing (EP), atherectomy, laser, and stenting, because each of these procedures requires specialized skills beyond those obtained for cardiac catheterization. Requirements for these have been reported previously by both the Society of Cardiac Angiography and Intervention and the ACC-AHA Task Force on Cardiac Catheterization.[11–15]

A process of ongoing review of performance and recertification is also important for proper operation of a cardiac catheterization laboratory. The physician director is responsible for obtaining this information and forwarding it to the credentials committee on a timely basis. In general, a physician should perform 150 cases per year, and if that physician works in more than one laboratory, at least 50 cases should be performed in each facility. Certain physicians who have extensive experience may be able to perform procedures at a lower number without compromising safety.

General Procedural Issues

Indications and Contraindications

The general purpose of cardiac catheterization is to define physiologic and anatomic cardiac abnormalities in patients in whom the diagnosis is unclear and in whom a more accurate diagnosis is important to their subsequent care.[16-17] A list of the common indications for cardiac catheterization is shown in Table 3-2. Patients with valvular heart disease and congenital heart disease, who have evidence of severe abnormalities, need hemodynamic and angiographic assessment to determine their nature and severity, as well as associated abnormalities. Patients in whom optimal treatment would be improved by further knowledge of their cardiovascular disorder should also be considered for cardiac catheterization. Most commonly, patients with valvular or congenital heart disease undergo cardiac catheterization prior to surgical or interventional therapy. There are certain exceptions to this, however. Patients who are young, who have no evidence of coronary artery disease, and whose cardiac abnormality is well defined by noninvasive testing may not need to undergo cardiac catheterization. An example might be a young person with congenital aortic stenosis.

Patients who have unexplained congestive heart failure, particularly if heart failure is of recent onset, may benefit from cardiac catheterization to assess the etiology of their heart failure. This may be particularly important in patients who are diabetic and have normal or only moderately impaired left ventricular function, because many of these patients have significant coronary artery dis-

Table 3-2   Indications for Cardiac Catheterization

1. Valvular and congenital heart disease
    a. To assess the severity of the abnormality for optimal preparation
    b. To assess the need for surgical or interventional therapy
    c. To exclude other associated abnormalities (e.g., CAD)
2. Congestive heart failure
    a. To determine the cause of CHF of unknown etiology
    b. To assess the patient for cardiac transplantation
3. Coronary artery disease
    a. To assess recurrent chest pain of uncertain etiology
    b. To assess the extent of CAD in high-risk patient subgroups
        1. Post MI
        2. Severe ischemia as shown by a markedly positive ECG or other provocative test
        3. Sudden cardiac death or recurrent VT/VF
        4. Evidence of ischemia and undergoing high-risk noncardiac surgery
    c. Prior to coronary revascularization with PTCA or CABG

Abbreviations: CAD, coronary artery disease; CHF, congestive heart failure; MI, myocardial infarction; VT, ventricular tachycardia; VF, ventricular fibrillation; PTCA, percutaneous transluminal coronary angioplasty; CABG, coronary artery bypass surgery.

ease as an explanation of their heart failure. All patients under consideration for cardiac transplant have cardiac catheterization prior to being listed for transplant.

The most common reason for undergoing cardiac catheterization in the United States is for the assessment of coronary artery disease. Patients who continue to have recurrent typical or atypical chest pain of uncertain origin and for whom diagnostic tests are not conclusive in excluding or including the disease, often undergo cardiac catheterization to clarify their coronary anatomy. In addition, patients who are at high risk for coronary artery disease or for cardiac complications also often undergo coronary angiography. This includes patients who are post–myocardial infarction, patients with markedly positive exercise tests or with other evidence of severe ischemia, patients who have had sudden cardiac death or who have recurrent ventricular tachycardia or fibrillation that is suspected to be due to coronary ischemia, and patients with evidence of ischemia who are undergoing high-risk noncardiac surgery, for example, aortic aneurysm repair. Most commonly, however, patients undergo coronary angiography prior to revascularization procedures such as angioplasty or bypass surgery.

Contraindications for cardiac catheterization are relative and should be individually determined for each patient, because the acuity of the medical problem may necessitate a higher risk procedure. Some commonly accepted relative contraindications include a recent stroke (within 1 month), progressive renal failure, active gastrointestinal bleeding, fever that may be due to infection, severe anemia, severe uncontrolled systemic hypertension, severe electrolyte abnormalities, severe systemic or psychological illness in which the prognosis is doubtful, extreme physiologic age, refusal to consider subsequent therapy such as angioplasty, bypass or valve surgery, severe digitalis intoxication, and documented anaphylactoid reaction to contrast media.

The ACC-AHA Ad Hoc Task Force has suggested that only low-risk patients undergo ambulatory catheterization to minimize the risk of the procedure.[1] They suggested that patients who live more than 1 hour away from the laboratory; who are being considered for an interventional therapeutic procedure; who are infants; who have had a recent stroke; who are suspected of having pulmonary hypertension, severe peripheral vascular disease, or severe diabetes; and who have had noninvasive testing suggesting severe ischemia be excluded from ambulatory catheterization. Other relative contraindications to cardiac catheterization include a history of contrast allergy, being older than 75, severe obesity, severe dementia, frequent premature ventricular contractions, and renal insufficiency (serum creatinine more than 2 mg/dL). It is optimal to treat patients with unstable angina, recent myocardial infarction, significant congestive heart failure, or who have severe ischemia in hospital-based laboratories, because these patients are more likely to have cardiac complications during cardiac catheterization.

Precatheterization Orders, Premedication, and Informed Consent

In nonemergency situations, the physician should meet with the patient and family members prior to the catheterization to properly explain the procedure, its indications, and its potential complications. During this meeting, the physician should obtain the informed consent of the patient for the procedure, and this informed consent should include all potential procedures that the patient might undergo during the cardiac catheterization. If an interventional procedure is planned in the same sitting, then a more detailed consent process is necessary to inform the patient and family of all potential risks of the procedures. Consent should be obtained prior to any premedication and is optimally done in a more casual setting, such as the physician's office prior to the procedure.

The patient should be fully evaluated by the attending physician, as well as by the physician[5] who will perform the cardiac catheterization. This should include a detailed history, physical examination, laboratory data that include complete blood count, coagulation parameters, electrolytes, renal function, chest x-ray, and ECG, as well as any other special test that may be germane to the patient's particular problem(s). Assessment of peripheral pulses and access site needs to be determined and if the femoral artery is not to be utilized, the risk and complications of alternative sites need to be explained to the patient. Ideally, the patient should be seen by one of the cardiac catheterization laboratory nurses or technicians prior to the procedure.[18] The patient should receive precatheterization orders. For hospitalized patients, this should be placed on the chart the day prior to the procedure and for outpatients, should be written for the patient at the time of their admission to the outpatient catheterization facility. Examples of routine pre- and postprocedure orders from our institution are shown in Fig 3-3 and Fig 3-4 A–C. In general, patients should receive nothing by mouth from midnight to the time of the procedure, except for the use of sips of water to take scheduled medication. Patients should be allowed to have an evening sedative if they feel anxious prior to the procedure or if they are already hospitalized and have given informed consent. The outpatient should be brought to the hospital by a family member or friend in ample time to be seen and prepared in the precatheterization facility. In general, all medications are continued the morning of the procedure, particularly in diabetics, who should be given one half of their morning dose of long-acting insulin, but regular insulin should be withheld. If they are on oral agents, these also should be discontinued and an IV started, supplemented with D5W along with electrolyte solution. Diuretics are usually withheld on the morning prior to the procedure, unless the patient has severe congestive heart failure, in which case a modified dose of diuretics may be given. Prior to the procedure, it is advisable to give the patient mild sedation. The usual regimens include diphenhydramine 25 to 50 mg PO or IV, promethazine 25 to 50 mg PO or IV, and di-

DATE	TIME	"GENERICALLY EQUIVALENT DRUG MAY BE DISPENSED UNLESS BOX IS CHECKED."	☐ ORDER #

Please line through any orders which do not pertain to your patient.

1. ADMIT TO CARDIOLOGY. _____ Attending _____ M.D.
   Telemetry   yes/no (circle one)
2. DIAGNOSIS: _____
   OBTAIN CONSENT for _____
   by _____ M.D.
3. CONDITION: _____
4. VITAL SIGNS: Per Nursing Routine or _____
5. ACTIVITY: _____
6. ALLERGIES: _____
7. DIET: Cardiac diet
8. NPO after midnight except for medications with sips of water.
9. Saline lock to left/right (circle one) arm. Flush q shift. Begin IV with
   $D_5 \frac{1}{2}$ / NS (circle one) at _____ cc/hr beginning at _____ AM/PM.
10. ON CALL TO CATH LAB:
    A. Patient to void.
    B. Benadryl _____ mg IV
    C. Reglan _____ mg IV
11. CHEST PAIN PROTOCOL:
    A. Give NTG 0.4 mg (1/150 gr) SL, stay at bedside, may repeat x 2 at
       5 minute intervals if no relief.
    B. EKG STAT
    C. Page H.O. covering or Attending for all episodes of pain
       _____ (beeper).
    D. O_2 2 L by nc PRN chest pain or shortness or breath
    E. Morphine _____ mg IV x _____ PRN chest pain (not to exceed 2 mg).

12. MEDICATIONS: Tylenol 1-2 tabs PO q 4-6 hrs PRN headache
                          Serax _____ mg PO q _____ hrs and qhs PRN anxiety or insomnia
                          MOM 30 cc PO BID PRN constipation
                          Mylanta 30 cc PO QID PRN indigestion
                          NTG 0.4 mg (1/150 gr) SL PRN chest pain
                          Colace 100 mg PO BID PRN constipation

           Ca++ Channel Blocker: _____
           Beta Blocker: _____
           Nitrates: _____
           Enteric ASA: _____
           Other Meds: _____
           _____
           _____
           _____

13. ADMISSION TESTS: CBC, PT/PTT, Chem 7, Type & Screen, EKG, PA & Lat CXR.

PRINT	PHYSICIAN SIGN	TIME/DATE NOTED	U S SIGN
TIME/DATE CHART CHECK	NURSE SIGN	TIME/DATE NOTED	NURSE SIGN

A

Figure 3-3 (A) Precardiac catheterization orders, circa 1996, University of Southern California Hospital.

azepam 5 to 10 mg PO or IV. Preprocedural hydration is important, particularly for patients at risk for contrast-induced renal failure. However, it should be given cautiously to patients who are in congestive heart failure. It is not necessary to discontinue antiplatelet agents prior to cardiac catheterization, and it is mandatory to have the antiplatelet agents continued if the patient is being considered for an interventional procedure. It is also not necessary to discontinue nitroglycerin, calcium channel blockers, or beta blockers prior to the procedure, and it is usually advisable to have these medications present to reduce the potential for ischemia during the procedure. If the patient is on heparin for the

DATE	TIME	*GENERICALLY EQUIVALENT DRUG MAY BE DISPENSED UNLESS BOX IS CHECKED*	☐ ORDER #

Please line through any orders which do not pertain to your patient.

1. Admit / Return / Transfer to _____ Attending _____ M.D. Telemetry   yes / no (circle one)

2. DIAGNOSIS: _____

3. VITAL SIGNS: q 15 minutes x 4, q ½ hour x 4, q 1 hour x 4 then q 4 hours until stable.

4. ACTIVITY: Bedrest until 6 hours after sheath removed.

5. DIET: Diet as tolerated. Advance to Cardiac diet.

6. Encourage PO fluids to _____ liters for the next 8 hours.

7. IV Fluids: NS / D₅ ½ NS (circle one) at _____ cc / hr for a total of _____ liters.

8. Total PO and IV fluids should equal _____ liters during the next 12 hours.

9. Do not elevate head of bed more than 30 degrees x 4 hours.

10. Sandbag to right / left groin for four (4) hours post cath.

11. Check right / left ped.ⁿ / brachial pulses with vital signs.

12. Check right / left femoral / brachial artery for bleeding, hematoma with vital signs.

13. PRESSURE DRESSING AND NO BLOOD PRESSURE R / L BRACHIAL ARTERY X 48 HOURS FOR ARM CATH.

14. RESTRAINT TO LEG TO PREVENT BLEEDING / SANDBAG DISLODGEMENT PRN.

15. EKG: Upon arrival to floor post procedure and in AM.

16. Blood work in AM: CBC, Chem 7.

17. Pain Medication:_____

18. CALL CARDIOLOGY OR PAGE H.O. _____ (beeper) FOR SYSTOLIC BP < _____, BLEEDING OR CHEST PAIN.

19. CONTACT ATTENDING OF RECORD FOR ADDITIONAL ORDERS.

20. Other: _____
           _____
           _____
           _____

PRINT	PHYSICIAN SIGN	TIME/DATE NOTED	U.S. SIGN
TIME/DATE CHART CHECK	NURSE SIGN	TIME/DATE NOTED	NURSE SIGN

B

Figure 3-3   (**B**) Postcardiac catheterization order.

treatment of unstable angina or postmyocardial infarction, it can be handled in a number of ways. If the patient is stable, the medication can be discontinued at least 2 hours prior to the procedure, allowing the ACT or PTT to return to near normal. A value of less than 150 seconds for the ACT would be considered safe for arterial puncture. In patients in whom unstable angina continues to be a symptomatic problem or in those who are within 72 hours of acute myocardial infarction, reduction of the heparin dose to one half of normal for 2 hours is an alternative method for obtaining arterial access. In those patients who need a constant complete dosage of heparin, arterial catheterization can be performed safely, if done by a skilled operator using a single walled approach. Patients should be advised of the increased risk of groin bleeding in this setting. Like-

DATE	TIME	"GENERICALLY EQUIVALENT DRUG MAY BE DISPENSED UNLESS BOX IS CHECKED "	☐ ORDER #

Please line through any orders which do not pertain to your patient.

1. Admit to DOU/CICU (circle one). Attending _____ M.D.
    Telemetry on DOU yes/no (circle one).
2. DIAGNOSIS: _____
    OBTAIN CONSENT for _____
    by _____ M.D.
3. CONDITION: _____
4. VITAL SIGNS: Per Nursing Routine or _____ .
5. ACTIVITY: _____
6. ALLERGIES: _____
7. DIET: Cardiac diet.
8. NPO after midnight except for medications with sips of water.
9. Saline lock to left/right (circle one) arm. Flush q shift. Begin IV with
    D5↓ NS / NS (circle one) at _____ cc/hr beginning at _____ AM/PM.
10. Heparin _____ Units IVP and _____ Units/hour continuous infusion.
    Check PTT q 6 hours for 24 hours and adjust infusion per Cardiology Heparin Dosing Protocol.
11. Foley catheter / Condom catheter (circle one) in AM.
12. ON CALL TO CATH LAB:
    A. Patient to void.
    B. Benadryl _____ mg IV
    C. Reglan _____ mg IV
13. CHEST PAIN PROTOCOL.
    A. Give NTG 0.4 mg (1/150 gr) SL, stay at bedside, may repeat x 2 at 5 minute intervals if no relief.
    B. STAT EKG
    C. Page H.O. covering or Attending for all episodes of pain _____ (beeper).
    D. Morphine _____ mg IV x _____ PRN chest pain (not to exceed 2 mg).
    E. O₂ at 2 L per nc PRN chest pain or shortness of breath.
14. MEDICATIONS: **Soluble aspirin** (not enteric coated) 325 mg po now and q 12 hours.
        Ranitidine 150 mg po BID
        Dipyridamole 75 mg po TID, first dose **now**
        Colace 100 mg PO BID constipation
        Tylenol 1-2 tabs PO q 4-6 hrs PRN headache
        Serax ___ mg PO q___ hrs and qHS PRN anxiety or insomnia
        MOM 30 cc PO BID PRN constipation
        Mylanta 30 cc PO QID PRN constipation
        NTG 0.4 mg (1/150 gr) SL PRN chest pain

    Ca++ Channel Blocker: _____
    Beta Blocker: _____
    Nitrates: _____
    Other Meds: _____
    _____
    _____
    _____
    _____

15. Cardiac Surgery consult pre-procedure (STAT for AM admits) yes/no (circle one).
16. ADMISSION TESTS: CBC, Chem 7. PT, PTT, Type & Screen, Lipid profile, EKG, PA & Lat CXR.
17. Hold furosemide (Lasix), hydrocholorothiazide, and potassium if ordered the morning of the procedure.
18. Give 1/2 the usual dose of NPH insulin, and no regular insulin the AM of the procedure.

PRINT	PHYSICIAN SIGN	TIME/DATE NOTED	U S SIGN
TIME/DATE CHART CHECK	NURSE SIGN	TIME/DATE NOTED	NURSE SIGN

A

Figure 3-4 (**A**) Cardiac interventional procedure admission order.

wise, patients who receive thrombolytic agents within 24 hours have increased risk of groin complications and should be warned of the potential of this problem. A preprinted standardized precatheterization order sheet is optimal to assure that all medications are given prior to the procedure. During the procedure, pain medication should be prescribed liberally so that the patient can be as comfortable as possible. Most commonly, back pain complicates the procedure, and oxycodone, meperidine, morphine, or midazolam are commonly used to relax the patient. These medications can also be given prior to the procedure in extremely anxious patients.

DATE	TIME	GENERICALLY EQUIVALENT DRUG MAY BE DISPENSED UNLESS BOX IS CHECKED.	□ ORDER #

Please draw a line through any orders which do not pertain to your patient.

1.   Admit/Return/Transfer to _____ Attending _____ M.D.
                                              Fellow: _____ M.D.

2.   ALLERGIES:

3.   VITAL SIGNS: q 15 minutes x 4, q 1/2 hour x 4, q 1 hour x 4 then q 4 hours until stable.

4.   Check right/left pedal/brachial pulses with vital signs.

5.   Check right/left groin for bleeding and hematoma with vital signs.

6.   PRESSURE DRESSING AND NO BLOOD PRESSURE R/L BRACHIAL ARTERY X 48 HOURS FOR ARM CATH.

7.   ACTIVITY: Bedrest until 6 hours after sheath removal.

8.   Do not elevate HOB > 30 degrees until 6 hours post sheath removal.

9.   DIET: Diet as tolerated. Advance to Cardiac diet.

10. Encourage PO fluids to ___ liters for the next 8 hours.

11. IV Fluids: NS / D_5 ½ NS (circle one) at ____ cc/hr for a total of ____ liters.

12. Heparin flush through arterial sheath until arterial and venous sheaths are pulled.

13. Cardiology fellow to DC sheaths at _____ AM/PM.

14. Femstop to right / left (circle one) groin. Maintain at ___mm Hg x ___ hours.

15. Continue to keep right/left leg straight for total of 6 hours after sheath removal.

PRINT	PHYSICIAN SIGN	TIME/DATE NOTED	U.S. SIGN
TIME/DATE CHART CHECK	NURSE SIGN	TIME/DATE NOTED	NURSE SIGN

B

Figure 3-4   **(B)** Postcardiac interventional procedure order.

16.   Total CPK & CPK-MB at _____ and in AM.

17.   EKG now and in AM.

18.   Blood work in AM: CBC, Chem 7.

19.   MEDICATIONS: Tylenol 2 tabs PO q 4-6 hours PRN headache
                     Serax ___ mg PO q___ hours and qhs PRN anxiety or
                     insomnia
                     MOM 30 cc PO BID PRN constipation
                     Mylanta 30 cc PO QID PRN indigestion
                     NTG 0.4 mg (1/150 gr) SL PRN chest pain
                     Colace 100 mg PO BID PRN consitpation

Enteric coated aspirin: _____
Pain medication: _____
Ca^{++} Channel Blocker: _____
Ticlid: _____
IV NTG at _____ mcg/min and adjust to BP of _____ mm Hg.
IV Heparin: _____ unit bolus and then _____ units/hr through
venous sheath.
                     DC Heparin at _____ AM/PM
                              OR
                     1/2 dose Heparin at _____ AM/PM. Increase
                     Heparin to full dose 2 hours after sheaths are
                     removed.
Other: _____
_____
_____
_____

20.   CONTACT ATTENDING OF RECORD FOR ADDITIONAL ORDERS.

21.   CALL CARDIOLOGY OR PAGE H.O. _____ (beeper) FOR
      SYSTOLIC BP < _____, BLEEDING OR CHEST PAIN.

PRINT	PHYSICIAN SIGN	TIME/DATE NOTED	U.S. SIGN
TIME/DATE CHART CHECK	NURSE SIGN	TIME/DATE NOTED	NURSE SIGN

Figure 3-4   **(B)** *Continued.*

DATE	TIME	"GENERICALLY EQUIVALENT DRUG MAY BE DISPENSED UNLESS BOX IS CHECKED"	☐ ORDER #

Please draw a line through any orders which do not pertain to your patient.

1. Admit/Return/Transfer to CICU. Attending _____ , M.D.
   Fellow _____ , M.D.
2. DIAGNOSIS: _____
3. VITAL SIGNS: q 15 minutes x 4, q 1/2 hour x 4, q 1 hour x 4 then q 4 hours until stable.
4. ACTIVITY: Sheaths removed/to be removed at _____ AM/PM, _____ (date).
   0-24 hours post sheath removal: strict bedrest, may elevate head of bed to 30°.
   24-48 hours post sheath removal: Bedrest, may sit on edge of bed. Commode chair only in late afternoon.
   48-72 hours post sheath removal: Out of bed to chair, ambulate in room, bathroom privileges.
   >72 hours post sheath removal: Ambulate ad lib.
5. DIET: Diet as tolerated. Advance to Cardiac diet.
6. Encourage PO fluids to _____ liters over the next 8 hours.
7. IV Fluids: NS / D₅ ½ NS (circle one) at _____ cc/hr for a total of _____ liters.
8. RESTRAINT TO RIGHT/LEFT LEG TO PREVENT BLEEDING, SANDBAG OR SHEATH DISLODGEMENT PRN.
9. Check right/left groin for bleeding or hematoma and check right/left pedal pulses with vital signs.
10. Hold all venipuncture sites for 5 min., no IM injections.
11. Heparin flush through arterial sheath until sheath removal.
12. EKG upon arrival to unit and q AM x 3.
13. Labs: CBC, PT, Chem 7 in AM. Total CPK & CPK-MB at _____ and in AM.
    PTT q 6 hours while on Heparin.
    CBC, PT QD.
14. PRN MEDICATIONS: Tylenol 1-2 tabs PO q 4-6 hours PRN pain
    Tylenol #3 1-2 tabs PO q 4-6 hours PRN pain
    Serax _____ mg PO q _____ hours and qhs PRN anxiety or insomnia
    MOM 30cc PO BID PRN constipation
    Mylanta 30cc PO QID PRN indigestion
    NTG 0.4 mg (1/150 gr) SL PRN chest pain
15. Docusate sodium 100 mg PO BID.
16. Soluble aspirin (not enteric coated) 325 mg po q 12 hours.
17. Dipyridamole 75 mg po TID.
18. Coumadin _____ mg po now and _____ mg po tomorrow. Call MD for daily dose.
19. Ca++ Channel Blocker: _____
20. IV NTG at _____ mcg/min and titrate to SBP of _____ mm Hg.
21. Dextran 40 10% 50 cc/hr IV continuous Infusion.
22. Urokinase 1 million units in 250 cc NS. Infuse via coronary infusion catheter at _____ cc/hr. DC at _____ AM/PM.

PRINT	PHYSICIAN SIGN	TIME/DATE NOTED	U S SIGN
TIME/DATE CHART CHECK	NURSE SIGN	TIME/DATE NOTED	NURSE SIGN

C

Figure 3-4 (**C**) Postintracoronary stent placement orders.

DATE	TIME	*GENERICALLY EQUIVALENT DRUG MAY BE DISPENSED UNLESS BOX IS CHECKED *	☐ ORDER #

23. IV Heparin:_____ unit bolus and then_____ units/hr continuous infusion through venous sheath.

24. Sheath Removal: Choose A or B.
    ____ A. Same day sheath removal: DC heparin upon leaving cath lab.

    ____ B. Next day sheath removal: DC heparin at_____ AM.

    When heparin DC'd follow the orders below:

    1. Check ACT q 1/2 hour.
    2. Fellow to remove sheath when ACT < 150 sec.
    3. Have atropine 1 mg ampule, 1% lidocaine, 5 mg IV Morphine Sulfate at bedside for sheath removal.
    4. Continue Dextran 40 10% at 50 cc/hr.
    5. Draw PTT at time of sheath removal.
    6. One hour post sheath removal give heparin as per following protocol, base on PTT drawn at time of sheath removal:

PTT Result	Action
PTT > 80	Start heparin drip at 1000 U/hr.
PTT 65-79	Give 1000 U heparin IV bolus and start drip at 1000 U/hr.
PTT <64	Give 2000 U heparin IV bolus and start drip at 1000 U/hr.

    This protocol is only for restarting heparin post sheath removal.

    7. Check groin for bleeding or hematoma q 1/2 hr x 4.
    8. Draw PTT 2 hr. after restarting heparin drip and adjust as per Cardiology Heparin Dosing Protocol.
    9. Check PTT q 6 hours while on heparin.
    10. DC Dextran when PTT > 55 for 2 consecutive PTTs after sheath removal.

25. FemoStop to right/left groin for 2 hours post sheath removal, then sandbag for next 6 hours. Keep right/left leg straight for 24 hours post sheath removal. Restrain right/left leg PRN to prevent bleeding or device dislodgement.

26. CONTACT ATTENDING OF RECORD FOR ADDITIONAL ORDERS.

27. CALL CARDIOLOGY OR PAGE H.O. _____ (beeper) FOR SYSTOLIC BP < _____, BLEEDING OR CHEST PAIN.

28. CALL CARDIOLOGY OR PAGE H.O. _____ (beeper) FOR ANY PTT < 55 or > 90 ON ANY STENT PATIENT.

PRINT	PHYSICIAN SIGN	TIME/DATE NOTED	U S SIGN
TIME/DATE CHART CHECK	NURSE SIGN	TIME/DATE NOTED	NURSE SIGN

Figure 3-4 (**C**) *Continued.*

DATE	TIME	*GENERICALLY EQUIVALENT DRUG MAY BE DISPENSED UNLESS BOX IS CHECKED*	☐ ORDER #

(Post-Interventional Procedure, Post-Stent Placement, Post-Thrombolytic Therapy, Unstable Angina and R/O Myocardial Infarction)

1.   Maintain PTT in 45-80 range.

2.   Draw PTT 2 hours after patient return from cath lab or 2 hours after completion of thrombolytic infusion and adjust as per protocol:

PTT Result	Action
PTT > 100	Decrease infusion rate by 200 units/hr. **Report PTT result to MD, recheck in 3 hours.**
PTT 80-100	Decrease infusion rate by 100 units/hr.
PTT 45-80	**Desired range**
PTT 40-45	Increase infusion rate by 200 units/hr.
PTT 35-40	Give 1,000 units IV bolus and increase infusion rate by 200 units/hr.
PTT 30-35	Give 2,000 units IV bolus and increase infusion rate by 200 units/hr. **Report PTT result to MD, recheck in 3 hours.**

3.   Recheck PTT q 6 hours while Heparin is infusing and readjust infusion as per above protocol.

PRINT	PHYSICIAN SIGN	TIME/DATE NOTED	U.S. SIGN
TIME/DATE CHART CHECK	NURSE SIGN	TIME/DATE NOTED	NURSE SIGN

D

Figure 3-4   (**D**) Heparin dosing protocol order.

Standardized Catheterization Protocols and Research Protocols

The catheterization laboratory should have a procedural manual that details all the procedures that are done in the laboratory for reference for the physicians and technical staff. Likewise, all research protocols that are approved by the institutional review board and are currently active within the catheterization laboratory should be carefully spelled out with the individuals who are responsible for overseeing the research protocol. The catheterization laboratory personnel should have an inservice on all research protocols prior to the initiating the project in the laboratory.

Patients should be scheduled prior to the procedure by a scheduling secretary or other catheterization laboratory personnel who are assigned this task. The daily schedule should be clearly visible to all staff. One technique commonly used to display the daily catheterization schedule is a large chalkboard placed in the outer hallway or anteroom before the procedure room, on which each patient is listed along with diagnosis and attending physician for each case. Patients who have special problems can be highlighted on the board, and those who are undergoing research protocols also can be so indicated. The scheduling process should be flexible enough to allow changing the schedule on basis of emergencies. Within the cardiac catheterization laboratory, a separate chalkboard is advisable, on which the details of each patient are noted, including diagnosis, laboratory data, and catheterization protocol. This allows the catheterization laboratory staff setting the room up to be aware of the patient's particular needs and the order in which the procedures will be undertaken.

Complications

The list of major complications of cardiac catheterization is shown in Table 3-3.[19] The most common complication is local groin hematoma at the site of catheter entry. Other commonly observed complications include numbness or weakness in the extremity or arterial insufficiency. These complications are higher when using the brachial approach than when using the femoral approach. More serious complications include stroke, acute myocardial infarction, distal embolization of atherosclerotic material from the aorta, contrast-induced renal failure, congestive heart failure, or drug reactions such as from protamine.

Table 3-3   Major Complications
of Diagnostic Catheterizations

	Number	*Percent*
Death	65	0.11
Myocardial infarction	30	0.05
Neurologic	41	0.07
Arrhythmia	229	0.38
Vascular	256	0.43
Contrast	223	0.37
Hemodynamic	158	0.26
Perforation	16	0.03
Other	166	0.28
Total (patients)	1021	1.7

Source: Modified from Noto TJ, Johnson LW, Krone R, et al. Cardiac catheterization 1990: a report of the Registry of the Society for Cardiac Angiography and Interventions (SCA&I). Cathet Cardiovasc Diagn 1991; 24:75–83.

High-Risk Patients

A list of risk factors for increased complications during cardiac catheterizations is shown in Table 3-4.[20] In these patients, special attention should be taken in preparing the patient and in performing the procedure. In addition, patients with significant associated problems should be monitored carefully during the procedure. A few specific areas of special note include patients with renal insufficiency. It has been suggested previously that these patients receive adequate oral or IV hydration prior to catheterization. Some authors have suggested the use of mannitol 20% at 20 ml/hr beginning immediately following the catheterization for 6 hours, while others have suggested Lasix immediately following the procedure and replacing urine output with IV fluid. A recent randomized study suggested that preoperative hydration is the most effective to reduce contrast-induced renal failure.[21] The risk of renal failure is proportional to the baseline serum creatinine level, and therefore, greater care should be taken with the patient whose creatinine level exceeds 2 mg/dL.

Patients who have had prior contrast reactions are at higher risk for developing a second repeat reaction and should be specifically identified in order to institute prophylactic therapy.[22] Two types of patients are recognized to be at increased risk of contrast-induced anaphylactoid reactions: those who have had

Table 3-4 Multivariate Predictors of MCOMP

Variable	Coefficient	OR (95% CI)
Moribund	−1.902	10.22 (3.77, 27.76)
NYHA class	−0.151	
I		1.00
II		1.15 (0.94, 1.41)
III		1.32 (0.92, 1.51)
IV		1.52 (1.16, 1.74)
HTN	−0.375	1.45 (1.22, 1.73)
Shock	−1.086	6.52 (4.18, 10.18)
AVD	−0.356	2.72 (2.02, 3.66)
Out/inpatient	0.336	0.63 (0.52, 0.76)
Renal insufficiency	−0.431	3.30 (2.39, 4.55)
Unstable angina	−0.244	1.42 (1.16, 1.74)
MVD	−0.301	2.33 (1.76, 3.08)
Acute MI < 24 hrs	0.975	4.03 (2.61, 6.21)
CHF	−0.319	2.22 (1.71, 2.90)
CM	0.787	3.29 (2.23, 4.86)

Abbreviations: AVD, aortic valve disease; HTN, hypertension; MVD, mitral valve disease; CHF, congestive heart failure; CM, cardiomyopathy; OR, odds ratio; CI, confidence interval; NYHA, New York Heart Assocation; MCOMP, major complications.
Source: Modified from Laskey W, Boyle J, Johnson LW, and The Registry Committee of the Society for Cardiac Angiography & Interventions. Multivariable model for prediction of risk of significant complication during diagnostic cardiac catheterization. Cathet Cardiovasc Diagn 1993;30:185–190.

prior anaphylactoid reactions and allergic patients. Repeat anaphylactoid reactions to conventional contrast medium have been reported in 16% to 44% of patients. Patients who have a history of atopy and asthma have a twofold increase in anaphylactoid reactions. However, because anaphylactoid reactions to contrast media are rare (0.23%), these patients are only at minimal increased risk for serious complications. For patients with prior anaphylactoid reactions, it is generally recommended that steroids and H_1 blockers be administered prior to the procedure. In general, prednisone 50 mg PO should be administered 13, 7, and 1 hour before the procedure, with diphenhydramine 50 mg 1 hour before. In addition, an H_2 blocker is often used if IgE-mediated antigen/antibody reactions are involved. Even if this is not entirely clear, due to their low risk, these agents are frequently used to help reduce further complications. Also, low-osmolality non-ionic contrast media have been used, because reported studies indicate that reactions are fewer with their use than with ionic contrast medium. While these measures do not completely prevent reactions, they reduce them to a minimum (less than 1%), making it feasible to consider repeat cardiac catheterization in these individuals.

Patients who demonstrate hemodynamic instability are also at high risk of cardiac complications during catheterization. In particular, patients who are in congestive heart failure should be treated prior to the procedure, because contrast medium is known to expand plasma volume by at least 20% and has negative inotropic effects that can result in worsening of the congestive heart failure. In these patients, minimal doses of x-ray contrast agents should be administered, and the use of low osmolar contrast agents and careful monitoring of right heart pressures, particularly pulmonary capillary wedge pressure, are important. If catheterization is essential and the patient remains hemodynamically unstable, consideration of placement of an intra-aortic balloon should be made with postprocedural monitoring of the pulmonary pressure.

Patients with acute myocardial infarction are also at increased risk of cardiac catheterization complications. If the procedure is being done for primary revascularization, the benefits of procedure clearly outweigh the small increase in risk attendant to the procedure. However, cardiac catheterization during an acute myocardial infarction should be avoided unless it will lead to a significant change in therapy that will benefit the patient. It appears that the risk of cardiac catheterization falls off significantly between 24 and 48 hours following acute myocardial infarction, and procedures may be done more electively at these times.[16]

Sterile Procedures

While the risk of infection during cardiac catheterization is extremely low, care still needs to be exercised to avoid infectious complications.[22] Cardiac catheterization is generally considered to be a clean surgical procedure unless it involves the implantation of prosthetic material, such as would occur during placement of a pacemaker. In general, the patient should be properly prepped, with removal of hair and cleaning of the skin. Antibiotics are not routinely advised, unless the patient has a known ongoing local infection at the site of puncture. The patient should be draped with nonporous drapes and operator personnel should wear sterile gloves and gowns. The overall incidence of infection with percutaneous cardiac catheterization has been reported to be 0.06%. The incidence rises tenfold, however, with the use of arterial cutdown. Although many laboratories do not require caps and masks, this should be routine procedure if arterial cutdown procedures are performed. It is generally recommended that caps and masks be used for percutaneous procedures in which the sheaths may be left in the patient for a prolonged period. It also is recommended that the operators wear caps and masks for percutaneous procedures involving acutely ill patients, patients undergoing interventional cardiology procedures, pacemaker placement, intra-aortic balloon insertion, or those in whom there was entry through a femoral arterial graft. Personnel in the room also should be cognizant of the sterile procedures, and the operator and ancillary personnel need to be particularly careful when dealing with patients with AIDS or hepatitis.

Prevention of Clot Formation

While the use of heparin anticoagulation during routine cardiac catheterization continues to remain controversial, it has become a standard and routine component of interventional cardiology procedures. In general, if the procedures are prolonged and multiple catheters are used, systemic anticoagulation is indicated. During routine cardiac catheterization, particularly in an outpatient setting, routine use of heparin may not be necessary. However, care should be taken in preparation of the catheters, solutions used for flushing should contain a small amount of heparin (3000 units/liter), and care should be taken in carefully wiping guidewires and catheters with proper aspiration and flushing before and after use. During interventional procedures, adequate heparinization should be given to prolong the ACT to greater than 300 seconds, and this level should be maintained during the procedure by periodic administration of heparin or a continuous infusion of heparin with measurement of ACT levels.

Prevention of Hematoma

One of the most neglected areas of cardiac catheterization patient management is proper removal of catheters to prevent development of hematoma or pseudoaneurysms.[23] Manual compression offers the greatest safety in the prevention of these complications. In patients on anticoagulation, however, such as those receiving intracoronary stent, the use of prolonged compression of the femoral access site with use of a compression device—C-clamp, Femstop (Bard,

Billerica, MA)—is necessary. Increased complications may occur due to patient motion. Proper training of ancillary personnel involved in sheath removal will help reduce subsequent complications.

Postcatheterization Orders and Procedures

A standardized postcatheterization and angioplasty order form should be available (see Figs 3-2 and 3-3). It should clearly delineate the procedure the patient has undergone, requirements for vital sign monitoring, laboratory tests, medications, and special monitoring requirements. In general, the femoral artery and/or venous sheath should be removed immediately following a diagnostic procedure or when the ACT is less than 150 seconds for interventional procedures and less than 100 seconds for diagnostic cardiac catheterization procedures. Patients' legs should be kept straight for 4 hours in a diagnostic procedure, but up to 8 hours following an interventional procedure. The groin should be checked regularly by the nursing staff for signs of bleeding, hematoma development, or pseudoaneurysm. Patients should be allowed to move several hours after removal of the sandbag or compression device. Most patients can be discharged from the hospital the same day as their cardiac catheterization if the procedure was performed on an elective basis. In most cases, patients are discharged the day following an elective interventional procedure.

Radiation Monitoring

All states have standard radiation protection requirements, and in some states, such as California, all individuals involved in the use of radiation must pass a qualifying examination and have their certificates prominently displayed in the radiology facility. Monitoring of radiation exposure is also mandated by law, and all operators must wear radiation badges under a lead apron to monitor for incidental radiation exposure.[4] In addition, many angiographers wear additional badges in the areas of the thyroid, eyes, or hands to monitor radiation to unprotected areas. Maximum permissable doses for occupational exposure have been published previously and are 5 rems per year for whole body exposure, including the lens of the eyes, gonads, and marrow. The radiation protection office in the hospital is responsible for monitoring and providing badges to all personnel involved in cardiac catheterization procedures.

Quality Assurance

It is the responsibility of the physician director of the cardiac catheterization laboratory to establish and maintain a quality assurance program for the laboratory.[24] In addition, the director is responsible for a continuous quality improvement process, which involves identification of quality indicators, risk adjustment for factors known to affect outcome, development of a data collection system, a process for evaluation of the outcomes, and feedback to the physicians and personnel involved in patient care to improve quality and reduce complications. Also, the problem should then be reevaluated to assure that the complications have been reduced by the changes made in the cardiac catheterization procedure. The laboratory director should be aware of the cost-effectiveness of the procedures and monitor closely the use of cardiac catheterization equipment. This aspect is particularly important in this current era of managed care and cost containment. In some laboratories, feedback to the physician operators on cost of equipment is a useful means of making each operator aware of the cost involved in the individual procedures.

Special Laboratories

Outpatient, Free-standing, and Mobile Catheterization Laboratories

As indicated, outpatient cardiac catheterization is now performed routinely with low complications, and as many as 50% of patients undergoing cardiac catheterization have the procedure in this setting. Low-risk patients need to be selected for outpatient cardiac catheterization procedures.[1] More strict criteria need to be applied for other nontraditional laboratory settings, such as the free-standing cardiac catheterization laboratory.[1] A free-standing lab is one that provides catheterization services but is not physically attached to the hospital.[25] Because access from this facility to a hospital may delay access to emergency services, greater care needs to be made in selecting patients for this type of procedure. Mobile cardiac catheterization laboratories are single or multiple units that are transported by land, sea, or air. Most typically, this is a cardiac catheterization laboratory that is in a large van, which is moved by truck from one location to another.[1,26,27] Again, because the facility is small and access to a hospital in the setting of an emergency may be difficult, great care must be taken in selection of patients for procedures in this type of setting. In addition, while the catheterization laboratory may be mobile, the physician and support staff assigned to the laboratory need to be experienced and meet all the standards necessary for optimal operation, as itemized for a hospital-based laboratory. It is not advisable to perform interventional procedures in a mobile catheterization laboratory.

Electrophysiology Laboratory

There are special requirements for electrophysiology studies. While the x-ray facility may be the same, a high-quality electrophysiology recorder and computer system are essential, along with a properly trained and experienced electrophysiology technician and nursing staff that are experienced in handling patients having these procedures. It is optimal to have a separate cardiac catheterization suite dedicated to electrophysiology studies, so that movement of the equipment in and out of the laboratory can be minimized.

Interventional Laboratory

While many of the requirements of a cardiac catheterization laboratory are the same for an interventional laboratory, extremely high quality cineangiography, digital imaging, and digital roadmapping are essential for interventional procedures.[3] Biplane angiography is desirable, though not necessary, with a high-quality C-arm system that can be rapidly moved to obtain optimal views of the treated artery. Again, the proper support equipment, access to surgical suites if necessary, and a full array of interventional catheters, including new interventional devices such as bailout stenting, are essential for operation of an interventional laboratory.

Pediatric Laboratory

Pediatric catheterization is optimally done in a biplane facility by trained pediatric nurses, technicians, and physicians. It is optimal that the pediatric facility be separate from the diagnostic cardiac catheterization laboratory, given the unique needs of the pediatric patient. In some circumstances, however, a shared cardiac catheterization laboratory is feasible, as long as the personnel are experienced in the performance of all types of procedures.

SELECTED READINGS

1. American College of Cardiology/American Heart Association Ad Hoc Task Force on Cardiac Catheterization. ACC/AHA guidelines for cardiac catheterization and cardiac catheterization laboratories. J Am Coll Cardiol 1991;18:1149–1182.
2. McCracken MJ, Chapman MJ. The cardiac catheterization suite. In: Bashore TM, ed. Invasive cardiology: principle and technique. Toronto: Decker, 1990:5–17.
3. Tcheng JE, Stack RS, Roubin AS. Design of the interventional cardiac catheterization laboratory. In: Roubin AS, Califf RM, O'Neill W, et al., eds. Interventional cardiovascular medicine—principles and practice. New York: Churchill Livingstone, 1994:401–407.
4. Laboratory Performance Standards Committee, Society for Cardiac Angiography and Interventions. Guidelines for radiation protection in the cardiac catheterization laboratory. Cathet Cardiovasc Diagn 1984;10:87–92.
5. Johnson LW, Moore RJ, Balter S. Review of radiation safety in the cardiac catheterization laboratory. Cathet Cardiovasc Diagn 1992;25:186–194.
6. Balter S and members of the Laboratory Performance Standards Committee, Society for Cardiac Angiography and Interventions. Guidelines for personnel radiation monitoring in the cardiac catheterization laboratory. Cathet Cardiovasc Diagn 1993;30:277–279.
7. Judkins MP. Guidelines for electrical safety in the cardiac catheterization laboratory. Cathet Cardiovasc Diagn 1984;10:299–301.
8. Laboratory Performance Standards Committee, Society for Cardiac Angiography and Interventions. Guidelines regarding qualifications and responsibilities of a catheterization laboratory director. Cathet Cardiovasc Diagn 1983;9:619–621.
9. Hill JA, Lambert CR, Pepine CJ. Aspects of catheterization laboratory administration. In: Pepine CJ, Hill JA, Lambert CR, eds. Diagnostic and therapeutic cardiac catheterization. 2nd ed. Baltimore: Williams & Wilkins 1994:37–51.
10. Laboratory Performance Standards Committee, Society for Cardiac Angiography and Interventions. Guidelines for professional staff privileges in the cardiac catheterization laboratory. Cathet Cardiovasc Diagn 1990;21:203–204.
11. Committee on Interventional Cardiology, Society for Cardiac Angiography and Interventions. Guidelines for credentialing and facilities for performance of coronary angioplasty. Cathet Cardiovasc Diagn 1988;15:136–138.
12. Cowley MJ, Faxon DP, Holmes DR. Guidelines for training, credentialing, and maintenance of competence for the performance of coronary angioplasty: A report from the interventional cardiology committee and the training program standards committee of the Society for Cardiac Angiography and Interventions. Cathet Cardiovasc Diagn 1993;30:1–4.
13. Interventional Cardiology Committee, Subcommittee on Peripheral Interventions, Society for Cardiac Angiography and Interventions. Guidelines for performance of peripheral percutaneous transluminal angioplasty. Cathet Cardiovasc Diagn 1990;21:128–129.
14. Lau FY, Ruiz C. Guidelines for balloon valvuloplasty: credentials and training. Cathet Cardiovasc Diagn 1990;21:135–136.
15. Ryan TJ, Bauman WB, Kennedy JW, et al. Guidelines for percutaneous transluminal coronary angioplasty. A report of the AHA/ACC Task Force on Assessment of Diagnostic and Therapeutic Cardiovascular Procedures (Committee on Percutaneous Transluminal Coronary Angioplasty). Circulation 1993;88:2987–3007.
16. American College of Cardiology/American Heart Association Task Force on Assessment of Diagnostic and Therapeutic Cardiovascular Procedures (Subcommittee on Coronary Angiography). Guidelines for coronary angiography. Circulation 1987;76:963A–977A.
17. Hanley P, Vlietstra RE, Fisher LD, et al. Indications for coronary angiography: changes in laboratory practice over a decade. Mayo Clin Proc 1986;61:248–253.

18. Owens P, Bashore TM. The preparation and care of the patient and the laboratory. In: Bashore TM, ed. Invasive cardiology: principle and technique. Toronto: Decker, 1990:19–39.
19. Noto TJ, Johnson LW, Krone R, et al. Cardiac catheterization 1990: a report of the Registry of the Society for Cardiac Angiography and Interventions (SCA&I). Cathet Cardiovasc Diagn 1991;24:75–83.
20. Laskey W, Boyle J, Johnson LW, and The Registry Committee of the Society for Cardiac Angiography and Interventions. Multivariable model for prediction of risk of significant complication during diagnostic cardiac catheterization. Cathet Cardiovasc Diagn 1993;30:185–190.
21. Goss JE, Chambers CE, Heupler FA, and members of the Laboratory Performance Standards Committee, Society for Cardiac Angiography and Interventions. Systemic anaphylactoid reactions to iodinated contrast media during cardiac catheterization procedures: guidelines for prevention, diagnosis, and treatment. Cathet Cardiovasc Diagn 1995;34:99–104.
22. Heupler FA, Heisler M, Keys TF, et al. Infection prevention guidelines for cardiac catheterization laboratories. Cathet Cardiovasc Diagn 1992;25:260–263.
23. Garber GR. Patient preparation and periprocedural management. In: Faxon DP, ed. Practical angioplasty. New York: Raven 1994:21–33.
24. Heupler FA, AL-Hani AJ, Dear WE, and members of the Laboratory Performance Standards Committee, Society for Cardiac Angiography and Interventions. Guidelines for continuous quality improvement in the cardiac catheterization laboratory. Cathet Cardiovasc Diagn 1993;30:191–200.
25. Society for Cardiac Angiography and Interventions, Laboratory Performance Standards Committee. Guidelines for freestanding cardiac catheterization laboratories. Cathet Cardiovasc Diagn 1992;26:88–89.
26. Holmes DR and the Trustees of the Society for Cardiac Angiography and Interventions. The mobile catheterization laboratory: should we pick it up and move it? Cathet Cardiovasc Diagn 1992;26:69–70.
27. Goss JE, Cameron A, for Society for Cardiac Angiography and Interventions, Laboratory Performance Standards Committee. Mobile cardiac catheterization laboratories. Cathet Cardiovasc Diagn 1992;26:71–72.

4

ACCESSING VASCULAR STRUCTURES

Bart G. Denys
Barry F. Uretsky
Kenneth Baughman
Marc J. Schweiger

Planning Vascular Access

PLANNING THE ACCESS site on the basis of the patient's history, physical examination, and anticipated cardiovascular diagnosis reduces procedure time and vascular complications. For instance, if the patient is suspected of having a cardiomyopathy or other condition with marked dilation of the right ventricle, right heart catheterization with a Swan-Ganz catheter is much easier using the right internal jugular vein versus the femoral vein. If the brachial artery approach is chosen for catheterization, standard Judkins-type catheters can be used from the left arm, but not from the right arm. Injection of the left internal mammary artery is usually easier from the ipsilateral brachial artery than from the femoral artery, particularly in patients with tortuosity of the iliac arteries or abdominal aorta, or widening of the aortic arch. Vascular history should include the question of claudication or past surgical vascular procedures such as vena cava ligation, Greenfield filter, or vascular bypasses. Past operative reports are invaluable as they will indicate the type of corrective procedure, insertion site and nature of vascular grafts (vein vs. Dacron), and the severity and anatomy of the treated vasculature. A preprocedure vascular examination should be documented and include BP difference between the left and right arms if present, presence and strength of pulses, presence of bruits, and other pertinent findings such as skin color, trophic changes, and ulcerations. Body habitus, such as extreme obesity, may dictate the use of the brachial artery instead of the femoral artery. As a rule of thumb, access should be directed to the artery with the strongest pulse, if appropriate for the procedure planned.

Choice of Accessing Needle

Needles for vascular access are of two major types: open-bore or Seldinger type (Fig 4-1). Open-bore needles have the advantage of demonstrating blood return immediately; in general, they are easy to manage. Seldinger needles have an obturator, frequently with a tiny lumen to show the operator when the anterior arterial wall has been penetrated. At that point, the operator may remove the obturator, and brisk pulsatile flow should be observed. Open-bore needles may become plugged by subcutaneous fat and other tissue; use of the Seldinger obturator may prevent this problem.

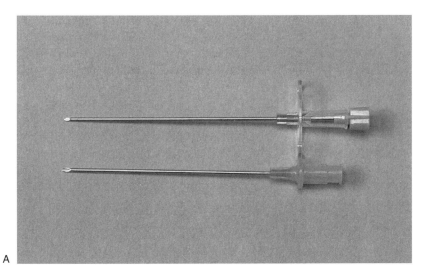

A

Figure 4-1 Many different needles are available to access vessels. They are essentially of two types: open-bore needles and needles with stylet (Seldinger). (**A**) The Seldinger needle with stylet in place.

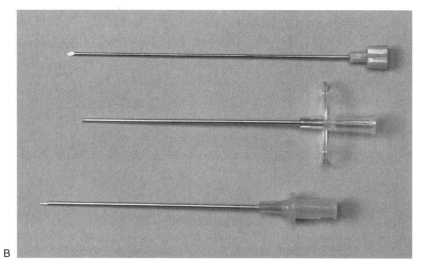

Figure 4-1 (**B**) Seldinger needles without stylet in place.

Choice of Wire

After obtaining arterial or venous access with the needle, a guidewire is threaded through the needle into the vessel. The operator should have decided prior to the procedure the type of wire to be used, the shape of the wire tip, and the length and the thickness of the wire shaft.

Many guidewires are made with stainless steel, usually coated with Teflon to decrease friction between the wire and the needle, sheath, or catheter. Other materials used for wires include Nitinol and an elastic alloy core coated with a hydrophilic plastic polymer (Terumo Corp, Medi-Tech, Watertown, MA). The hydrophilic "slippery" wire is particularly helpful in negotiating diseased and tortuous peripheral vessels. Some types of wires use stainless steel without a coating. These include wires used for rotational atherectomy (Boston Scientific, Boston, MA) and the wire used for manipulation in the left atrium during mitral valvuloplasty using the Inoue valvuloplasty balloon (Toray Co., Tokyo, Japan).

Wires are manufactured in many lengths, but are of three general types. A short wire (15–30 cm) may be used to place a sheath. A 125- to 150-cm length may be used to thread a catheter to the central aorta or great vein. A 250- to 300-cm wire may be used for catheter exchanges without moving the wire tip. Wire tips may be straight or J-tipped. With both types, the wire tip is "soft" or "flexible," that is, easily deformable. For most access cases and catheter exchanges, a J-tip is preferable, because there is general consensus that a J-tip wire is less likely to produce dissection of the artery than a straight-tipped wire. On the other hand, a straight-tipped wire is particularly useful in crossing the aortic valve in patients with aortic stenosis (see Chapter 13). A straight-tipped wire may be useful in cannulating smaller arteries, such as the brachial or radial.

Wire tips have either a fixed core or a movable core. A straight wire with a movable core can be converted to a J-tip by pulling the movable core back. Wire diameters used vary widely from 0.018″ to 0.063″. The smallest sizes (0.018″, 0.021″, 0.025″) may be used with a Swan-Ganz catheter to increase its stiffness, so as to more easily negotiate curves from right atrium to the pulmonary artery position. Difficulty typically occurs in patients with an enlarged right atrium or ventricle. The 0.032″ wire is often used in the brachial artery and for intra-aortic balloon placement. The 0.035″ to 0.038″ wires are the "workhorse" wires for routine diagnostic left heart cases, and for insertion of most guiding catheters used in interventional cases. An 0.063″ wire is occasionally used for interventional cases, particularly if larger sheath and catheter sizes are used (10 Fr and larger).

Vascular Sheath

Twenty years ago, most left-sided catheterizations were performed using tapered-tip catheters and no sheaths. Today, most catheterizations are performed with a sheath (Fig 4-2), with the possible exception of the multipurpose catheter approach from the leg and Sones cutdown technique from the right brachial artery (see Chapter 7). Sheaths have the following characteristics: a tube through which catheters may be passed; a diaphragm that, when a catheter

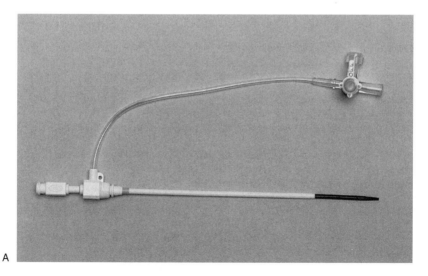

A

Figure 4-2   (A) A typical sheath is shown. The sheath is a tube with a rubber diaphragm distally and a side-arm through which pressure can be measured or drugs infused.

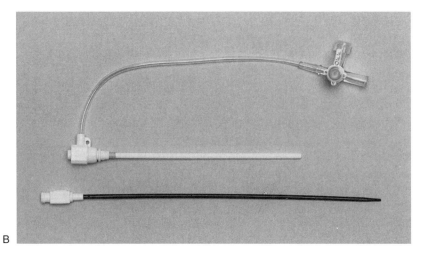

B

Figure 4-2 (**B**) The components of the sheath.

is in place, does not leak blood or allow air to pass into the sheath; and a side-arm to measure pressure or infuse drugs. Sheaths range in diameter from 4 Fr to 22 Fr (used in percutaneous cardiopulmonary bypass). Sheaths used in diagnostic catheterization range from 5 Fr to 8 Fr. If measuring arterial pressure from the side-arm is desired, the sheath should be one Fr size larger than the catheter within it. Typically, sheaths are 20 to 35 cm long. Longer sheaths are particularly useful in straightening the tortuous ileofemoral vessels to improve torque control. Operator sheath preference is usually related to the following parameters: the quality of the diaphragm, the degree of friction between the sheath and the catheter being passed through it, and the propensity of the catheter to kink within the sheath.

Femoral Artery and Vein

The common femoral artery is preferred for percutaneous arterial cannulation because it is large, easily compressible, and accessible. After the right groin area is prepped and draped, the femoral artery is located by the operator by palpation. When drawing an imaginary line between the anterior superior iliac spine and the pubis, the arterial pulsation is near or at the midpoint of the line. With the palm of the hand resting on the anterior iliac crest, the tip of the index finger will be positioned approximately over the correct site for puncture. Ideally, the femoral artery is to be entered about 1 to 2 cm below the inguinal ligament (Fig 4-3). Some individuals rely on the inguinal crease for selection of the puncture site. However, the distance from the inguinal ligament to the inguinal crease is very variable, particularly in obese patients. Cannulating the artery too low will increase the chance of entering the superficial femoral artery rather

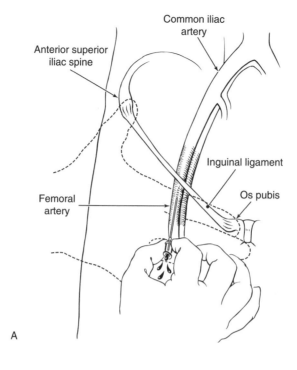

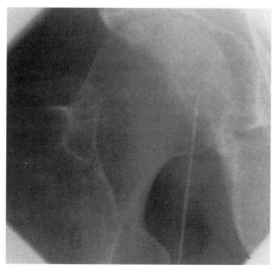

Figure 4-3 Accessing the femoral artery. **(A)** An imaginary line between the superior anterior crest and the pubis is constructed. This imaginary line usually corresponds to the location of the inguinal ligament. The place on this line where there is arterial pulsation is an excellent place to obtain access. As such, the needle should enter approximately 1 cm below the imaginary line while advancing at a 30- to 60- degree angle. **(B)** An excellent method of localizing the place to access is to fluoroscope the femoral head. The needle point should be over the lower inner quadrant.

than the common femoral artery. This entry site may predispose to dissection, arterial occlusion, pseudoaneurysm, bleeding, and arteriovenous fistula formation. When in doubt, position can be checked under fluoroscopy. The needle tip should be in the inner lower quadrant of the femoral head (see Fig 4-3). Entering the artery above the inguinal ligament may make catheter advancement difficult, lead to problems in compressing the artery, increase the risk of hematoma formation, and favor intraperitoneal or retroperitoneal bleeding.

After the arterial puncture site has been localized, the overlying skin is anesthetized, typically with 1% lidocaine intradermally. Injection of the skin after localizing the artery enables the operator to more accurately inject the skin area. Especially in patients with weak pulses, pulse localization can be more difficult after the skin is infiltrated. The subcutaneous tissue is also injected, taking care that lidocaine is not injected into a vascular structure. Attempts at anesthetizing the periosteum in the region of the femoral artery and vein are worthwhile but usually not completely successful. In summary, the generous use of lidocaine can often make the difference between a happy patient and an unhappy one.

The femoral vein runs parallel and medial to the femoral artery at the inguinal ligament area. The femoral vein is usually larger in diameter than the artery. The vein is compressible and cannot be palpated. When accessing both the artery and vein at the same site, the vein should ideally be accessed about 1 cm medially and below the arterial puncture site. This separation probably decreases the likelihood of developing a postprocedure arteriovenous fistula. After anesthetizing the skin, two 2- to 4-mm skin incisions are made with a surgical blade over the vein and artery. A subcutaneous "tunnel" may be made with a hemostat. This tunnel will allow the arterial and/or venous sheaths to encounter less resistance on entering the vascular structure. We find it easiest to puncture the vein with an open-bore needle (e.g., Cook, Bloomington, IN) attached to a 10-ml syringe. The needle is advanced through the skin opening at an angle of less than 45 degrees (the angle is that formed by the needle and skin plane) to a depth of 2 to 3 cm. While negative pressure is applied to the syringe, the needle is slowly advanced until blood freely enters the syringe. The needle is held steady, the syringe removed, and the appropriate guidewire advanced. Whenever resistance is experienced, progress of the guidewire should be checked under fluoroscopy. The needle is then withdrawn over the guidewire while digital pressure is applied over the puncture site. The sheath/dilator assembly can then be gently advanced with a twisting motion over the wire and into the vein, and the wire and dilator removed. The side-arm of any sheath should not contain air. To ensure this, blood is aspirated from the side-arm and a saline flush ($\sim$ 2–5 ml) is injected.

Arterial access can be achieved with the same needle. In all cases, a single (anterior) wall stick should be the goal. The needle should be grasped in the right hand, using the first three fingers. The needle should be advanced gently through the skin opening until a vigorous, pulsatile blood return is achieved.

Most textbooks recommend entering the vessel at a 30- to 45- degree angle. Experience has shown that most operators use an even more acute angle. This approach locates the artery entry point away from the skin opening and may complicate postprocedural hemostasis. Using a less acute angle (> 45 degrees) does not usually result in adverse effects but does shorten the length of the subcutaneous needle track and moves the entry point closer to the skin opening. If extravascular bleeding occurs, it will be detected earlier and subcutaneous infiltration will be less likely to occur, because blood can readily exit through the skin opening. When using the right inguinal area, the artery is palpated with the second and third fingers of the left hand. When using the left groin, it is most preferred, particularly for the relatively inexperienced operator, to lean across the patient and use the same technique.

It should be emphasized that the operator must be certain that the landmarks have been correctly identified. Some operators prefer to straddle the artery with their fingers, vertically identifying the point between their fingers as the artery's center. Others place both second and third fingers above and perpendicular to the vessel. The important aspect is to have "control" of the artery, that is, to be able to manually compress the artery for hemostasis if necessary. The operator should try to feel at the needle hub the pulsation transmitted from the anterior wall of the femoral artery, and then the needle should be slowly advanced. Pulsatile blood return through the obturator with the Seldinger-type needle or large volume flow through the open-bore needle signifies that the needle has entered the vessel through the anterior wall. If possible, effort should be made to avoid advancing the needle through the back wall of the artery. If blood return is not obviously pulsatile, however, it may be necessary to advance the needle further. If the needle is partially through the anterior arterial wall, advancement results in true pulsatile flow. If the needle is against the posterior wall, further advancement typically results in loss of flow and discomfort when the periosteum is touched by the needle. The operator will then know that needle retraction will result in brisk pulsatile flow with re-entry of the needle tip in the lumen. If no pulsatile flow occurs with this maneuver, it is likely that the needle either has grazed the side of the artery or has entered a small branch. In these cases, the needle should be removed and digital compression applied for at least 2 to 4 minutes.

Once the needle is in the vessel, the needle angle may be made more acute as long as pulsatile flow through the needle continues. A guidewire will usually pass without difficulty. Fluoroscopy may be used to observe movement of the guidewire tip and should be used whenever the slightest resistance is felt. It is important to emphasize that the guidewire should be introduced only if there is brisk pulsatile flow exiting the accessing needle. After needle access, a guidewire may be inserted into the vessel and sheath placement may then proceed after needle removal. In cases in which a sheath is not used, a long (130–150 cm) wire is required. After the wire tip is at the level of the diaphragm in the descending aorta, the dilator is removed over the wire, pressure applied with the first three fingers of the left hand, the wire wiped with sterile saline and the catheter advanced over the guidewire. When the catheter tip approaches the skin (usually being advanced by an assistant), the wire is pulled backward into the catheter until it exits the distal end of the catheter. It is important to emphasize that while only the guidewire is in the artery, the hole in the artery is larger than the guidewire. If adequate pressure is not applied proximal to the hole, blood loss through the skin or subcutaneous bleeding with development of a hematoma is likely. Thus the operator should have control of the vessel, as shown in Figure 4-4.

Potential complications from femoral artery cannulation include development of a subcutaneous or retroperitoneal hematoma, producing severe anemia or hypotension from persistent blood loss. Pseudoaneurysm, arteriovenous fistulas, or thrombus formation with leg ischemia also may occur. In general, for diagnostic procedures, the incidence of these complications should be no higher than 0.5–1.0%. Risk factors for hematoma development probably include use of intravenous (IV) heparin postprocedure, larger sheath sizes, and peripheral vascular disease. If the needle is advanced too far laterally, it may encounter the lateral femoral cutaneous nerve, producing immediate severe pain and, rarely, a chronic dysesthesia syndrome.

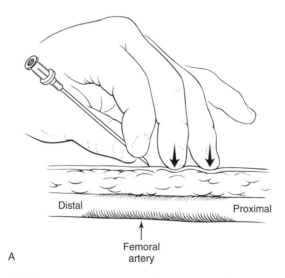

Distal

Proximal

Femoral
artery

A

Figure 4-4   **(A)** The femoral artery has been entered by a large bore needle with backflow of blood. Note the operator's finger positions. As soon as the needle passes into the vessel through the anterior wall, brisk pulsatile flow occurs. This technique is called the "one wall stick." It prevents occult bleeding through the posterior wall.

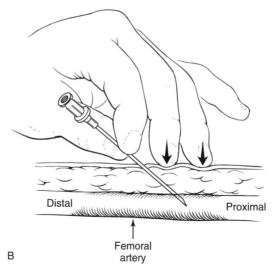

Distal   Proximal

Femoral
artery

B

Figure 4-4 **(B)** A wire is then passed through the needle into the vessel. The needle is removed, and a sheath is inserted.

Brachial Artery Cannulation

Percutaneous Technique

The operational anatomy of the brachial fossa is shown in Figure 4-5. If the use of Judkins catheters is planned, the left brachial artery should be used. The brachial artery is palpated at the elbow crease after the antecubital fossa has been prepped and draped. A towel may be placed under the elbow to maximally straighten the arm and fixate somewhat the position of the brachial artery. The overlying skin and subcutaneous area are infiltrated with a local anesthetic, typically lidocaine. The skin is incised with a scalpel (No. 11 blade). The artery is palpated (with the right hand for the left brachial artery), utilizing the second and third fingers. We prefer palpating the artery just proximal to the skin incision. An open-bore or Seldinger-type needle is then advanced slowly at an angle of approximately 60 degrees, attempting to feel the artery moving the needle before vessel entry. Once there is blood return, a J-tipped or straight-tipped guidewire (0.035″ or 0.038″, at least 44 cm in length) is advanced into the vessel through the needle. The needle is then removed and the sheath advanced as described previously for the femoral approach. Should the needle traverse too medially, it may hit the brachial vein with consequent bleeding in the brachial compartment, making subsequent attempts at brachial artery access more difficult. If the needle is directed even more medially, it may impinge

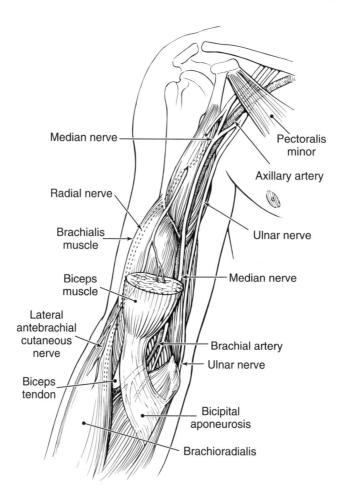

Figure 4-5 Anatomy of the brachial fossa. The aponeurosis above the brachial artery and deep vein has been removed in this diagram. The deep vein is medial and deep to the brachial artery and is not shown. (Reprinted with permission from Basmajian JV, Slonecker CF, eds. Grant's method of anatomy. 11th ed. Baltimore: Williams & Wilkins, 1986. Copyright © 1986, Williams & Wilkins Co.)

on the median nerve, which will produce a sensation of severe electric shocks down the arm and into the hand.

Brachial Artery Cutdown

The arm is placed on a board and taped at the wrist to maintain anatomic landmarks during the procedure. A towel may be placed under the elbow to maximally straighten the arm and fix landmarks. After the skin is prepped and draped, the brachial artery is palpated. Lidocaine is injected, initially intradermally using a fine needle (typically 25 gauge), then deeper using a somewhat larger (20–22 gauge) and longer needle. A transverse incision (15–20 mm) is made just proximal to the crease overlying the palpable artery (Fig 4-6A). When venous cannulation is required, the incision should extend medially. Good exposure is crucial to a safe cutdown; thus, the length of the incision is mandated by the quality of the exposure. If it is appreciated during cutdown that structures are not adequately seen, the incision should be extended. Tissues are separated by blunt dissection using a curved hemostat. The median nerve should be studiously avoided. The median nerve lies posteromedially to the brachial artery. To improve exposure retractors, either self-retaining or Army-Navy retractors held by an assistant may be used in performing the dissection. It should be emphasized that the "roof" above the brachial artery and vein and median nerve is a dense fascia (Fig 4-6B). This structure must be dissected to isolate the vessels. The operator may choose a small curved hemostat to gently dissect the fascial plane around the vessels and to isolate these structures (Fig 4-6C). When the artery is visualized, it may be brought to the surface with a curved hemostat. The proximal and distal portions of the exposed artery are secured with cloth umbilical or silastic tapes or thick (No. 1 or 2) silk sutures, and the artery is cleaned of fascia (1–2 cm), adjacent nerves, and veins by using fine forceps and hemostats (Fig 4-6D). This step is important in successful brachial artery cannulation. Removing fascia and overlying tissue allows the artery more freedom of movement by the operator. It also allows for an easier artery repair after the procedure. Vascular ("bulldog") clamps may be applied distally to prevent backbleeding (Fig 4-6E). They may be placed both proximally and distally during arteriotomy repair. Appropriate tension on the proximal and distal umbilical tapes are applied and a small (1-mm) transverse incision is made in the artery with a scalpel (Fig 4-6F). It should be large enough only to admit the tip of the catheter. The vessel is then intubated by a catheter by opening the artery with a small "right-angle" forceps (Fig 4-6G) and the proximal vascular clamp removed and the proximal tape loosened. The catheter chosen is then advanced a short distance into the artery. The catheter is aspirated, flushed, and connected to the manifold. A similar approach can be employed to cannulate the brachial vein or the superficial, medially located basilic vein. Because of the diminutive size of the brachial artery, relatively low flow distal to the arteriotomy, and direct control of the artery, heparinization to a therapeutic PTT or ACT is recommended. At the end of the procedure, vascular clamps are placed to allow suturing in a bloodless field after confirmation of vessel patency by observing blood flow from both proximal and distal sides of the arteriotomy (Fig 4-6H). The artery can be closed with 6.0 Prolene sutures with a continuous suture or simple interrupted suture (Fig 4-6I). For a continuous suture, a stay or anchor suture should be placed immediately outside the arteriotomy at both ends. The continuous suture is begun immediately adjacent to the arteriotomy. The edges of the arteriotomy should approximate without "gaps." The running suture is tied to the distal stay suture. Very gentle digital pressure is applied to

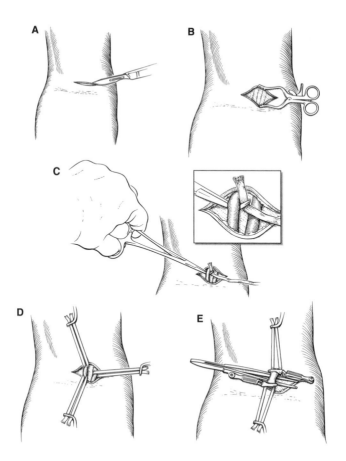

Figure 4-6 Brachial cutdown technique. **(A)** An incision (10–20 mm) is made over the brachial artery. It should be extended (by 5–10 mm) medially if the brachial vein is to be used for a right heart catheterization. **(B)** The skin has been incised. The subcutaneous tissue has been dissected. A dense fascia has been encountered. The brachial artery and vein are below it. **(C)** The dense fascia has been separated. The operator has dissected adjoining vessels and nerves away from the brachial artery. The artery has been cleared to the adventitia approximately 10 mm in length. Then, the operator has placed a small hemostat under the brachial artery. The hemostat is holding an umbilical tape that will be passed under the vessel. **(D)** The artery has two umbilical tapes in place, with hemostats at the end for control. The arteriotomy will be made between the two tapes. The vein has been isolated and retracted to prevent it from being injured. In this example, it will not be used. **(E)** Vascular clamps are placed distally and proximally. The vessel should be straight and slightly on stretch. A small forceps may be placed under the vessel for this purpose. If the vessel is too loosely held, controlling the arteriotomy incision is difficult. If the vessel is too taut, the arteriotomy will be unintentionally extended. An alternative method of creating a bloodless field may be performed without the vascular clamps. The umbilical tapes are pulled tight by an assistant or twisted to prevent bleeding and obscuring the view. **(F)** A 1- to 2-mm arteriotomy is made with a No. 11 blade on the anterior surface of the artery. The anterior wall can be held up by a "right-angle" forceps to limit the possibility of inadvertently perforating the posterior wall with the blade. **(G)** A right angle is placed in the vessel to maximize the hole opening and ensure there is an opening from the outside of the vessel. The proxi-

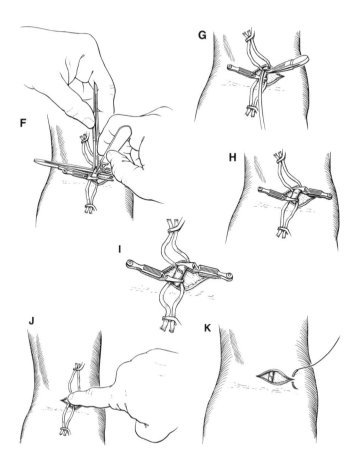

mal umbilical tape or vascular clamp may be loosened to demonstrate bleeding through the hole. This finding ensures that the anterior incision is a through-and-through cut. The catheter is then inserted, typically without a wire. The proximal umbilical tape is loosened or the vascular clamp removed. A straight wire also may be used to lead into the vessel. Note that the catheter has a tapered tip. The shaft of the catheter will stretch the brachial artery incision. After catheter removal, the intrinsic elasticity of the vessel will decrease the size of the hole and make for a smaller repair. (**H**) At the end of the procedure, vascular clamps may be used to maintain a bloodless field for repair. If only umbilical or other types of strings are used, the vessel will be stretched, making vascular repair more difficult and increasing the possibility of sutures pulling through the incision. Before suturing the arteriotomy incision, the vascular clamp proximally should be loosened to demonstrate brisk flow and that clot is not present. The same maneuver should be performed distally. The distal flow may not be pulsatile because the flow will be coming from collaterals. If no flow is present, threading a Fogarty catheter distal to remove clot should be performed. (**I**) The arteriotomy may be closed by simple interrupted sutures, or a continuous suture. (**J**) Very gentle digital pressure is applied to the arteriotomy site. Note that the vascular clamps have been removed, but the umbilical tapes remain. (**K**) The vessel is pulsatile without blood leaking at the suture line. The circulating nurse or technician has ascertained that the radial pulse is strong. At that point, the umbilical tapes are removed and the vessel is returned to its normal anatomic site. Silk sutures (2.0, 3.0, 4.0) may be used to suture the skin.

the arteriotomy site if there is leakage at the suture line (Fig 4-6J). If there is no leak between sutures and the radial pulse is present, the umbilical tapes are removed and the skin is sutured with 2.0 to 4.0 silk sutures (Fig 4-6K). If bleeding persists at the suture line, the incision should be inspected carefully to determine whether either an additional suture or a revision of the suture line is required. If there is no pulse distally, the suture line must be taken down and a Fogarty catheter inserted proximally and/or distally to remove clots. If distal flow cannot be restored, consultation with a vascular surgeon is often very helpful.

Internal Jugular Vein Cannulation

The internal jugular vein is positioned lateral to the carotid artery, medial to the external jugular vein, and usually just lateral to the outer edge of the medial head of the sternocleidomastoid muscle. To identify landmarks, patients are instructed to lie supine without a pillow under the head, and in the case of the right internal jugular, with the head turned 30 degrees to the left. Patients with low venous pressures may be placed in the Trendelenburg position or perform a Valsalva maneuver, thus engorging the extrathoracic jugular vein. In the supine position, even patients with normal venous pressures will show pressure transients including a and v waves.

There are several reasonable approaches to internal jugular vein access. Some physicians (BGD, BFU) have utilized ultrasound to guide access to the internal jugular vein. This method has been documented to reduce complications, procedure times, and patient discomfort. Although it is recognized that ultrasound is not routinely available in most laboratories, it has provided invaluable information on the technique of jugular vein access and mechanism of complications such as pneumothorax or puncture of the carotid artery. A high anterior approach from the top of the triangle formed by the two heads of the sternocleidomastoid muscle and clavicle is recommended. This location moves the puncture site as far away as feasible from the upper lung tip. Especially in obese patients, it can be difficult to localize the triangle correctly. In these cases, it is helpful to put a finger in the suprasternal recess and move to the right (for right internal jugular access). The first elevation palpated is the medial head of the sternocleidomastoid muscle. The finger should be moved over the medial head and follow the edge superiorly until the top of the triangle is palpated. With the head slightly rotated to the contralateral side, the skin is anesthetized with 1% lidocaine solution. The skin is nicked with a surgical blade with care not to cut the external jugular vein, which crosses the same area superficially. An open-bore needle with a 10-ml syringe is inserted through the skin, pointing slightly toward the ipsilateral nipple. A steeper angle (> 45 degrees) rather than the more shallow one often recommended in textbooks is used. The needle is gently advanced 1.5 to 2.5 cm. Ultrasound has demonstrated that the center of the internal jugular vein is universally between 1.5 to 2.0 cm below the skin. Advancing the needle more than 2.5 cm greatly increases the risk of pneumothorax.

The needle is withdrawn while aspirating the syringe. Because using this technique virtually eliminates the risk of pneumothorax, it is helpful to let the patient perform a Valsalva maneuver (Fig 4-7). This greatly increases the diameter of the internal jugular vein, facilitating puncture. When the first attempt is unsuccessful, the needle angle may be more acute and parallel to the long axis of the body. The urge to introduce the needle deeper than 2 cm should be resisted. If the carotid artery can be palpated along its length, the needle can be aimed 1 cm laterally and parallel to the carotid artery. Ultrasound has also shown that anatomic variations are relatively rare. The so-called lateral vein occurs in less than 1% of patients (Fig 4-8). Patients who have had multiple jugular vein cannulations or long-term indwelling catheters may demonstrate occlusion or scarring of the vein, increasing the difficulties in accessing the vein, even with the aid of ultrasound (Fig 4-9). Most of these patients will, however, have normal venous anatomy on the other side.

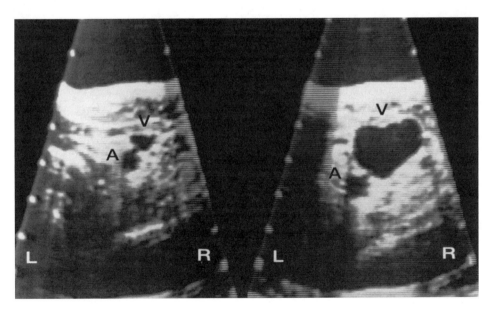

Figure 4-7 Ultrasound of internal jugular vein at baseline (left panel) and during a Valsalva maneuver (right panel). Note the carotid artery below and slightly medial to vein (V). This view is a transverse section looking from caudal to cranial.

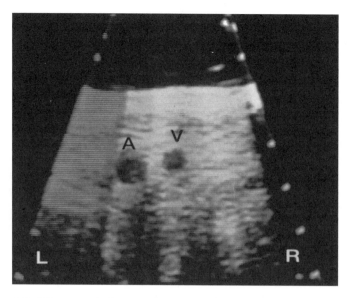

Figure 4-8 Ultrasound demonstrates a truly laterally displaced internal jugular vein (V). (A), in carotid artery.

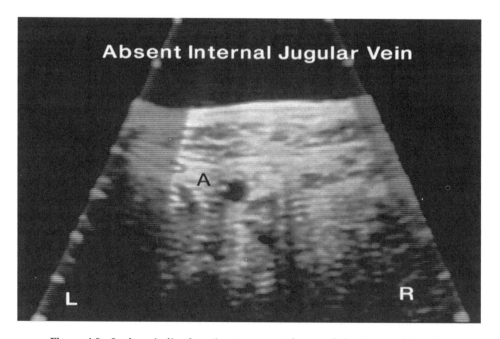

Figure 4-9 In hospitalized patients, repeated use of the internal jugular vein can result in its occlusion or severe scar formation. This picture shows occlusion of the right internal jugular vein. Note that the carotid artery (A) is well seen.

Another technique to access the internal jugular vein is the method utilized at Johns Hopkins University Hospital (by KB). It employs a small (25-gauge) "finder" needle to determine the location of the vein. This needle is inserted through the course of previously instilled lidocaine in the anticipated direction of the vascular structure to be entered. The angle between the syringe and skin is 30 to 45 degrees. If greater than 7-Fr sheath is used for vascular access, a small incision is made in the skin with a No. 11 blade, and the skin and subcutaneous tissues are separated gently with mosquito forceps to ensure ease of access of the sheath. Either an Amplatz or micropuncture needle attached to a syringe with a small amount of saline flush is then used to follow the course of the finder needle into the vein. Once blood is aspirated, the syringe is separated from the needle and a 0.025″ wire guide is inserted through the needle into the vein. The needle is removed, and a larger bore dilator (4 Fr) or the Teflon Amplatz is advanced over the guidewire. The 0.025″ wire is removed and replaced by a 0.032″ wire. The Teflon 4-Fr introducer can then be removed. A larger sheath, usually 7 Fr, 8 Fr, or 9 Fr, is passed into the vessel over the wire. One must have a segment of wire longer than the sheath outside the skin to prevent inadvertent loss of the wire in the central veins. Once the sheath is adequately placed, the central dilator is removed and the sheath system is flushed.

Severe complications from internal jugular vein cannulation should be < 1%. The most concerning are pneumothorax and trauma to the carotid artery. The latter can be disastrous if unrecognized with inappropriate placement of a sheath in this vessel. Other complications that occur rarely are brachial plexus injury, recurrent laryngeal nerve trauma, and hemothorax.

Subclavian Vein Cannulation

Cannulation of the subclavian vein has been utilized most frequently in hospitalized patients, particularly those in intensive care units. This large vein is used for infusion of drugs, nutrition, and temporary pacing. This vein, both right and left, is the preferred route for implanting a permanent pacemaker wire, with a "pocket" made caudal to the vein.

Pertinent operational anatomy is shown in Figure 4-10. The proximal subclavian vein and artery are hidden behind the first rib, proximal clavicle, and sternum. The vein is the more superficially located vessel. The vessels emerge at approximately the midpoint of the clavicle. The vein is relatively accessible after that point. Toward its lateral margin, the vessel is extrathoracic and travels in a somewhat deeper location.

There is no technique that has been universally accepted as standard. One method is to consider the clavicle as divided into three equal-length sections (see Fig 4-10). The medial end of the most lateral section will be the place

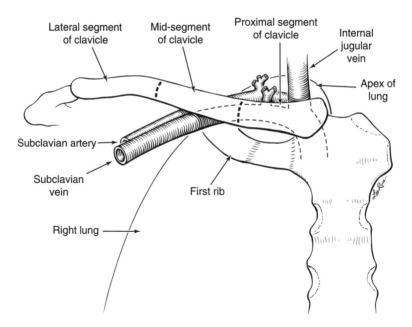

Figure 4-10   Operational anatomy for accessing the right subclavian vein.

where the needle passes through the skin. The skin is anesthetized with 1% lidocaine. A small skin incision (2–4 mm) is made to allow the sheath to follow without resistance. The needle traverses the skin at or about 30 degrees. The needle should be directed at the sternal notch. The needle tip should be "hugging" (i.e., touching) the inferior surface of the clavicle. The needle should probably not enter the skin for more than 2 to 3 cm for fear of the needle hitting the lung, with consequent pneumothorax. If the vein is not entered on the first attempt, the needle angle may be changed to slightly more superior or inferior, with small changes in needle angle. Although the most lateral subclavian vein is extrathoracic, it is more difficult to access because it is somewhat deeper and has less well defined landmarks.

Complications in attempting to cannulate the subclavian vein include pneumothorax (0.3%–1.0%), puncture of the subclavian artery (0.5%–1.0%), bleeding into mediastinum (0.2%–0.5%), and injury to the phrenic nerve (< 0.01%). If the subclavian artery is entered inadvertently, it cannot be easily compressed. This complication is particularly dangerous in patients who are anticoagulated. Causing a pneumothorax has prevented this technique from becoming the clearly favored approach for central vein cannulation. The use of ultrasound may allow entry more laterally and thereby decrease the risk of inducing a pneumothorax.

Hemostatic Methods After Cardiac Catheterization

General Comments

Hemostasis by some method is required after catheterization. This procedure may be performed by a physician, nurse, or cardiovascular technician. Whoever performs this procedure should have had formal training and proctorship before working independently. Vascular problems including bleeding requiring transfusion or increase in hospital length of stay, pseudoaneurysm, and arteriovenous fistula formation continue to have the highest incidence of all catheterization-related complications. As such, each individual who performs compression should be experienced in this technique.

For arterial sites, distal flow past the point of compression should be ascertained by the presence of a distal pulse by either palpation or Doppler. Venous compression may be applied for 5 to 10 minutes with much less pressure because the vein is highly compressible and has a very low hydrostatic pressure.

Manual Compression

Digital compression should be considered the gold standard for compressive methods. Performed properly, it can prevent bleeding and maintain distal perfusion. It has the advantage of second-to-second modulation of vascular compression with continuous observation. It has the disadvantage of necessitating that a staff member be unavailable for procedures during the holding period. Pressure may be applied with the middle finger on the puncture site, the fourth finger above the site, and the second finger below the hole. Alternatively, all three fingers may compress at the site and above it. Digital pressure should be applied by fingertips only, such as that applied by a musician to the keys of a piano or the strings of a violin (Fig 4-11).

Prior to hemostatic compression, one pulsation without pressure should be allowed to send blood preferentially through the skin. It has been claimed that such a maneuver will favor blood loss through the skin, if the vascular entry site should open. Typically, "firm" pressure, but one in which the distal pulse is present, may be applied for 10 minutes, less firm for 2 to 5 minutes, and "light" for 2 to 5 minutes. At the end of the allotted time, the site should be viewed. One should resist the temptation of "peeking." If bleeding continues, another 15 to 20 minutes of pressure should be applied.

Risk factors for prolonged bleeding include patients with severe atherosclerosis at the puncture site. In this case, there is loss of elasticity, without approximation of vessel edges when catheter and sheath are removed. Continuation of IV heparin or administration of a thrombolytic agent will make it difficult to remove the sheath and have adequate hemostasis. In general, the

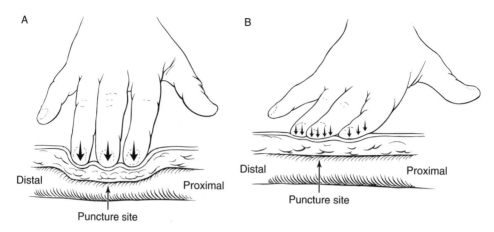

Figure 4-11 Application of digital pressure. **(A)** This is the correct technique, because all of the pressure is transmitted in a very small area. **(B)** This panel shows poor technique, because pressure is spreading throughout entire fingers, so that pressure (pressure = force/area) is less in each place due to the larger area covered. Arrows represent points of compression.

larger the catheter or sheath inserted, the higher the incidence of vascular complication. For example, in "low-risk" patients (see Chapter 16), using a 6-Fr diagnostic catheter with no heparin may have a vascular complication rate of less than 1%. Conversely, patients who have 9- to 10-Fr sheaths during interventional procedures and continued IV heparin have been reported to have a vascular complication rate 50 to 100 times greater (5%–10%). Other risk factors for bleeding include (1) elevated blood pressure, (2) obesity, (3) patients who move about after catheterization despite orders to the contrary, and (4) elderly patients.

Application of a pressure dressing may be useful in some patients, particularly those whom the physician believes will move the affected limb. Unfortunately, with such a dressing, significant blood loss may occur before the problem is recognized. For that reason, we do not use a pressure dressing routinely.

C-Clamp

A vascular clamp may be substituted for manual compression (Fig 4-12). This approach has the advantage of freeing up personnel for other functions. In addition, it provides pressure over a relatively small area. Its limitations include the inability to modulate pressure easily, some discomfort from the device, and the possibility that a hematoma may occur without observation, even by a trained individual. Disposable equipment is limited to the disk applied at

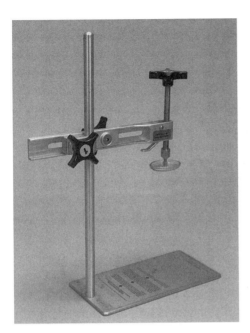

Figure 4-12 A C-clamp. The disk that applies pressure rests on the patient's entry point. The disk is the only disposable part of the apparatus.

the site; as such, this method is quite economical, particularly when one includes the cost of a catheterization laboratory staff member freed up to do other tasks. It is our practice to utilize the C-clamp for routine diagnostic and interventional cases.

Femo-Stop

The Femo-Stop (USCI, Billerica, MA) (Fig 4-13) utilizes a fluid-filled clear plastic compression bag that molds to skin contours. It is held in place by straps passing around the hip. The amount of applied pressure may be modulated and observed with a sphygmomanometer gauge. It allows visualization of the skin incision site. A major limitation for routine use is the relatively high cost of disposables. We reserve the use of this device for patients in whom prolonged compression is anticipated or if bleeding persists despite prolonged digital compression or C-clamp use.

Vasoseal

The Vasoseal (Datascope, Inc., Fairfield, NJ) (Fig 4-14), recently approved for clinical use by the Food and Drug Administration, places a processed animal collagen plug on the adventitial side of the vessel to promote rapid thrombosis. Collagen should not be in contact with the circulating blood if applied correctly. This device has undergone human studies with reasonable short-term

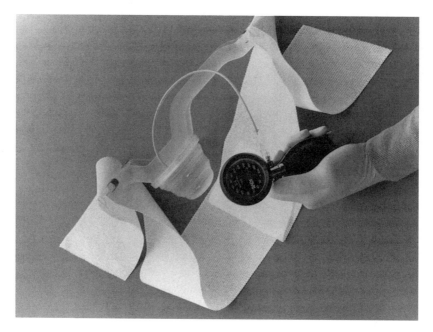

Figure 4-13   The Femo-Stop. The clear plastic bag over the incision allows visual inspection of entry site. The straps and bag are for one use only. (Courtesy of USCI.)

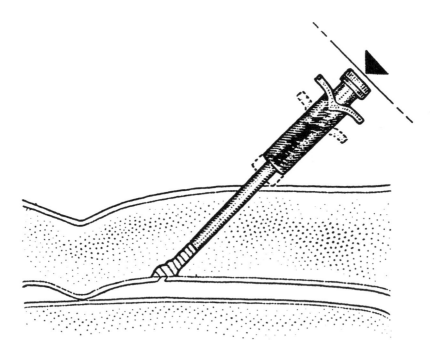

Figure 4-14   The Vasoseal. This system applies collagen to the outside of the vessel promoting arterial hemostasis. (Courtesy of Datascope, Inc.)

results. It offers the possibility of decreasing vascular complications while also decreasing compression time and bed rest postprocedure. The long-term local effects are unknown.

Angio-Seal

The Angio-Seal (Quinton, Inc., Seattle, WA) (Fig 4-15), recently approved by the FDA, is somewhat different from Vasoseal, although it also applies collagen outside the vessel. With this device, an "anchor" with material identical to absorbable sutures is pushed through the arterial sheath into the vessel itself. This anchor is attached to an absorbable suture, which is brought outside the body. A collagen plug is "tamped" onto the outside of the vessel. By tying the suture tightly, the anchor will adhere to the endothelial surface and the collagen to outside the vessel. This device has undergone clinical testing. It holds the promise, as does Vasoseal, of decreasing vascular complications and allowing rapid patient mobilization.

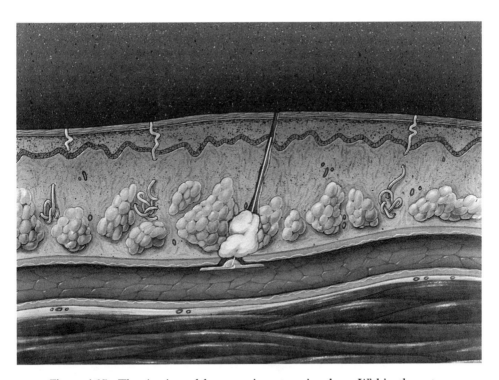

Figure 4-15   The Angio-seal hemostatic system in place. Within the artery itself is an "anchor" composed of the same material as absorbable sutures, and immediately tied down to the outside of the vessel is a collagen plug. Holding this system together is resorbable suture. (Courtesy of Quinton, Inc.)

SELECTED READINGS

Agarwal SK, Roubin GS. Percutaneous vascular acess for cardiac interventions. In: Roubin G, Califf R, Stack R, et al., eds. Interventional cardiovascular medicine: principles and practice. Churchill Livingstone, 1994:687–207.

Denys BG, Uretsky BF, Reddy PS. Ultrasound-assisted cannulation of the internal jugular vein. Circulation 1993; 87:1557–1562.

Grossman W. Cardiac catheterization by direct exposure of artery and vein. In: Grossman W, ed. Cardiac catheterization and angiography. Philadelphia: Lea & Febiger, 1976:13–24.

Tilkian AG, Daily EK. Cardiovascular procedures. Diagnostic technique and therapeutic procedures. St. Louis: Mosby, 1986:32–82.

5

HEART PRESSURES AND CATHETERIZATION

Peter A. McCullough
James A. Goldstein

H
EMODYNAMIC ASSESSMENT BY measurement of intracardiac pressures and determination of cardiac output is a fundamental component of invasive cardiac evaluation. This chapter considers the principles of pressure measurement and their application to evaluation of the pathophysiology and hemodynamic status of patients with cardiovascular disease.

Pressure is defined as force per unit area. Force expressed through liquid is a transmitted pressure wave. Pressure waves reflect dynamic mechanical events over time, resulting in fluctuating cycles per second, termed the *fundamental frequency*. Cardiac pressures are measured with devices whose intrinsic physical properties influence the data obtained. Transduction is the conversion of pressure waves into electrical signals. The sensitivity of the device refers to the relationship of the input signal (fluctuation in force/area) to the output signal (movement of a manometer membrane). This relationship, considered over a range of frequencies, is termed the *frequency response* of the system. Damping is the dissipation of energy in the system due to friction. Desirable properties of any pressure measurement system include adequate sensitivity for the expected range of input signals with respect to amplitude and frequency and optimal damping of unwanted energy in the system. The type of catheter used also influences pressure measurements. The frequency response of fluid-filled catheter systems is directly proportional to the lumen radius of the catheter and inversely related to its length and compliance. Catheters are typically connected to a manifold, which transmits the pressure wave through connecting tubing to the pressure transducer, which in turn generates an electrical signal output proportional to movement of the transduction membrane. This signal is displayed and recorded on the physiologic recorder.

Potential sources of error and artifact must be recognized in all pressure measurement systems. The transducer must be properly positioned at the zero-reference mid-chest level; positioning above this level underestimates pressure, and below this level overestimates pressure. Deterioration in the frequency response (damping) is most commonly due to air bubbles in the manifold and/or tubing or thrombus within the catheter. Motion of the tip of the catheter within the heart causes motion of the column of fluid within the catheter and tubing, thus creating a catheter whip artifact, which may account for significant pressure swings. Summation of reflected waves from the great vessels may result in peripheral vessel amplification, which may elevate peak peripheral arterial (femoral or brachial) pressure, a phenomenon that may be observed by simultaneous measurement of central aortic and femoral pressure.

It is essential to appreciate the physiologic implications of measured pressures, particularly in assessment of chamber diastolic properties. Systolic pressures are conceptionally obvious, representing the contractile force generated to propel blood. Diastolic pressure interpretation is somewhat more complex. Measured filling pressure is a function of the blood volume distending the walls

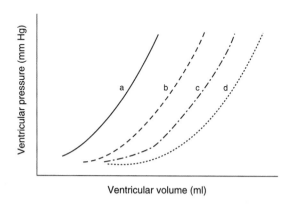

Figure 5-1   Fundamental to the understanding of diastolic pressures is the concept of chamber stiffness (i.e., the change in pressure for a given change in volume). Thus, in this example, chamber *a* is the stiffest ventricle. The reciprocal of stiffness is compliance, that is, change in volume for a given change in pressure. Thus, *a* is the least compliant chamber, *b* and *c* are intermediate, and *d* is the most compliant or least stiff.

of the chamber measured, the intrinsic compliance of that chamber, and the extrinsic effects of neighboring structures (contralateral ventricle, pericardium). Therefore, diastolic pressures must be considered in terms of the actual pressure exerted within the chamber (the true transmural distending pressure), which provides insight into chamber "preload" or chamber volume (Fig 5-1). Elevated diastolic pressures may confirm the presence and severity of "backward failure" (pulmonary or systemic venous congestion). However, elevated diastolic pressures do not necessarily indicate increased chamber volume, but may instead be a reflection of altered stiffness (hypertrophy, ischemia) or extrinsic influences (pericardial constraint). Thus, we measure pressure both because it is convenient and because it determines the extent of backward failure, but we should not equate diastolic pressure as necessarily equivalent to chamber volume or preload.

Right Heart Catheterization: Catheters and Techniques

Right heart catheters may be introduced through several venous approaches, including femoral, brachial, jugular, and subclavian veins (see Chapter 4). In general, in patients undergoing left heart catheterization, the same site employed for arterial access is most often utilized (femoral or brachial). If right heart catheterization alone is performed, the access site depends on whether there is intent to leave the catheter indwelling for hemodynamic monitoring (e.g., patients with congestive heart failure), in which case internal jugular and subclavian approaches may allow for a more stable position and less of an infection risk than the femoral approach. On the other hand, hemorrhagic diathesis and mechanical ventilation recommend the femoral approach.

The vast majority of right heart catheterizations are performed with an 8-Fr multilumen balloon-tipped flotation catheter with thermodilution cardiac output capability (e.g., Swan-Ganz type). These catheters are inserted through a venous access sheath and then advanced antegrade toward the right heart with the balloon inflated, optimally under fluoroscopic monitoring. Using femoral access, the catheter is initially positioned in the inferior vena cava (IVC) and pressure recorded, then advanced into the mid-right atrium (RA), to the superior vena cava (SVC), and then back in the RA, with pressures recorded and oxygen saturation samples often obtained at each site. The catheter is then advanced across the tricuspid valve into the right ventricle (RV), obtaining pressure and oximetry samples. If difficulty is encountered advancing the catheter into or through the RV, the catheter may be retracted into the IVC and, with the balloon deflated, directed into the hepatic vein, which "shapes" the catheter into a gentle curve and facilitates advancement across the tricuspid valve

(Fig 5-2A). Alternatively, the catheter may be "banked" off the lateral RA wall by deflating the balloon, orienting the catheter tip toward the lateral RA, advancing the catheter against the RA wall to initiate a loop, and inflating the balloon, which then points toward the tricuspid valve, allowing easier passage of the catheter into the RV (Fig 5-2B). Once in the RV, the catheter can be advanced into the pulmonary artery (PA) by positioning the catheter tip in the body of the RV and slowly rotating the catheter clockwise until the catheter tip is seen to "snake" upward toward the RV outflow tract, at which point the catheter can be advanced into the PA (Fig 5-2C). If this maneuver is unsuccessful, forming a loop in the RA, as described, is usually successful. In difficult cases, and particularly with severe pulmonary hypertension and/or tricuspid regurgitation (TR), utilization of a stiffening guidewire (0.018″–0.025″) may facilitate catheter advancement. In all cases, prior to advancement of the catheter into the RV, the ECG should be checked to exclude left bundle branch block, which increases the risk for transient heart block when the catheter encounters the interventricular septum, along whose right endocardial surface runs the vulnerable right bundle branch. Once PA pressure has been measured and oximetry samples obtained, the catheter is advanced into the "wedge" position, confirmed by forward motion of the balloon tip to a stationary position associated with diminution of the pressure pulse to a characteristic atrial waveform. Optimal wedge position can be confirmed by oximetry and subsequently balloon release. Once repositioned in the PA, thermodilution cardiac output determinations can be obtained.

Other catheters are occasionally utilized for right heart catheterization. The Berman flotation catheter is stiffer and somewhat more maneuverable than the Swan-Ganz, but lacks thermodilution capabilities and an end hole to measure wedge pressure. Non-balloon catheters include those with multiple side holes and a closed end (e.g., Lehman catheter) designed for right heart angiography. Stiffer end-hole catheters (e.g., Cournand catheter) may be used to obtain a truer wedge pressure (i.e., less damping than a Swan-Ganz catheter).

Excluding access site problems, there should rarely be a clinical complication from insertion and manipulation of the Swan-Ganz catheter in the catheterization laboratory. Fluoroscopic, hemodynamic, and electrocardiographic monitoring should optimize patient safety. In addition to an occasional problem at the access site, other rare complications include development of right bundle branch block (complete heart block in a patient with preexisting left bundle branch block), ventricular irritability, and very rarely sustained ventricular tachycardia or atrial antiarrhythmias, particularly atrial fibrillation. Death should be exceedingly rare and should be limited to patients brought to the catheterization suite *in extremis*.

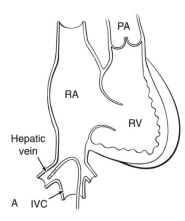

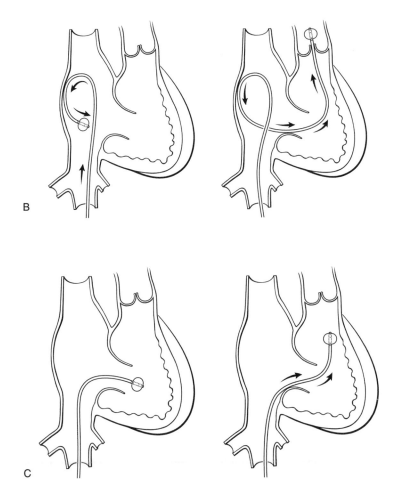

Figure 5-2 Techniques to facilitate catheter into the right ventricle in difficult cases. (**A**) Directing the catheter into the hepatic vein produces a curve that, when advanced, may direct the catheter tip across the tricuspid valve. (**B**) The balloon is deflated, with the catheter directed toward the lateral wall and advanced until a loop has been developed with the catheter tip pointing toward the tricuspid valve. The balloon is inflated and the catheter advanced across the tricuspid valve. The catheter can usually be advanced to the PA without difficulty. (**C**) Once in the RV, the catheter can be rotated in a clockwise manner. The loop will be enlarged with this maneuver, so the catheter should be gently retracted to maintain the same loop size. As the catheter tip points upward in the outflow tract, the catheter should be advanced across the pulmonary valve. RA, right atrium; PA, pulmonary artery; RV, right ventricle; IVC, inferior vera cava.

Interpretation of Right Atrial Pressure Waveforms

Normal Contours

Normal pressure contours for the RA, RV, PA, pulmonary capillary wedge (PCW), and left ventricle (LV) are depicted in Figure 5-3, and normal values are listed in the Appendix. The SVC and proximal IVC waveforms mirror that of the RA. Under physiologic conditions, the RA waveform has four major components, consisting of two positive and two negative waves for each cardiac

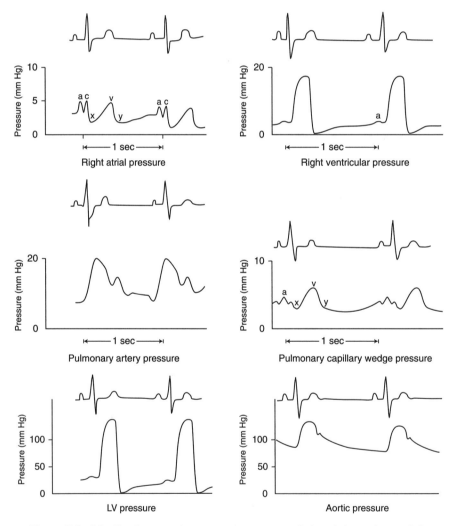

Figure 5-3   Idealized normal pressure contours of the right atrium, right ventricle, pulmonary artery, pulmonary capillary wedge, left ventricle, and aorta are shown.

cycle. These waveform components are best timed relative to both simultaneous ECG and concomitant systolic pressure (aortic, LV, RV, or PA), the latter of which definitively establishes the phases of the cardiac cycle. The RA deflection termed the *a wave* is a positive deflection seen immediately after the P wave on the ECG. It precedes ventricular systole. The upstroke and amplitude of the a wave reflect the strength of RA contractility and RV compliance. The x descent, the negative deflection following the a wave during early ventricular systole, is determined by two mechanical events, with the initial phase of the x descent reflecting active atrial relaxation, and the latter portion of the descent attributable to systolic intrapericardial depressurization as pericardial volume (i.e., intracardiac volume) is reduced during ventricular emptying. The c wave, a positive deflection during early ventricular systole, corresponds to tricuspid closure and represents upward movement of the tricuspid valve or early TR resulting in a brief rise in RA pressure. When present, the c wave divides the x descent into x and x′ components, the initial x component reflecting RA relaxation and the x′ descent associated with systolic intrapericardial depressurization. The v wave is a positive wave during ventricular systole and corresponds to passive atrial filling during ventricular ejection. The y descent is the downward slope following the v wave and represents atrial emptying during ventricular systole.

The Respiratory Cycle and Right Atrial Pressure

There is a reciprocal relationship between RA pressure and flow. Venous return to the atria is biphasic, with two flow peaks associated with the dual dips in atrial pressure during the nadirs of pressure corresponding to the x and y descents. Filling of the RV occurs primarily during the "passive" inflow phase (y descent), with a "booster" contribution at end-diastole attributable to atrial contraction (a wave). Under physiologic conditions, right heart flows, volumes, and pressure are influenced by respiratory oscillations in intrathoracic pressure (ITP). Inspiration increases the magnitude of negative ITP, which augments venous return from the extrathoracic cavae to the right heart, resulting in a decrease in caval pressures. Although right heart volumes and flows increase with inspiration, the more negative ITP surrounding the heart causes measured diastolic chamber pressures in the RA and RV to decrease. Inspiration also results in a normal oscillation in measured aortic pressure, inducing a decrement of 10 to 12 mm Hg in aortic systolic pressure. There are several mechanisms underlying this normal physiologic inspiratory drop in aortic pressure. Augmentation of right heart filling results in diminished LV volume due in part to septal shifting toward the LV. Additionally, negative ITP increases afterload to the LV by requiring it to overcome this negative pressure as well as extrathoracic vascular resistance. Finally, negative ITP favors pooling of blood in the lungs, decreasing LV diastolic volume.

Assessment of Right Atrial Pressure Abnormalities

Elevated systemic venous pressure in clinical right heart failure most commonly manifests as elevated neck veins, peripheral edema, hepatomegaly, and ascites. The hemodynamic differential diagnosis of systemic venous hypertension may be considered from an anatomic pathophysiologic tour through the right heart following the path taken by a catheter. Systemic venous congestion may result from vena caval obstruction (tumors, thrombus) and therefore not truly reflect right heart abnormalities. Vena caval obstruction will be evident hemodynamically as elevated central venous pressures, blunted x and y descents in the SVC/IVC waveforms reflecting impaired inflow and a pressure gradient between the affected cava and RA. In the absence of caval obstruction, elevated jugular venous pressure is synonomous with RA hypertension. Right atrial pressure elevation may result from arrhythmias, including tachyarrhythmias (most commonly atrial fibrillation with rapid ventricular response) and bradyarrhythmias (most commonly complete heart block). Elevated RA pressure is more commonly related to space-occupying lesions, pressure or volume overload, intrinsic atrial myocardial disease, or extrinsic compression or restraint (pericardial and other interactions). Right atrial pressure overload may be due to tricuspid valve obstruction or RV diastolic dysfunction. Tricuspid valve obstruction may result from rheumatic tricuspid stenosis, primary or secondary tumors, bulky vegetations, and, rarely, carcinoid valve involvement. Regardless of the cause, tricuspid obstruction is characterized hemodynamically by elevated mean RA pressure with an augmented a wave and x descent reflecting enhanced RA contraction and relaxation, a blunted y descent indicative of impaired atrial emptying, and a diastolic gradient (often only a few mm Hg) between RA and RV during simultaneous tracings with a persistent gradient at end-diastole (i.e., not simply an early diastolic flow gradient) (see Chapter 14). Right ventricular diastolic dysfunction may be caused by RV hypertrophy, RV myocardial infiltrative diseases, or myocardial ischemia. Resultant RA pressure demonstrates a prominent a wave and x descent reflecting enhanced atrial contraction and relaxation into a poorly compliant RV.

Atrial masses (tumors, clots) increase RA pressure, both through space-occupying effects as well as through potential obstruction to atrial inflow (caval obstruction), atrial outflow (tricuspid valve obstruction), and occasionally by inducing tricuspid valve incompetence (prolapsing myxoma). Atrial masses generally demonstrate hemodynamic features similar to tricuspid valve obstruction, with elevated mean RA pressure and a blunted y descent. However, the augmented atrial contraction and relaxation may not be as evident; consequently, the a wave and x descent may be less impressive. Right atrial volume overload often results from TR, atrial septal defect, anomalous venous return, or RV systolic or diastolic dysfunction. Regardless of the cause, TR transmits RV pressure to the RA, augmenting the RA pressure secondary to volume overload. There is a relatively rapid y descent reflecting early brisk emptying of the engorged RA. As TR becomes more severe, the v-wave amplitude increases and occupies a greater duration of systole, causing large systolic waves with relative obliteration of the intrinsic c wave and x descent. In wide-open TR, the RA pressure trace mirrors the RV pressure because there is functionally a common RA/RV chamber. This can be best appreciated by simultaneous RA and RV tracings (Fig 5-4). Functional TR may occur from RV dilatation and/or diastolic or systolic dysfunction. In this situation, for any given degree of TR, the RA pressure may be higher compared with a normally functioning RV. Atrial septal defect or anomalous venous return results in a left-to-right shunt with RA and RV volume overload. The RA pressure contour will be determined in large part by the magnitude of the shunt, the severity of RV systolic and diastolic dysfunction, the presence of secondary pulmonary hypertension, and the degree of

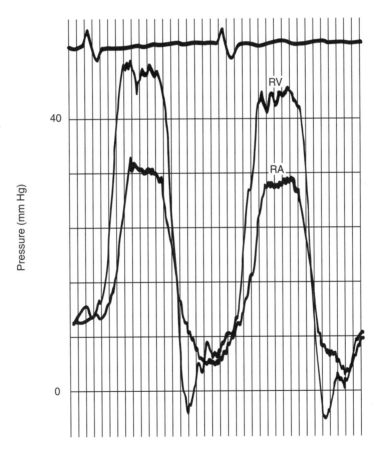

Figure 5-4   Right atrial and RV pressure tracings in severe tricuspid regurgitation. RA, right atrial; RV, right ventricular. (Kindly supplied by Dr. James A. Shaver.)

functional TR. Mean RA pressure may be elevated in these congenital heart problems, but the RA waveform, particularly the x and y descent, may be decreased as a result of RV systolic failure. These hemodynamic findings are not specific, and may be seen in other conditions that provoke elevations in pressure- or flow-mediated work, such as dilated cardiomyopathy. Accordingly, the presence of an atrial septal defect requires documentation of an oxygen saturation "step-up" (see Chapter 10). Atrial cardiomyopathic processes virtually always occur in the setting of concomitant ventricular dysfunction. Nevertheless, the additional effects of intrinsic impairment of atrial contraction (from ischemia, cardiomyopathy, or myocarditis) and compliance (from ischemia, fibrosis, infiltration, myocardial hypertrophy) may influence the hemodynamic findings for any given degree of ventricular involvement. Atrial dysfunction also exists in the transplanted heart, in which a severely dilated, poorly compliant, poorly contractile, and electromechanically dyssynchronous atrial chamber is created by surgical hybridization of the recipient and donor atria. Accordingly, such hearts typically manifest elevated mean RA pressure with decreased a wave and x descent reflecting impaired atrial contraction and relaxation. Such abnormalities are exacerbated by unresolved postoperative pulmonary hypertension and episodes of rejection. Additionally, in the early postoperative period ($< 6-8$ weeks), a pattern resembling restrictive cardiomyopathy may be seen, usually but not always, related to acute rejection.

The RA is an intrapericardial structure and both it and the RV are thin, compressible, and exquisitely sensitive to the external resistance of the pericardium. Increases in intrapericardial pressure (IPP) are directly and proportionately transmitted to the RA. Accordingly, the pathophysiology of the pericardial process is reflected in the RA waveform. The pathophysiology of pericardial disorders and their hemodynamic manifestations in the RA and RV are discussed subsequently.

Interpretation of Right Ventricular Pressure Waveforms

Normal Contours

The normal RV pressure contour is characterized by a monophasic systolic wave (with an occasional early systolic notch associated with tricuspid closure coincident with the c wave on the RA trace). As with the LV, the maximal rate of rise of the RV pressure (dp/dt) is directly related to the RV contractile state. The RV diastolic pressure contour reflects early relaxation and passive filling followed by active atrial transport, thereby inscribing a progressive rise followed by an end-diastolic "kick" (see Fig 5-3). Because the RV is thinner and more compliant than the LV, its filling pressure is normally lower. Furthermore, the more compressible nature of the RV and its dynamic diastolic relationship with the LV across their shared interventricular septum render RV diastolic properties (and therefore measured pressures) exquisitely sensitive to the extrinsic effects of the pericardium, as well as of the LV.

Assessment of Right Ventricular Pressure Abnormalities

Right ventricular hemodynamic abnormalities can be categorized pathophysiologically as primary pressure- or volume-overload states or cardiomyopathic processes. Furthermore, abnormalities may be described as either acute or chronic in nature, with hemodynamic events that are usually quite different. Right ventricular pressure overload may result from outflow obstruction (infundibular, pulmonic valvular, or postvalvular stenosis) or increased pulmonary vascular resistance (precapillary, capillary, or postcapillary). Increased RV afterload, whether from pulmonary outflow obstruction or elevated pulmonary vascular resistance (PVR), results in an elevated peak RV systolic pressure. The level of increased RV systolic pressure relates to the severity and acuity of the process. The RV is a thin-walled chamber designed as a "volume pump" and is relatively less well equipped to generate high pressure. Thus, challenged by a large acute increase in RV afterload, for example in the setting of massive pulmonary embolus, the RV may not be able to respond with an an adequate increase in RV systolic pressure, with resultant RV systolic failure, low forward cardiac output, and systemic hypotension. In response to a less severe but chronic increase in afterload, however, the RV can hypertrophy and generate systemic and even super-systemic pressure. If increased afterload is due to obstruction to RV outflow, pullback from the PA to the RV will determine if the lesion is postvalvular, valvular, or prevalvular. A very narrowed outflow lesion may preclude passage of the inflated balloon flotation catheter, which usually can be traversed with the balloon deflated. When RV and PA peak systolic pressures are elevated but equal, delineation of the source of pulmonary hypertension is dependent on further analysis of PCW pressure and calculation of PVR (to be discussed). Right ventricular pressure overload increases RV myocardial wall stress, resulting in compensatory RV hypertrophy. Patients with RV hypertrophy typically manifest RV diastolic dysfunction, with elevated RV filling pressure and an augmented end-diastolic pressure rise associated with enhanced atrial transport.

Acute RV volume overload may be due to acute TR (secondary to endocarditis or ruptured chordae) or a sudden increase in volume (such as in an acquired ventricular septal defect after acute myocardial infarction). Chronic TR may occur as a result of rheumatic heart disease, carcinoid syndrome, or as a sequela of endocarditis. Chronic RV volume overload may result from congenital heart disease (e.g., atrial septal defect, anomalous venous return, ventricular septal defect). Pressure changes from RV (as well as LV) volume overload are directly proportional to the acuity of its development, its severity, and the compliance of the RV. At one end of the spectrum, sudden severe acute volume overload will produce significant increases in RV diastolic pressure because of the relatively small size of the RV, with the pressure increasing disproportionately as the ventricle reaches its elastic limit. Contrast this situation with chronic TR, in which chronic ventricular remodeling allows a significant increase in RA and RV volume and consequently a much lower RV end-diastolic pressure than in acute volume overload.

Myopathic processes also produce changes in RV pressures. Acute depression of systolic function (e.g., from myocarditis) is often manifested by a disproportionately high (relative to systolic) diastolic pressure. This phenomenon is due at least in part to the normal size of the ventricle. If a myopathic process becomes chronic, dilation of the involved chamber will develop and despite poor systolic function of that chamber, diastolic pressures may actually become lower than acutely.

An important and frequently encountered abnormality of RV function is due to RV ischemia and infarction in patients with acute inferior myocardial infarction. Acute right coronary artery occlusion proximal to the RV branches impairs global RV performance in nearly 50% of patients with acute transmural inferior-posterior infarction, resulting in a spectrum of hemodynamic derangements. Acute ischemia leads to RV free-wall dyskinesis and global RV systolic dysfunction, which produces a decrease in transpulmonary flow and results in diminished LV preload and decreased cardiac output despite relatively preserved global LV performance in many cases. Right ventricular ischemia induces severe RV diastolic dysfunction. Depressed RV systolic performance results in RV dilatation and ischemia, which impairs both early RV relaxation and decreases RV compliance. These abnormalities result in a progressive pandiastolic impedance to RV filling, manifest in the RV waveform as a rapid rise in diastolic pressure to an elevated plateau ("dip and plateau" or "square root sign") and in the RA waveform by elevated mean RA pressure with a blunted y descent (Fig 5-5). The status of RA function is an important determinant of cardiac performance under conditions of acute RV free-wall dysfunction. In the setting of acute RV ischemia, RV diastolic dysfunction imposes increased preload and afterload on the RA, resulting in elevated mean RA pressures with a blunted y descent indicative of impaired RV filling. These loading conditions stimulate augmented RA contraction, reflected in the RA waveform by increased a wave amplitude, with associated enhanced RA relaxation manifest as a prominent x descent ("W" pattern). In such patients, augmented RA contraction enhances RV filling and contributes to hemodynamic stability. These important compensatory contributions are emphasized by the adverse effects of concomitant RA ischemic dysfunction associated with proximal occlusion of the right coronary artery that compromises the right atrial branches, resulting in ischemic depression of RA function manifest as elevated mean RA pressure but with depressed a wave and x descent ("M" pattern) and associated with more severe hemodynamic compromise (see Fig 5-5). Right ventricular diastolic dysfunction adversely affects LV diastolic properties, because acute RV dilation and elevated diastolic pressure may alter LV filling and compliance through diastolic ventricular interaction-mediated reversal of the curved interventricular septum. Acute RV dilation within the noncompliant pericardium elevates intracardiac pressure, the resultant pericardial constraint further impairing both RV and LV compliance and filling. The effects of pericardial constraint contribute to the pattern of progressive pan-diastolic resistance to RV filling, elevated RA pressure, and the phenomenon of equalized diastolic filling pressures. Under conditions of RV free-wall dysfunction, RV systolic performance is dependent on LV/septal contractile contributions transmitted by systolic ventricular interactions mediated by septal thickening and paradoxical septal motion. These interactions may result in a bifid RV systolic pressure waveform (Fig 5-6), the initial peak corresponding to early paradoxical septal bulging and the later peak to maximal LV septal contraction during peak systolic pressure generation.

Right ventricular systolic myopathy may be seen with various nonischemic processes. With the exception of RV dysplasia, such cardiomyopathic processes virtually always affect the LV to some extent. In a minority of cases, RV involvement may predominate clinically. The primary RV effect of the cardiomyopathy in addition to RV systolic dysfunction is elevated RV diastolic pressure. Right atrial pressure is typically elevated, owing to RV volume overload (a compensatory mechanism to maximize myocardial stretch), and may be further increased by functional TR. Secondary pulmonary hypertension usually results from the effects of cardiomyopathy on the left heart. This increased afterload further exacerbates RV dysfunction.

Restrictive cardiomyopathies are characterized by pathophysiologic processes that result in predominant diastolic dysfunction with little or lesser impairment of systolic performance. Common etiologies of restrictive cardiomyopathy include amyloidosis, hemachromatosis, radiation, sarcoidosis, and scleroderma. These diseases are systemic and virtually always affect both ventricles to some extent, resulting in clinically apparent left, right, or biventricular diastolic dysfunction. Typically, RA mean pressure is elevated. However, unless the RA itself is involved by the infiltrative process and rendered dysfunctional, there is augmented RA contraction and relaxation, manifested as a prominent a wave and sharp x descent. Right ventricular diastolic pressure is itself elevated, but often in a pattern in which there is a rapid rise in mid-diastole to an elevated plateau, inscribing a dip and plateau or square root sign in the RV diastolic pressure trace. Pulmonary capillary wedge pressure is also typically elevated, reflecting left heart diastolic dysfunction. There may be equalization of diastolic filling pressures as seen in primary pericardial diseases (constriction and tamponade, to be discussed later). More usual, however, is some difference

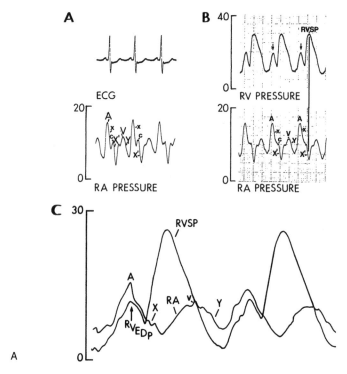

Figure 5-5   **(A)** Right atrial (RA) and right ventricular (RV) tracings with RV infarction with well-functioning RA ("W" pattern). Hemodynamic recordings from a patient with a W pattern. Peaks of W are formed by prominent A waves, and most prominent right atrial (RA) descent occurs just before T wave of ECG (panel A). Simultaneous RA and RV pressures (panel B) demonstrate that this prominent descent coincides with peak RV systolic pressure (RVSP) and is therefore an X' systolic descent, followed by a comparatively blunted Y descent. Peak RVSP is depressed, RV relaxation is prolonged, and there are a dip and a rapid rise in RV diastolic pressure. Prominent RA A waves are reflected in the right ventricle as an augmented end-diastolic pressure (EDP) rise (arrows). These waveform relations are confirmed by simultaneous superimposed RA/RV pressure recordings (panel C).

in the elevated diastolic pressures; left-sided pressures are often somewhat greater than right-sided ones and may be further separated by increasing ventricular filling time (e.g., post–premature ventricular contraction) or increasing systemic volume by a fluid challenge. Typically, the greater intrinsic stiffness of the left ventricle compared with the right separates end-diastolic pressure with a higher LV end-diastolic pressure. It should be pointed out that, at least in theory, if the RV takes the major brunt of the infiltrative process, it is possible to have a higher RV than LV diastolic pressure. The separation in diastolic pressures (typically > 5 mm Hg) is an important criterion for suspecting restrictive myopathy rather than constrictive pericardial disease. As the right-sided chambers become less distensible, the respiratory swings in pressure diminish. In its

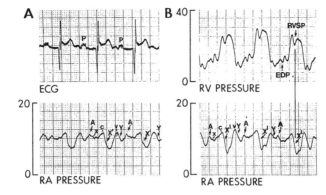

Figure 5-5 **(B)** Tracing of RA with ischemia in patient with acute inferior myocardial infarction ("M" pattern). Tracings of M pattern of RA pressure. When timed by ECG (panel A), the most prominent negative deflection in RA is coincident with T wave, suggesting a diastolic Y descent. In contrast, its relation to RV pressure (panel B) demonstrates that this prominent descent coincides with peak RVSP, indicating a systolic X′descent, whereas diastolic Y descent is blunted. M pattern comprises a depressed A wave, X descent before a small C wave, a prominent X′ descent, a small V wave, and a blunted Y descent. Peak RVSP is depressed and bifid (arrow), with delayed relaxation and an elevated EDP. (All pressures are measured in mm Hg). (Reproduced by permission from the American Heart Association, Inc., from Goldstein JA, Barzilai B, Rosamond TL, et al. Determinants of hemodynamic compromise with severe right ventricular function. Circulation 1990; 82:359–368.)

ultimate form, there is no respiratory variation, with an unchanged mean or even elevated pressure and a more pronounced a wave during inspiration.*

Relationship of Intrapericardial Events and Intracardiac Pressures

Elevated IPP is a major mechanism by which the pericardium exerts adverse hemodynamic effects, limiting chamber filling and thereby forward output (systolic limitations) and increasing diastolic pressures, resulting in diminished chamber preload with elevated filling pressures. Elevated IPP may result from accumulation of fluid within the pericardium culminating in clinical tamponade (see Chapter 15). The RA waveform inscribes a prominent a wave, owing to augmented RA contraction into the stiff RV; the x descent is sharp, attributable to enhanced atrial relaxation as well as systolic intrapericardial depressurization; and the y descent is blunted, reflecting pan-diastolic impairment of RV filling (Fig 5-7). Cardiac tamponade is a condition that emphasizes the

---

*Kussmaul's sign—an inspiratory increase in mean RA pressure—is rare. Only a few unequivocal cases have been presented in the medical literature. Its rarity, even if a real phenomenon, should be recognized by the invasive cardiologist.

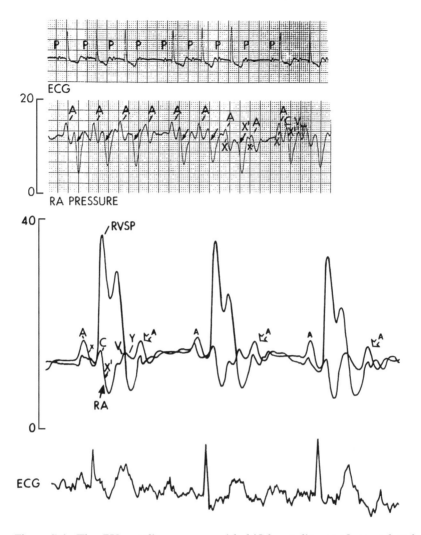

Figure 5-6   The RV systolic pressure with bifid systolic waveform related to ventricular interdependence. Hemodynamic recordings from a patient with a W pattern and severe low cardiac output precipitated by 2-degree atrioventricular block (upper panel). Recording of RA pressure and ECG (upper panel) demonstrates augmented A waves and prominent X' and blunted Y descents, confirmed by simultaneous superimposed RA and RV pressure recordings (lower panel). Presence of both X and X' descents, delineated in conducted beats only (upper panel), demonstrates an additional problem with identification of components of RA pressure waveform. Right ventricular systolic pressure (RVSP) morphology is bifid, and a diastolic dip and plateau pattern are evident. Slight variation in timing of simultaneous superimposed RA/RV pressure recordings may be due to differences in maximal frequency response. RVEDP, RV end-diastolic pressure. (Reproduced by permission from the American Heart Association, Inc., from Goldstein JA, Barzilai B, Rosamond TL, et al. Determinants of hemodynamic compromise with severe right ventricular function. Circulation 1990;82:359–368.)

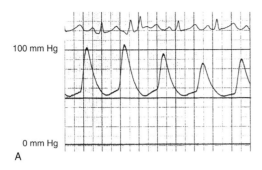

A

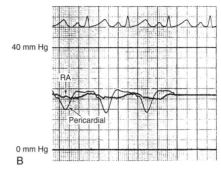

B

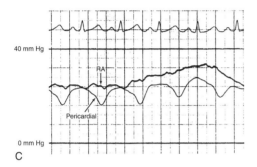

C

Figure 5-7 Cardiac tamponade. The patient was a 38-year-old woman who was intubated and hypotensive. **(A)** A 30-mm Hg pulse difference (pulsus paradoxus) is apparent on the arterial tracing. **(B)** The right atrial (RA) pressure is elevated; the mean RA and pericardial pressures are equal. **(C)** After only 70 ml of pericardial fluid was removed, pericardial pressure fell below RA. **(D)** After 550 ml was removed, pulsus paradoxus decreased to 12 mm Hg. **(E)** At the end of the case, RA contours were apparent, with a slight decrease in RA pressure and a more marked decrease in pericardial pressure. However, pericardial pressure was quite elevated, suggesting the possibility of residual pericardial fluid or an element of pericardial constriction.

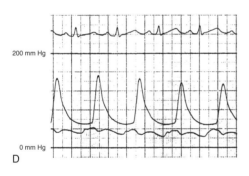

D

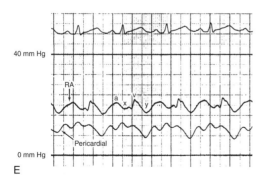

E

limitations of extrapolating true chamber preload from measured filling pressure; despite elevated filling pressures, the chambers in tamponade are volume-deprived due to the increase in pericardial pressure. The fluid-filled catheter not only measures the true transmural pressure generated by the intracardiac volume distending the chambers, but also includes the intrapericardial pressure. The uniform pressure exerted by the pericardium on all chambers leads to "equalization" of diastolic pressures in the RA, RV, PCW, and LV. In patients breathing spontaneously and in normal sinus rhythm, cardiac tamponade typically results in a prominent pulsus paradoxus (inspiratory decrement in aortic systolic pressure greater than 12 mm Hg), due to intact inspiratory augmentation of RV filling within the distended pericardium, resulting in abrupt reductions in LV preload as the RV expands and further compresses the volume-starved LV through septal-mediated diastolic interaction and pooling of blood in the lungs.

Constrictive pericarditis occurs when a thick inelastic pericardium encases the heart and restricts filling of both ventricles. In contrast to tamponade, this process is typically slowly progressive and develops over several months to years. Constriction alters chamber compliance, resulting in biventricular diastolic dysfunction manifested clinically as predominant chronic right heart failure (elevated venous pressure, enlarged liver, peripheral edema). As in tamponade, constriction is manifested in the RA waveform as elevated mean pressure with both a prominent a wave and sharp x descent reflecting enhanced atrial contraction into the stiff RV with subsequent accelerated atrial relaxation. However, there are important differences in the diastolic abnormalities produced by tamponade and constriction. In contrast to the pan-diastolic impairment of filling characteristic of cardiac tamponade, in constriction early ventricular filling is relatively unaffected. Thus, the y descent is sharp, which serves as an important differentiating characteristic from tamponade (blunted y descent) (Fig 5-8). However, as the ventricles fill in constriction, they rapidly reach the resistance of the stiff pericardial shell, at which time filling pressures rapidly rise to an elevated plateau. A distinctive RV waveform characterized by a dip and plateau or square root pattern reflects rapid RV relaxation, with a sharp increase in filling pressure as the expanding ventricle meets the constraints of the pericardium. The LV pressure waveform often exhibits a dip and plateau pattern similar to that seen in the RV. Right atrial, RV, PCW, and LV filling pressures are elevated and equalized, reflecting the common resistance of the pericardium to these chambers (see Chapter 15). In contrast to tamponade, in which ITP is transmitted through the pericardium and inspiratory augmentation of venous return and right heart filling are intact (resulting in a prominent paradoxical pulse), in constrictive pericarditis the inelastic pericardial shell does not allow inspiratory augmentation of right heart filling. Therefore, patients with constrictive pericarditis do not typically manifest large swings in peak systolic pressure during the respiratory cycle. Instead, the inspiratory gradient

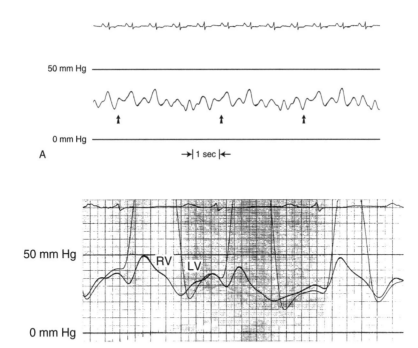

Figure 5-8   Lack of respiratory variation in (**A**) the mean (light line) right atrial (RA) pressure tracing and (**B**) equalization of right ventricular (RV) and left ventricular (LV) diastolic pressures in a patient with severe constrictive pericarditis. After pericardiectomy, RA and RV systolic pressures normalized and respiratory variation in RA and RV pressures were present (data not shown). Arrows represent onset of inspiration.

created between the extrathoracic great veins and intrathoracic but extrapericardial great vessels, combined with the increased intra-abdominal pressure associated with deep inspiration, induces a surge of blood rushing back to the thoracic cage that is precluded from entering the heart by the constricted pericardium, resulting in an inspiratory unchanged or increased in jugular venous pressure, a phenomenon termed *Kussmaul's sign.* Kussmaul's sign can best be demonstrated when, with the tip of the right heart pressure catheter in the SVC, a frank increase or lack of inspiratory decrease with increased a wave excursion in pressure is evident (see Fig 5-8). When pericardial effusions are combined with thickened inelastic pericardial layers (typically postsurgical hemorrhagic effusions, radiation-induced changes), effusive-constrictive hemodynamics may develop, a hybrid with features that span the spectrum of tamponade and constriction. The hallmark is biventricular diastolic dysfunction with elevated and equalized filling pressures, a right atrial y descent that may be either sharp or blunted depending on the pattern of pericardial compliance, and either a pulsus paradoxus or a lack of inspiratory atrial pressure decline, depending on whether inspiratory augmentation of venous return has been impeded by abnormalities of pericardial compliance.

It should be emphasized that many of the hemodynamic phenomena described, including elevated equalized diastolic filling pressures and dip and plateau are somewhat nonspecific hemodynamic findings. For example, equalized filling pressures may be seen in patients with RV ischemic dysfunction and restrictive cardiomyopathies. Patients with abrupt chamber dilatation of the left heart (e.g., acute severe mitral regurgitation), in which sudden increases in LV volume result in elevated IPP, and diastolic ventricular interactions that impact RV compliance, may also show equalization of diastolic pressures. Conversely, preexisting pathologic conditions may preclude equalization of filling pressures that would otherwise be present in pericardial disease in the aforementioned conditions. Specifically, conditions associated with intrinsic cardiac disease may result in disproportionate elevation of filling pressures in one side of the heart versus the other, which may impact the manifestations of external pericardial resistance induced by restriction, tamponade, and so forth. Tamponade, constriction, restriction, and RV infarction share several pathophysiologic features, hemodynamic characteristics, and clinical manifestations that can lead to diagnostic mistakes if not appreciated. Although elevated equalized diastolic filling pressures may be observed in all of these conditions, careful examination of the RA and RV waveforms and correlation with noninvasive studies, particularly echocardiography, should help to differentiate these conditions. For example, although cardiac tamponade and RV infarction are both low-output states, have clear lung fields, and disproportionate elevation of RV filling pressures with elevated mean RA pressure and blunted y descents, echocardiography clearly differentiates these conditions through documentation of RV dilatation and dysfunction in patients with ischemic RV involvement, and prominent effusion with chamber collapse in those with cardiac tamponade. Although constriction and RV infarction both result in disproportionate elevation of right heart filling pressures with RV dip and plateau, and a peak systolic-to-diastolic pressure ratio of less than 3:1, the sharp RA y descent in constriction reflecting rapid unimpeded RV filling in the first third of diastole is in clear contrast to the blunted y descent in RV infarction indicative of the early component of pan-diastolic impedance to RV inflow. Echocardiography can differentiate these two conditions, with RV dilatation and dysfunction characteristic of ischemic RV involvement and the lack of RV systolic impairment or LV ischemic involvement characteristic of constrictive pericarditis. However, constriction and restriction may be indistinguishable by clinical, hemodynamic, and echocardiographic assessment. In such cases, endomyocardial biopsy may be helpful in excluding infiltrative restrictive processes (e.g., amyloid, iron deposition disease, etc.), particularly when noninvasive studies (echo, CT, MRI) do not reveal prominent increases in pericardial thickness.

Interpretation of Pulmonary Artery Pressure Waveforms

The PA pressure waveform reflects transmitted systolic pressure from the RV following opening of the pulmonic valve, with a diastolic pressure component determined by PVR. Because pulmonary diastolic pressure is typically greater than RV diastolic pressure, catheter passage from the wide pressure pulse RV waveform to the PA is characterized by transition to a narrower pressure pulse with equivalent systolic peak but higher diastolic pressure. The most commonly observed abnormality in the PA waveform is pulmonary hypertension (see Chapter 17), reflecting elevated pulmonary vascular (arteriolar) resistance. Pulmonary vascular resistance is calculated as

$$PVR = \frac{\text{Mean PA pressure} - \text{mean PCW pressure}}{\text{Cardiac output}}$$

Pulmonary vascular resistance may be expressed as "Wood Units" (preceding formula without units). Another and more commonly used parameter is obtained by multiplying this Wood unit by 80; the value is expressed as dynes-sec-cm^{-5}. Eliminating the term PCW from the numerator allows calculation of the total pulmonary resistance. This parameter is useful in considering the resistance the RV must overcome to generate forward flow.

Elevated PVR may be precapillary, attributable to pulmonary emboli or primary pulmonary hypertension; capillary, secondary to obstructive or restrictive lung diseases; or postcapillary, related to elevated PCW pressure or, rarely, obstructive pulmonary veno-occlusive disease. Measurement of the "transpulmonary gradient," the difference between the mean PA diastolic and PCW pressures, may help differentiate these resistance locations, with an elevated gradient (>12–15 mm Hg) suggesting either precapillary pathology or capillary intrinsic lung disease, whereas a lower gradient with elevated PCW suggests postcapillary left heart failure. There are, however, patients with LV dysfunction who have large elevations in this gradient, so conclusions regarding resistance location must be made cautiously. Documentation of the presence or absence of left heart pressure elevation and pathology, as well as determinations of primary lung and PA abnormalities, may be necessary to delineate the underlying mechanism of pulmonary hypertension, which in some cases may be multifactorial. The response of pulmonary pressures to therapeutic interventions (treatment of left heart failure, underlying chronic obstructive pulmonary disease) and attempts to vasodilate the pulmonary resistance vessels (e.g., with nitroprusside, PGE-1, nitric oxide) may provide insight into both mechanism and reversibility (see Chapter 17).

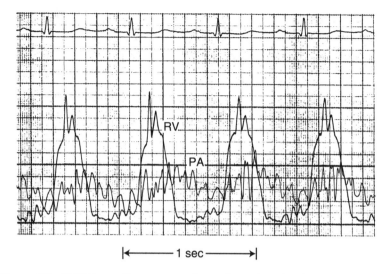

1 sec

Figure 5-9 RV/PA gradient across the pulmonic valve in congenital pulmonic stenosis. In this example, rigid catheters were used to measure pressure. Note the underdamping pressure tracing with large swings in pressure (see discussion at beginning of chapter).

Right heart catheterization of patients with severe pulmonary hypertension may be technically challenging and associated with an increased incidence of complications. The severe right heart dilation and functional TR typically encountered render passage of soft balloon flotation catheters more difficult, especially from the femoral approach. Consideration should be given to right heart catheterization from the jugular, subclavian, or left brachial approach, which exploits the natural curve of such catheters and can be more easily banked off the lateral RA across the tricuspid valve, along the floor of the RV, and into the PA. When employing the femoral approach, maneuvers to form an inverse J in the RA are often necessary to gain sufficient support to advance the catheter through the right heart. Utilization of a stiffening wire (0.018″–0.025″) through the catheter may facilitate its passage in difficult cases. In all such patients, contact with the RA or RV may induce tachycardias, which are usually poorly tolerated.

Pulmonic outflow obstruction is diagnosed by the presence of a systolic gradient between the RV and PA. This abnormality is best documented both during antegrade catheter advancement and by using a catheter pullback technique. To perform the pullback maneuver, following measurement in the wedge position, the catheter tip is demonstrated fluoroscopically to be distal to the pulmonic valve, then pulled back into the RV. An alternative approach utilizes a double-lumen catheter with the two lumens straddling either side of the stenotic area to obtain instantaneous peak measurements to identify a gradient. Figure 5-9 demonstrates a prominent gradient across the pulmonic valve in a patient with congenital pulmonic stenosis. Pulmonic regurgitation is most commonly due to severe pulmonary hypertension, and less commonly to intrinsic valvular abnormalities (endocarditis, congenital heart disease). Pulmonic insufficiency induces RV/RA volume overload, resulting in elevated filling pressures, which are typically superimposed on the preexistent effects of severe pulmonary hypertension on the right heart. The hemodynamic findings are therefore nonspecific, with significant regurgitant flow most easily discernible by ultrasound.

Interpretation of Pulmonary Capillary Wedge Pressure Waveforms

The PCW pressure is a delayed and somewhat damped measurement of left atrial (LA) pressure transmitted through the pulmonary capillary and venous system to an end-hole catheter "wedged" in the PA and "looking" downstream (Fig 5-10). The normal PCW tracing mirrors LA events and therefore, as in the

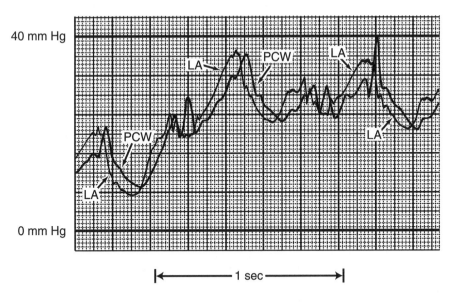

Figure 5-10 Simultaneous pulmonary capillary wedge (PCW) and left atrial (LA) pressure. Note that the mean pressure is identical, but the PCW wave contours are delayed. Transmission of the LA pressure through the pulmonary vascular tree accounts for the delay. A typical Swan-Ganz catheter will produce a relatively damped tracing because of the relatively small lumen and high compliance of the catheter. In this example, a larger lumen (7-Fr) catheter with increased stiffness (Goodale-Lubin) accounts for the PCW tracing resembling the LA tracing, except for the delay.

RA, reflects atrial contraction and relaxation as well as passive filling and emptying. On fluoroscopy, the catheter—which moves back and forth with each systolic pulsation when freely floating in the PA—is seen to advance with the balloon tip wedged and immobile. Optimal wedging may be confirmed by careful and slow aspiration of blood for oximetric sampling, which should demonstrate an arterialized ($\geq 95\%$) saturation.

Excepting the rare entities of pulmonary veno-occlusive disease and LA obstruction due to cor triatriatum, the PCW reliably estimates mean LA pressure. Accordingly, elevated PCW virtually always indicates LA hypertension, which may be due to mitral valve disease (stenosis, regurgitation), or LV diastolic dysfunction (secondary to LV hypertrophy, primary volume overload, infiltration, ischemia, etc.), or secondary to LV systolic dysfunction. Mitral valve obstruction (valvular due to rheumatic stenosis, orificial due to tumors or clots) results in a pan-diastolic gradient between the LA and LV, documented by simultaneous PCW (or LA pressure) and LV diastolic pressure recordings (Fig 5-11). Because increased flow across the mitral valve (e.g., severe mitral regurgitation [MR]) can lead to an early diastolic "flow" gradient, it is essential to determine that such gradients are present at end-diastole to confirm obstruction.

When mitral obstruction results in chronic LA hypertension, pulmonary hypertension commonly results. Although a v wave may be expected to indicate

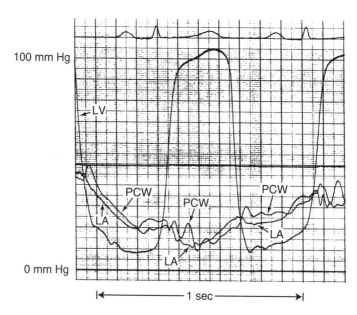

Figure 5-11   Left ventricular, PCW, and LA pressure tracings in a patient showing moderate mitral stenosis. It can be seen that the gradient is almost the same with both LA and PCW tracings.

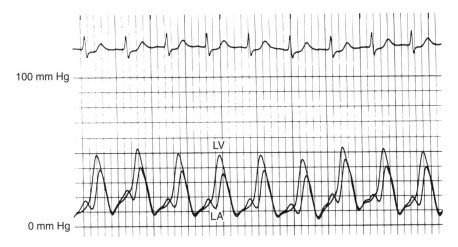

Figure 5-12 Severe acute mitral regurgitation. The LV and PCW tracings are shown. The "regurgitant" wave may be transmitted back to the PA, showing a bifid or "rabbit ear" waveform (not shown in this example).

more significant MR, the dilated LA commonly seen in mixed mitral stenosis–MR may "absorb" the regurgitant wave and mask the severity of the MR. It should be noted that tricuspid and/or aortic valve disease may coexist with rheumatic mitral disease and influence the hemodynamic findings. Mitral regurgitation induces left heart volume overload. Mitral regurgitation may be due to primary valvular abnormalities (mitral valve prolapse, myxomatous degeneration, rheumatic mitral disease, endocarditis) or secondary to functional incompetence due to subvalvular tethering and annular dilatation associated with LV cardiomyopathy or ischemic papillary muscle dysfunction. The major hemodynamic findings are elevated PCW pressure with prominent v wave and elevated LV filling pressure (Fig 5-12). In severe MR, the v wave may be transmitted back to the PA, resulting in a bifid or "rabbit ear" waveform. The magnitude of elevation of PCW pressure and v wave amplitude is influenced by the volume and acuity of the regurgitant jet, rate of forward pulmonary venous return into the atrium, LA compliance, and LV afterload and contractility.

Interpretation of Left Ventricular Pressure Waveforms

The LV pressure waveform consists of a rapidly rising systolic upstroke, whose peak rate of pressure rise (+dp/dt) reflects in part the intrinsic LV contractile state. Isovolumic contraction ends as the aortic valve opens and ejection begins, inscribing a notch just prior to the systolic pressure peak (see Fig 5-3). As blood is ejected, the pressure peaks and then declines. When LV pressure falls below aortic pressure, ejection ceases and the aortic valve closes, inscribing another notch in the waveform, termed the *incisura*. The subsequent decline in LV systolic pressure represents active LV relaxation. As LV pressure falls below LA pressure, the mitral valve opens and LV filling begins. There is a slow early rise in diastolic pressure that is a summation of inflow volume, which would be expected to increase LV pressure, and LV relaxation, which would be expected to decrease LV pressure. A prominent end-diastolic increase reflects atrial contraction.

Left ventricular pressure is typically measured by employing a single-lumen pigtail-shaped catheter with both end hole and side holes, the latter of which facilitates high-pressure dye injection for LV cineangiography. This catheter is advanced retrograde from the aortic root toward the LV with the aid of a J-tipped guidewire (0.035″–0.038″), with the wire tip initially retracted into the catheter. In the right anterior oblique projection (30–45 degrees), the pigtail is oriented parallel to the septal plane (open toward the LV apex) and slowly advanced across the valve over the wire into the LV apex. In cases in which the aorta is severely dilated or the aortic valve obstructed, utilization of a straight wire (0.035″–0.038″) may be necessary to enter the LV. Especially in cases of aortic stenosis, it is essential that the wire be positioned superior to the volcano-shaped stenotic orifice, and the multiple gentle forward-thrusting motions of the wire to cross the valve be spent "knocking at the door," not banging against the "sides" in the aortic sinuses (see also Chapter 13). The pigtail catheter (or alternatively a Judkins right coronary or multipurpose catheter) can be advanced or retracted within the aortic root to facilitate optimal positioning of the wire at the valve orifice. Once the catheter has entered the LV, it should be moved toward the apex in a position that does not induce ectopy and in which the catheter can be seen to move freely within the LV with each beat. Left ventricular pressure should be measured before and after LV cineangiography. Finally, a pullback pressure measurement is performed to determine the presence of LV outflow tract or aortic valve obstruction. If there is clinical suspicion of a sub- or supravalvular gradient, a catheter with a single end hole should be employed. A slow fluoroscopically monitored pullback from the LV apex through the outflow tract, subaortic valve region, and supra-aortic valve region will effectively determine the presence and location of obstructive lesions. Figure 5-13 shows pressure tracings in the case of subaortic and aortic stenosis. Caution should be employed in interpretation of such gradients, for artifactual intraventricular gradients can occur when the catheter becomes entrapped in a hypertrophic or hypercontractile ventricle. Contrast LV angiography and correlation with echocardiography usually suffice to clarify the significance of such gradients. In cases of suspected obstruction, a double-lumen pigtail catheter may be employed with two pressure measurement systems for simultaneous recording of LV and aortic pressure. This method may be preferable to simultaneous measurements utilizing the side-arm of the femoral artery access sheath, both because the indwelling catheter typically obstructs the sheath and because

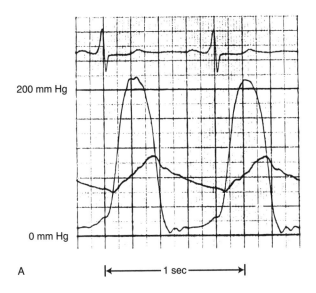

200 mm Hg

0 mm Hg

A |← 1 sec →|

Figure 5-13 Obstruction to outflow at the **(A)** valvular and **(B)** left ventricular (LV) outflow tract is shown. Note the difference in contour of the aortic pressure (Ao) with prolonged upstroke and delayed peak in aortic stenosis and "spike-and-dome" contour in subaortic stenosis. Findings in hypertrophic obstructive cardiomyopathy include dynamic outflow gradient and bifid or spike-and-dome arterial contour, and the decrease in pulse pressure after a long pause (Braunwald-Brockenbrough sign). PVC, premature ventricular contraction. (IHSS tracing kindly provided by James A. Shaver, M.D.)

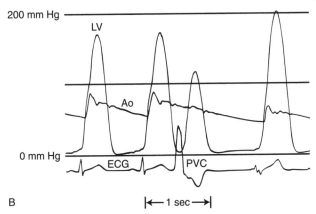

200 mm Hg

0 mm Hg

B |← 1 sec →|

of the phenomenon of peripheral amplification whereby diminished central aortic pressures become enhanced "downstream" owing to elasticity effects in the periphery and the "summation" of pressure waves. Should arterial pressure be recorded from the side-arm of a femoral sheath, the sheath should be one Fr size larger than the catheter in the sheath. To gauge the magnitude of pressure difference, central aortic (before entering the LV) and femoral pressures should be measured and recorded simultaneously. Although peak systolic pressures may not be identical, the mean pressures should. If this is not the case, a check of all aspects of the measuring system should be performed to determine the site of the technical problem. In most cases, any measured "simultaneous" gradient should be confirmed by pullback from the LV to the aorta.

The LV is affected by conditions that induce pressure and/or volume overload and cardiomyopathic processes, as well as extrinsic influences from the pericardium and the RV via diastolic interactions. Pressure overload may be acquired from long-standing systemic hypertension, or fixed sub-aortic, aortic, or supra-aortic obstruction. Hypertension results in concentric LV hypertrophy with a noncompliant LV characterized by high filling pressure with an exaggerated end-diastolic "kick" and absence of an LV-aortic gradient. Prolonged untreated hypertension and concentric LV hypertrophy produce diastolic dysfunction, with later systolic dysfunction developing if hypertension is severe and poorly controlled. Aortic obstruction is characterized by a gradient between the LV and the aorta. In fixed aortic stenosis, peak gradients obtained by the pullback method should be compared with the mean gradient, which is less affected by beat-to-beat variations in pressure. Furthermore, because peak gradient measurements by pullback are sequential and not instantaneous, such gradients may not correspond precisely with the instantaneous systolic gradient. Atrial fibrillation and other rhythms with substantial beat-to-beat variability limit the validity of the pullback gradient method. The double-lumen pigtail method facilitates measurement of both peak instantaneous and mean gradients. Hypertrophic cardiomyopathy may be characterized by concentric hypertrophy or asymmetric septal hypertrophy and a noncompliant LV, without or with variable degrees of dynamic LV outflow obstruction at the mid-cavity level (cavity obliteration between the hypertrophic septum and posterolateral walls) or in the outflow tract (septum and anterior mitral leaflet). Obstruction is dynamic throughout the cardiac cycle, with early systolic ejection unimpeded, peak obstruction evident in mid-systole, and later ejection often relatively unimpaired (see Fig 5-13). Accordingly, the aortic systolic pressure is typically bifid, with an early systolic peak followed by a mid-systolic dip and then a second later systolic peak.

Other hemodynamic findings seen in hypertrophic cardiomyopathy include pulsus alternans and the Braunwald-Brockenbrough sign in the arterial tracing. This sign shows the postpremature ventricular contraction increase in gradient and consequent decrease in aortic pulse pressure. This sign develops because of an increased end-diastolic volume, transient increase in contractility (post–extrasystolic potentiation), and lowering of arterial diastolic pressure. One hallmark of hypertrophic obstructive cardiomyopathy is the lability of the obstruction and gradient. The presence and magnitude of obstruction is influenced by LV volume, contractility, heart rate, and peripheral resistance. Accordingly, because the gradient is not always present at rest, provocative maneuvers may be required. The Valsalva maneuver may be employed or amyl nitrate administered, both of which reduce preload and exacerbate obstruction. Dynamic obstruction further intensifies excess afterload and LV diastolic dysfunction, resulting in elevated LV filling pressure with exaggerated LV end-diastolic pressure. The PCW pressure may be elevated with a large a wave. In some patients with hypertrophic cardiomyopathy, LA hypertension may result in pulmonary hypertension, particularly if there is significant MR with the obstruction. Furthermore, some patients manifest elevated RV diastolic pressures owing to hypertrophy of the septum, with a subset of patients with dynamic RV outflow gradients.

Primary LV volume overload occurs with intrinsic MR, aortic insufficiency (AI), and left-to-right shunts at the ventricular level (VSD, PDA). The hemodynamic effects of MR and AI are influenced by the severity of the leak and acuity of development of the accompanying volume overload. (Mitral regurgitation has already been discussed.) The hallmark of chronic AI is a widened aortic pulse pressure (>40 mm Hg) with reduced end-diastolic difference between aortic and LV pressures (normally at least 70 mm Hg). This reduction in the aorta-LV end-diastolic gradient is depicted in Figure 5-14. As AI becomes more severe, the aortic pulse pressure widens further and LV diastolic pressure steadily increases. In patients with bradycardia and a noncompliant vascular tree (e.g., in the elderly), a widened pulse pressure may mimic AI. When LV contractility is intact, systemic vascular resistance is low and cardiac output is elevated. It should be noted, as previously emphasized, that thermodilution cardiac output underestimates forward flow across a leaky valve. In acute AI (endocarditis, aortic dissection), the LV has less time to accommodate to the volume overload, resulting in more severe LV diastolic dysfunction and therefore increased LV diastolic pressure for any given degree of leak. There is also more

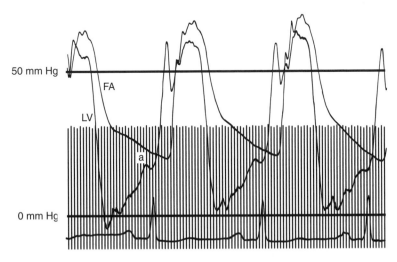

Figure 5-14 Severe acute aortic regurgitation (see text). FA, femoral artery pressure. (Kindly provided by James A. Shaver, M.D., with permission from Shaver JA, Cardiac auscultation: a cost-effective diagnostic skill. Curr Probl Cardiol, 1995;20(7):441–532.)

severe low output and vasoconstriction due to "systolic limitations," because the ability of the LV to acutely dilate and increase stroke volume to compensate for the leak is limited. Under these conditions, aortic and LV diastolic pressure may equilibrate in mid-diastole and the mitral valve closes prematurely. Severe chronic AI ultimately leads to systolic dysfunction with elevated filling pressures and low output. Quantitation of the severity of AI is best established by aortic angiography.

Left ventricular cardiomyopathy may be classified as restrictive, hypertrophic (usually restrictive as well), or dilated (see Chapter 17). Restrictive cardiomyopathies, as previously discussed, induce LV diastolic dysfunction with preserved contractility, resulting in elevated LV end-diastolic pressure and near-equalization of filling pressures between the LV, RA, RV, and PCW. A dip and plateau may be seen in the LV pressure trace similar to that observed in the RV. Careful simultaneous pressure recordings at high gain (40 mm Hg) should be made separately of the LV and RA, LV and RV, and LV and PCW. Following volume loading (300–500 ml) diastolic pressures may increase and "separate" the LV from the RA and RV pressures, thereby pointing toward restriction rather than constriction (but not definitively differentiating these conditions). Dilated cardiomyopathy may be primary (ischemic or nonischemic) or secondary to severe pressure overload (hypertension, aortic stenosis) or volume overload (MR, AI, ventricular septal defect). Regardless of the cause, such cardiomyopathic hearts usually manifest both LV systolic and diastolic dysfunction, evidenced hemodynamically as a diminished systolic upstroke and peak LV systolic pressure, with delayed relaxation and elevated diastolic pressure. Pulmonary hypertension is frequently present as a result of chronic LA hypertension, particularly if there is functional MR, a common mechanical complication of dilated cardiomyopathy.

SELECTED READINGS

1. Braunwald E, et al. Idiopathic hypertrophic subaortic stenosis. Circulation 1964; 30:78.
2. Brockenbrough EC, Braunwald E, Morrow AG. A hemodynamic technique for the detection of hypertrophic subaortic stenosis. Circulation 1961;23:189–194.
3. Cannon RO, Schenke WH, Bonow RO, et al. Left ventricular pulsus alternans in patients with hypertrophic cardiomyopathy and severe obstruction to left ventricular outflow. Circulation 1986;73:276.
4. Cresci SG, Goldstein JA. Hemodynamic manifestations of ischemic right heart dysfunction. Cathet Cardiovasc Diagn 1992;27:28–33.
5. Cresci S, Goldstein JA, Cardona H, et al. Impaired left atrial function after cardiac transplantation: disparate contribution of donor and recipient atrial components studied on-line by quantitative echocardiography. J Heart Lung Transplant 1995; 14:647–653.
6. Frank S, Braunwald E. Idiopathic hypertrophic subaortic stenosis. Clinical analysis of 26 patients with emphasis on the natural history. Circulation 1968;37:759.
7. Frye DL. Physiologic recording by modern instruments with particular reference to pressure recording. Physiol Rev 1960;40:753.
8. Fuchs RM, Henser RR, Yin FCP, Brinker JA. Limitations of pulmonary wedge v waves in diagnosing mitral regurgitation. Am J Cardiol 1982;49:849–854.
9. Goldstein JA. Pathophysiology of hemodynamically severe right ventricular infarction. Coronary Artery Dis 1990;1:314–327.
10. Goldstein JA, Barzilai B, Rosamond TL, et al. Determinants of hemodynamic compromise with severe right ventricular function. Circulation 1990;82:359–368.
11. Goldstein JA, Weddell JF, Barzilai B, et al. Right atrial ischemia exacerbates hemodynamic compromise associated with experimental right ventricular dysfunction. J Am Coll Cardiol 1991;18:1564–1572.
12. Gordon JB, Folland ED. Analysis of aortic valve gradients by transseptal technique: implications for non-invasive evaluation. Cathet Cardiovasc Diagn 1989;17:144–151.
13. Grose R, Strain J, Cohen MW. Pulmonary arterial V waves in mitral regurgitation: clinical and experimental observations. Circulation 1984;69:214.
14. Grossman W, Baim DS. Cardiac catheterization angiography and intervention. 4th ed. Philadelphia: Williams & Wilkins, 1991.
15. Meaney E, Shabetai R, Bhargava BE, et al. Cardiac amyloidosis, constrictive pericarditis, and restrictive cardiomyopathy. Am J Cardiol 1976;38:543–556.
16. Morgan BC, Able FL, Mullins GL, Guntheroth WG. Flow patterns in cavae, pulmonary artery, pulmonary vein and aorta in intact dogs. Am J Physiol 1966; 210:903–909.
17. Murgo JP. The hemodynamic evaluation in hypertrophic cardiomyopathy: systolic and diastolic hypertension. Cardiovasc Clin 1988;19:193.
18. Murgo JP, Westerhof N, Giolma JP, Altobelli S. Aortic input impedance in normal man: relationship to pressure wave forms. Circulation 1980;62:105–116.
19. Reddy PS, Curtiss EI, O'Toole JD, Shaver JA. Cardiac tamponade: hemodynamic observations in man. Circulation 1978;58:543–556.
20. Ross J Jr, Brauwald E, Gault JH, et al. The mechanism of the intraventricular pressure gradient in idiopathic hypertrophic subaortic stenosis. Circulation 1966;34:558–578.
21. Schapira JN, Harold JG (eds). Two-dimensional echocardiography and cardiac Doppler. 2nd ed. Baltimore: Williams & Wilkins, 1990:599.
22. Shabetai R, Fowler NO, Fenton JC, Massangkay M. Pulsus paradoxus. J Clin Invest 1965;44:1882–1898.

6

CARDIAC ANGIOGRAPHY

Marvin A. Konstam
Richard D. Patten
Carey D. Kimmelstiel
Neil J. Halin
Jan B. Namyslowski
Alan J. Greenfield

Radiographic Principles

THE AMOUNT OF radiographic exposure on a cine frame is determined by the exposure duration, the current used in generating the x-ray beam (measured in milliamperes or mA), and the distribution of x-ray energies (number of x-rays at each kiloelectron volt [keV]) employed. The maximum x-ray energy is determined by the generator kilovoltage (kVp). Typical cineradiographic exposure times used during cardiac cineradiography are kept below 8 milliseconds to minimize motion blurring. The automatic brightness control monitors the intensity of x-rays reaching the image intensifier and adjusts both mA and kVp, according to a preset algorithm, to achieve and maintain a fixed optimal image brightness. (Some newer cineradiographic systems also adjust the camera iris). Increased kVp not only increases the penetrating power of the x-ray beam, but also influences the contrast level of the radiographic exposure by determining the relative x-ray absorption of various adjacent body parts.

In the case of angiography, the key determinant of diagnostic contrast is the relative absorption between iodine-containing and non–iodine-containing structures. Examining changes in x-ray absorption by iodine with increasing x-ray energy, there is a jump in absorption, designated the "K-edge," at approximately 33 keV. Therefore iodine contrast is maximal using an x-ray beam with the maximum number of x-ray energies slightly above 33 keV. This effect typically occurs for generator voltage in the 70- to 80-kVp range. Image contrast declines for x-rays above this energy, because more energetic x-rays are more penetrating and are less differentially absorbed. As kVp increases above the 70- to 80-kVp range, as mandated by the automatic brightness when thick body parts must be penetrated, iodine contrast declines, resulting in a loss of vascular definition within surrounding tissues.

Cine Film Versus Digital Imaging

X-rays that penetrate the patient are transformed into visible light by the input phosphor located at the face of the image intensifier. The image intensifier then amplifies the light energy for visualization and recording. With conventional film cineradiography, the amplified light images are recorded in rapid sequence onto individual frames of film by a cine camera. Many catheterization laboratories are now converting to digital angiography, in which light images are captured by a television camera interfaced to a computer, which acquires and stores the images on a digital matrix. Digital imaging may be employed to reduce the amount of contrast media used during angiography or ventriculography, for facilitating automated quantitative analysis of arterial luminal dimensions or of ventricular volumes, and to enhance the diagnostic quality of the radiographic images. Following acquisition, images may be processed using such techniques as image subtraction, background subtraction, contrast enhancement, and edge enhancement to improve image quality. As opposed to film, where image brightness and contrast are set during development, digital images may be displayed in any desired gray scale, with the option of continuous adjustment of brightness and contrast. Processing and display may thereby "correct" for suboptimal x-ray technique. Adequate images for volumetric and functional analysis may be performed using injection of smaller amounts of contrast media. These advantages may reduce the risks associated with angiography. Furthermore, compared with film storage, image archiving on a digital storage medium is likely to be more efficient in terms of space, accessibility, and cost.

Digital images facilitate quantitative geometric and functional analyses. The same computer system used to process and display images usually houses analytic software. Edge-detection algorithms, based on the rates of change in image contrast, can map vascular and cardiac contours and calculate structural dimensions (incorporating distancing information relevant to magnification or comparing dimensions to those of a known structure, such as the catheter). Such programs automate and standardize calculation of arterial stenosis severity and ventricular volumes. In addition to conventional geometric volumetric analysis (discussed later), digital imaging permits assessment of ventricular volumes by densitometry. The density of contrast media within the ventricular cavity (calculated as image density in the ventricular region minus image density prior to contrast injection) is directly proportional to ventricular volume during any portion of the cardiac cycle. The technique is most suitable to estimating relative changes in volume and thereby calculating ejection fraction (EF). The accuracy of absolute volume estimates is more questionable. Densitometric analysis offers the advantage of not relying on geometric assumptions. Errors may result from inaccurate identification of ventricular boundaries or from inaccurate estimation of "background" density—image density that is not contributed by the contrast media bolus. Because relative volumes are estimated by integrating the image density over the entire ventricular region, only a single projection is needed. Densitometric volume analysis is best performed in the right anterior oblique (RAO) projection, confining measurements to the time prior to entrance of significant amounts of contrast media into the circulation.

Digital subtraction permits enhancement of contrast within vascular structures. A "mask image" is recorded prior to injection of contrast material and is subtracted from subsequent contrast-containing frames. This technique enhances vascular or ventricular visualization, by subtracting image contrast arising from extravascular structures. It permits imaging with more dilute concentrations or more peripheral injection of contrast media.

With digital imaging, the capabilities of the computer limit the rate of data acquisition, resulting in a trade-off between acquisition rate and the information content of each image. The matrix size is an expression of the number of picture elements composing each image and is a limitation of image resolution. For example, a matrix size of 256×256 indicates that each image comprises 256 rows, each row containing 256 picture elements. A matrix size of 256×256 is usually adequate for ventriculography, although the improved resolution afforded by matrix sizes of 512×512 or even 1024×1024 may be needed for adequate definition of small blood vessels during angiography. For a given computer system, the greater the number of picture elements or the greater the information content (gray scale) of each picture element, the slower the limit of image acquisition. Adequate frame rates for ventricular functional analysis are discussed later. Thus, during vascular imaging, one might reduce the framing rate to achieve optimal image resolution, whereas during ventriculography, one might sacrifice resolution to achieve adequate framing rate for functional analysis.

Radiographic Contrast Material

All intravascular radiographic contrast agents in present use employ iodine as the x-ray–absorbing atom. There are two general groups of contrast agents: ionic and non-ionic.

Ionic contrast agents are salts of triiodinated benzoic acid derivatives, such as diatrizoate. The cation is usually sodium or meglumine (e.g., sodium meglumine diatrizoate). The osmotic load associated with the administration of these agents can cause clinical deterioration in patients in whom baseline ventricular filling pressures are high.

One means of limiting the osmolality of ionic agents is to double the iodine content per particle in solution. These low ionic agents (e.g., sodium meglumine ioxaglate) are dimers that allow the delivery of an equal iodine concentration at a reduced osmolality compared with standard ionic agents.

Non-ionic contrast agents (e.g., iohexol, iopamidol, ioversol) reduce both the osmotic load and toxicity associated with contrast angiography. These agents are fully substituted triiodinated benzene derivatives. In each case, a single non-ionic molecule contains three iodine atoms per molecule.

Adverse consequences of intracardiac or intracoronary administration of contrast material include electrophysiologic effects, hemodynamic effects, allergic-like reactions, and nephrotoxic effects. Electrophysiologic effects may include suppression of sinus node and atrioventricular node function and alteration of repolarization. Changes in automaticity, refractoriness, and conduction velocity may produce bradyarrhythmias. Repolarization abnormalities frequently produce T-wave alterations and may be responsible for ventricular arrhythmias. The rare occurrence of ventricular fibrillation is thought to be due to calcium sequestration by chelating agents as well as the anionic moiety present in contrast media. Improvements in both ionic and non-ionic agents have reduced the incidence of life-threatening ventricular arrhythmias. Low and non-ionic formulations produce less adverse electrophysiologic reactions. However, there exists no concrete evidence proving that these differences result in improved patient outcome.

Intracardiac or intracoronary injection of contrast material results in a variety of hemodynamic alterations resulting from a combination of vasodilation and reduced myocardial contractility. These actions produce systemic hypotension and variable effects on left and right heart filling pressures, which are usually short-lived. However, lasting adverse effects may occur in patients with compromised ventricular function and in patients with severe ischemic heart disease. Effects may be perpetuated by induction of ischemia and by the subsequent influence of the osmotic load. The incidence of all adverse hemodynamic effects of contrast material administration is markedly reduced by the use of low or non-ionic agents.

Allergic-like reactions complicate contrast administration in 1% to 2% of cases. The most usual manifestation is urticaria. More severe reactions are unusual and include reactions simulating anaphylaxis and pulmonary edema. These reactions are not truly allergic but result from direct complement activation and release of histamine and other vasoactive and inflammatory mediators from mast cells and basophils. It appears that low or non-ionic formulations are associated with a lower frequency of allergic-like reactions, although contrast-associated differences in the incidence of the more severe reactions have not been proven.

Contrast administration can cause renal dysfunction, especially when antecedent renal impairment is present, particularly in the presence of diabetic nephropathy or intravascular volume depletion. The precise mechanisms involved in contrast-mediated nephrotoxicity are not certain but are thought to involve direct tubular injury and renal vasoconstriction, causing reduced renal blood flow and ischemic injury, especially in the renal medulla. Some clinical trials have suggested less nephrotoxicity when non-ionic contrast is used in patients with preexisting renal insufficiency. A recent meta-analysis has suggested that there may be a lower incidence of nephrotoxicity in patients with pre-existent renal dysfunction given non-ionic versus ionic agents; on the other hand, in patients with normal renal function, no differences in the incidence of renal dysfunction after contrast were found. Probably more important than the choice of contrast agents in preventing contrast-induced nephrotoxicity is the liberal use of fluids prior to the procedure.

In patients with increased risk for allergic-like reactions to contrast media (e.g., those with prior allergic-like reactions, atopic individuals, asthmatics), risk is reduced by appropriate premedication. Such treatment consists of several doses of prednisone or methylprednisolone. Two recommended regimens are 30 mg of methylprednisolone at least 12 hours and then again 2 hours prior to contrast administration, or prednisone 50 mg, every 6 hours for 3 doses beginning 13 hours before contrast administration. H_1- and H_2-receptor blockers have also been advocated in these patients. Typical regimens include the administration of diphenhydramine 50 mg and cimetidine 300 mg 1 hour prior to contrast administration. Compared with high-osmolality contrast agents, low-osmolality agents reduce the incidence of allergic-like reactions. Steroid and antihistamine treatment prior to administration of ionic contrast material has been reported to reduce the incidence of contrast-associated morbidity approximately to the level observed after non-ionic contrast administration. In patients with previous reactions to contrast media, current recommendations are for premedication combined with the use of a low-osmolality contrast agent.

Nausea and vomiting may be treated with 5 to 10 mg of intravenous (IV) prochlorperazine. Urticaria may be treated with parenteral diphenhydramine alone or in combination with H_2 blockers. Bronchospasm should be treated immediately with subcutaneous (0.1–0.2 mg) or IV epinephrine (0.1 mg). This therapy must be applied cautiously in patients with coronary disease or left ventricular dysfunction, especially in those patients treated with β-adrenergic blockers, given the potential for unopposed α-adrenergic agonism. Protracted wheezing can be effectively treated with inhaled bronchodilators. Hypotension in the setting of sinus rhythm is treated primarily with fluid resuscitation, with addition of vasoconstrictor agents if needed. Intravenous atropine 0.5 to 1.0 mg should be given when a bradycardic rhythm is present. In patients with acute hypotension, excess vagal tone should be suspected and atropine administration considered, even in the presence of a normal heart rate (i.e., absence of an appropriate tachycardic response to hypotension). Ventricular fibrillation is treated with emergent electrical defibrillation.

No specific precautions are required for the prevention of contrast nephropathy in patients with normal renal function. In patients with compromised renal function, hydration with 0.45% saline (1 mL/kg/hr) starting 12 hours before and continuing until 12 hours after the procedure is recommended. Low-osmolality agents are suggested in these patients. Pretreatment with either mannitol or diuretic is of no proven benefit. Prior to angiographic study, medications that can aggravate contrast nephrotoxicity (e.g., nonsteroidal anti-inflammatory agents) should be withheld.

Non-ionic agents are reported to have fewer anticoagulant and antiplatelet effects when compared with standard contrast media. Low ionic contrast agents appear to more closely approximate standard contrast material with respect to these effects. The clinical importance of these reports is unclear, especially because most catheterization laboratories employ heparin anticoagulation during left heart catheterization.

The major drawback to the routine use of low and non-ionic contrast material is the cost of these agents. Newer formulations may represent an increase of up to 20-fold in cost compared with standard contrast material. Routine use of non-ionic contrast material during catheterization would add an estimated $200 million to annual health care expenditures in the United States.

Current recommendations are to use lower osmolar contrast agents in selected patients judged to be at high risk for complications during catheterization. Such patients include those with prior allergic-like reactions during the administration of contrast agents, heart failure, shock, severe valvular disease, and preexisting renal dysfunction, particularly due to diabetes.

Left Ventriculography

Indications, Contraindications, Risks

Radiographic left ventriculography is indicated for assessment of regional and focal left ventricular (LV) size, shape, and performance; for identifying and quantifying mitral regurgitation; and for identifying and localizing ventricular-level left-to-right intracardiac shunts. Given the ability of noninvasive imaging modalities to accomplish many of these goals, performance of left ventriculography in the catheterization laboratory is generally reserved for those cases in which coronary angiography is indicated or in which noninvasive techniques are not sufficient to fully assess valvular or congenital disease.

Contraindications to left ventriculography result from risks related to intraventricular injection of contrast material and to catheter manipulation within the ventricle. The possibility of pregnancy is a strong relative contraindication to all angiographic procedures employing ionizing radiation.

Excessive susceptibility to the nephrotoxic, negative inotropic, or arrhythmogenic potential of contrast material or prior history of contrast-induced allergic-like reactions should be considered a relative contraindication to ventriculography. When such conditions exist, the risk may be reduced by optimizing selection of the agent used (discussed earlier). Furthermore, the likelihood of complication may be reduced by minimizing the volume of contrast injected. Use of digital angiographic techniques may assist in achieving this goal (discussed earlier).

Left ventricular pressure should be recorded and end-diastolic (ED) pressure should be noted following catheter insertion into the LV prior to contrast injection and again following ventriculography. Although clinical heart failure induced by left ventriculography is unusual, LV end-diastolic (LVED) pressure in excess of 20 mm Hg prior to ventriculography should alert the operator to the possibility of inducing pulmonary edema due to a combination of the osmotic load and acute negative inotropic action of contrast material. Under such conditions, contrast volume should be kept to a minimum and consideration should be given to pretreatment with nitrates and to use of low-osmolar contrast agents (discussed earlier). Active myocardial ischemia and critical left main coronary artery stenosis should also be considered relative contraindications to contrast left ventriculography. If LVED pressure rises above 25 mm Hg following ventriculography, consideration should be given to treatment with nitrates or diuretics.

The known presence of intracardiac thrombus is a relative contraindication to ventriculography because of the potential for dislodgment and embolization, although the risk is probably low with sessile thrombi associated with myocardial infarction that is more than 6 months old.

Prior to injection of the full contrast load, test injection should be performed to ensure a free intracavitary catheter position. During contrast injection, the operator should be prepared to withdraw the catheter rapidly in the event of myocardial staining or sustained ventricular tachycardia. Intramyocardial contrast injection may result in life-threatening ventricular arrhythmia and myocardial injury. Left ventricular perforation represents a rare but life-threatening complication, resulting in cardiac tamponade. Perforation with tamponade should be considered in the differential diagnosis of sudden hypotension and tachycardia. The appearance of pulsus paradoxus may be an important clue. This complication is rare with the use of a multiholed pigtail catheter (discussion follows).

Ventricular premature contractions and nonsustained ventricular tachycardia are common during left ventriculography. These arrhythmias result primarily from mechanical stimulation by the catheter and by the contrast stream. Their occurrence is minimized by use of catheters with multiple side holes, particularly a multiholed pigtail catheter (discussion follows), and by attention to placement of the catheter in a nonarrhythmogenic position prior to full-dose contrast injection. A defibrillator should be close at hand while manipulating a catheter within the left ventricle and during contrast injection. Although unusual, the operator must be alert to the occurrence of sustained ventricular tachycardia or ventricular fibrillation during contrast injection. If these life-threatening arrhythmias occur, the catheter should be withdrawn rapidly, and the patient should be expeditiously cardioverted or defibrillated.

Catheters

Because of the potential for catheter recoil and for intramyocardial contrast injection, left ventriculography should never be performed with a catheter containing a single end hole. Rather, a catheter containing multiple side holes, with or without an end hole, should be employed. A multihole pigtail catheter (Fig 6-1) is probably associated with the lowest likelihood of arrhythmic and traumatic complications and is therefore considered the catheter of choice in most laboratories. A straight or angled multiple side-holed catheter without an end hole, such as the Eppendorf, Berman, or NIH catheters, is an alternative, although these do not permit guidewire-assisted insertion or exchange. A multipurpose catheter (see Fig 6-1) containing both an end hole and side holes may be used. This catheter accommodates a guidewire, but the straight-tipped side hole increases the arrhythmic potential and the potential for intramyocardial injection or perforation.

Multiple side-hole pigtail catheters may be either angled or straight. The angled pigtail facilitates placement and positioning in the majority of patients by conforming to the orientation of the LV outflow tract and aortic root. However, it may carry a disadvantage in a minority of patients with a small or horizontally oriented left ventricle, in whom the catheter's angle does not coincide with the anatomy. In these cases and in others in which the aortic valve is difficult to cross, the greater pushability of the non-angled catheter offers an advantage. Also, for ventricles in which a nonarrhythmogenic catheter position is difficult to achieve, the nonangled catheter may be rotated on its axis to alter its orientation, whereas the angled pigtail does not offer this option.

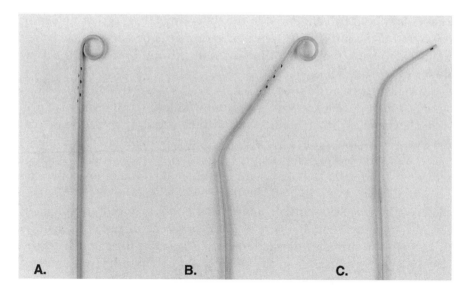

Figure 6-1 Commonly used catheters for left ventriculography. **(A)** Non-angled multihole pigtail catheter; **(B)** angled pigtail catheter; **(C)** multi-purpose catheter.

Catheter Insertion and Positioning

The pigtail catheter is advanced from the femoral artery over a 0.038" J-tipped guidewire to the level of the diaphragm. At this point, the guidewire is withdrawn and the catheter is aspirated with a syringe (approximately 5 mL of blood) to remove any air, connected to the manifold, and flushed with heparinized saline. The pigtail is then advanced to the aortic valve. While viewing the catheter in the RAO view, the pigtail is torqued such that the curl at the distal end of the catheter points upward, giving a "number six" configuration. It is then advanced to the aortic valve, forcing the end against the valve. If the catheter does not readily cross the valve, it should be withdrawn, torqued slightly, and advanced again. In the presence of an atypical anatomic configuration or sclerocalcific valve, in which crossing is impeded, catheter placement is facilitated by a guidewire. The guidewire may first be employed within the body of the catheter to stiffen it, but if this maneuver is insufficient, a straight, floppy guidewire may be advanced across the valve, to be followed by the catheter. Advancement and withdrawal of the catheter alters the position of the wire to achieve proper positioning for crossing.

The catheter should be positioned in the mid-body of the LV. It should be free of the LV wall and of the mitral valve–chordal apparatus to reduce the likelihood of (1) serious arrhythmia, (2) intramyocardial injection, and (3) catheter-induced mitral regurgitation. A test injection of approximately

5 mL of contrast material at the same flow rate as the subsequent LV angiography should be performed to screen for these potential problems.

Projections

Biplane left ventriculography for assessing ventricular performance and mitral regurgitation is usually performed using RAO (approximately 30 degrees) and left anterior oblique (LAO) (45–60 degrees) projections (Fig 6-2). (Single-plane ventriculography is generally performed in the RAO view.) Cranial angulation (approximately 15–20 degrees) of the x-ray beam (from a posterior source) optimizes visualization of the LV in the LAO projection by reducing foreshortening. The exact angulation should be adjusted based on rotation of the ventricle in an individual patient and the degree of its relative horizontal or vertical orientation. The goals in choosing the exact projections to be used are (1) to view the ventricle approximately perpendicular to its long axis and (2) to minimize overlap with the spine. The RAO view permits visualization and functional assessment of the anterior wall, apex, and inferior wall. The cranially angulated LAO projection views the interventricular septum, apex, lateral wall, and posterior wall. In both projections, the image intensifier (generally employed in a large-field [e.g., 9″] mode) should be positioned to visualize the entire LV and a sufficient area of the left atrium to adequately assess mitral regurgitation. In the RAO view, the lateral margin of the field should be positioned

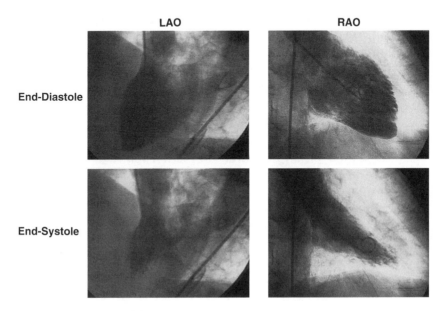

Figure 6-2 Normal left ventriculogram. LAO, left anterior oblique; RAO, right anterior oblique.

just lateral to the LV apex, while minimizing lung exposure. Optimal operation of the automatic brightness control requires fairly uniform tissue density throughout the field of view. A semi-opaque diaphragm, incorporated in most cineradiographic systems, should be positioned over any portion of the lung that is within the field to achieve more uniform density.

Contrast Injection and Frame Rate

The rate and volume of injection of radiographic contrast media should be chosen to achieve complete mixing with blood within the ventricle, thereby permitting visualization of the entire LV cavity through two or three cardiac cycles. In an adult, this goal is usually achieved by injection of 25 to 30 mL of contrast media at a rate of approximately 14 to 16 mL/sec. The exact volume and rate used should be determined during test injection of approximately 5 mL of contrast, which will permit subjective assessment of the size of the ventricle and the rate of emptying. Smaller contrast volumes may be used in the presence of a small left ventricle or low cardiac output state. Circumstances that require larger injection volumes and injection rates (up to 40 mL and 25 mL/sec in an adult) include those in which the ventricle empties rapidly, such as high cardiac output states and aortic regurgitation. A dilated ventricle per se does not necessarily mandate larger than normal contrast boluses. Where large volumes are needed to fully opacify the ventricle, consideration can be given to diluting the contrast media, thus permitting full mixing within the ventricle without employing excessive amounts of contrast media.

A gradual rise in flow rate over 0.5 to 1.0 second reduces the likelihood of inducing ventricular arrhythmia due to the physical impact of contrast injection. In addition to the remote possibility of inducing sustained ventricular tachycardia, ventricular premature beats (VPBs) preclude meaningful analysis of ventricular function and of the presence and severity of mitral regurgitation. (Mitral regurgitation induced during VPBs has no functional significance.)

Power injectors in present use exert sufficient pressure to deliver the pre-set flow rate, up to a given pressure limit. Pressure limits of 450 to 1000 pounds per square inch are typically employed during left ventriculography. Pressure limits serve to prevent catheter rupture during injection, a rare occurrence with present-day catheters.

The framing rate chosen for cineventriculography is a trade-off between radiation dose and temporal resolution. At given radiographic settings and frame size, total radiation dose during cine filming is directly proportional to the number of frames exposed. Table 6-1 indicates the temporal resolution achieved, expressed as frames per cardiac cycle, at various heart rates and framing rates ranging from 15 to 60 frames/sec. For clinical purposes, the frame rate should be sufficient to assure reasonably accurate depiction of the left ventricle at end-diastole and end-systole. At heart rates below 90 beats per minute, a

Table 6-1 Temporal Resolution (Frames per
Cardiac Cycle) During Ventriculography
at Various Heart Rates and Framing Rates

Heart rate (min^{-1})	15 frames/ sec	30 frames/ sec	45 frames/ sec	60 frames/ sec
60	15	30	45	60
100	9	18	27	36
120	7.5	15	22.5	30
150	6	12	18	24

framing rate of as low as 15 frames/sec is probably adequate for this purpose. At higher heart rates, faster framing rates (usually 30 frames/sec) should be employed. Faster framing rates are needed for measurement of time-dependent parameters of ventricular function, including ejection rate and peak filling rate. They are also needed for examining the relationship between pressure and volume changes through the cardiac cycle, including construction of LV pressure-volume loops. Such analyses are not commonly performed in clinical practice but are valuable for investigational assessment of contractility, relaxation, and compliance characteristics of the ventricle and may require frame rates sufficient to achieve at as many as 30 frames per cardiac cycle.

Volume Calculations

Techniques and concepts for assessing LV systolic and diastolic function from the left ventriculogram are based on ejection-phase and filling-phase indices, derived from calculation of LV volume. Estimates of absolute LV end-diastolic volume (EDV) and end-systolic volume (ESV) represent valuable indicators of prognosis and of the need and timing of surgical intervention in the presence of valvular regurgitant lesions.

Ejection fraction, the ratio of stroke volume to EDV [EF = EDV/(EDV −ESV)], is the most commonly measured index of systolic performance. It is influenced by LV preload and afterload, as well as by contractility. Measurement of absolute ESV has an advantage as an indicator of contractility, being independent of preload. It is linearly related to afterload within physiologic ranges. It has, therefore, been preferred by some investigators and clinicians over EF for assessing contractile function, particularly in the setting of valvular regurgitation. In a multivariate analysis of patients with myocardial infarction, ESV was found to be the strongest predictor of subsequent mortality.

Combined analysis of LV pressure and volume through the cardiac cycle provides a powerful tool for analyzing LV contractile function and diastolic compliance. Such analysis is carried out by sampling instantaneous pressure, using a micromanometer-tipped catheter, during ventriculography. At fixed timepoints during ejection, LV volume changes linearly with changes in LV pressure, within a physiologic range and at a constant level of contractility. Changes in the maximal slope of the relation between systolic pressure and volume at any fixed time-point (E_{max}), usually taken at end-systole, is a sensitive indicator of changes in contractile state. Left ventricular stiffness (the inverse of compliance) may be defined as the rate of change in LV pressure with a given change in volume during the terminal phase of diastolic filling.

Formulas for calculating LV volume were initially derived using biplane left ventriculography. Formulas that are applied to single-plane ventriculograms, performed in the RAO projection, assume a constant relation between the two minor dimensions of the left ventricle. All volumetric formulas are only as accurate as the underlying assumptions regarding LV shape. Thus, atypically or irregularly shaped ventricles, as may result from myocardial infarction, reduce the accuracy of volume calculations, particularly when using single-plane ventriculography. Nevertheless, commonly used formulas, both single-plane and biplane, if carefully applied, usually provide reasonably accurate volume calculation for clinical purposes.

Left ventricular volume may be estimated by either (1) utilizing Simpson's rule (Fig 6-3), which divides the ventricle into a series of slices of an assumed planar configuration and sums the volumes of all slices; or (2) assuming the left ventricle to have a given three-dimensional shape.

Chapman et al. applied Simpson's rule, assuming the ventricle to be composed of a series of 1-mm-thick elliptical slices with dimensions determined from biplane ventriculograms. The volume (V) of each slice is calculated as

$$V = \pi\, h\, (D_1 \times D_2/4)$$

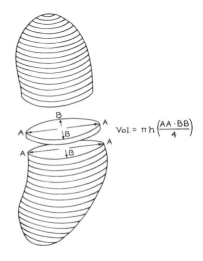

Figure 6-3 Method for calculation of LV volume using Simpson's rule. AA and BB represent the two axes of an ellipse; h is the height of each respective slice. (Reproduced by permission from the American Heart Association, Inc. from Chapman CB, Baker O, Reynolds J, Bonte FJ. Use of biplane cinefluorography for measurement of ventricular volume. Circulation 1958; 18:1105–1117.)

where h is slice thickness and D_1 and D_2 are the axes of the ellipse derived from two perpendicular projections. Application of Simpson's rule to single-plane (RAO) ventriculograms requires assuming a constant relationship between the two axes, D_1 and D_2. The most common assumption is that $D_1 = D_2$; that is, that the LV is circular in cross-section:

$$V = \pi\, h\, (D^2/4)$$

Computerized analysis of digital angiograms has made application of Simpson's rule less tedious and more feasible in clinical practice.

Dodge and others have estimated volume more simply, assuming the LV configuration to resemble that of a prolate ellipsoid (area-length method):

$$V = \frac{4\,\pi}{3}\, \frac{Lmax}{2}\, \frac{M}{2}\, \frac{N}{2}$$

or

$$V = (\pi/6)\, Lmax\, M\, N$$

where Lmax is the length of the major axis (i.e., the longest measured dimension) and M and N are the respective lengths of the two perpendicular minor axes. Although some investigators have measured the minor axis of the LV directly, at the midpoint of the long axis, the more commonly applied method derives each minor axis length from the planimetered ventricular area (A) of each respective perpendicular projection:

$$A_M = \pi\, M\, L/4$$

or

$$M = 4\, A_M/(\pi\, L),$$

where A_M and M are the respective planimetered area and minor axis length in a given projection. Substituting, LV volume may be calculated directly from the two planimetered areas, A_M and A_N and the maximal dimension in either projection, Lmax:

$$V = \pi/6\, Lmax \cdot 4\, A_M/\pi L_M \cdot A_N/\pi L_N$$

or

$$V = 0.849\, Lmax \cdot (A_M/L_M) \cdot (A_N/L_N)$$

Measured lengths and areas must be corrected for magnification that results from radiographic beam divergence. The degree to which a linear segment (L) is magnified ($L_{measured}/L_{true}$) is directly proportional to the ratio of the distances (1) from the x-ray tube to the image intensifier (distance X-I) to (2) from the x-ray tube to the left ventricle (distance X-V).

A correction factor [CF = $L_{true}/L_{measured}$ = 1/magnification ratio = distance X-V/distance X-I] for magnification may be derived by measuring these distances. Such measurement is facilitated by biplane imaging systems. Approximating the location of the LV centerpoint in one plane permits measurement of distances in the perpendicular plane. Modern biplane systems employ an isocenter system, such that by positioning the table-top height to center the left ventricle in the lateral projection, the ventricle is automatically placed at the vertex of rotation for each imaging system. Most systems, then, compute the distances from which CF may be derived.

The CF may be directly measured by comparing lengths or areas (A) within the radiographic image to those of a known object positioned at the level of the left ventricle. One approach is to image an external radio-opaque grid and compare measured and known areas ($CF^2 = A_{true}/A_{measured}$). Alternatively, the measured diameter of the contrast-filled LV catheter, on the image, may be compared with its known dimension.

The formula for LV volume calculation then becomes

$$V = 0.849\, Lmax\, (CFmax) \cdot (A_M/L_M)(CF_M) \cdot (A_N/L_N)(CF_N)$$

where CFmax is the CF for magnification in the projection in which Lmax is measured. Or,

$$V = 0.849\, (CFmax) \cdot A_M(CF_M) \cdot A_N(CF_N)/Lmin$$

where Lmin = L_M or L_N, whichever is shorter.

Actual volume differs from calculations, based on the preceding formulas, because of variance of LV shape from that of an ellipsoid. Papillary muscles and muscular trabeculae contribute to this variance. A number of laboratories have derived regression relations between calculations (V_{calc}) and actual measurements (V_{act}) made by postmortem injection of known amounts of contrast media into LV cavities. Dodge et al. derived the following regression equation for biplane (posteroanterior and lateral) left ventriculograms:

$$V_{act} = 0.928\, V_{calc} - 3.8\ ml$$

The biplane area-length method of calculating LV volume has been successfully applied using RAO and cranially angulated LAO views, as well as to posteroanterior and lateral views.

Dodge also has validated the area-length method for single-plane ventriculograms. Assuming (1) that the long axis of the ventricle is seen in the projection employed and (2) equivalence of the two perpendicular minor axes, the preceding equation becomes

$$V = 0.849 \times A^2 \, (CF)^3 / L$$

The inaccuracy of the two assumptions required for single-plane volumetric measurement results in greater error for this technique. Additionally, single-plane volume measurements generally exceed those obtained using biplane images. The following regression formula has been derived from experimental observations:

$$V_{act} = 0.951 \, V_{calc} - 3.0 \text{ ml}$$

Left ventricular volume calculation using the area-length method requires inclusion of the entire LV image within the planimetered area. This requirement is most problematic at end-systole, when trabeculations have maximally thickened and contrast volume has been reduced along the perimeter of the ventricle. Viewing the ventriculogram during motion facilitates identifying the outermost limits of contrast density to be drawn on the stopped-motion end-systolic frame. Underestimating the extent of the LV perimeter at end-systole results in underestimating ESV and overestimating EF.

Function and Viability

Analysis of regional LV wall motion assists in assessment of regional myocardial viability; the latter is a key determinant of the potential gain to be derived from revascularization in the presence of coronary obstructive disease.

It has been recognized recently that motion and viability are not synonymous. Retention of wall motion implies viability. A dysfunctional myocardial segment, however, may still be partially or wholly viable due to "stunning," related to recent ischemic insult, or "hibernation," related to ongoing severe ischemia. Where regional systolic dysfunction has been identified within a viable myocardial segment, revascularization often produces functional recovery. Numerous methods have been employed to assess viability in dysfunctional myocardium. These include analysis of contractile augmentation during post-extrasystolic potentiation or during infusion of an inotropic agent. During dobutamine infusion, wall motion may be analyzed using contrast ventriculography or, more commonly, echocardiography. An alternative, and probably more sensitive, approach to analyzing viability is myocardial perfusion imaging. Thus, assessment of potential benefit from revascularization often requires analysis of both wall motion and viability.

Regional Wall Motion and Ventricular Aneurysms

Wall motion is most often graded subjectively (Figs 6-4 and 6-5):

Hypokinetic: reduced systolic motion
Akinetic: absent motion
Dyskinetic: outward motion during systole

A ventricular aneurysm is a discrete LV region containing the entire thickness of ventricular wall, but devoid of viable myocardium, manifesting dyskinetic motion. It predisposes the patient to clinical heart failure, beyond that produced by a comparably sized akinetic segment. It serves as an ejection sink, reducing forward stroke volume, and increases diastolic wall stress, thereby acting to accelerate hypertrophy and adverse remodeling of the residual viable myocardium. Ventricular aneurysms are also associated with high-grade ventricular arrhythmia and with thromboembolism. Left ventricular aneurysms may occur anywhere in the ventricle, but are most commonly apical.

Figure 6-4 Ventriculographic images in RAO projection, showing inferior wall hypokinesis (arrow).

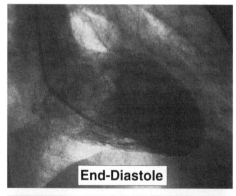

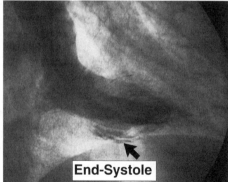

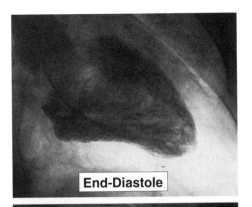

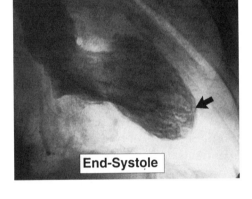

Figure 6-5 Ventriculographic images in RAO projection, showing anterior akinesis and apical (arrow) dyskinesis.

It is useful to attempt to distinguish a true aneurysm from a false aneurysm, because the latter is predisposed to rupture. A false aneurysm is far less common and represents a sealed-off ventricular rupture. Unlike a true aneurysm, a false aneurysm is not bounded by full-thickness ventricular wall. It is often more clearly demarcated from the normal wall, with which it often forms an acute angle. It may not be possible, however, to definitively distinguish between a true and a false LV aneurysm on the basis of ventriculography.

Left ventricular thrombus is frequently associated with aneurysm formation and may be detected by left ventriculography as a smooth, sometimes pedunculated filling defect. It is most often observed at the apex, in association with a wall motion abnormality.

Qualitative assessment of regional wall motion is characterized by substantial intra- and interobserver variability. A number of methods have been formulated to assess wall motion objectively and quantitatively using contrast left ventriculography. One method examines changes in planimetered areas, from end-diastole to end-systole, of LV chamber segments. External reference markers should be used to correct for any translational or rotational motion occurring during the cardiac cycle. In the RAO view, the LV cavity may be divided into three areas by utilizing the long axis (midpoint of the aortic valve to the apex) and a perpendicular minor chord drawn one-fourth of the distance from the apex to the aortic valve. This minor chord divides the LV into apical and basilar segments. The base is further divided along the long axis into anterior and inferior segments. Regional function is defined as change in segment area from diastole to systole.

A second method for quantifying regional wall motion examines fractional shortening of segments drawn from the endocardial surface to the central long axis. The LV long axis is divided into equal segments by three or four perpendicular chords. An additional apical segment may be taken along the long axis, although shortening fraction of a longitudinally oriented apical segment has shown considerable normal variation. Correction must be made for translational motion. Correction may be achieved by superimposing the long axes on the ED and ES silhouettes. Alternatively, a coronary sinus catheter and the aortic–mitral valve junction have been used as translational reference markers.

The preceding methods have a number of potential pitfalls. First, delineation of the long axis and its perpendicular chords may be associated with significant intra- and interobserver variability. Second, contraction of the left ventricle is not symmetrical about a long axis but is multicentric. An alternative approach examines regional wall motion relative to the ventricular center of gravity, or "centroid." The endocardial surface is identified by computerized detection of the rate of change in contrast density. Rotational motion must be corrected by use of reference markers. One technique employs 128 radial grids drawn from the center of gravity to the endocardial borders. Fractional shortening along the various axis segments, from end-diastole to end-systole, may be plotted for the entire LV circumference. Although an advance above the hemi-axis method, this method is based on the incorrect assumption that wall motion of all segments proceeds toward a center of gravity.

The centerline method constructs a curve connecting all points that are equidistant from the endocardial margins of the superimposed ED and ES images (Fig 6-6). A series of shortening segments is drawn perpendicular to this equidistant curve, radially around the LV silhouette, from the ED to the ES margin. The length of each regional shortening segment is expressed as a fraction of the ED circumference. Segmental shortening may be plotted against the position of the segment along the LV perimeter to create a circumferential functional profile, which may be compared with the distribution of values from a normal population. The centerline method offers the substantial advantage that it does not require correction for translational motion, and it has been found to be highly reproducible. It may be applied to single-plane, RAO ventriculogram, or to biplane studies. It has gained considerable acceptance in investigations of regional ventricular function.

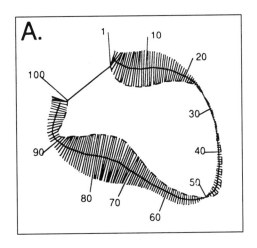

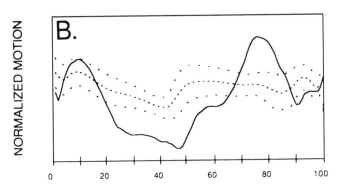

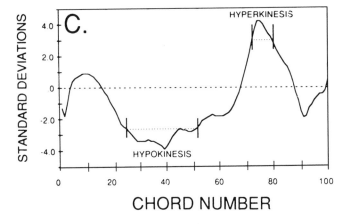

Figure 6-6 Centerline method for quantitating regional wall motion. **(A)** The ventricle with both ES and ED silhouettes, and the centerline drawn between them. Chords are drawn radially between these outlines, perpendicular to the centerline. **(B)** Normal range for chord lengths adjusted for heart size, dividing chord length by the ED circumference (dotted lines). The adjusted chord lengths are shown by the solid line. **(C)** Adjusted chord lengths expressed as units of SD from the normal mean (zero line). See text for details.

Regurgitant Volume: Assessment of Mitral Regurgitation

Mitral and aortic regurgitation can be quantified by measuring LV volumes, at end-diastole and end-systole, and forward cardiac output, by the Fick or thermodilution method. Forward stroke volume (SV_F) and total LV stroke volume (SV_{LV}) are calculated by

$$SV_F \text{ (mL)} = \text{cardiac output (mL/min)/heart rate (min}^{-1})$$

$$SV_{LV} = EDV - ESV$$

Regurgitant volume (RV) and regurgitant fraction (RF) are then calculated by

$$RV = SV_{LV} - SV_F$$

$$RF = RV/SV_{LV}$$

In the presence of both mitral and aortic regurgitation, RV and RF, calculated in this manner, relate to total regurgitant flow and do not permit quantitation of either lesion alone.

Assessment of mitral regurgitation is more commonly performed by qualitative assessment of the amount of contrast media ejected into the left atrium following LV injection (Fig 6-7):

1+ Faint opacification of the atrium, with clearing during each subsequent beat

2+ Opacification of the atrium that does not clear but is not as intense as the LV

3+ Atrial opacification equal to that of the ventricle

4+ Immediate opacification of the entire atrium, with reflux into the pulmonary veins

In addition to identifying and quantifying mitral regurgitant flow, the left ventriculogram may provide additional information relevant to the etiology of valvular dysfunction. Although better identified by echocardiography, mitral valve prolapse may be observed by left ventriculography. The mitral leaflets form the inferior aspect of the posterior border of the left ventricle in the RAO projection. In the presence of mitral valve prolapse, either of valvular origin or due to chordal rupture or papillary muscle dysfunction, one or both leaflets may be seen to bow posteriorly into the left atrium. In the presence of 3+ to 4+ regurgitation, the posterior mitral leaflet may be visualized as a curvilinear radiolucent structure, delineated by contrast media on either side. Under these conditions, valve motion may be easily tracked.

The presence and distribution of calcium also may aid in the diagnosis. Mild to moderate mitral regurgitation may be an accompaniment of mitral annular calcification. Mitral annular calcium may be identified as a C-shaped or

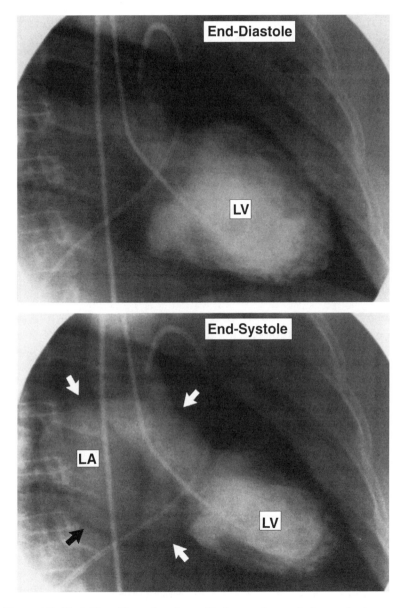

Figure 6-7   End-diastolic and end-systolic frames from a left ventriculogram, performed in the RAO projection in a patient with severe mitral regurgitation. The left atrium (arrows) is opacified during systole. LA, left atrium; LV, left ventricle.

U-shaped rim of calcium that encircles the valve. This pattern differs from that of rheumatic disease, in which the calcification predominates centrally at the tips of the valve leaflets.

Findings in Hypertrophic Disease and Measurement of Left Ventricular Mass

In patients with chronic LV pressure overload (e.g., hypertension, aortic stenosis), concentric LV hypertrophy occurs and serves to limit increases in systolic wall stress. Left ventriculography in such cases may reveal a supranormal (>65%) EF, often with associated partial cavity obliteration. The LV cavity is commonly altered from its normal elliptical configuration, with systolic apex-to-base shortening, into a more cylindrical configuration, with loss of apex-to-base shortening and contraction toward the cylindrical centerline.

In hypertrophic cardiomyopathy, LV hypertrophy occurs without identifiable hemodynamic stimulus. Although hypertrophy may be symmetrical, in this setting it is more commonly localized or asymmetrical. Left ventriculography (Fig 6-8) frequently shows obliteration of a portion of the LV cavity adjacent to the area of hypertrophy. When asymmetrical hypertrophy occurs in the basal septum, it may result in dynamic outflow tract obstruction and mitral regurgitation, which are provoked or exacerbated by maneuvers that augment contractility or reduce systolic or diastolic load. The anterior leaflet of the mitral valve is drawn toward the septum during systole due to high-velocity blood flow in the subaortic region. Easily recognized by echocardiography, systolic anterior mitral valve motion may also be seen by ventriculography. It is best observed in the LAO projection, using caudal angulation. Patterns of midcavity or apical LV cavity obliteration also may be observed. The latter pattern, most commonly described in Japan, results in a spade-shaped LV contour.

Although uncommonly measured for clinical application, LV mass can be estimated from the left ventriculogram, according to the method devised by Rackley et al. Ventricular chamber volume is calculated using the biplane area-length method described previously. The outer margin of the LV wall is outlined in the posteroanterior or RAO projection, and a 4-cm segment of the free wall (at the juncture of the apical and mid-portion) is selected. The area of this segment is measured by planimetry, and the average wall thickness over this area is calculated area divided by length. This value for wall thickness is corrected for magnification (see previous discussion). The total volume (V) of the left ventricular chamber (c) plus muscle wall (w) is calculated using the formula

$$V_{c+w} = 4/3 \cdot \pi [M/2 + h] \cdot [N/2 + h] \cdot [Lmax/2 + h]$$

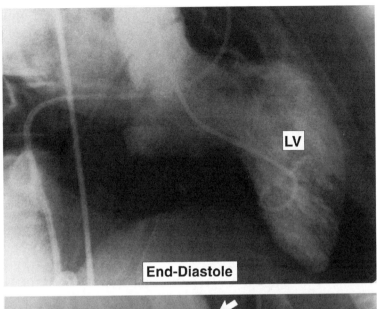

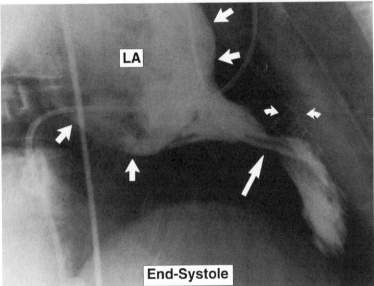

Figure 6-8 Left ventriculogram in the RAO projection in a patient with hypertrophic cardiomyopathy. The ES frame shows cavity obliteration (long arrow) and intramyocardial contrast trapping (curved arrows). There is severe mitral regurgitation. LA, left atrium; LV, left ventricle.

where Lmax is the length of the major axis (i.e., the longest measured dimension), M and N are the respective lengths of the two perpendicular minor axes, and h is wall thickness. Left ventricular mass is then calculated by the equation

$$(V_{c+w} - V_{act}) \cdot 1.050$$

where V_{act} is the corrected LV chamber volume, as derived in the preceding equation; 1.050 represents the specific gravity of heart muscle. Because postmortem studies have shown overestimation of ventricular mass by approximately 2% to 3% using this method, calculated values may be multiplied by a CF of 0.97. The upper limit of normal, as determined by Kennedy, is $119 \, \text{g/m}^2$. At present, the most accurate estimates of human LV mass are probably obtained by either rapid CT scanning or MRI.

Right Ventriculography

Indications, Contraindications, Risks

Assessment of right ventricular (RV) function can provide important, clinically relevant, pathophysiologic information for a variety of disease states, including ischemic, myopathic, valvular, congenital, and pulmonary vascular disease. Documentation of RV systolic dysfunction may indicate the presence of RV ischemia or infarction. Among patients with left heart failure, RV systolic function has been found to correlate with survival, as well as with functional status. In severe pulmonary hypertension, RV systolic function is usually impaired due to abnormal systolic load. Indices of RV performance have been found to roughly correlate with pulmonary artery pressure in patients with valvular or congenital disease, LV failure, or primary pulmonary or pulmonary vascular disease. In the setting of an acute ventricular septal defect, RV systolic function has been found to be a major predictor of survival following surgical repair. Likewise, in patients with congenital heart disease, assessment of RV systolic performance may provide important physiologic insight and may help to guide therapy and anticipate surgical outcomes. Altered RV function may represent the explanation for continued functional impairment following repair of such congenital anomalies as atrial and ventricular septal defects, transposition of the great arteries, pulmonic stenosis, and tetralogy of Fallot. When RV systolic functional impairment occurs in the presence of normal loading conditions, such abnormality may be due to coronary artery obstructive disease, involvement of the right ventricle with a myopathic process, or RV dysplasia.

Nevertheless, right ventriculography is performed infrequently in the adult cardiac catheterization laboratory, primarily because much of the information to be derived may be obtained or inferred from other data, including hemodynamic, echocardiographic, or radionuclide ventriculographic findings.

Right ventriculography is relatively safe and carries less risk than left heart catheterization with left ventriculography. Uncommon complications include right heart perforation with cardiac tamponade, pulmonary embolism, and right bundle branch block. Pulmonary embolism due to catheter-derived thrombus is rarely clinically relevant. Right bundle branch block is generally self-limited. However, it occurs with sufficient frequency to warrant rapid accessibility to ventricular pacing in patients with a baseline left bundle branch block. Ventricular arrhythmias occur almost universally during RV catheterization, but rarely result in sustained ventricular tachycardia. In addition to the usual potential adverse effects of intravascular administration of contrast media, abrupt hemodynamic deterioration may occur following right heart contrast administration in patients with severe pulmonary hypertension. In such patients, right ventriculography should be either avoided or performed using reduced volumes of contrast media.

Technique

Right ventriculography is performed during chamber opacification by injection of radiographic contrast media into the vena cava, right atrium, or right ventricle. Contrast media are generally injected via a catheter with multiple side holes, such as a pigtail, Eppendorf, or Berman (balloon-tipped with side holes) catheter, in volumes of 25 to 45 ml in adults. Typical injection rates range from 15 to 25 ml/sec. The total dose and injection rate for contrast media must be based on the nature of the underlying pathology, with higher doses and injection rates required in the presence of RV volume overload. Final selection of dose and injection rate is made following inspection of the appearance of the ventricle during a test injection.

Measurement of EF requires that images be obtained at near-maximal (diastolic) and near-minimal (systolic) RV volumes. The frame rate necessary to achieve this goal depends on heart rate. For clinical measurement of EF, recording at a rate of 15 frames per cardiac cycle is sufficient for approximating minimal and maximal volumes. A slower framing rate may result in underestimation of EF. Rates of 30 to 40 frames per cardiac cycle are necessary to assess time-dependent indices of ventricular systolic and diastolic performance, such as ejection and filling rates, and to construct volume curves through the cardiac cycle.

In contrast to the left ventricle, the complexity of RV shape obviates adequate estimates of RV volume from single-plane ventriculography. Biplane ventriculography is generally performed in either (1) posteroanterior and lateral projections or (2) RAO and LAO projections. Visualization of the right ventricle in the posteroanterior or LAO view is optimized by cranially angulating the radiographic beam approximately 15 to 20 degrees to reduce foreshortening of the RV cavity and improve separation of the RV outflow tract from the pulmonary artery.

Assessment of Right Ventricular Volumes and Function

The configuration of the right ventricle makes functional assessment based on volumetrics inherently more difficult and less precise than the corresponding measurements for the left ventricle. The RV shape is complex and does not readily lend itself to any simple geometric approximation. Unlike the left ventricle, the right ventricle comprises anatomically (and embryologically) distinct inflow (sinus) and outflow (conus) portions. These two portions of the right ventricle are separated by the crista supraventricularis. Mechanical systole proceeds from the inflow to the outflow regions, with contraction of the inflow region normally preceding that of the outflow region by 25 to 50 milliseconds. Attempts at geometric approximation of RV volume are further confounded by the coarse myocardial trabeculations of the RV free wall and right side of the interventricular septum. A large muscle bundle, known as the moderator band, extends from the inferior aspect of the interventricular septum to the free wall, where it attaches to the anterior papillary muscle. More than the left ventricle, the right ventricle changes its shape substantially from diastole to systole and under conditions of pressure and volume overload. The pattern of contraction of the normal right ventricle may be likened to movement of the sides of a bellows, with two approximately parallel (but in the case of the right ventricle, curved rather than flat) walls moving toward and away from each other, rather than concentric movement toward a common central axis. However, in the volume-overloaded right ventricle, this pattern may be substantially altered as the interventricular septum becomes concave toward the RV cavity during diastole, and systolic contraction is more concentric. These inherent difficulties must be considered when assessing RV function.

Difficulties in RV volumetric measurement and variability in methodologies have resulted in disagreement regarding normal RV EF. Estimates of the lower limits of normal for RV EF have ranged from approximately 0.40 to 0.50.

One of two approaches may be employed for estimation of RV volume: (1) assumption of a geometric approximation of the overall RV shape and (2) use of Simpson's rule. Several models may be employed for approximating the overall RV shape, including (1) a combination of an ellipsoidal body and a cylindrical outflow tract; (2) a pyramid; (3) a prism, with rectangular frontal and lateral planes and a triangular horizontal plane; and (4) a prolate ellipsoid. The dimensions of these various models are generally derived from biplane ventriculograms. Simpson's rule methodology entails dividing the ventricle into a series of thin slices, presuming the shape of each slice, calculating its volume accordingly, and summing the various volumes. This technique probably provides for more accurate volumetric estimation. Using Simpson's rule, each cross-sectional RV slice has been likened in shape to either an ellipse, a triangle, or a rectangle. Good agreement between radiographic geometric calculations and direct volumetric measurement has been found with application of these techniques to postmortem radio-opaque RV casts. Because RV configuration changes substantially through the cardiac cycle and with differences in distension pressure, it is questionable whether postmortem cast findings are applicable to ES volume or to ED volume in the setting of altered loading conditions. Nevertheless, Simpson's rule analysis probably provides reasonably accurate estimation of RV volumes in vivo.

Aortography

Indications and Contraindications

In the cardiac catheterization laboratory, aortography is performed most frequently for one of the following indications: (1) to detect and assess the severity of aortic insufficiency; (2) to evaluate suspected aortic pathology, including aneurysm, dissection, or coarctation; and (3) to identify the course of an anomalous coronary artery or saphenous vein graft. Other indications include evaluation of trauma with suspected aortic injury and vasculitides, particularly Takayasu's aortitis.

There are few contraindications to aortography. Renal insufficiency and severe heart failure with elevated ventricular filling pressures represent relative contraindications to administration of radiographic contrast media.

Catheters and Technique

The most commonly employed catheter for aortography is the multihole pigtail catheter, which minimizes the risk of intimal dissection or perforation during power injection. Removing the guidewire and "double flushing" the catheter (aspiration, discarding, and flushing) within the descending aorta minimize the risk of cerebral thromboembolism. For ascending aortography, the catheter is usually positioned 1 to 2 cm above the aortic valve to minimize the likelihood of interfering with valve competence.

Biplane cineangiography is most commonly performed with approximately 30-degree RAO and 60-degree LAO angulation. The latter is optimally performed using 10 to 20 degrees of cranial angulation (the posterior x-ray source is angled cranially). The LAO view with cranial angulation affords optimal "unwrapping" of the aortic root and arch, eliminating overlap between the ascending and descending aortic segments. Typically, large-sized image intensifiers (e.g., 7″ diameter) are employed during aortography to achieve an adequate field of view. Field positioning depends on the indication for aortography. For example, detection of and grading aortic regurgitation or mapping the route of an anomalous coronary artery or bypass graft requires inclusion of the left ventricle in the field, or panning from the aorta to the left ventricle. Where indications are purely related to aortic pathology, the field should be centered in the area of suspected pathology.

A several-milliliter test injection should be performed to assure proper catheter position. Typical injection parameters during aortography are 30 to 50 mL over approximately 2 seconds. Injection at these rates (15–25 mL/sec) may result in catheter recoil, which may be prevented by manually stabilizing the catheter during injection. Cineangiography facilitates assessment of aortic regurgitation. Alternatively, cut-film aortography, typically obtained at a rate of approximately 6 images per second affords improved resolution for other indications, including detection of aortic dissection.

Aortic Regurgitation

The assessment of aortic regurgitation represents the most common indication for aortography in the cardiac catheterization laboratory. Several subjective grading systems have been proposed for the semiquantitative assessment of aortic regurgitation. The following is one such scheme:

1+ Regurgitant stream evident with absent or minimal opacification of the left ventricle

2+ Regurgitant stream evident with faint or incomplete opacification of the left ventricle

3+ Complete opacification of the left ventricle but with less density than the aorta

4+ Complete opacification of the left ventricle to an extent greater than or equal to that of the aorta

Which method is "correct"? When compared with more objective methods of quantitating aortic regurgitation—regurgitant volume and regurgitant fraction, derived from comparison of LV and forward stroke volumes (see previous discussion)—the correlation with such qualitative schemes is not consistent. One difficulty results from the fact that concomitant mitral regurgitation influences the calculation of regurgitant fraction and volume, which does not permit direct quantitation of the relative contribution of each lesion. In one study, the correlation between the two methods of quantitating aortic regurgitation was found to be better where LV volume was relatively large (LVEDV > 100 mL), whereas another study found the opposite.

It should be recognized that the various approaches to quantify aortic regurgitation, including those based partly or wholly on ventriculographic findings, examine the lesion from differing physiologic as well as methodologic perspectives. For example, regurgitant volume is the absolute volume of regurgitant flow. Regurgitant fraction is regurgitant flow as a fraction of total LV stroke volume. Semiquantitative assessment of regurgitant severity based on inspection of aortographic images is not directly analogous to either of these two measurements, because it is influenced not only by regurgitant volume but also by LV volume. That is, for a given regurgitant volume, the severity of regurgitation will appear less in the presence of a larger LVEDV. Thus, semiquantitative assessment of regurgitant grade may be more analogous to Doppler quantitation of aortic regurgitation, which examines the relative volume of the regurgitant jet within the ventricle.

Some authors have advocated quantitating the ratio of regurgitant volume to LVEDV as a logical means of determining the likelihood of clinical benefit from surgical repair of aortic regurgitation. For a given magnitude of regurgitant flow, there is less likelihood of benefit in the presence of a severely dilated ventricle, compared with a less dilated ventricle. This ratio is analogous to the semiquantitative aortographic assessment, which depends both on regurgitant flow and on LV diastolic volume. Thus, although subjective, assessment of aortic regurgitation by aortography offers useful information in guiding the recommendation for valve replacement.

Ascending Aortic Aneurysms

Aortography affords a means for delineating the extent, nature, and severity of the gross pathology in the setting of ascending aortic aneurysm. These may be atherosclerotic, inflammatory, or degenerative in nature. Of the degenerative lesions, the most common cause is cystic medial necrosis associated with Marfan's syndrome. The severity and extent of the aneurysm influences the operative and non-operative risks, and hence the decision for surgical repair. Aortography now represents part of the diagnostic armamentarium serving this purpose, with other useful tests including ultrasound, magnetic resonance imaging (MRI), and computed tomography (CT). Non-operative risk increases as an aneurysm enlarges. Some authors have reported that in patients with Marfan's disease, the risk of spontaneous dissection increases substantially with aortic root dilatation beyond a 6-cm diameter. Others have suggested that aortic dissection occurs more frequently in Marfan's when the aortic diameter enlarges to twice that of the uninvolved distal aorta. Aneurymsal involvement of the arch vessels requires more complex and intricate surgical repair, resulting in substantially higher risk. Although considerable information regarding the anatomy of aortic aneurysms may be derived via noninvasive imaging modalities, prior to surgical repair, coronary arteriography is generally required to evaluate coronary involvement and the possibility of concomitant coronary artery disease. The latter is a significant cause of late morbidity and mortality among patients with aortic aneurysms. In addition, aortic root angiography provides information regarding the presence and severity of aortic insufficiency, which often occurs as a consequence of aortic root dilatation.

Aortic Dissection

Acute aortic dissection represents a life-threatening condition. Rapid diagnosis is crucial. There are two general classification schemes for aortic dissection. The scheme proposed by De Bakey et al. classifies dissections into types I to III. Types I and II involve the ascending aorta, with type I extending from the arch into the distal aorta, and type II being confined to the ascending aorta. Type III dissections are confined to the descending aorta. The Stanford system classifies as type A or proximal those dissections involving the ascending aorta. Those sparing the ascending aorta are classified as type B. De Bakey type I and II dissections are both classified as type A under the Stanford scheme. Current recommendations suggest immediate surgery for acute type A dissections and medical therapy for uncomplicated type B dissections.

The goals of diagnostic imaging in patients with suspected aortic dissection are to determine the presence and extent of the dissection, confirm involvement of the ascending aorta, localize the site of intimal tear and reentry (if present), quantify aortic regurgitation, and diagnose involvement of aortic branch vessels, including the coronary arteries. Aortography has been considered the gold standard for the diagnosis of aortic dissection. More recently, less invasive modalities, specifically CT, transesophageal echocardiography (TEE), and MRI, have been evaluated in the diagnosis of aortic dissection. No modality fulfills all diagnostic goals.

Computed tomography has a reported sensitivity of 82% to 100% and specificity of 90% to 100% for diagnosis of aortic dissection. Limitations include the need for contrast administration and the inability to provide hemodynamic data or information concerning involvement of coronary arteries and degree of aortic insufficiency. Computed tomography is poor at identifying intimal flaps or sites of dissection entry. Transesophageal echocardiography has been reported to have a high sensitivity and specificity. However, two recent reports documented specificities of only 68% and 77% for this technique. The advantages of TEE include its rapidity, portability, lack of need for contrast, and its ability to quantitate aortic valvular regurgitation and LV systolic function. It is only fair in determining branch vessel involvement. Magnetic resonance imaging has been found to be highly sensitive and specific in the diagnosis of aortic dissection. However, it cannot be performed in patients with certain metallic prostheses and is time consuming. The latter is an important restriction in hemodynamically unstable patients. During MRI, a patient is inaccessible, again posing logistic problems in unstable patients.

The sensitivity of aortography in detecting aortic dissection ranges from 90% to 100%, with specificity approaching 100%. False-negative results may occur if flow through the false lumen is vigorous enough to obscure visualization of the intimal flap. In addition to providing a diagnosis, aortography also provides important information regarding the location of the intimal tear, communication channels between true and false lumens, involvement of the coronaries and arch vessels, and detection of aortic regurgitation. This added information is of vital importance to the surgeon in deciding the operative approach.

In suspected aortic dissection, the initial aortogram should be performed with contrast injection 1 to 2 cm above the aortic valve to evaluate the ascending aorta and the arch. Depending on the results of these images, an injection into the descending aorta also should be performed. Previously, large cut-film angiography had been utilized for the evaluation of aortic dissection. However, despite slight reduction in resolution, cineangiography may offer advantages of shorter procedure time and improved evaluation of aortic insufficiency and the coronary ostia. Arciniegas et al. compared biplane cut-film angiography with biplane cineangiography and found the latter to be superior to cut-film in defining morphologic characteristics of the intimal tear.

Aortography in the presence of aortic dissection is accompanied by risks, the most important being the possible propagation of the dissection if power contrast injection is introduced into the false lumen. Generally, aortography in experienced hands is safe and rarely contributes to clinical deterioration. Disastrous consequences can be avoided by careful hand injections if false lumen cannulation is suspected.

Congenital Abnormalities

Coarctation constitutes the most common indication for aortography in adult patients with congenital heart disease. If coarctation is suspected or known, pressures must be monitored carefully during a slow pullback of the pigtail catheter to document the gradient across the coarctation. Other possible indications in those with congenital disease include supravalvular stenosis, subaortic membrane, and patent ductus arteriosus.

Aortography can aid in diagnosing sinus of Valsalva aneurysm. This abnormality is most frequently congenital but also is associated with Marfan's syndrome, syphilis, and bacterial endocarditis. Congenital aneurysms most frequently involve the right or noncoronary sinus. Sinus of Valsalva aneurysms may cause aortic insufficiency. Rupture often causes left-to-right shunting, usually into the right atrium or ventricle. Aortography confirms the diagnosis and localizes the aneurysm and shunt, if present.

Pulmonary Angiography

Indications, Contraindications, Risks

The most common indication for pulmonary angiography is suspected pulmonary embolism. Rarely in an adult, pulmonary angiography is performed for suspected congenital disease, such as branch pulmonary arterial stenosis. Initial evaluation of a patient with suspected pulmonary embolism should usually be a radionuclide ventilation-perfusion lung scan. In the setting of high clinical suspicion of pulmonary embolism, a "high probability" lung scan is usually sufficient to institute therapy. Likewise, in the setting of a "normal" or "low-probability" lung scan with low clinical level of suspicion, the post-test probability for pulmonary emboli is sufficiently low to avoid additional testing. Pulmonary angiography is indicated when definitive diagnosis of acute pulmonary embolism is needed and one of the following criteria is met:

1. Discordant lung scan and clinical assessment
2. Intermediate (indeterminate) probability lung scan
3. Suspicion of pulmonary embolism with a contraindication to anticoagulation
4. When the clinical condition warrants consideration of thrombolytic treatment, embolectomy, or vena cava interruption

Multiple chronic pulmonary emboli must be distinguished from primary pulmonary hypertension. In the setting of unexplained pulmonary hypertension, ventilation-perfusion lung scanning may be performed as an initial screening tool for pulmonary emboli. Any uncertainty of the diagnosis based on these findings indicates the need to perform pulmonary angiography.

Relative contraindications to pulmonary angiography include elevated left or right heart filling pressure, pulmonary hypertension (particularly if mean pulmonary artery pressure exceeds 40 mm Hg), renal insufficiency, and prior allergic-like reaction to intravascular radiographic contrast media (see section on contrast material). Because passage of a catheter through the right ventricle may provoke right bundle branch block, a transvenous pacing wire should be placed prophylactically in patients with left bundle branch block to avoid inducing complete heart block.

Risks of pulmonary angiography are similar to those of right ventriculography, as previously described. There is an additional risk of pulmonary arterial rupture, particularly with excessive guidewire manipulation or wedge pulmonary arteriography (discussion follows).

Stein et al. reported a mortality rate of 0.5% during pulmonary angiography, a 1.0% incidence of nonfatal major complication, and a 5.0% incidence of minor complication (Table 6-2). Complication rates were not related to age, except for an increase in contrast-induced acute renal failure in the elderly. This

Table 6-2   Complications of Pulmonary
Arteriography During the PIOPED Study

Death (0.5%)
Nonfatal major complications (1.0%)
    Respiratory distress requiring CPR and/or intubation
    Renal failure requiring dialysis
    Puncture-site hematoma requiring transfusion
Minor (5.0%)
    Respiratory distress not requiring ventilation support
    Transient renal dysfunction
    Angina
    Hypotension
    Pulmonary congestion (CHF)
    Urticaria, itching
    Hematoma not requiring transfusion
    Cardiac dysrhythmia
    Subintimal injection
    Narcotic overdose
    Nausea and vomiting
    Right bundle branch block

Abbreviations: PIOPED, Prospective Investigation of Pulmonary
Embolism Diagnosis; CPR, cardiopulmonary resuscitation; CHF,
congestive heart failure.
SOURCE: Stein PD, Athanasoulis C, Alavi A, et al. Complications and validity of pulmonary angiography in acute pulmonary embolism. Circulation 1992;85:462–468.

study failed to show a correlation between complication rate and pulmonary arterial pressure, although this negative finding may have been influenced by selection bias within their study population. Three percent of pulmonary angiograms were nondiagnostic. Other studies have shown higher major complication rates, possibly due to inclusion of patients with more severe hemodynamic derangement and injection into the main pulmonary artery. The latter technique has been abandoned.

Pulmonary artery pressure should be measured prior to angiography, both to aid in the diagnosis and to assess the risk of a large-volume contrast material injection. The risk of inducing severe hemodynamic compromise increases with increasing degrees of pulmonary hypertension, presumably due to vasoactive effects of contrast material. Risks are reduced by minimizing the volume of contrast material used and avoiding main pulmonary artery injection.

Catheters and Insertion Technique

Catheters currently used for pulmonary angiography fall into two broad categories: pigtail catheters and flow-directed catheters (Table 6-3). The older Eppendorff and NIH catheters are less desirable because of a higher rate of cardiac and pulmonary outflow tract perforation associated with their use.

Table 6-3   Catheters Used in Pulmonary Angiography

Catheter Type	Description	Advantages	Disadvantages
NIH	Closed end hole, straight		High risk of cardiac perforation or dysrhythmia
Grollman	Pigtail (ring-up*), 3-cm 90-degree bent arm, small diameter ring	Easy passage into right heart and PA, pre-formed shape, ring-up shape allows guidewire use to select PA from RV	Length of primary catheter curve may be too short in enlarged RA/RV; 2-degree curve in unmodified Groll-man catheter pre-vents insertion from upper body
Other curved pigtail	Large diameter ring, ring-up or down, varying length of 90-degree bent arm	Longer bent arm may help facilitate pas-sage in enlarged right heart	Ring-down** pigtail makes guidewire passage difficult and dangerous (possible cardiac perforation)
Straight pigtail	Standard straight-body pigtail	Unformed bent arm allows individual patient tailoring of catheter shape	Requires either tip deflector or bent-wire to direct into heart and PA, requires greater operator skill
Flow-directed balloon catheter	1. Swan-Ganz–type: end hole, proximal balloon, not multi-holed	Flow directed, may be passed without fluoroscopy (bed-side) (Swan-Ganz only)	Poor segmental selec-tivity, small vascular bed imaged each injection, risk of PA rupture during in-jection (Swan-Ganz only) Risk of PA rupture during balloon inflation (both catheters)
	2. Berman type: closed end, distal balloon, multiple proximal holes	Atraumatic (no guidewire), allows subsegmental injections	

Abbreviations: PA, pulmonary artery; RV, right ventricle; RA, right artery.
*Superior-pointing. ** Inferior-pointing.

Larger-sized catheters (7 to 8 Fr) are relatively easy to steer and advance and are relatively resistant to recoil during injection. Recent improvements in catheter material have permitted adequate rates of contrast injection with catheters as small as 5 Fr. Although less stiff than larger-diameter catheters, 5-Fr catheters offer lower profile (helpful in cases of valvular stenosis) and allow for smaller vascular punctures. Smaller catheters, however, have a greater ten-dency to recoil during injection, falling back into the main or contralateral pul-monary artery, and potentially resulting in vascular injury.

Venous access for pulmonary angiography may be achieved from the femoral, jugular, or brachial approach. Using the femoral approach, the right common femoral vein presents a relatively straight course into the inferior vena cava. The left common femoral vein forms a tighter angle with the inferior vena cava, reducing torque transmission to the catheter tip. Use of the right common femoral vein facilitates placement of a device for caval interruption, if such an intervention is indicated. Non–balloon-directed catheters are generally advanced into the inferior vena cava with the aid of a J-tipped guidewire (0.035″ or 0.038″, depending on catheter internal diameter) under fluoroscopic control. If there is any difficulty in advancing the catheter, hand injection of contrast material should be performed to determine venous patency and the presence of thrombus. Identification of venous thrombus may be sufficient to guide therapy, mandating anticoagulation, without proceeding to pulmonary angiography. If pulmonary angiography remains indicated (e.g., due to suspicion that venous thrombus is old, or need to document recurrent emboli for additional intervention), an alternative access site should be chosen.

With an angled catheter (e.g., Grollman) in the right atrium, the guidewire should be withdrawn, allowing the primary bend in the catheter to reform. The catheter may then be advanced through the tricuspid valve and rotated to direct it toward the pulmonary outflow tract and main pulmonary artery. Depending on the size of the right heart, it may be necessary to straighten the primary catheter curve using the stiff end of the guidewire. Under no circumstances should the stiff end of the guidewire be allowed to deform the actual pigtail tip or to protrude from the end hole of the catheter, risking perforation. If the catheter is of a pigtail ring-up variety, and advancement into the pulmonary outflow tract is difficult, the soft end of a 3-mm J-wire may be advanced through the end hole, providing guidance to the catheter into the pulmonary artery. Once in the main pulmonary artery, the catheter can be directed into the right or left pulmonary artery using direct catheter torque or using the guidewire to direct the tip.

Straight pigtail catheters may be directed into the pulmonary artery using a curved wire or a specialized tip-deflecting wire, the curve of which may be controlled by the operator. The deflector should never be advanced to straighten the pigtail or to protrude from the catheter end hole. The wire is first deflected to direct the catheter toward the tricuspid valve, and the catheter is advanced over the wire deflector, keeping the latter fixed as a guide. After the catheter crosses the tricuspid valve, the wire should be relaxed and the catheter withdrawn slightly to allow it to straighten and engage the pulmonary outflow tract. The relaxed wire can be used to stiffen and support the catheter as it is advanced into the main pulmonary artery, then deflected to assist in selecting the right or left pulmonary artery.

Flow-directed balloon catheters with multiple side holes (e.g., Berman catheter; Arrow International, Inc., Reading, PA) are available with sufficient strength and lumenal diameter for pulmonary angiography. The distal balloon follows blood flow, facilitating placement in the pulmonary artery. When placed from the femoral approach, clockwise rotation while the catheter is just across the tricuspid valve usually diverts it cranially for advancement into the pulmonary outflow tract. Although it may be difficult to direct into the arterial segments of interest, some selectivity in positioning a balloon-tipped catheter may be achieved by varying the volume of air used to inflate the balloon during passage, or by turning the patient onto his or her side. Pulmonary angiography is performed with the catheter free in a large vascular branch and the balloon deflated. A Swan-Ganz (Baxter Healthcare Corp., Irvine, CA) catheter may be used for segmental and subsegmental occlusion pulmonary angiography, performed with the balloon inflated. However, care must be taken to inject only small volumes of contrast media at slow injection rates, because excessive injection may result in Swan-Ganz catheter rupture or rupture of the occluded pulmonary arterial segment.

Contrast Injection and Imaging

Typical initial contrast injection rates for unilateral left main or right main pulmonary arteriography are 20 to 25 mL/sec for a total of 40 to 50 mL. Injection rates should be tailored to the individual patient. For example, lesser injection rates and total volumes should be used in patients with reduced cardiac output. Subsequent injection rates are adjusted based on initial visualization and the degree of selectivity of the injection. For wedge pulmonary angiography, gentle hand injection is performed during imaging, monitoring the image and limiting contrast injection to that needed to fill the arterial segment. The balloon should be deflated immediately upon completion of imaging, and contrast clearance should be verified.

Pulmonary angiography is most commonly performed using rapid-sequence cut-film imaging. A typical filming sequence is 3 films/sec × 3 seconds; 1 film/sec × 4 seconds; and 1 film every other second for 6 seconds. Cineangiography is generally less desirable, because it does not provide for comparable resolution with a sufficiently large field of view. For example, standard cut-film systems with high-speed image-intensifying screens typically provide resolution of 6 to 8 line-pairs per mm (lpm). A 9-inch image intensifier in a cineradiographic unit typically provides resolution of only 3.5 to 4.0 lpm. A 9-inch image intensifier provides marginal field size for single-lung pulmonary angiography. Improved resolution is available with smaller image intensifiers, but with unacceptable sacrifice in field size.

The suspected side of the pulmonary embolism should be studied first, with injections performed in at least two projections. Initial biplane imaging may typically be performed by using the ipsilateral posterior oblique projection and either the opposite oblique or an anteroposterior projection. Targeted magnification runs may then be performed in areas of special interest, based on findings on initial runs or on lung scan, for better visualization of small vessels, using selective contrast injection and smaller focal spot imaging. In the absence of clinical contraindications, both lungs should be imaged, providing a baseline for future studies. Documentation of baseline findings is important when a patient represents with the presumptive diagnosis of recurrent pulmonary embolism, and inferior vena cava filter or interruption is being considered.

Interpretation

Emboli as small as 1 mm can be detected on serial radiographs when selective injections are performed. Interobserver agreement of interpretation of pulmonary angiograms ranges from 80% to 95%, with most disagreement occurring with pulmonary emboli in subsegmental vessels.

Radiographic signs of acute pulmonary embolism include acute, abrupt cutoff of branching vessels and intraluminal filling defects (Fig 6-9) outlined with a shell of contrast ("railroad tracks"). Massive central emboli and "saddle"

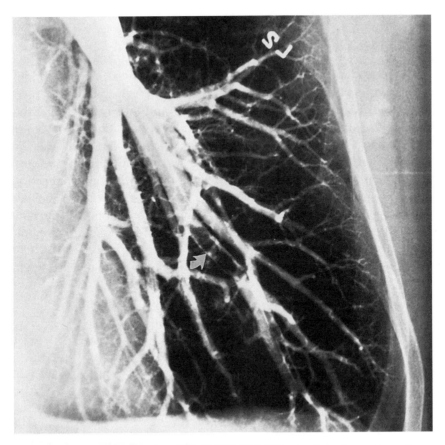

Figure 6-9 Pulmonary angiogram showing evidence of a pulmonary embolus (filling defect, arrow).

emboli (emboli occluding the main pulmonary artery from right to left) are more easily, but less commonly, seen. The so-called secondary signs of pulmonary embolism, such as reduced regional vascularity, are not reliable.

Several common findings must be recognized as artifacts and distinguished from pulmonary emboli: (1) layering artifacts due to layering of contrast media along posterior vessel walls with unopacified blood flowing above; (2) streaming artifacts due to inflow of unopacified blood into a contrast-filled vessel (i.e., from collateral vessels); (3) overlapping and parallel vessels, with differences in contrast density, creating "pseudo" emboli; (4) atelectasis causing vascular crowding; and (5) normal hypovascularity about the lingula, left mid-lung, and right minor fissure.

Diagnosis of chronic pulmonary emboli is more difficult. Auger et al. described the following signs of chronic pulmonary emboli: "pouching" of the pulmonary artery; webs or bands across lobar or segmental arteries; intimal irregularity secondary to thrombus lining pulmonary artery walls; abrupt vessel narrowing due to recanalization effects; concentric mural thrombus, appearing as contraction of the pulmonary artery; and frank vessel obstruction.

Digital Subtraction Pulmonary Angiography

A number of attempts have been made to perform pulmonary angiography using peripheral injection of contrast material and digital subtraction angiography (see preceding section). With digital angiography, the resolution of the image is limited by the image matrix. Digital subtraction studies performed using a 512×512 matrix and injection of contrast material into the vena cava or right atrium reliably detected pulmonary emboli only within the first three pulmonary arterial branchings. Small vessel visualization may be enhanced using edge-enhancement algorithms. Images may be substantially degraded by motion, resulting in misregistration between the contrast-containing image and the mask. The diagnostic potential of digital subtraction angiography should be enhanced by newer technology permitting matrix sizes of 1024×1024 or greater, although clinical data are not yet available to validate this presumption.

SELECTED READINGS

Radiographic Principles

Moore RJ. Imaging principles of cardiac angiography. Rockville, MD: Aspen, 1990.

Radiographic Contrast Material

American College of Cardiology Cardiovascular Imaging Committee. Use of nonionic or low osmolar contrast agents in cardiovascular procedures. J Am Coll Cardiol 1993; 21:269–273.

Barrett BJ, Carlisle EJ. Metaanalysis of the relative nephrotoxicity of high- and low-osmolality iodinated contrast media. Radiology 1993;188:171–178.

Barrett BJ, Parfrey PS. Prevention of nephrotoxicity induced by radiocontrast agents. N Engl J Med 1994;331:1449–1450. Editorial.

Benotti JR. The comparative effects of ionic versus nonionic agents in cardiac catheterization. Invest Radiol 1988;23(suppl 2):366–373.

Bettmann MA. Radiographic contrast agents—a perspective. N Engl J Med 1987; 317:891–893.

Brezis M, Epstein FH. A closer look at radiocontrast-induced nephropathy. N Engl J Med 1989;320:179–181. Editorial.

Bush WH, Swanson DP. Acute reactions to intravascular contrast media: types, risk factors, recognition, and specific treatment. Am J Roentgenol 1991;157:1153–1161.

Greenberger PA, Patterson R. The prevention of immediate generalized reactions to radiocontrast media in high-risk patients. J Allergy Clin Immunol 1991;87:867–872.

Hill JA. Issues in selecting a contrast agent for the cardiac catheterization laboratory. Invest Radiol 1991;28(suppl 4):5–10.

Lasser EC, Berry CC, Talner LB, et al. Pretreatment with corticosteroids to alleviate reactions to intravenous contrast material. N Engl J Med 1987;317:845–849.

Lieberman P. Anaphylactoid reactions to radiocontrast material. Ann Allergy 1991; 67:91–100.

McClennan BL. Adverse reactions to iodinated contrast media: recognition and response. Invest Radiol 1994;29(suppl 1):46–50.

Porter GA. Contrast medium-associated nephropathy: recognition and management. Invest Radiol 1993;28(suppl 4):11–18.

Solomon R, Werner C, Mann D, et al. Effects of saline, mannitol, and furosemide on acute decreases in renal function induced by radiocontrast agents. N Engl J Med 1994;331:1416–1420.

Tommaso C. Selection of angiographic contrast media: nonionic vs. ionic. Primary Cardiol 1993;19:11–18.

Weisberg LS, Kurnik PB, Kurnik BRC. Risk of radiocontrast nephropathy in patients with and without diabetes mellitus. Kidney Int 1994;45:259–265.

Left Ventriculography

Als AV, Paulin S, Aroesty JM. Biplane angiographic oblique and half-axial left anterior oblique technique. Radiology 1978;126:511–514.

Arvidsson H. Angiocardiographic determinations of left ventricular volume. Acta Radiol [Diagn] 1961;56:321–339.

Bhargava V, Warren S, Vieweg WVR, Shabetai R. Quantitation of left ventricular wall motion in normal subjects: comparison of various methods. Cathet Cardiovasc Diagn 1980;6:7–16.

Brower RW. Evaluation of pattern recognition rules for the apex of the heart. Cathet Cardiovasc Diagn 1980;6:145–157.

Chaitman BR, Bristow JD, Rahimtoola SH. Left ventricular wall motion assessed by using fixed external reference systems. Circulation 1973;48:1043–1054.

Chaitman BR, DeMots H, Bristow JD, et al. Objective and subjective analysis of left ventricular angiograms. Circulation 1975;52:420–425.

Chapman CB, Baker O, Mitchell JH, Collier RG. Experiences with a cinefluorographic method for measuring ventricular volume. Am J Cardiol 1966;18:25–30.

Chapman CB, Baker O, Reynolds J, Bonte FJ. Use of biplane cinefluorography for measurement of ventricular volume. Circulation 1958;18:1105–1117.

Clayton PD, Jeppson GM, Klausner SC. Should a fixed external reference system be used to analyze left ventricular wall motion? Circulation 1982;65:1518–1521.

Dodge HT, Sandler H, Ballew DW, Lord JD. The use of biplane angiocardiography for the measurement of left ventricular volume in man. Am Heart J 1960;60:762–776.

Dodge HT, Sandler H, Baxley WA, Hawley RR. Usefulness and limitations of radiographic methods for determining left ventricular volume. Am J Cardiol 1966; 18:10–24.

Fujita M, Sasayama S, Kawai C, et al. Automatic processing of cineventriculograms for analysis of regional myocardial function. Circulation 1981;63:1065–1074.

Gelberg HJ, Brundage BH, Glantz S, Parmley WW. Quantitative left ventricular wall motion analysis: a comparison of area, chord, and radial methods. Circulation 1979; 59:991–1000.

Goodyer AVN, Langou RA. The multicentric character of normal left ventricular wall motion. Implications for the evaluation of regional wall motion abnormalities by contrast angiography. Cathet Cardiovasc Diagn 1982;8:225–232.

Greene DG, Carlisle R, Grant C, Bunnell IL. Estimation of left ventricular volume by one-plane cineangiography. Circulation 1967;35:61–69.

Grossman W. Assessment of regional myocardial function. J Am Coll Cardiol 1986; 7:327–328.

Ingels NB, Daughters GT, Stinson EB, Alderman EL. Evaluation of methods for quantitating left ventricular segmental wall motion in man using myocardial markers as a standard. Circulation 1980;61:966–972.

Leighton RF, Wilt AA, Lewis RP. Detection of hypokinesis by a quantitative analysis of left ventricular cineangiograms. Circulation 1974;50:121–127.

Lopez JF, Hanson S, Orchard RC, Tan L. Quantification of mitral valvular incompetence. Cathet Cardiovasc Diagn 1985;11:139–152.

Mathey DG, Sheehan FH, Schofer J, Dodge HT. Time from onset of symptoms to thrombolytic therapy: a major determinant of myocardial salvage in patients with acute transmural infarction. J Am Coll Cardiol 1985;6:518–525.

McDonald IG. The shape and movements of the human left ventricle during systole. Am J Cardiol 1970;26:221–230.

Rackley CE. Value of ventriculography in cardiac funtion and diagnosis. In: Brest AN, ed. Cardiovascular clinics: diagnostic methods in cardiology. Philadelphia: F.A. Davis, 1975:283–296.

Rogers WJ, Smith RL, Bream PR, et al. Quantitative axial oblique contrast left ventriculography: validation of the method by demonstrating improved visualization of regional motion and mitral valve function with accurate volume determinations. Am Heart J 1982;103:185–194.

Sandler H, Dodge HT. The use of single plane angiocardiograms for the calculation of left ventricular volume in man. Am Heart J 1968;75:325–334.

Sandler H, Dodge HT, Hay RE, Rackley CE. Quantitation of valvular insufficiency in man by angiocardiography. Am Heart J 1963;65:501–513.

Sasayama S, Nonogi H, Fujita M, et al. Analysis of asynchronous wall motion by regional pressure-length loops in patients with coronary artery disease. J Am Coll Cardiol 1984;4:259–267.

Sheehan FH, Bolson EL, Dodge HT, et al. Advantages and applications of the centerline method for characterizing regional ventricular funtion. Circulation 1986; 74:293–305.

Sheehan FH, Mathey DG, Schofer J, et al. Effect of interventions in salvaging left ventricular function in acute myocardial infarction: a study of intracoronary streptokinase. Am J Cardiol 1983;52:431–438.

Sheehan FH, Stewart DK, Dodge HT, et al. Variability in the measurement of regional left ventricular wall motion from contrast angiograms. Circulation 1983;68:550–559.

Slager CJ, Hooghoudt TEH, Serruys PW, et al. Quantitative assessment of regional left ventricular motion using endocardial landmarks. J Am Coll Cardiol 1986;7:317–326.

Sniderman AD, Marpole D, Fallen EL. Regional contraction patterns in the normal and ischemic left ventricle in man. Am J Cardiol 1973;31:484–489.

Tzivoni D, Diamond G, Pichler M, et al. Analysis of regional ischemic left ventricular dysfunction by quantitative cineangiography. Circulation 1979;60:1278–1283.

Wexler LF, Lesperance JL, Ryan TJ, et al. Interobserver variability in interpreting contrast left ventriculograms. Cathet Cardiovasc Diagn 1982;8:341–355.

Zir LM, Miller SW, Dinsmore RE, et al. Interobserver variability in coronary angiography. Circulation 1976;53:627–632.

Hypertrophic Disease and Measurement of Left Ventricular Mass

Adelman AG, McLoughlin MJ, Marquis Y, et al. Left ventricular cineangiographic observations in muscular subaortic stenosis. Am J Cardiol 1969;24:689–697.

Braunwald EB, Morrow AG, Cornell WP, et al. Clinical, hemodynamic and angiographic manifestations. Am J Med 1960;29:924–945.

de Simone G, DiLorenzo L, Costantino G, et al. Supernormal contractility in primary hypertension without left ventricular hypertrophy. Hypertension 1988;2:457.

Kennedy JW, Baxley WA, Figley MM, et al. Quantitative angiocardiography I. The normal left ventricle in man. Circulation 1966;34:272–278.

Leman RB, Spinale FG, Dorn GW, et al. Supernormal ejection performance is isolated to the ipsilateral congenitally pressure-overloaded ventricle. J Am Coll Cardiol 1989; 13:1314.

Maron BJ, Bonow RO, Cannon RO, et al. Interrelations of clinical manifestations, pathophysiology, and therapy. N Engl J Med 1987;316:780–789.

Rackley CE, Dodge HT, Coble YD, Hay RE. A method for determining left ventricular mass in man. Circulation 1964;29:666–671.

Simon AL, Ross J, Gault JH. Angiographic anatomy of the left ventricle and mitral valve in idiopathic hypertrophic subaortic stenosis. Circulation 1967;36:852–867.

Right Ventriculography

Arcilla RA, Tsai P, Thilenius O, Ranniger K. Angiographic method for volume estimation of right and left ventricles. Chest 1970;60:446–454.

Baker BJ, Wilen MM, Boyd CM, et al. Relation of right ventricular ejection fraction to exercise capacity in chronic left ventricular failure. Am J Cardiol 1984;54:596.

Cohen M, Fuster V. What do we gain from the analysis of right ventricular function? J Am Coll Cardiol 1984;3:1082–1084.

Cohen M, Monsen C, Francis X, et al. Comparison of single plane videodensitometry-based right ventricular ejection fraction in right and left anterior oblique views to biplane geometry-based right ventricular ejection fraction. J Am Coll Cardiol 1987; 10:150–155.

Ferlinz J. Measurements of right ventricular volumes in man from single plane cine-angiograms. Am Heart J 1977;94:87–90.

Ferlinz J. Right ventricular function in adult cardiovascular disease. Prog Cardiovasc Dis 1982;25:225–267.

Ferlinz J, Gorlin R, Cohn PF, Herman MV. Right ventricular performance in patients with coronary artery disease. Circulation 1975;52:608–615.

Gentzler RD, Briselli MF, Gault JH. Angiographic estimation of right ventricular volume in man. Circulation 1974;50:324–330.

Goldman ME. Emerging importance of the right ventricle. J Am Coll Cardiol 1985; 5:925–927.

Horn V, Mullins CB, Saffer SI, et al. A comparison of mathematical models for estimating right ventricular volumes in animals and man. Clin Cardiol 1979;2:341–347.

Konstam MA, Cohen SR, Salem DN, et al. Comparison of left and right ventricular end-systolic pressure-volume relations in congestive heart failure. J Am Coll Cardiol 1985; 5:1326–1334

Konstam MA, Idoine J, Wynne J, et al. Right ventricular function in pulmonary hypertensive adults with and without atrial septal defects. Am J Cardiol 1983;51: 1144–1148.

Konstam MA, Pandian N. Assessment of right ventricular funtion. In: Konstam, MA, Isner JM, eds. The right ventricle. Boston: Kluwer Academic, 1988:1–15.

Lange PE, Budach W, Radtke W, et al. Right ventricular imaging with digital subtraction angiocardiography using intraventricular contrast injection. Am J Cardiol 1984; 54:839-842.

Morrison D, Goldman S, Wright AL, et al. The effect of pulmonary hypertension on systolic function of the right ventricle. Chest 1983;84:248–257.

Polak JF, Holman BL, Wynne J, Colucci WS. Right ventricular ejection fraction: an indicator of increased mortality in patients with congestive heart failure associated with coronary artery disease. J Am Coll Cardiol 1983;2:217–224.

Rappaport E, Wong M, Ferguson RE, et al. Right ventricular volumes in patients with and without heart failure. Circulation 1965;31:531–541.

Aortography

Adachi H, Omoto R, Kyo S, et al. Emergency surgical intervention of acute aortic dissection with the rapid diagnosis by transesophageal echocardiography. Circulation 1991;84(suppl III):14–19.

Arciniegas JG, Soto B, Little WC, Papapietro SE. Cineangiography in the diagnosis of aortic dissection. Am J Cardiol 1981;47:890–894.

Arvidsson H, Karnell J. Quantitative assessment of mitral and aortic insufficiency by angiocardiography. Acta Radiol [Diagn] 1964;2:105–119.

Ballal RS, Nanda NC, Gatewood R, et al. Usefulness of transesophageal echocardiography in assessment of aortic dissection. Circulation 1991;84:1903–1914.

Baron MG. Angiocardiographic evaluation of valvular insufficiency. Circulation 1971;43:599–605.

Beachley MC, Ranniger K, Roth F-J. Roentgenographic evaluation of dissecting aneurysms of the aorta. Radiology 1974;121:617–625.

Blanchard DG, Kimura BJ, Dittrich HC, DeMaria AN. Transesophageal echocardiography of the aorta. JAMA 1994;272:546–551.

Carlsson E, Gross R, Holt G. The radiological diagnosis of cardiac valvar insufficiencies. Circulation 1977;55:921–933.

Cigarroa JE, Isselbacher EM, DeSanctis RW, Eagle KA. Diagnostic imaging in the evaluation of suspected aortic dissection: old standards and new directions. N Engl J Med 1993;328:35–43.

Ciobanu M, Abbasi AS, Allen M, et al. Pulsed Doppler echocardiography in the diagnosis and estimation of severity of aortic insufficiency. Am J Cardiol 1982;49:339–343.

Crawford ES. The diagnosis and management of aortic dissection. JAMA 1990;264:2537–2541.

Crawford ES, Svenson LG, Coselli JS, et al. Surgical treatment of aneurysm and/or dissection of the ascending aorta, transverse aortic arch, and ascending aorta and transverse aortic arch: factors influencing survival in 717 patients. J Thorac Cardiovasc Surg 1989;98:659–674.

Croft CH, Lipscomb K, Mathis K, et al. Limitations of qualitative angiographic grading in aortic or mitral regurgitation. Am J Cardiol 1984;53:1593–1598.

Dailey PO, Trueblood HW, Stinson EB, et al. Management of acute aortic dissections. Ann Thorac Surg 1970;10:237–247.

De Bakey ME, Henly WS, Cooley DA, et al. Surgical management of dissecting aneurysms of the aorta. J Thorac Cardiovasc Surg 1965;49:130–149.

DeSanctis RW, Doroghazi RM, Austen WG, Buckley MJ. Aortic dissection. N Engl J Med 1987;317:1060–1067.

Eagle KA, DeSanctis RW. Diseases of the aorta. In: Braunwald, ed., Heart disease, a textbook of cardiovascular medicine. Philadelphia: Saunders, 1988:1546–1576.

Eagle KA, Quertermous T, Kritzer GA, et al. Spectrum of conditions initially suggesting acute aortic dissection but with negative aortograms. Am J Cardiol 1986;57:322–326.

Erbel R, Börner N, Steller D, et al. Detection of aortic dissection by transesophageal echocardiography. Br Heart J 1987;58:45–51.

Godwin JD, Herfkens RL, Skiöldebrand CG, et al. Evaluation of dissections and aneurysms of the thoracic aorta by conventional and dynamic CT scanning. Radiology 1980;136:125–133.

Gott VL, Pyeritz RE, Magovern GJ, Jr, et al. Surgical treatment of aneurysms of the ascending aorta in the Marfan syndrome: results of composite-graft repair in 50 patients. N Engl J Med 1986;314:1070–1074.

Gutierrez FR, Gowda S, Ludbrook PA, McKnight RC. Cineangiography in the diagnosis and evaluation of aortic dissention. Radiology 1980;135:759–761.

Hart WL, Berman EJ, LaCom RJ. Hazard of retrograde aortography in dissecting aneurysm. Circulation 1963;27:1140–1142.

Hunt D, Baxley WA, Kennedy JW, et al. Quantitative evaluation of cineaortography in the assessment of aortic regurgitation. Am J Cardiol 1973;31:696–700.

Khandheria BK. Aortic dissection: the last frontier. Circulation 1993;87:1765–1768. Editorial.

Landtman M, Kivisaari L, Standertskjöld-Nordenstam CG, Taavitsainen M. Computed tomography in pre- and postoperative evaluation of aortic dissection. Acta Radiol [Diagn] 1986;27:273–278.

Lehman JS, Boyle JJ, Debbas JN. Quantitation of aortic valvular insufficiency by catheter thoracic aortography. Radiology 1962;79:361–369.

Levine HJ, Gaasch WH. Ratio of regurgitant volume to end-diastolic volume: a major determinant of ventricular response to surgical correction of chronic volume overload. Am J Cardiol 1983;52:406–410.

Mohiaddin RH, Longmore DB. Functional aspects of cardiovascular nuclear magnetic resonance imaging: techniques and application. Circulation 1993;88:264–281.

Nienaber CA, Spielmann RP, von Kodolitsch Y, et al. Diagnosis of thoracic aortic dissection: magnetic resonance imaging versus transesophageal echocardiography. Circulation 1992;85:434–447.

Nienaber CA, von Kodolitsch Y, Nicolas V, et al. The diagnosis of thoracic aortic dissection by noninvasive imaging procedures. N Engl J Med 1993;328:1–9.

Perry GJ, Helmcke F, Nanda NC, et al. Evaluation of aortic insufficiency by Doppler color flow mapping. J Am Coll Cardiol 1987;9:952–959.

Pressler V, McNamara JJ. Thoracic aortic aneurysm, natural history and treatment. J Thorac Cardiovasc Surg 1980;79:489–498.

Pressler V, McNamara JJ. Aneurysm of the thoracic aorta, review of 260 cases. J Thorac Cardiovasc Surg 1985;89:50–54.

Pyeritz RE, McKusick VA. The Marfan syndrome: diagnosis and management. N Engl J Med 1979;300:772–777.

Reimold SC, Ganz P, Bittl JA, et al. Effective aortic regurgitant orifice area: description of a method based on the conservation of mass. J Am Coll Cardiol 1991;18:761–768.

Sandler H, Dodge HT, Hay RE, Rackley CE. Quantitation of valvular insufficiency in man by angiocardiography. Am Heart J 1963;65:501–513.

Sellers RD, Levy MJ, Amplatz K, Lillehei CW. Left retrograde cardioangiography in acquired cardiac disease. Technic, indications and interpretations in 700 cases. Am J Cardiol 1964;14:437–477.

Shuford WH, Sybers RG, Weens HS. Problems in the aortographic diagnosis of dissecting aneurysm of the aorta. N Engl J Med 1969;280:225–231.

Soto B, Harman MA, Ceballos R, Barcia A. Angiographic diagnosis of dissecting aneurysm of the aorta. Radiology 1972;116:146–154.

Svensson LG, Crawford S, Coselli JS, et al. Impact of cardiovascular operation on survival in the Marfan patient. Circulation 1989;80(suppl I):233–242.

Thorsen MK, San Dretto MA, Lawson TL, et al. Dissecting aortic aneurysms: accuracy of computed tomographic diagnosis. Radiology 1983;148:773–777.

White RD, Lipton MJ, Higgins CB, et al. Noninvasive evaluation of suspected thoracic aortic disease by contrast-enhanced computed tomography. Am J Cardiol 1986;57:282–290.

Pulmonary Angiography

A Collaborative Study by the PIOPED Investigators. Value of the ventilation/perfusion scan in acute pulmonary embolism: results of the Prospective Investigation of Pulmonary Embolism Diagnosis (PIOPED). JAMA 1990;263:2753–2759.

Auger WR, Fedullo PF, Moser KM, et al. Chronic major-vessel thromboembolic pulmonary artery obstruction: appearance at angiography. Radiology 1992;182:393–398.

Baltaxe HA, Levin DC. A modified technique of pulmonary arteriography. Radiology 1987;100:425–427.

Beachley MC, Tisnado J, Konerding K, Vines FS. Alternate technique for pulmonary arteriography. Am J Roentgenol 1980;134:195–196.

Bookstein JJ. Segmental arteriography in pulmonary embolism. Radiology 1969;93:1007–1012.

Bookstein JJ, Feigin DS, Seo KW, Alazraki NP. Diagnosis of pulmonary embolism. Radiology 1980;136:15–23.

Grollman JH Jr, Gyepes MT, Helmer E. Transfemoral selective bilateral pulmonary arteriography with a pulmonary-artery-seeking catheter. Radiology 1970;96:202–204.

Novelline RA, Baltlarwich OH, Athanasoulis CA, et al. The clinical course of patients with suspected pulmonary embolism and a negative pulmonary arteriogram. Radiology 1978;126:561–567.

Pond GD. Pulmonary digital subtraction angiography. Radiol Clin of North Am 1985;23:243–260.

Quinn MF, Lundell CJ, Klotz TA, et al. Reliability of selective pulmonary arteriography in the diagnosis of pulmonary embolism. Am J Roentgenol 1987;149:469–471.

Reilley RF, Smith CW, Price RR, et al. Digital subtraction angiography: limitations for the detection of pulmonary embolism. Radiology 1983;149:379–382.

Sostman HD, Rapoport S, Gottschalk A, Greenspan RH. Imaging of pulmonary embolism. Invest Radiol 1986;21:443–454.

Stein PD, Athanasoulis C, Alavi A, et al. Complications and validity of pulmonary angiography in acute pulmonary embolism. Circulation 1992;85:462–468.

Tempkin DL, Ladika JE. New catheter design and placement techniques for pulmonary arteriography. Radiology 1987;163:275–276.

7

CORONARY ARTERIOGRAPHY

Marc J. Schweiger

T HE MOST FREQUENTLY performed procedure in the catheterization laboratory is coronary arteriography. Basic principles and techniques for this procedure are presented in this chapter. We offer one caution: Although there are some technical approaches that are accepted universally, most catheterization laboratory operators have developed unique practical approaches for optimally performing the procedure. Most catheterization laboratories also have developed certain "tried and true" protocols for optimizing efficacy in their particular setting. This diversity emphasizes the fact that more than one technical approach to coronary arteriography may be effective. Thus, the practical suggestions in this chapter represent only some of many acceptable approaches.

Precatheterization Evaluation

All patients require a thorough history and physical examination prior to angiography. Symptoms of claudication, together with the physical examination, influence the site of arterial access. The severity of the patient's symptoms may influence the order in which the procedure is performed and the contrast agent used (see Chapter 16). For patients on heparin, the decision to discontinue it prior to the procedure, decrease the dose, or continue at full dose depends to a great extent on the index of suspicion of critical coronary disease.

Knowledge of allergies to medicines and contrast agents is mandatory. Ideally, in patients previously studied, the coronary angiogram should be reviewed. If that is not possible, the catheterization report should be read, searching particularly for any technical difficulties encountered (e.g., difficulty in seating a standard catheter). The patient should be asked about the feasibility of lying in the supine position for several hours during and after the catheterization. Potential difficulties that may be anticipated include severe lower back pain and inability to void in the supine position.

The physical examination should be thorough, with specific attention paid to the cardiovascular examination and aspects that may pose technical problems. Any signs of valvular, congenital, or myopathic disease must be evaluated carefully. Blood pressure should be obtained in both arms, carotid arteries auscultated for bruits, the abdomen palpated for aortic aneurysm, brachial and femoral pulses palpated and auscultated as potential access sites, and other peripheral pulses (radial, dorsalis pedis, posterior tibial) palpated to compare postcatheterization with this baseline examination.

Laboratory tests that should be performed prior to coronary angiography include a complete blood count, electrolytes, BUN, and creatinine. Prothrombin time (PT) and partial thromboplastin time (PTT) should be obtained if there are any questions regarding the patient's bleeding risk. An ECG should be performed proximate (within 2–4 weeks) to an elective procedure, and a chest x-ray, if not previously obtained.

It is the physician's responsibility to discuss the procedure with the patient. Patients are typically anxious prior to catheterization. Although risks of the procedure must be frankly and clearly discussed, an attempt should also be made to reassure patients. It is useful to remind patients that they will be awake, although sedated, and that any problems that may arise should be brought to the attention of the laboratory staff. Patients should be told that they may be asked to cough during coronary injections. They should be instructed on the coughing technique prior to the actual procedure. Telling them the procedural volume of the laboratory and operator tends to reinforce the routine nature of the procedure and often helps to allay anxiety.

Before beginning the procedure, it is important to document in the medical record the indication for the procedure. When the operator is not the patients' primary cardiologist, he or she must assume the consultant's role in concurring that the procedure is truly indicated.

Technical Plan for Coronary Arteriography

A number of technical decisions need to be made prior to each procedure. These include site of vascular access (arm vs. leg), cutdown or percutaneous approach (if the brachial approach is used), sheath or sheathless vascular access, type of contrast agent, the order of the procedure (e.g., coronary arteriography first or after left ventriculography), catheter size, need for a right heart catheterization, and need to insert a temporary pacemaker.

Arm (Brachial Artery) or Leg (Femoral Artery) Approach?

This decision is often based on the experience of the operator and the laboratory. Both the percutaneous femoral (Judkins) approach and cutdown of the brachial artery (Sones) are acceptable methods if no contraindication exists in a particular individual. Patients with symptoms of leg claudication require careful auscultation of femoral pulses and palpation of distal pulses. In general, the triad of claudication, femoral bruit, and absent distal pulses in the affected limb precludes a femoral approach. A palpable femoral pulse with a bruit and present distal pulses in a patient with claudication do not necessarily preclude a femoral approach, but should increase the level of operator caution. The presence of an aorto-bifemoral graft does not rule out a percutaneous Judkins approach, but usually requires use of multiple dilators to gain satisfactory access. Patients with a femoral-popliteal graft usually cannot be approached via that limb. In many of these patients, an arm approach is preferable. Consultation with a vascular surgeon is often useful in these situations.

When approaching a patient from the arm, there are additional decisions to make. The operator experienced in the Sones technique will usually perform the procedure via the patient's right arm, utilizing a cutdown. The physician experienced in the femoral approach must decide which arm to use and whether to perform the procedure percutaneously or by cutdown. Approaching via the left arm allows the use of preformed catheters utilized for the standard femoral Judkins technique. Most laboratories, however, are set up as right-handed, and techniques for moving the table and monitor placement must be established beforehand to avoid confusion during the procedure itself. The techniques utilizing the right arm involve different catheters and more catheter manipulation. Physicians primarily experienced in the Judkins technique can, and probably should, perform their arm cases percutaneously to diminish the likelihood of vascular injury. It should be noted that in the era of outpatient catheterization, the arm approach allows patients to ambulate more quickly than the leg approach.

Sheath Versus Sheathless?

Most laboratories routinely use an arterial sheath to facilitate catheter exchange and minimize patient discomfort. In obese patients, the use of a sheath minimizes the risk of catheter kinking while going through the skin or subcutaneous tissue. Using direct vascular exposure (cutdown on the brachial artery) obviates, in most cases, the need for a sheath. Using a single catheter for the entire procedure (e.g., a multipurpose catheter for both coronaries and left ventricular injection) decreases the need for an arterial sheath.

Which Contrast Agent?

The operator must decide whether to utilize a standard ionic (high-osmolality) contrast agent or a low-osmolality agent, many of which are also non-ionic. The low-osmolality agents have been shown to decrease mild and moderate adverse reactions, including patient discomfort, with less derangement of electrocardiographic and hemodynamic parameters (see Chapter 6). They have not, however, been shown in most studies to affect long-term outcome, including adverse renal effects. They are considerably more expensive. There is also some concern that the non-ionic agents may be somewhat thrombogenic. We reserve use of low-osmolality agents for patients at high risk for adverse reactions, including patients with high-risk unstable angina, poor left ventricular function, older patients, and patients expected to receive a large volume of contrast agents. Angiography of internal mammary conduits is less uncomfortable with low-osmolality agents. These agents may be useful in the patient with a history of previous contrast sensitivity.

When to Use a Temporary Pacemaker?

The rule of thumb is to consider utilizing a temporary pacemaker upon entering the contralateral ventricle when a conduction delay is present. Therefore, a temporary pacemaker may be useful in a patient who has a right bundle branch block and is undergoing left ventriculography. Because the right coronary catheter will occasionally enter the left ventricle, it is often prudent to establish temporary pacemaking when performing coronary angiography in patients with a right bundle branch block. Patients with Mobitz 2 atrioventricular (AV) block and complete (third-degree) block should usually have a temporary pacemaker in place. In patients who cannot vigorously cough (somnolent, elderly, weak), use of nonionic dye or pretreatment with atropine also should be considered.

When to Perform a Right Heart Catheterization?

Right heart catheterization is usually not necessary in evaluating the patient with suspected or known coronary disease. The routine use of right heart catheterization with coronary angiography has been discouraged in the present health care environment, where rapid throughput and lowering of costs have gained increased importance. Right heart catheterization and cardiac output determination are indicated in coronary patients with poor left ventricular (LV) function and/or concomitant valvular, congenital, or myopathic heart disease.

What Order of the Procedure?

The clinical situation dictates whether coronary arteriography or left ventriculography is performed first. When severe three-vessel disease, left main, left main "equivalent," or other high-risk anatomy is suspected; when LV function is known to be highly impaired, as ascertained by noninvasive methods; or when the primary purpose of the catheterization is to visualize the coronary arteries, coronary arteriography should probably be performed first (see Chapter 16). Using a Judkins right coronary catheter, the operator may enter the left ventricle (LV) prior to coronary arteriography, permitting measurement of LV end-diastolic pressure. In the early days of coronary angiography, it was felt that left ventriculography should be performed first so that LV hemodynamics would not be affected by the contrast agent used in coronary injections and to observe regional wall motion prior to performing coronary angiography. This approach is often unnecessary in many patients in whom adequate noninvasive evaluation of ventricular function (e.g., echocardiography, radionuclide ventriculography) has been performed prior to catheterization.

Which Catheter Size?

The choice of catheter size is often a matter of physician experience and comfort. Larger-bore catheters (7 Fr or 8 Fr) are easier to manipulate in tortuous anatomy and may provide better coronary artery visualization under conditions of high flow (e.g., in patients with aortic insufficiency). Smaller catheters (5 and 6 Fr) probably decrease access-site vascular complications. As such, smaller catheters should be used routinely unless there is a good clinical reason to do otherwise.

Which Catheters to Use?

The choice of catheters depends on whether the case is being performed via the leg or arm (Fig 7-1). In patients undergoing catheterization from the leg or left arm, preformed Judkins catheters are often initially used. The primary bend is defined as the angle from tip to first bend. The secondary bend is the second bend from the tip. The primary bend on both left and right Judkins catheters is 90 degrees. The secondary bend is 180 degrees for the left and 30 degrees for the right. The left 4 catheter has a 4.2-cm arm between the primary and secondary bend, the 5 catheter has a 5.2-cm arm, and the 6 catheter has a 6.2-cm arm. The 4 size is typically used first and will successfully cannulate most vessels. In patients whose aortic root is known to be enlarged, the physician may choose a Judkins catheter with a larger secondary curve, either a 5 or 6 catheter. In patients with a smaller aortic root diameter, a catheter with a smaller arm between the primary and secondary bend, such as a Judkins 3.5, will often cannulate the vessel. The Judkins right 4 catheters are often success-

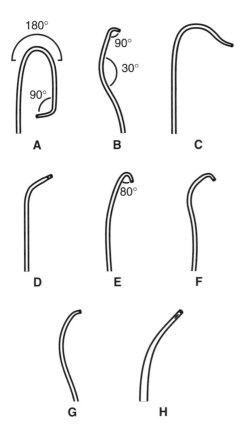

Figure 7-1 Shapes of commonly used catheters for coronary arteriography (see text for description of their uses). **(A)** Left Judkins catheter. The primary curve is 90 degrees and the secondary is 180 degrees. The difference in the length of the straight portion determines its number (3.5, 4, 5, 6). **(B)** Right Judkins catheter. The primary bend is 90 degrees and the secondary bend is 30 degrees. **(C)** Amplatz catheter. The prototypical shape is shown. The size of the secondary curve determines the number (AL1-AL3, AR1-AR3). The Castillo family of catheters (not shown) have a shape similar to the Amplatz but have a shorter shaft (80 cm) to be more easily used from the arm. **(D)** The multipurpose A2 (Schoonmaker-King) catheter has an end-hole and two side holes very close to the catheter tip. The A1 is identical, except that it has only a single end-hole. **(E)** Internal mammary catheter. **(F)** Left bypass graft catheter. **(G)** Right bypass graft catheter. **(H)** Sones catheter tip. The original Sones catheters were constructed with woven Dacron, which softens over time and allows the catheter to be shaped for an individual patient. These catheters are now available in plastics used in other catheters.

ful, even in cases in which a larger left Judkins catheter is needed. The Amplatz family of catheters are preformed alternatives and have progressively larger secondary curves. They are particularly useful in cannulating coronary ostia that are out of plane or have a high takeoff. They are useful in vessels with a short left main or separate ostia of the circumflex (CX) and left anterior descending (LAD). The Amplatz catheters can be used to cannulate both the left and right coronary artery (RCA). The catheters have a tendency to "dive" forward if the operator retracts the catheter after the vessel has been intubated. As a result, the coronary near or at its ostium may be injured or dissected. Thus, this type of catheter should be used only by experienced operators. Sones catheters, which are not preshaped, are used from the right arm and should be used by physicians experienced in the Sones technique. These catheters are usually not effective from the leg because they lose torque control after the turn in the aortic arch. The multipurpose catheter (Schoonmaker-King) may be used from the arm or the leg. It has the advantage of being able to be used for ventriculography as well as coronary arteriography. Considerable experience in catheter manipulation is necessary to use this catheter appropriately.

Patients with previous coronary bypass grafting may require use of additional catheters, though the Judkins right coronary catheter is frequently successful in cannulating venous and internal mammary conduits. The right coronary bypass graft–seeking catheter (which has a larger angle to the primary curve than the right Judkins catheter) is often successful in cannulating grafts when the right Judkins is unsuccessful. Amplatz and multipurpose catheters also may be used in difficult-to-cannulate grafts. The multipurpose catheter is particularly useful for the saphenous vein graft to the RCA because of the angle of the catheter and typical location of the saphenous vein takeoff on the right anterior aspect of the aorta. The internal mammary catheter has a longer tip and less of a primary bend (80 degrees) than the right Judkins catheter (90 degrees), and is generally the catheter of choice for internal mammary conduits. With use of these catheters, upwards of 98% of all patients requiring coronary arteriography will be successfully studied. Occasionally, a specialty catheter is required. The approach to angiography in patients with previous coronary bypass grafting is discussed in greater detail later in this chapter.

Coronary Anatomy and Angiographic Views

Knowledge of coronary anatomy, radiographic conventions (Fig 7-2), and the expected configuration of the vessel in various angiographic views is essential for the performance of coronary angiography. Views are described based on the position of the image intensification tube relative to the patient. Thus, if the tube is rotated to the left, the view is a left anterior oblique (LAO). If, for example, the tube is rotated so that it is above the level of the heart toward the left shoulder, it is classified as a cranial. The RCA emerges from the right coronary sinus, which is on the anterior surface of the aorta, and runs caudally and posteriorly in the atrioventricular sulcus between the right atrium and right ventricle (Figs 7-3 and 7-4 on pages 204–212). The first branch of the RCA is the conus branch. This vessel emerges at the level of the pulmonary valve and in about 50% of cases has a separate ostium located just anterior to the right coronary orifice. The conus branch is a frequent contributor of collaterals to the LAD and must be identified in cases in which the LAD appears occluded. The sinus node artery, which arises from the proximal RCA in approximately 60% of cases, is an atrial branch coursing superiorly and posteriorly. Alternatively, it may arise from the proximal CX artery in most of the remaining 40%. Multiple right ventricular (RV) branches (acute marginals) of the RCA course anteriorly. An RV branch at the distal end of the mid-RCA has been called the acute marginal (AM). The RCA is the dominant vessel in approximately 90% of cases. Dominance is defined by the vessel that supplies the posterior descending branch in the posterior interventricular groove and the posterolateral branches supplying the posterior left ventricle. When the RCA is dominant, it supplies

(text continues on page 213)

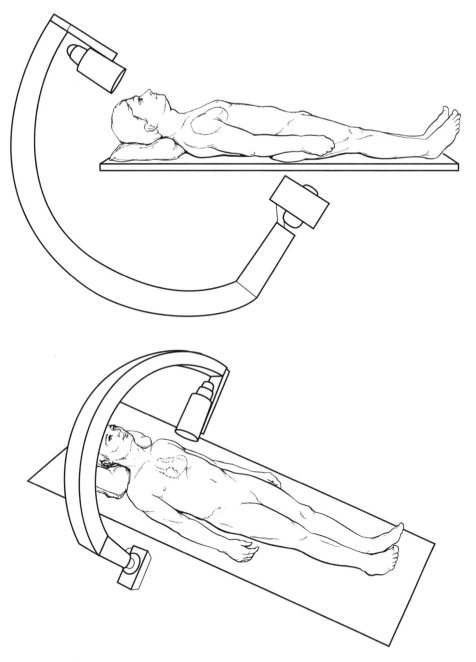

Figure 7-2 Radiographic conventions for angiography in the catheterization laboratory. The view is defined by the position of the image intensification (II) tube relative to the patient's heart (i.e., where the II tube "sees"
the heart). Thus, the right anterior oblique approach has the II tube on the
patient's right, and the left anterior oblique approach has the II tube on
the patient's left. Cranial angulation has the II tube angulated above the
heart, and caudal projection has the II tube below the heart.

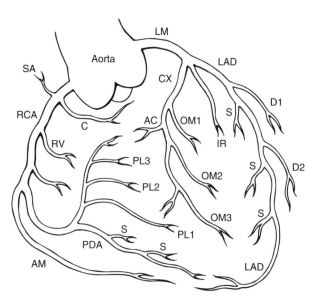

Figure 7-3 Coronary arteries in a right dominant circulation in an anteroposterior projection. The right coronary artery (RCA) trunk has 3 major divisions: proximal, mid, and distal. Proximal RCA originates at the ostium and ends after the first curve; the mid begins after the first curve and ends with the second curve and is usually considered the straight segment in right anterior oblique (RAO) view, and the distal RCA is the remainder of the trunk in the atrioventricular (AV) groove. The distal can be further subdivided into the segments before and after the branching of the posterior descending coronary artery (PDA). In a right dominant circulation, the posterior LV wall is vascularized by the posterolateral branches (PL), numbered sequentially. The sinus node artery (SA) arises from the RCA in approximately 60% of cases. It courses superiorly and to the right in this projection. Right ventricular branch(es) supply the free wall of the RV, and the RV branch(es) near the junction of mid- and distal RCA is also known as the acute marginal branch(es) (AM). Some have utilized the term *RV branches* to denote all vessels including the AM. The first LV branch of the RCA is the PDA, followed by the PLs (usually three). The conus (C) branch crosses the outflow tract of the RV. The left coronary artery (LCA) bifurcates after only a few millimeters in most individuals. This proximal part defines the left main (LM). The segment that travels in the left AV groove is defined as the circumflex (CX). Branches that supply the left lateral heart are named obtuse marginals (OM), which are numbered sequentially regardless of size. If the left coronary is dominant, then the first three LV branches from the CX are defined as OMs and the more distal branches are the PLs, with the posterior interventricular branch also named PDA. The segments of the CX may be named as proximal (up to and including the origin of the first large OM and distal CX past that point). The CX also usually supplies the left atrium. The left anterior descending (LAD) travels in the anterior interventricular groove and typically terminates at the apex. Proximal LAD may be defined as the segment from the LAD origin to the first septal perforator, even if this distance is short. This demarcation makes physiologic sense, because coronary occlusion before the first septal is typically more severe than after this branch. The distal point of the mid-LAD is less rigorously defined and is typically the location where the LAD dips downward on an RAO view. Alternatively, the distance between the distal point of the proximal LAD and the apex may be divided into two, defining the mid- and distal LAD. Branches of the LAD that supply the LV free wall are named "diagonals" and are numbered sequentially (D1, D2 . . .). If the LM trifurcates, the middle vessel, which typically runs a similar course to the first diagonal, is known as the ramus intermedius (IR). Septal perforators (S) arise from the LAD at right angles and are numbered sequentially (S1, S2 . . .).

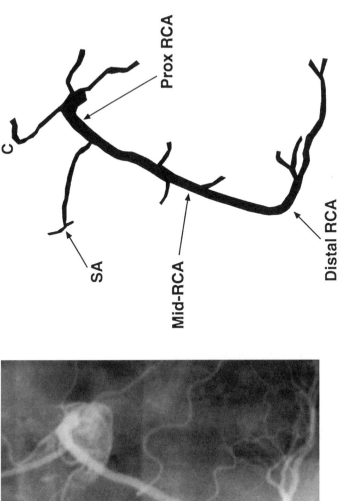

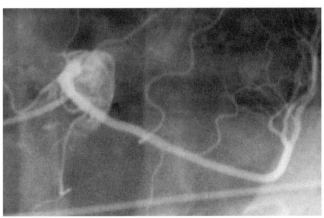

Figure 7-4 Angiographic appearance of the RCA. The angiographic frame is on the left and the schematic is on the right. Figure 7-4A: RAO (30 degrees). This angulation provides excellent visualization of the mid-RCA. This vessel appears angiographically normal with smooth walls without focal narrowing and tapering from the proximal to distal vessels. The LV branches are laid out in this view. Please note that in this and subsequent diagrams of the RCA, not all vessels are included or labeled. C, conus; SA, sinus node artery.

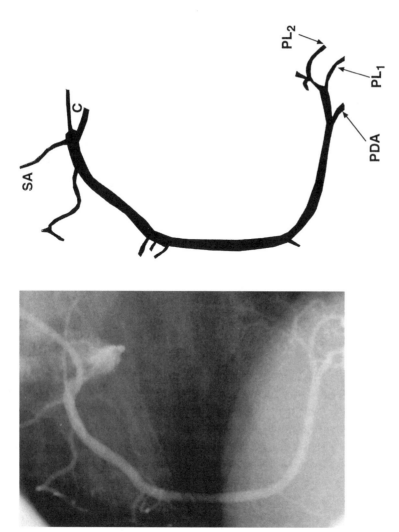

Figure 7-4B   The LAO (45 degrees) projection can clearly show the RCA itself. The LV branches themselves are often foreshortened and may be better appreciated on the RAO or LAO cranial. In this example, the RCA is not quite normal. The mid-RCA appears slightly narrower than the distal RCA. PDA, posterior descending artery; PL, posterolateral branch.

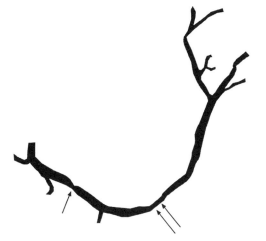

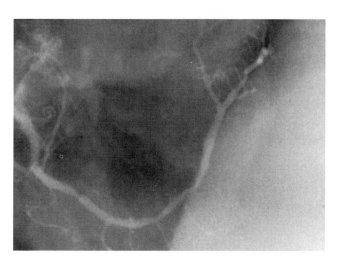

Figure 7-4C The LAO (45 degrees) cranial (30 degrees) is particularly good for locating the origins of the RCA branches and examining their courses. In this example, the RCA is "diffusely" diseased, with a roughened appearance to the lumen from proximal to distal RCA. The origins of the LV branches are well seen. The worst lesion is a 50% focal mid-RCA lesion (one arrow) and a longer (15–20 cm) 50% mid- to distal lesion (double arrows).

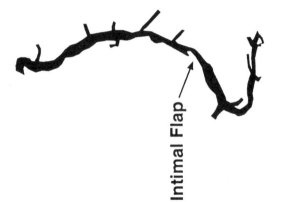

Intimal Flap

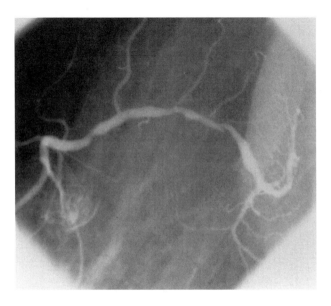

Figure 7-4D   RAO (80 degrees) in the same patient as Figure 7-4C. This special view was employed to demonstrate the impressive eccentricity of the lesion. Note that the more proximal lesion appears similar to the one in Figure 7-4C, but the more distal area shows a more impressive lesion with an intimal flap observed (arrow).

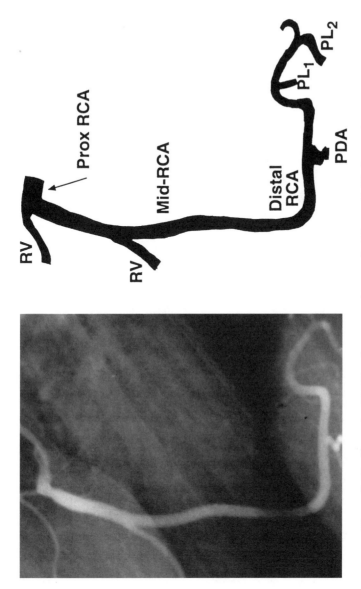

Figure 7-4E Lateral of RCA of same patient as in Figure 7-4B shows the RCA well to the crux.

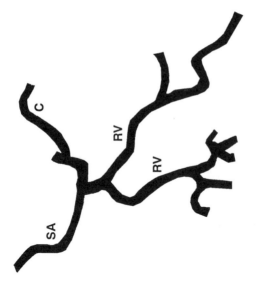

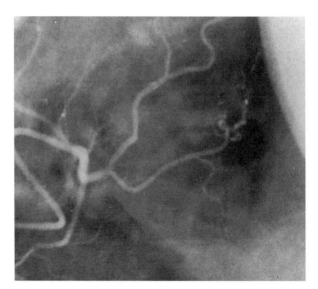

Figure 74F RAO of a nondominant RCA and (Fig 7-4G) LAO of nondominant RCA in the same patient. Note that the RCA terminates before the expected crossing of the interventricular and atrioventricular grooves.

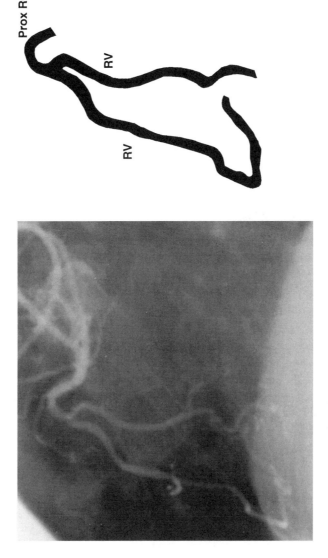

Prox RCA

RV

RV

Figure 7-4 G LAO of nondominant RCA in the same patient as shown in Fig 7-4F.

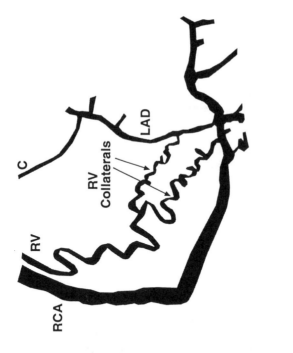

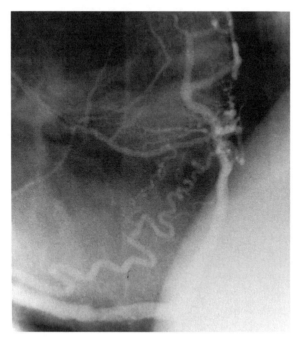

Figure 7-4H The RCA provides collaterals to the LAO via the conus (C) branch and an RV branch. Note the serpiginous configuration of the RV collateral. Such arterial curviness is typical for well-developed collaterals.

the posterior descending branch and continues to supply the posterior LV branches as well as the AV nodal artery. When the RCA is nondominant, it tapers and does not reach the crux of the heart (where the atrioventricular and interventricular sulcus cross). In a co-dominant system, portions of the posterior descending are supplied by both the RCA and CX coronary arteries, or the RCA supplies the posterior descending artery as its terminal branch. The CX supplies the posterolateral branches. The posterior interventricular septum may have a dual blood supply, with part of the posterior groove artery arising from the distal CX (supplying the interventricular septum at the crux) and the distal aspect supplied as a terminal branch of the RCA in a co-dominant system.

The proximal RCA as well as the posterior LV branches are usually well visualized in the LAO (typically 30- to 60-degree) projection (see Fig 7-4). Adding cranial angulation to the LAO brings out the bifurcation of the RCA into the posterior descending and LV branches (see Fig 7-4B). The right anterior oblique (RAO) (typically 30- to 60-degree) projection often clearly shows the mid-RCA and the posterior descending (see Fig 7-4C). Adding cranial angulation to the RAO lays out the area between the acute margin and crux. A left lateral view is often helpful in delineating the RCA up to the crux of the heart. It should be emphasized that although stereotyped angles may be performed on all patients, modified views may be required to optimally visualize a particular segment.

The left main coronary artery emerges from the left coronary sinus, which is on the left and somewhat lateral aspect of the aorta. The left main has a variable length (usually 1–10 mm), has no side branches, and bifurcates into the LAD and CX. Occasionally, there is no functional left main, and the LAD and CX arise from separate ostia. The LAD runs in the interventricular sulcus and generally terminates after curving around the apex of the heart. Occasionally, the LAD terminates proximal to the apex in patients with a long posterior descending artery from the RCA or CX. Conversely, in patients with a short posterior descending, the LAD may supply more of the inferoposterior interventricular septal surface of the heart. The LAD gives off diagonal branches that supply the free wall of the anterior left ventricle (Figs 7-3 and 7-5) and septal perforators that course deep into the interventricular septum (to the left in the LAO view and perpendicular in the RAO view). These branches are numbered sequentially from proximal to distal. The left main occasionally trifurcates with the middle branch supplying a part of the anterior wall of the left ventricle. This branch is known as the intermediate ramus.

The CX travels along the atrioventricular sulcus between the left atrium and left ventricle. If it reaches the crux of the heart to supply the posterior descending, it is classified as left dominant. If the CX supplies the posterior wall and the RCA provides a vessel in the posterior interventricular groove, the coronary circulation is considered co-dominant. Generally, the CX will be closer to

(text continues on page 222)

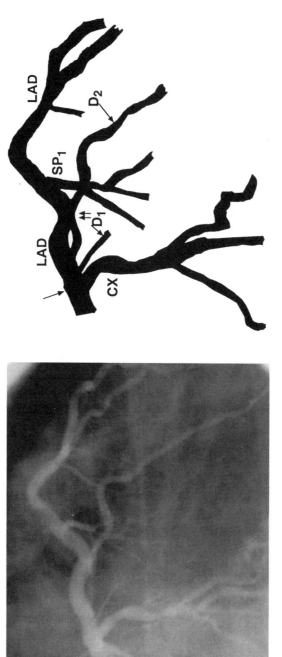

Figure 7-5 Angiographic appearances of the left coronary artery. Figure **7-5A: RAO.** This view may show the proximal and mid-LAD and the obtuse marginals (OMs). It tends to foreshorten the proximal CX. In this example, the mid-LAD is visualized without vessel overlap, but the proximal LAD is less unambiguously seen because the second diagonal (D₂) crosses the proximal LAD (single arrow) and obscures somewhat more distally the inferior border of the LAD (double arrows). There are vessel lesions in the proximal CX in at least two sites. Please note that in this and subsequent drawings, not all vessels are shown or labeled. SP1, first septal perforator artery.

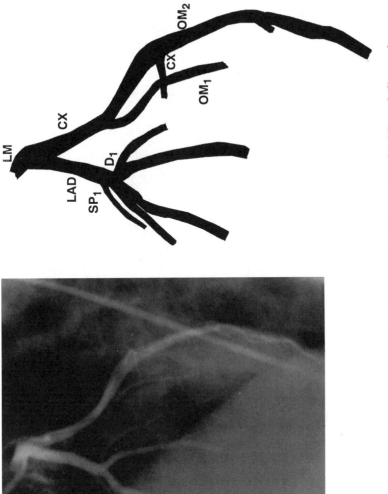

Figure 7-5B LAO with cranial tilt shows the proximal LAD and diagonal (D) branches, proximal intermediate branch (when present), and OMs. In this example, the proximal LAD, except for the ostial LAD, is well shown. Note that the diaphragm obscures the mid- and distal LAD. LM, left main.

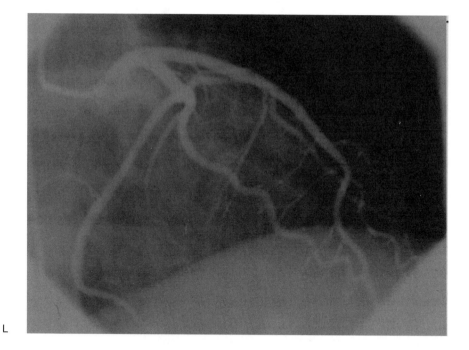

L

R

Figure 7-5C   A normal left system in the RAO view (30 degrees) with caudal angulation (25 degrees). This view is excellent for showing the CX and, often, the proximal LAD.

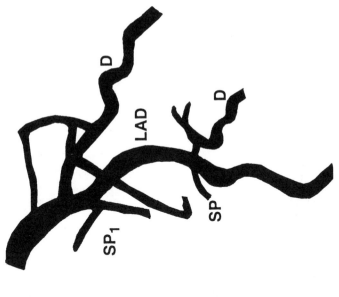

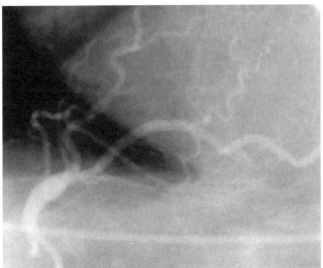

Figure 7-5D   The anteroposterior (AP) with cranial tilt shows the LAD and its diagonal (D) branches, with vessel overlap limited to the very proximal LAD and one area of the mid-LAD.

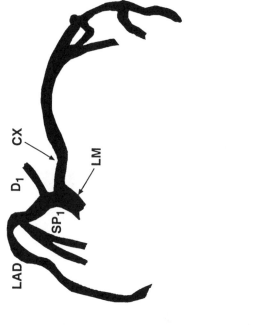

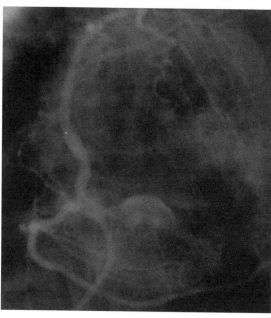

Figure 7-5E The LAO with caudal tilt ("spider view") is excellent in some cases to show the left main (LM) and origins of the CX and LAD. In this example, there are luminal irregularities but no high-grade lesion of LAD and CX. There is a small first diagonal very close to the LAD origin.

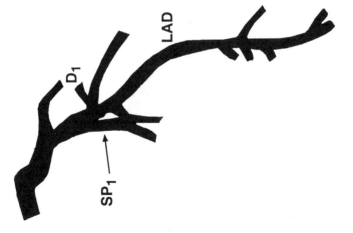

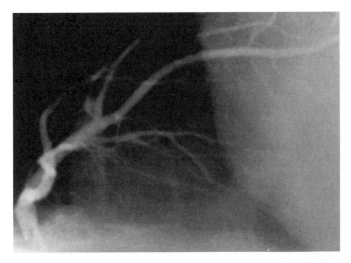

Figure 7-5F   RAO with cranial tilt may bring out LAD and the origin and course of diagonal branches. In this example, a normal CX and LAD overlap. After the first septal perforator (SP) and first diagonal, the LAD is well seen without vessel overlap or foreshortening.

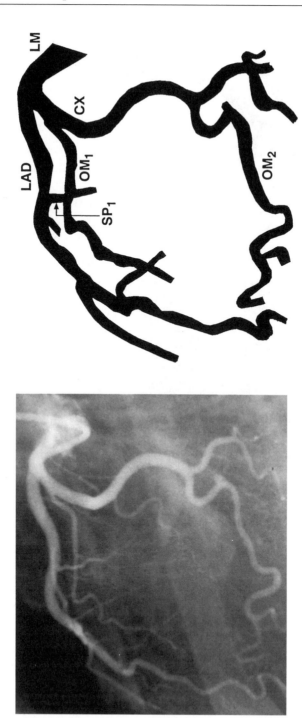

Figure 7-5G   The left lateral projection may show the mid-LAD well.

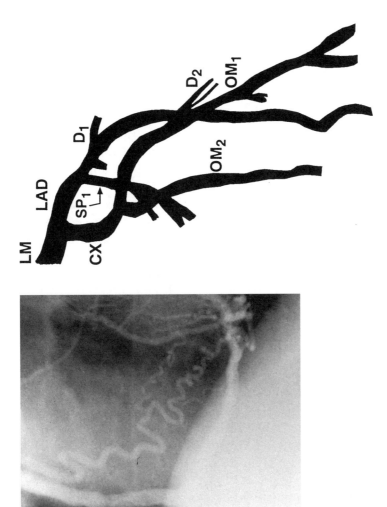

Figure 7-5H   The straight anteroposterior shows the mid-LAD and CX well.

the spine than the LAD when viewed in standard LAO and RAO projections. Branches of the CX supply the lateral surface of the left ventricle and are termed *obtuse marginal* branches. They are numbered sequentially from proximal to distal. The portion of the CX in the AV groove is generally called the AV groove CX. If the CX is dominant or co-dominant, its first three branches are denoted obtuse marginals (first, second, third) and subsequent branches, typically three, are named as posterolateral branches (first, second, third). Atrial branches arise from the CX and are seen to travel posteriorly in the RAO projection. The sinus node artery arises from the CX approximately 40% of the time.

In general, the left main coronary artery may be viewed in a shallow RAO or LAO projection, a straight or angulated posteroanterior projection, or an LAO projection with cranial or caudal angulation. The angiographer should be certain prior to terminating the case that adequate visualization of the left main and its branches has been obtained. The proximal LAD is usually well seen in a straight RAO (see Fig 7-5A), LAO with cranial angulation (Fig 7-5B), LAO with caudal angulation (see Fig 7-5C), RAO with caudal angulation, and a posteroanterior with cranial angulation (see Fig 7-5D). The mid- and distal LAD are well seen in the RAO with cranial angulation (see Fig 7-5F), and posteroanterior with cranial angulation (see Fig 7-5D). The left lateral view is also a good view for the mid-LAD (see Fig 7-5G), as is the straight anteroposterior projection (see Fig 7-5H). The origin of the diagonals are also seen well in the LAO with cranial angulation (see Fig 7-5B). The origin of the ramus branch and CX is usually well seen in the LAO with caudal angulation (the "spider" view) (see Fig 7-5E). The mid-ramus is well seen in the LAO cranial view. The caudal RAO projection is often a good view for the proximal and distal CX. The LAO caudal may be useful to see the origin of branching marginals, as may the left lateral. In patients with a left dominant system, the LAO cranial and the straight RAO are good views for visualizing the posterior descending artery.

Finally, it must be emphasized that pre-set angles will not be effective in every patient. Body habitus and previous chest surgery are just two of the factors that determine the heart's position in the chest (horizontal, vertical, or usually somewhere in between).

Catheterization of the Femoral Artery and Vein

The technique of accessing the femoral artery and vein is described in Chapter 4. After accessing the artery, a 0.032″ to 0.038″ J-tipped guidewire is advanced through the needle at least 20 cm. The wire should advance very easily with no resistance. Fluoroscopy should be used to observe the tip of the guidewire. The needle is removed over the guidewire, with firm pressure applied to the puncture site with the first three fingers of the left hand. It is important to emphasize that although the guidewire alone is in the artery, the hole in the artery is larger than the guidewire. If adequate digital pressure is not applied proximal to the hole, blood loss through the skin or a subcutaneous hematoma may develop. Thus, the operator should have "control" of the vessel (see Fig 4-4, Chapter 4). Blood is removed from the wire by manually wiping the wire with a saline-soaked gauze sponge. A dilator (of the same Fr size as the angiographic catheters chosen) is advanced over the wire (with or without a sheath). The dilator (and sheath) are advanced into the artery while holding the dilator as close to the skin as possible. A rotating motion helps to advance the dilator. The dilator is then removed with the wire (leaving the sheath in place). The side-arm of the sheath should then be aspirated and flushed with heparinized saline. In cases in which a sheath is not used, the dilator is removed over the wire, pressure is applied with the first three fingers of the left hand, the wire is wiped with sterile saline, and the catheter is advanced over the guidewire. When the catheter approaches the skin (usually being advanced by an assistant), the wire is pulled backward into the catheter until it exits the distal end. In cases in which a sheath is used, the wire may be preloaded into the catheter. In either circumstance, the catheter is then advanced, the J-tipped guidewire leading, under fluoroscopic guidance, around the aortic arch. The guidewire is removed and wiped with a saline-soaked gauze pad. A syringe is attached to the end of the catheter and 3 to 4 ml of blood is withdrawn. A second syringe filled with sterile saline is then attached to the end of the catheter. Blood is again withdrawn and when viewed in the syringe, the syringe is then injected to flush the catheter. The catheter is then attached to the manifold for pressure monitoring. After all sheaths are in place, heparin is generally administered in doses varying between 2000 and 5000 units, depending on the preference of the laboratory and the expected duration of the procedure. For routine diagnostic coronary arteriography, some operators do not give heparin in order to minimize bleeding complications. Such an approach requires meticulous attention to maintaining catheters and wires free of thrombus. Continuous arterial monitoring is important (typically, the pressure tracing will "damp" as a thrombus develops). In addition, free aspiration of blood through the catheter followed by saline infusion should be performed at intervals. Minimizing the time of the procedure and the time the guidewire is in the vessel probably further decreases the possibility of thrombus formation. Heparinization is preferred for patients in whom it may be expected that the procedural time will be relatively long.

In patients with aorto-iliac disease or extreme vessel tortuosity, the guidewire may not pass easily. It is important *not* to push the wire if it is not moving freely. The wire position should be ascertained by fluoroscopy. If the wire is not exiting the needle, it should be removed and the presence of pulsating blood return ascertained. If there is strong pulsatile return, the needle should be redirected (e.g., different angle to skin) and the wire reinserted. If this maneuver

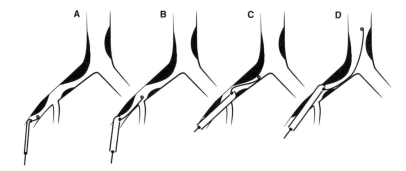

Figure 7-6 Maneuvering through a partially obstructing iliac artery. **(A)** A right Judkins catheter is advanced over a J-tipped wire. **(B)** The catheter is pointing medially and the wire is advanced past the first obstruction. **(C)** The catheter is advanced over the wire and rotated to face the lateral artery wall. **(D)** The guidewire is advanced past the obstruction into the abdominal aorta. **(E)** The catheter is advanced into the aorta, past the obstruction.

does not solve the problem, the needle may be slightly withdrawn, while ascertaining when blood return becomes brisk. The wire is then reinserted. If this does not allow for wire entry into the vessel, consideration should be given to trying a different location (typically slightly higher). The needle may have found a branch or branch point preventing adequate wire movement. Should the wire exit the needle but meet resistance in the iliac, the first step is to remove the wire to ascertain vigorous blood flow. A coated hydrophilic "glide" wire (e.g., Terumo wire, Medi-Tech, Watertown, MA) will often navigate the vessel in which a Teflon-coated wire has failed. Alternatively, a 0.032″ to 0.038″ wire with a very tapered tip (0.014″–0.018″) may be employed. If this maneuver is not successful, we have had success using either a right Judkins catheter or a 5-Fr "red rubber" catheter, pointing the wire in one direction or other (Fig 7-6). Contrast injections can be made through these catheters. The right Judkins catheter can be used to direct the wire, whereas the "red rubber" is particularly useful in tortuous anatomy. Once the wire is advanced to the central descending aorta, it is important to perform all catheter exchanges as centrally as is technically feasible. A long (280- to 300-cm) exchange-length wire should be used to minimize risk of arterial trauma and problems in navigating the difficult ilio-femoral anatomy.

In patients undergoing concomitant right heart catheterization or pacemaker insertion, femoral venous puncture is performed as described in Chapter 4. When the guidewire is advanced approximately 10 to 15 cm, it should be visualized fluoroscopically. It should lie to the operator's left (patient's right) of the patient's spine. The needle should be removed, the wire cleaned with saline, the sheath advanced over the wire, and the wire and dilator removed as previously described. The side-arm of any sheath should not contain air. To ensure this, blood is aspirated from the side-arm and saline (3–5 ml) is injected.

Cannulation of the Left Coronary Artery: The Judkins Approach

The left Judkins catheter allows cannulation of the left coronary artery with minimal manipulation, manual dexterity, or experience. The appropriately sized catheter can intubate the ostium without rotational manipulation. As Judkins first pointed out, the operator should allow the catheter do its job (Fig 7-7). The most common reason for an inexperienced operator to fail in cannulating the left coronary is excessive rotation of the catheter. The left Judkins catheter is advanced around the arch with the guidewire in place. The wire is removed, and the catheter is aspirated and flushed. The catheter is loaded with contrast and then advanced down into the ascending aorta, with the tip traveling leftward. The tip of the catheter is relatively horizontal until it cannulates the left coronary ostium. When the catheter enters the orifice, it should be advanced slightly. If the patient has an enlarged aortic root (e.g., from hypertension, aortic valve disease, intrinsic aortic disease), the Judkins 4 catheter may not reach the ostium and the Judkins 5 will be required. In situations in which the Judkins 4 catheter points superiorly just proximal to the left main, using a Judkins 5 catheter is usually effective. For a very large aortic root,

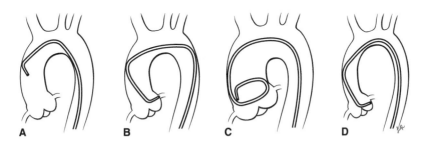

Figure 7-7 Cannulation of the left coronary with a Judkins catheter. **(A)** The catheter around the aortic arch. **(B)** The catheter is advanced and should easily intubate the left coronary artery. **(C)** If the catheter is relatively small for the aortic root, the catheter will fold on itself. **(D)** If the catheter is too large for the root, the tip often becomes fixed below the coronary ostium. (Adapted from Tilkian AG, Daily EK. Cardiac catheterization and coronary arteriography. In: Tilkian AG, Daily EK, eds. Cardiovascular procedures. St. Louis: Mosby, 1986:137.)

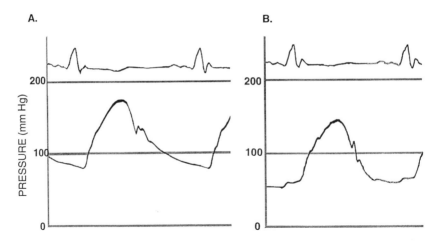

Figure 7-8   If the catheter partially obstructs flow, a damped or "ventricular-ized" pressure will occur. (**A**) Normal and (**B**) ventricularized pressures in the same patient are shown. If unappreciated and not corrected, this decrease in flow can produce hemodynamic instability.

a left 6 Judkins catheter may be needed. Occasionally, in patients with a narrow aortic root, the tip of the left Judkins 4 catheter may point inferiorly to the coronary ostium. In such circumstances, gentle pressure on the catheter, pushing it down into the left sinus, followed by pulling the catheter back, may cannulate the vessel. A left 3.5 Judkins catheter, an Amplatz catheter, or a multipurpose catheter may be useful if the vessel cannot be cannulated using this maneuver.

It is very important that the catheter be advanced slowly, with constant arterial pressure monitoring through the catheter itself. If the arterial pressure damps or "ventricularizes" in the coronary artery, the catheter needs to be withdrawn (Fig 7-8). When unsure of catheter position, a 1- to 2-ml contrast test injection is mandatory. The operator must know at all times where the tip of the catheter is. The operator should be fastidious in not overadvancing the catheter in the left main. A test injection under fluoroscopy should be performed. If this injection indicates subselective cannulation of the LAD or CX, the catheter should be withdrawn and another test injection performed. Occasionally, the operator will find that the patient has actually and/or functionally separate ostia of the two main branches. In such circumstances, selective angiography of each vessel may be necessary. When the LAD is cannulated, slight catheter withdrawal and clockwise rotation often cannulate the CX. When the CX is selectively cannulated, counterclockwise rotation together with slight catheter withdrawal often cannulates the LAD.

Cannulating the Right Coronary Artery: The Judkins Approach

There are two approaches for cannulating the RCA: approaching from below and approaching from above (Fig 7-9). These techniques are similar and the operator should probably be proficient in both. In both approaches, the catheter is advanced around the aortic arch with a J-tipped guidewire leading ahead of the catheter itself. Once in the ascending aorta, the wire is removed, the catheter is hand aspirated, connected to the manifold and flushed with dye. Under pressure monitoring, without torquing the catheter, the catheter is advanced to the aortic valve, with the tip facing the left shoulder (in the LAO projection). The catheter is withdrawn from the valve and slowly torqued in a clockwise manner. The catheter needs to turn as a unit, with the right hand turning the rotating adapter or distal catheter and the left hand facilitating turning of the catheter near the arterial sheath or skin (in a sheathless procedure). The most common error made by the inexperienced operator is over-vigorously torquing the catheter without observing under fluoroscopy concomitant turning of the catheter tip. As the catheter is withdrawn approximately

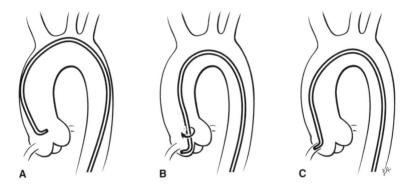

Figure 7-9 Technique for cannulating the right coronary artery. Cannulation of the right coronary artery may be performed by one of two methods (see text). This diagram demonstrates one technique for cannulating the right coronary with the Judkins catheter. The catheter tip is advanced to the right cusp, at which time the operator will feel resistance and observe lack of catheter tip movement on fluoroscopy. (**A**) The catheter is pulled above the valve leaflet under fluoroscopy approximately one rib interspace ($\sim$ 2 cm). (**B**) The catheter is torqued clockwise until it suddenly descends. Frequently, there is stored torque. If the operator waits, the catheter often continues its rotation. (**C**) When the operator feels that the catheter tip has come to rest, the catheter is rotated slightly clockwise (and withdrawn slightly), which usually intubates the vessel. (Adapted from Tilkian AG, Daily EK. Cardiac catheterization and coronary arteriography. In: Tilkian AG, Daily EK, eds. Cardiovascular procedures. St. Louis: Mosby, 1986:139.)

1 cm from the valve, the catheter should be torqued no more than a half turn. The catheter should continue to be withdrawn and turned. The catheter should turn every time the operator applies torque to it. A gentle withdrawal and catheter rotation less than or as great as 180 degrees most often cannulates the vessel. When the vessel is cannulated, if too much torque has been applied, it will be necessary to "back torque" the catheter slightly—a counterclockwise rotation to keep the tip in the right coronary ostium. When unsuccessful, the operator should try again, changing the speed of catheter withdrawal and the amount of torque slightly. Test contrast injections may help in locating the right coronary ostium.

An alternative approach is started with the catheter 1 or 2 cm above the left coronary ostium (approximately one rib interspace on fluoroscopy), with the tip pointing toward the left shoulder (LAO view). Once again, the catheter should be slowly torqued clockwise. The catheter will then descend into the right sinus. Occasionally, the tip turns into the right ostium. When the catheter has been excessively torqued, the catheter tip may continue to turn after it has dropped. Once the operator is convinced that no more turning is likely to occur, continued torquing should usually allow the catheter to enter the right coronary ostium. When unsuccessful, the operator should try again. If unsuccessful because the catheter tip is above the ostium, the same maneuver should be performed but with the tip somewhat lower than on the previous attempt. If the tip is too low on the first attempt, the procedure should be repeated, with the maneuver begun farther from the valve cusp.

Pressure monitoring should accompany all catheter maneuvers. When starting below the vessel, if the catheter is not withdrawn enough as torque is applied, the catheter may enter the left ventricle. Typically, ventricular ectopy occurs, and the catheter should be withdrawn immediately. When ectopy is not present, the more experienced operator may withdraw the catheter and apply clockwise torque at the same time, because this may facilitate cannulation of the right coronary ostium.

Cannulating the Left and Right Coronary Ostia: The Amplatz Technique

Left Amplatz catheters are occasionally chosen for patients with difficult to cannulate left coronary ostia (Fig 7-10). These catheters are somewhat more difficult to use than the Judkins catheters and may have a higher propensity for causing injury to the coronary artery. These catheters are probably not appropriate for the inexperienced operator. They are useful for vessel take-offs that are "out of plane," for high-take-off coronary ostia, and for patients with short left mains or separate take-offs of the LAD and CX. The Amplatz catheters come in different curve sizes (see Fig 7-1). The left Amplatz catheter can also

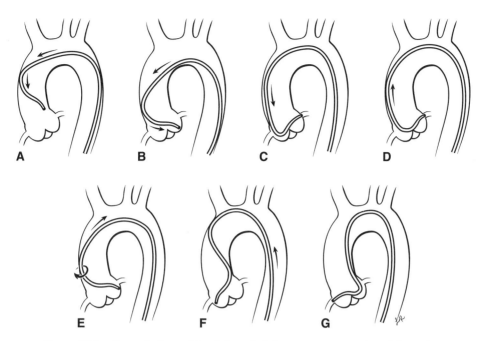

Figure 7-10   Cannulation of the left and right coronary arteries with an Amplatz catheter. **(A–D)** Left coronary maneuver. The catheter tip should "lead" around the arch to the left cusp. It should then be pushed ahead, and the tip should "climb" up the sinus to lodge in the left main. When the catheter is retracted by the operator, the tip has a tendency to "dive," which may damage the coronary. Arrows represent operator push or pull. **(E–G)** Right coronary maneuver. For cannulation of the right ostium, the catheter tip should lead, rotated clockwise. As it turns, the tip will have a tendency to rise above its curve. The catheter should be slowly withdrawn so that the tip continues to lead. A small advancement of the catheter usually intubates the vessel. (Adapted from Tilkian AG, Daily EK. Cardiac catheterization and coronary arteriography. In: Tilkian AG, Daily EK. Cardiovascular procedures. St. Louis: Mosby, 1986:141.)

cannulate the right coronary ostium, using a technique similar to that described for the right Judkins catheter. The left Amplatz is advanced around the arch, the guidewire is removed, and the catheter is aspirated and flushed. Under constant pressure monitoring, the catheter is advanced so that its tip points toward the left coronary ostium. The tip should be lower than the major curve of the catheter. The catheter tip will generally point to the left sinus, inferior to the ostium. With advancement, and slight rotation as necessary, the appropriately sized Amplatz will cannulate the left coronary ostium. At that point, withdrawal of the catheter may cause it to move forward, and advancement will cause it to move back in the vessel. If the Amplatz catheter appears too large to climb up the aortic wall into the ostium, a smaller loop Amplatz should be used. When the catheter tip advances past the ostium and points vertically, a larger curved Amplatz should be tried. It should be noted that the Amplatz catheters frequently require rotational manipulation to enter an out-of-plane coronary ostium.

Cannulation with the Multipurpose Catheter

The multipurpose (Schoonmaker-King) catheter can be used to perform both left and right coronary angiography. It has distal side holes and can accept relatively high contrast flow rates (10–15 ml/sec) and can be used for ventriculography, though requiring considerably more operator experience than for a pigtail catheter. Unlike the Judkins and Amplatz catheters, the multipurpose catheter requires significant manipulation to successfully cannulate the coronary ostia. There is no standard technique that is always successful.

One method for cannulating the left coronary artery is to perform catheter manipulation in the RAO projection. The catheter tip is pointed to the right, with a loop formed in the noncoronary cusp, while advancing and torquing clockwise. At this point, further clockwise torquing transports the tip to the left cusp, where advancing or retracting the catheter allows entry into the left coronary ostium (Fig 7-11).

An alternative technique for cannulating the left ostium is quite similar to the Sones technique from the arm. The operator may begin imaging in the LAO projection (approximately 30–45 degrees) (Fig 7-12). In this view, the left coronary sinus is on the patient's left, and the right coronary sinus is on the patient's right and somewhat lower than the left, with the noncoronary cusp lying posteriorly. The ideal method to cannulate the left coronary ostium is to form a small loop in the left sinus and gradually advance the catheter while injecting contrast to verify position. Frequently, catheter advancement with some rotation cannulates the vessel. Occasionally, an oversized loop will form, and the tip of the catheter will point superiorly above the ostium. In this circumstance, gentle retraction of the catheter with or without slight rotation may cannulate the vessel. Frequently, multiple attempts and maneuvers are required to cannulate the ostium. Having the patient take a deep breath may facilitate vessel intubation. There are also multiple techniques to advance the catheter into the left coronary sinus. With the catheter in the mid-ascending aorta, the catheter should be advanced with a gentle clockwise torque. If this maneuver is unsuccessful after a number of attempts, the catheter may be advanced with slight counterclockwise torque in an attempt to form a small loop in the noncoronary cusp. Advancing the catheter slightly while applying a gentle clockwise torque, in an attempt to bring the catheter around to the left coronary sinus, may succeed. In situations in which the catheter is in or above the right coronary sinus, rotation of the catheter counterclockwise may allow positioning in the left coronary sinus.

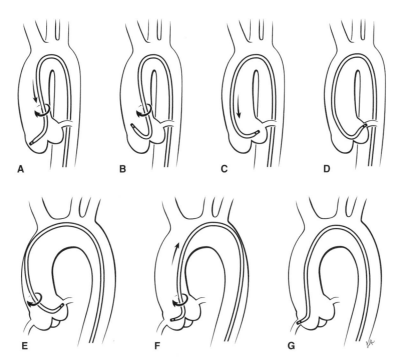

Figure 7-11 Cannulation of the left (**A–D**) and right (**E–G**) coronary with a multipurpose catheter. The RAO projection is used. The ostium of the right coronary is not shown for illustrative purposes in panels a – d. It would be facing directly forward above the right cusp. The catheter tip is pointed to the right. The catheter is turned clockwise, and a loop is made. Further turning will move the catheter tip into the left cusp. Advancement (in this case) or retraction of the catheter usually results in intubation of the left main. Cannulation of the *right* coronary begins with the catheter looped in the left coronary cusp and removed from the left ostium. The LAO view, as shown here, is often used. The catheter is torqued clockwise. This maneuver produces an increase in the size of the loop, so gentle withdrawal while torquing to maintain the size of the loop is required. The catheter tip will fall into the right cusp and often into the right ostium. If the tip is below the ostium, gentle advancement frequently intubates the artery. (Adapted from Pepine CJ, Lambert CR, Hill JA. Coronary angiography. In: Pepine CJ, Lambert CR, Hill JA, eds. Diagnostic and therapeutic cardiac catheterization. 2nd ed. Baltimore: Williams & Wilkins, 1994:258.)

Cannulation of the RCA (see Fig 7-11) with the multipurpose catheter also may require multiple maneuvers. The right coronary ostium lies inferior to the left coronary ostium. Forming a small loop in the left coronary sinus should be attempted. The catheter should be turned clockwise slowly in an attempt to bring the catheter anterior and rightward. Frequently, the tip of the catheter may become fixed in the left sinus and thus gentle retraction of the catheter

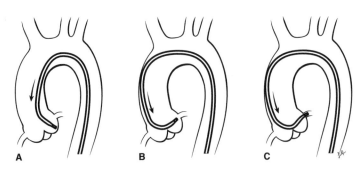

Figure 7-12 (**A–C**) An alternate method for cannulating the left coronary uses a modified Sones technique. The catheter is pointed to the left cusp and advanced to form a loop. The loop is increased in size. It may enter the left ostium. If not, clockwise torque and adjusting the loop size may be necessary.

may be necessary to rotate the tip. After gentle retraction, the tip may fall and point inferiorly. The "trick" is to maintain the configuration of the small loop, and after retracting, gentle advancement is often necessary while slowly rotating the catheter. Ultimately, the tip should drop and cannulate the right coronary ostium, provided the loop is of proper size. Frequent test injections are useful in localizing landmarks. When rotating the catheter from the left sinus is unsuccessful, the multipurpose type can frequently cannulate the right coronary ostium by having the tip climb up the right coronary sinus with the heel of the catheter in the left coronary cusp. The catheter should be advanced with slight clockwise rotation, attempting to have the tip point toward the right sinus, with the heel on the medial side of the aorta as viewed in the LAO projection. Often the catheter will prolapse in the ventricle with this technique. The "trick" is to anticipate this event and either pull back or torque the catheter just prior to catheter prolapse. Advancement of the catheter, with or without catheter rotation, is performed once the tip of the catheter is in the right sinus. The operator should be careful with down-going RCA, because the multipurpose catheter can "dive" into the vessel, increasing the risk of intimal dissection. Frequent test injections and constant pressure monitoring are essential.

Femoral Approach: Aftercare

At the completion of the procedure, the sheath (and/or catheter) is removed. Manual pressure using three fingers, beginning at and extending cephalad from the puncture site, may be applied. Alternatively, a clamp device or other compressive device may be used. Pressure is initially applied forcefully to obliterate the pulse and ensure that bleeding is prevented through the puncture site or into the soft tissues. Pressure is gradually reduced over the next 10 to 20 minutes, at which point it is removed entirely. The groin should then be viewed for 5 minutes prior to dressing the site and moving the patient. Distal pulses are checked before and after catheter removal. If there is a particular concern that bleeding from the catheterization site is likely, a pressure dressing may then be applied; otherwise, a small clear bandage may be used. Prior to sheath removal, protamine sulfate may be used to reverse heparin, except in patients with insulin-dependent diabetes, in which there is a reported increased incidence of severe reactions. The recommended dose is 10 mg of protamine for every 1000 units of administered heparin. Measuring the activated clotting time (ACT), both before and after protamine, provides a guide to the timing of catheter and sheath removal. Sheaths are removed when the ACT is less than 150 seconds. Laboratories that use low-dose heparin rarely administer protamine.

Patients are generally kept at bed rest for 5 to 6 hours, with the catheterized leg immobilized in a straight position. A rule of thumb is 1 hour of rest per catheter Fr size used (e.g., 6 Fr = 6 hours of bed rest). Newer hemostatic devices may allow earlier mobilization (see Chapter 4). Frequent vital signs are obtained (every 15 minutes for 1 hour, then every hour for 4 hours), with observation of the access site and evaluation of the peripheral pulse. Oral fluids are encouraged. Intravenous (IV) fluids also may be infused, because contrast agents have a potent osmotic diuretic effect. Nurses are instructed to notify the physician if there is no urine output after 2 hours. Only mild analgesia (e.g., acetaminophen) should be ordered, because in a routine case, there should be no significant discomfort from percutaneous catheterization. Patients are instructed to notify the nurse immediately and to self-administer femoral artery compression in the case of unexpected bleeding.

After 1 to 2 hours in the supine position, the head of the bed may be raised 30 to 45 degrees. At the end of 5 to 8 hours, patients are ambulated, initially with nurse's assistance. After 1 to 2 hours of ambulation, outpatients may be discharged, provided the incisional area is dry, distal pulses are intact, and the coronary anatomy and clinical picture are consistent with standards for same-day discharge.

Catheterizing the Brachial Artery

Percutaneous Versus Cutdown

The physician experienced in the Judkins technique may feel most comfortable employing a percutaneous technique of the left brachial artery. This technique is essentially the same as the Judkins femoral technique, except for different landmarks. In general, a small (5- or 6-Fr) sheath and catheters should be employed. Utilizing the left arm allows the use of preformed Judkins or Amplatz catheters. In many laboratories, such an approach is cumbersome because the laboratory layout favors use of the right side of the patient for vascular access. (For specific percutaneous and cutdown techniques, see Chapter 4.)

Catheter Advancement

The catheter chosen can be advanced with or without a leading guidewire. There may be difficulty in advancing the catheter into the ascending aorta. Under these circumstances, turning the patient's head in the other direction, removing the pillow, abducting the arm farther from the body, performing a Valsalva maneuver, or deep breathing may facilitate catheter advancement. The catheter should move as if sliding on butter and should not be forced. Not heeding this advice and forcefully pushing the catheter may produce an intimal dissection. It is frequently preferable to lead the catheter with a J-tipped guide wire (as opposed to a straight-tipped catheter).

Cannulating the Coronaries

The operator will most often be using either a multipurpose or Sones catheter from the right arm. Individuals who routinely use the multipurpose (Schoonmaker-King) catheter from the femoral approach may prefer it when performing brachial catheterizations. The techniques for vessel intubation for these catheters are similar to those described for the multipurpose catheter femoral artery approach. Castillo catheters, which are quite similar in shape to Amplatz catheters but somewhat shorter (80 cm), also may be used from the arm.

Brachial Artery Aftercare

With the percutaneous approach, aftercare is similar, though not identical, to removal of a catheter and sheath from the femoral artery. When the catheter and sheath are removed, bleeding may be allowed briefly prior to applying digital pressure. Digital pressure or pressure by an inflated sphygmomanometer cuff over a folded gauze should then be applied. The radial artery should have a palpable pulse while compression is performed. When a brachial cutdown has been used, repair may be accomplished as described in Chapter 4.

When patients are returned to their rooms, bed rest for 1 to 2 hours is recommended. They are allowed to sit up in bed. A mild analgesic may be ordered for pain as needed. Oral fluid intake is encouraged and IV fluids may be used as well. Ambulation may occur as early as 30 to 60 minutes after the procedure in asymptomatic patients. If there is no urine output within 2 hours, the physician should be called. Frequent vital signs and brachial and radial artery pulse checks are employed. After ambulation for 3 to 4 hours, patients may be discharged, provided their coronary anatomies and clinical conditions allow it.

Catheterization of Patients with Previous Bypass Surgery

Patients with previous coronary bypass graft surgery account for an increasing percentage of the population studied by coronary angiography. In this group of patients, it is necessary to review the operative report and to review the preoperative angiogram if at all possible.

An initial approach for catheterizing aortocoronary saphenous vein grafts is to use a right Judkins catheter, perform right coronary angiography, and then proceed to cannulate the bypass graft(s) with this catheter. The technique used for cannulating the grafts starts progressively higher in the aortic root until as many grafts as possible are visualized. An alternative approach is to consider the portion of the ascending aorta as a cylinder. The Judkins right catheter should be moved up and down the cylinder, typically from the second to the fourth sternal suture. If the catheter doesn't "snag" the graft ostium, the catheter is rotated 5 to 10 degrees, and the process repeated. Using either of these techniques, most grafts will be found. Some surgeons leave markers at the site of the graft anastomosis on the aorta, simplifying the hunt for the grafts. Often, there are no markers, but the surgical clips may give a hint as to the origin of the grafts. Most often, the proximal anastomosis of bypass grafts are on the most surgically accessible aspect (i.e., the anterior surface of the aorta). Frequently, all of the proximal anastomotic sites are very close together, often vertically or horizontally placed. Frequent test injections are mandatory, particularly when the catheter is not moving freely. Test injections may show a segment of a graft (a "nubbin" or "nipple") indicative of graft occlusion (Fig 7-13). When the operator cannot visualize all of the conduits with the right Judkins, another catheter should be used. A graft-seeking catheter is helpful, especially the right graft seeker for all venous grafts. Some physicians utilize a left graft seeker, which has a 90-degree primary bend, for left grafts (see Fig 7-1). (The left graft seeker is similar to the right Judkins, but has a more pronounced secondary bend).

When unable to visualize all of the venous bypass grafts, it is important to obtain as much information as possible from the native coronary arteries. Collateral flow from a native or graft vessel to the distal vessel subserved by the graft indicates an occluded or functionally occluded graft. Native coronary angiography may show retrograde graft filling or competitive distal flow (dye washout), indicating graft patency, or normal distal flow without graft filling, suggesting

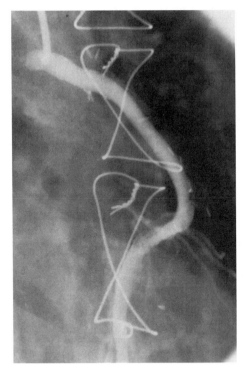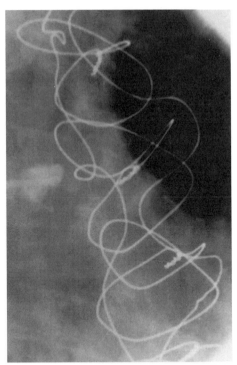

Figure 7-13 RAO projection of (left) patent and (right) occluded left saphenous vein bypass graft.

graft occlusion. When native coronary arteriography (and/or LV wall motion) suggests a patent graft that has not been visualized, another attempt to find the graft should be made using either an Amplatz or multipurpose catheter. The multipurpose catheter is particularly useful for the right coronary graft, which is typically at or near the right anterior aspect of the ascending aorta. If still unsuccessful, aortography may be performed in the proximal ascending aorta to determine graft patency and origin (see Chapter 6).

The internal mammary artery (IMA) is a frequently used, durable graft. The left internal mammary artery (LIMA), usually anastomosed to the LAD or, less frequently, a large diagonal or obtuse marginal, originates inferiorly and anteriorly from the subclavian artery between the superior thyrocervical trunk and the left vertebral artery (Fig 7-14). The right internal mammary artery (RIMA) usually arises anterior and inferior from the right subclavian between the superior thyrocervical trunk and right vertebral, but may arise from the brachiocephalic artery before the origin of the subclavian and the vertebral artery origin.

The catheters of choice for IMA cannulation are the internal mammary and right Judkins catheters. The internal mammary catheter has a configura-

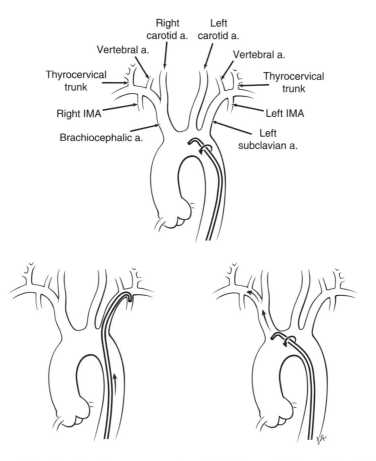

Figure 7-14 Functional anatomy and method of cannulation of the LIMA and RIMA areas. To enter the left subclavian, the right Judkins is torqued counterclockwise. The catheter should be advanced and engage the LIMA at the inferior surface of the left subclavian. If forward movement is not easy, a J-tipped wire should be advanced into the subclavian and the catheter advanced over it. The wire is removed and the catheter is retracted by the operator to "snag" the LIMA. If the right Judkins catheter is in the subclavian, but the primary angle needs to be more acute, an internal mammary catheter will usually succeed. An exchange-length guidewire allows the wire to be in the subclavian or axillary artery during catheter exchange. The maneuver is similar with cannulating the RIMA, except that the maneuver begins with the catheter in a more central location. (Adapted from Tilkian AG, Daily EK. Cardiac catheterization and coronary anteriography. In: Tilkian AG, Daily EK, eds. Cardiovascular procedures. St. Louis: Mosby, 1986:144.)

tion similar to the right Judkins catheter but has a longer tip length and a slightly shallower primary curve (see Fig 7-1). To cannulate the IMA, the LAO projection (40–60 degrees) may be utilized to cannulate the subclavian or brachiocephalic artery. In this view, a mediastinal soft-tissue density is formed with the left subclavian and right brachiocephalic arteries emanating from the left and right borders of this soft tissue shadow. The internal mammary catheter is advanced just proximal to the origin of the left subclavian (or right brachiocephalic), turned *counterclockwise,* and advanced slightly to facilitate vessel entry. Alternatively, the anteroposterior projection may be used. The catheter tip should be at the distal boundary of the aortic knob. The catheter should be rotated counterclockwise. If the catheter engages the left carotid, the catheter tip should be retracted and the maneuver repeated. The technique for entering the left subclavian or right brachiocephalic is one of the few in cardiovascular angiography that specifically requires a counterclockwise catheter movement. A J-tipped guidewire is then advanced down the subclavian artery to the axillary artery. The right coronary or IMA catheter is then advanced to the midsubclavian artery. The guidewire is withdrawn (in the anteroposterior projection for the LIMA and the LAO projection for the RIMA), the catheter is withdrawn into the proximal subclavian, and test injections are performed to identify the origin of the vessel. Non-ionic or low-osmolality ionic contrast agents may be used to minimize patient discomfort. After the origin of the vessel is identified, the catheter is advanced or withdrawn—the LIMA cannulated with counterclockwise rotation and the RIMA with clockwise rotation. Internal mammary angiography is then performed while watching carefully for pressure damping, because the IMA may be more prone to dissection due to their smaller caliber and sharp angle of origin.

When the RIMA or LIMA cannot be cannulated utilizing the aforementioned technique, alternatives include using a right Judkins catheter, using nonselective injection when the tip of the catheter is near the origin of the vessel (utilizing an inflated sphygmomanometer in the ipsilateral arm), or accessing the vessel via the appropriate brachial artery.

Technical Issues

Manifold, Injection Techniques, Framing, Panning

A number of different manifold systems are available. All have the same basic components. Figure 7-15 shows a three-component manifold with three stopcocks. The first stopcock is attached via a fluid-filled line to a transducer, the second is attached to dedicated flush line, and the third port is attached to contrast. Once the catheter has been inserted and the wire removed, the catheter is aspirated to ensure that no air is in the system. The contrast syringe, containing 1 or 2 ml of heparinized flush solution, is attached to the manifold and the flush is withdrawn slowly into the control syringe to avoid air bubbles. The pressure stopcock is then opened to withdraw blood into the contrast syringe. The blood is then flushed from the catheter. Contrast is then withdrawn slowly into

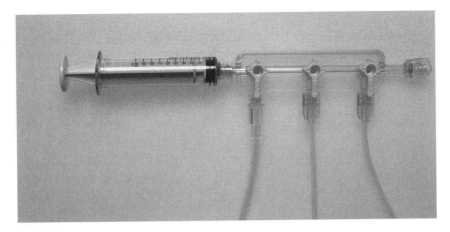

Figure 7-15 A typical manifold set-up for coronary arteriography. The proximal part is a dedicated pressure line attached distally to a pressure transducer. The middle port is a dedicated flush line attached to a saline flush bag under high pressure. The distal port is attached to contrast medium.

the syringe and 1 ml of dye is injected into the aortic root under fluoroscopic visualization.

Arterial pressure should be monitored continuously, except when injecting contrast. After cannulating the coronary ostium with no change in arterial pressure, coronary injections may commence. An initial test injection of approximately 1 ml to confirm catheter position is often useful. The patient is usually instructed to breathe deeply. The breathing maneuver should be visualized under fluoroscopy so that the vessels will be positioned to minimize panning. Once the view is appropriately framed, the patient is instructed to take a deep breath as the operator activates the cine foot peddle, and the injection is begun after the x-ray image appears on the television monitor. The operator should place the shutters within the field, even if it is only at the edge of the image. This technique will reduce scatter and improve image quality as well as decrease radiation exposure to the staff. In addition, the image intensifier should be as close to the patient as possible to optimize image quality. A common mistake of the inexperienced angiographer is to rush the injection without proper table centering so that excessive panning is required. This movement leads to the camera light meter adjusting to many different densities, which in turn may cause poor cineangiographic quality. Another common mistake is to begin injection prematurely so that the vessel territory is seen only with dye present; this makes it difficult to see calcification or retained dye, which could indicate dissection or thrombus. In general, the left coronary artery requires approximately 5 to 10 ml of dye, depending on the patient's size and underlying cardiac condition. (For example, coronary angiography in patients with severe aortic insufficiency or ventricular hypertrophy often requires upwards of 10 ml/left coronary injection). The RCA, in general, requires less contrast. The more experienced angiographer can modulate the injection based on the quality of the cine television image. In general, the artery should be injected vigorously to optimize opacification. A rapid but definite increase in manual pressure should be employed so that the catheter does not recoil from the ostium. Following injection, the operator should immediately view the ECG signal and turn the stopcock to visualize arterial pressure. The operator should learn to appreciate the heart beating during the injection so that heart rate slowing or ectopy may be detected as early as possible. Patients with hypertrophied ventricles (i.e., aortic stenosis, severe hypertension) or high flow states (e.g., anemia, aortic insufficiency) require more contrast per injection. Patients with smaller vessels (i.e., nondominant right coronary) require less. Relatively large amounts of injected contrast may lead to profound bradycardia or asystole. Thus, the less-experienced angiographer should err on the side of injecting somewhat less than an adequate amount until the technique of modulating the contrast injection is learned. The patient should be instructed in vigorous coughing ("cough CPR") until the dye effects wane (usually 5–20 sec).

In some laboratories, the physician performing the angiography also moves the table (pans). This approach is ideal with an experienced angiographer because he or she knows the objects of interest. The inexperienced operator should not consider simultaneous injecting and panning. Panning should be done slowly, generally in a circular motion, following the dye down to the end of the vessel and then moving the table to visualize any collateral circulation. As mentioned previously, proper positioning of the table should minimize the amount of panning necessary and optimize cine quality.

There is much more to performing a coronary angiogram than the technical aspects. It is imperative that the operator review the findings as the procedure proceeds. Are all vessels present and accounted for? Could there be an anomalous takeoff of a vessel or a flush occlusion? Does that segment without any apparent vessels move on ventriculography and if so, what then is its blood supply? Has the panning been adequate to identify all collaterals? Have all of the coronary segments been adequately and optimally visualized? The playback (either videotape or digital) should be utilized to ensure that all appropriate data are obtained before the patient's study is considered complete.

Pressure Damping and Ventricularization

It is imperative to constantly monitor pressure from the tip of the angiographic catheter. A decrease in catheter tip pressure occurs when coronary inflow is impeded. This may occur if the catheter is obstructing flow as it abuts on a critical stenosis, when the catheter tip is larger than the vessel (e.g., inhibiting nondominant RCA or conus branch), or when the tip of the catheter is impinging on the vessel wall. Pressure damping also may occur when the catheter is not in the coronaries if it has been overtorqued and is kinked, or if the catheter is up against the aortic wall. Ventricularization—the change in pressure contour from arterial to somewhat the appearance of a ventricular pressure contour—may occur when coronary flow is obstructed, as observed in Figure 7-8. When pressure damping or ventricularization occurs, the catheter should be withdrawn until the pressure normalizes. Test injections should be performed to ascertain if high-quality angiography is possible without ventricularization. When damping occurs repeatedly in the RCA and test injections have not been helpful, a small injection under cine with rapid removal of the catheter is appropriate. This injection verifies whether the catheter was in a conus branch or a nondominant RCA. Left coronary artery damping (or ventricularization) most often indicates left main pathology. Under these circumstances, injections in the left sinus are appropriate to try to visualize the left main and its proximal branches. Changing catheters may be necessary to facilitate good sinus injections with adequate visualization. The inexperienced operator should rarely, if ever, inject into a coronary artery when pressure is damped or ventricularized.

Iatrogenic Complications and Their Prevention

Practitioners have developed a number of different ways to perform coronary arteriography safely and effectively. This section describes the technical problems that may result in complications and the author's approach to their prevention. Some procedure-related complications (e.g., contrast-induced allergic reactions) have already been described; the reader should refer to the appropriate sections for these issues. Monitoring the patient during coronary arteriography may be likened to a firefighter's job. Most of the time no danger signs appear, but when they do, there must be a rapid and safe response to terminate the underlying problem.

Air Embolism

Injection of air into the coronary circulation can have catastrophic results, including myocardial infarction, hypotension, and sustained arrhythmias. Fortunately, the coronary circulation can often tolerate small amounts of air injected inadvertently. Air typically appears radiographically as small spherical or ovoid bodies surrounded by contrast. The prevention of this complication includes ascertaining that the manifold system has no leaks. This can be accomplished by placing a finger over the manifold outflow port (the connection to the catheter) and vigorously pushing forward the dye syringe filled with either contrast or saline. If there is a loose connection in the system, fluid will leak at that site. That connection should be tightened and the maneuver repeated. In addition, drawing back on the contrast syringe, with the finger over the outflow site, also will reveal if there is an air leak. If there are no loose connections, no air will enter the system. The operator is then ready to connect the manifold to the catheter. Additional stopcocks to the basic manifold system should be avoided to minimize the risk of a loose connection and consequent air leaks.

After the catheter has been advanced to the central aorta, blood should be allowed to drip back from the proximal catheter end and the catheter aspirated of 2 to 3 ml of blood. This ensures that no residual air is left in the catheter. The connection of the manifold should always be a fluid-to-fluid connection. Finally, it is likely a small amount (<1 ml) of air may be lodged in the contrast syringe. The contrast syringe should be held in a semivertical position and the syringe tapped so that the air rises to the back of the syringe. Leaving at least 2 to 3 ml of contrast in the injecting syringe further lessens the risk of injecting air. In most cases, small amounts of injected air will traverse the coronary circulation without event. In the case of a symptomatic state (often persistent chest pain and ECG changes, usually ST elevation), another injection should be made to ascertain if there is a very large lodged air collection preventing coronary flow. If this situation exists, emergency consultation, if feasible, with an experienced interventionist is recommended. A small (0.016″ to 0.024″) end-hole catheter may be advanced through a Y-connector (Tuohy-Borst) over a small steerable guidewire (0.014″–0.018″) into that arterial segment. The guidewire is then removed and aspiration can be performed to remove the retained air.

Thromboembolic Events

Iatrogenic thromboembolic events include myocardial infarction (in-situ catheter thrombus injected into the coronary artery) or stroke (in-situ thrombus injected into the ascending aortic arch and lodging intracranially). Thrombus formation can be substantially lessened by aspiration of blood from the catheter immediately after its entry and prior to its connection to the manifold. If aspiration is difficult or impossible, a clot may already be present within the catheter. The operator *should not flush the catheter.* The catheter should be withdrawn slightly to remove possible contact with the arterial wall. If blood cannot be aspirated after several maneuvers, the catheter should be removed and flushed outside the patient. Typically, a "stringy" clot will be flushed from the catheter tip.

If blood aspirates freely through the catheter, the catheter should be attached with a fluid-fluid connection to the manifold and the pressure tracing observed. This tracing should show a typical arterial contour. If there is evidence of damping, the system should be checked for air, and the catheter should be reaspirated to ascertain that the problem is not within the catheter itself. Any change in the arterial contour during the procedure may be due to clot formation within the catheter. As such, it is imperative to continuously monitor arterial pressure through the catheter, except when contrast injections are made. Risk of thromboembolic events is lessened by fastidious attention to detail, including careful cleaning of guidewires and minimizing the time each catheter is in the patient.

Finally, the use of heparin (2000- to 5000-unit bolus injection after access has been obtained) is probably helpful in maintaining a thrombus-free system. To minimize groin-site bleeding postcatheterization, the heparin effect may be reversed by injecting protamine in a dose of 25 to 50 mg (10 mg/1000 units of heparin + "fudge factor" [unknown constant] related to elapsed time from last heparin injection). Alternatively, low-dose heparin (1500–3000 units) may be given without protamine at the procedure's end. Protamine should probably not be used in insulin-dependent diabetics, because an increased incidence of serious reactions including anaphylaxis has been reported. Some angiographers have chosen to perform coronary arteriography without systemic anticoagulation to minimize postprocedure bleeding at the groin site. Obviously, meticulous attention to detail is mandatory.

Another probable cause of embolic events, particularly strokes, in a percentage of cases, is due to catheter dislodgement of atheromatous material in the central aorta. Care should be taken to minimize this occurrence by following several practical approaches. The catheter and leading guidewire should be observed fluoroscopically as they course peripherally to centrally. The guidewire should be observed to move freely, without evidence of the guidewire tip deforming or being stationary, which would suggest its fixation in a plaque. A J-tipped (as opposed to a straight-tipped) guidewire may further lessen the chance of lifting and dislodging a plaque. Fluoroscopy should follow the catheter movement to avoid inadvertent entry into the carotid vessels. In patients with tortuous, difficult-to-traverse peripheral vessels, where there is also likely to be significant central as well as peripheral plaque accumulation, a long (240- to 300-cm) guidewire may be used to exchange catheters in the central aorta without running the risk of scraping plaque while moving upward from the descending aorta, as may occur with the usual-length (140-cm) guidewire. It also should be noted that if excessive pressure is applied for hemostasis after catheterization, an in-situ thrombus may form distal to the site of compression. As such, a palpable or Doppler audible pulse should be present distally during arterial compression.

Bleeding from the Access Catheter Site Postprocedure

This complication can be minimized in several ways. The use of a "one-walled stick" should limit bleeding to an anterior accumulation rather than the possibility of a major but occult retroperitoneal bleed from a posterior wall bleed. Smaller diagnostic catheters (5–6 Fr), protamine postcatheterization in patients given heparin, or a heparinless procedure will probably further decrease bleeding risk. Prolonged (15- to 20-min) pressure hemostasis, either manually or using a compression device, will also further decrease the bleeding risk.

Coronary Artery Dissection Caused by Catheter

This rare complication is often poorly tolerated. It probably occurs in the proximal RCA more frequently than in the left main coronary artery. Because the incidence of this complication is very low ($< 0.01\%$), risk factors for its occurrence can be described only anecdotally. Most authorities feel that certain catheters that tend to "dive" into the artery, such as the Amplatz, multipurpose (Schoonmaker-King), and Sones catheters, may have a greater propensity to cause dissection, compared with the Judkins catheter. The angiographer should appreciate when the catheter does dive and decide whether its location is acceptable for further injections or whether it should be withdrawn. Factors to be considered include whether arterial pressure is damped (signifying either blood flow impedance by the catheter or impingement on or into the vessel wall), how far into the vessel the catheter has advanced, and the level of difficulty in accessing the vessel. Very small injections of contrast in the artery (if the arterial pressure contour shows no evidence of flow obstruction) may clarify whether contrast flows freely or a dissection has already occurred. The management of the dissection is dependent on its severity, the adequacy of distal blood flow, the risk territory of the artery involved, the status of the other vessels, and the patient's overall condition. For example, "watchful waiting" may be indicated for a small dissection with minimal contrast observed in a rather small vessel, or emergency surgery or coronary intervention (e.g., PTCA or stent) may be indicated if a very large artery with impaired flow subserving a large myocardial territory is involved.

To minimize the risks further, several manufacturers have employed a "soft-tip" feature, in which the catheter tip (~0.5–2.0 mm) is made of a relatively soft, compliant material. Whether this feature provides added protection is difficult to gauge because the complication of coronary dissection secondary to catheter manipulation is rare.

Catheter Knotting and Kinking

When a catheter becomes knotted or kinked somewhere in its shaft, it is not yet an adverse patient event. If the problem is not recognized, however, subsequent catheter movement may likely produce an adverse event. Typically, catheter manipulation produces kinking or knotting if a part of the catheter is fixed. For example, if the operator is torquing a right coronary catheter and the tip is fixed in an aortic plaque (which the operator does not appreciate), a kink may occur, producing damping or complete obliteration of the arterial pressure tracing. If the operator then pushes or pulls the catheter, vascular trauma may result. It is emphasized that the operator observe a one-to-one ratio between manual torquing and tip movement. If the problem is recognized, it may often be corrected by reversing the torquing movement to the original position. If catheter pressure remains damped or absent, the operator can cautiously advance a guidewire to the kink. After kink removal, preferably in the descending aorta, or lower (if possible) to avoid any CNS embolic risk, the straightened catheter should be removed, because its torquability has been seriously compromised at the kink site.

Bradycardia and Asystole

Long pauses or frank asystole may be produced after coronary injections, particularly of the RCA. In general, the longer the duration and the larger the amount of contrast, the higher the risk of sinus and AV node suppression. The technical solution is to inject (usually) 5 to 10 ml *rapidly* (1–2 sec) for the left system, 4 to 8 ml for the usual right dominant system, and 2 to 6 ml for a small nondominant right artery. Typically, there will be some degree of sinus slowing. If there is no sinus activity or the rate is very slow (<30 beats/min), vigorous coughing is useful to clear the dye and accelerate return of sinus rhythm. The mechanism for this favorable effect is unclear but is likely to be related at least in part to cough CPR. If an initial injection provokes an extremely prolonged period of the bradyarrhythmia (20–30 sec) or asystole in the *absence* of prolonged or excessive dye injection, consideration should be given to inserting a temporary RV pacer, using IV atropine (0.8–1.0 mg/dose) prophylactically and/or changing to non-ionic dye. Profound sinus bradycardia, usually with accompanying hypotension, may be caused by a vasovagal reaction. This event usually occurs during vessel accessing or vessel/sheath removal but may occur at any time during the procedure. Atropine (0.8–1.0 mg/dose) administered intravenously when there is a decrease in heart rate and BP is usually successful in treating a vasovagal reaction.

Ventricular Fibrillation

If a catheter occludes coronary flow and remains in place, ventricular fibrillation eventually follows. Likewise, if the catheter partially damps ventricular pressure, it is probable that coronary blood flow is compromised to some extent. If the operator then injects contrast, there is a higher than average likelihood that ventricular fibrillation will occur. Sometimes it is essentially impossible to obtain adequate coronary arteriography without catheter occlusion. Situations include severe ostial disease or a small (nondominant) RCA. To minimize adverse arrhythmic as well as hemodynamic sequelae, the catheter should be occlusive for as short a period of time as possible. A carefully planned cine run, including optimal framing, panning strategy, adequate contrast in the syringe, charged defibrillator, monitoring of ECG and arterial pressure, and a high state of preparedness of the circulating nurse and control room technologist should always be routine aspects of injection in any setting, but particularly in this situation. If there is damping when entering the left main, the catheter should be removed and a cusp shot taken to ascertain if significant left main disease is present. Even if this finding does not appear to be present, the catheter should be in the vessel for the minimal time, including minimal number of injections for diagnostic adequacy. Because occlusion of the left main produces widespread myocardial ischemia as well as ventricular fibrillation, defibrillation may be less effective in returning the patient to hemodynamic stability, despite conversion to a sinus rhythm. Prophylactic use of intra-aortic balloon pumping may be helpful. In addition, low-osmolality contrast agents may be used owing to their milder effect on myocardial contractility than that of ionic dye.

Hypotension

Hypotension occurs primarily in two laboratory situations. The first is in the patient who has a higher than average probability of developing hypotension because of an underlying cardiac condition. Such patients include those with severe coronary obstruction, a large acute myocardial infarction (with or without "impending" shock), and known poor ventricular function who present with either a sustained recurrent ventricular arrhythmia or severe ischemia or a new infarction. These patients may be treated based on their known underlying condition, which is beyond the scope of the chapter.

In the patient who develops unexpected hypotension, several causes should be considered, including vasovagal reaction, blood loss, myocardial ischemia either from coronary dissection or due to unsuspected but critical coronary disease or hypotension secondary to an arrhythmia. Most of these conditions are relatively easy to diagnose, with the exception of bleeding. Bleeding may occur retroperitoneally, resulting in major blood loss without physical signs. This route of bleeding is usually related to passing the accessing needle posteriorly, with blood loss through the posterior vessel wall. The development of hypotension from retroperitoneal bleeding is unusual while the patient is still in the laboratory, but it may occur in a lengthy case and should always be considered in the differential diagnosis of catheterization laboratory hypotension. Nicking a branch of the superficial femoral artery may produce sustained bleeding into the thigh, accumulating up to several hundred milliliters of blood without obvious signs or symptoms. If there is no evidence of vasovagal reaction, ischemia, or arrhythmia, volume expansion measures should be performed if no contraindications to volume loading exist while determining if bleeding is the problem. Swan-Ganz catheter placement is often helpful when the etiology to the hypotension remains uncertain.

Technical Mistakes and Their Prevention

Injection Errors

The goal of the injection technique is to fully visualize the luminal borders of the vessel. A hand injection that is not forceful enough will result in unclear border definition ("dye streaming"). The operator is required to see the catheter on the television monitor prior to injection and should inject the dye as close to a bolus as possible. A test injection is useful to ascertain if the vessel is framed correctly. The operator should appreciate the ECG and pressure data with the catheter intubating the vessel. If they are the same as baseline recordings, the operator may feel comfortable about proceeding. If there is damping, the operator should usually take a test injection cautiously to ascertain cause (e.g., tip inside branch, ostial stenosis, etc.) If the operator injects contrast very vigorously, the catheter may recoil and exit the coronary. A gentle (but rapid) increase in injection pressure usually prevents this problem.

Improper Framing and Panning

In most cases, the entire length of the coronary artery in question cannot be photographed without moving the table (panning). This being said, most of the arterial tree can be cined without panning. The automatic exposure control (AEC) system (see Chapter 2) provides the proper exposure settings at the onset of cine. Most of the arterial tree should be on the screen and recorded before panning. Panning completes visualization of the vessels in question and continues to visualize areas of collateralization to the contralateral vessel. If panning is excessive, with the camera moving predominantly over lung (increasing x-ray penetration), it may "fool" the AEC system and result in inadequate visualization of the coronaries.

To remove the diaphragm from the x-ray field and increase x-ray penetration and consequently improve detail of the angiogram, patients are instructed to breathe deeply and then stop breathing. In thin patients, this technique may not be critical for an adequate study. In the stocky patient, this approach is important. The inexperienced operator's command of "Take a deep breath and hold it, please!" often results in not only suspended breathing but also a marked Valsalva maneuver, pushing the diaphragm back into the picture. The operator should instruct the patient to continue to inspire, even when the patient feels that further inspiration is impossible. Commands may include such directions as, "Breathe in like you're sucking through a straw." It is helpful if the circulating nurse or operator demonstrates the maneuver.

Inadequate Visualization of Part of the Coronary Tree

The operator must be convinced that all segments of the coronary vasculature are seen adequately, preferably in orthogonal views. Thus, the playback system (analog tape or digital acquisition and playback) in the catheterization laboratory must allow for high-quality on-line review.

Angiographic Interpretation

Interpretation of coronary angiography should be described both quantitatively and qualitatively. To adequately interpret an angiogram, the physician should review the films, specifically looking at each coronary segment. Any area with a stenosis should be viewed in two perpendicular projections where there is no vessel overlap. The abnormal area of the vessel is compared with the "normal" segment and is most often expressed as percent diameter stenosis. Because lesions may not be concentric, an average of the stenosis obtained in two views should be expressed. If the stenosis is viewed only in one view, that fact should be stated. Cross-sectional area of a stenosis is an important determinant of blood flow (an 80% diameter stenosis in a 4-mm vessel will have different significance than an 80% diameter stenosis in a 2-mm vessel); thus, an attempt should be made to quantitate the vessel size (using the angiographic catheter as a reference) as well as the cross-sectional area. Likewise, lesion length has important flow implications and should be determined. Other characteristics of the lesion such as its shape—concentric versus eccentric, calcified versus noncalcified, tortuous versus straight—length of lesion, and the presence or absence of thrombus also should be noted (Fig 7-16).

Quantitation of Coronary Lesions

The most commonly employed quantitative method of coronary angiographic interpretation is the "eyeball" method. The interpreter visually estimates the degree of narrowing compared with a normal (reference) segment, expressed as percentage diameter stenosis. The eyeball method has the disadvantage of being an estimation. It has the advantage of being less time consuming as well as being time tested (see Chapter 16). The most important aspect in clinical decision making is not the method used to judge stenosis severity but the assurance that high-quality angiography is performed, taking all appropriate views, injecting adequate contrast, panning properly, developing the film optimally, and viewing it under ideal conditions (i.e., appropriate light source for cine film; excellent-quality super VHS player when viewing tape). In general, eyeball interpretation tends to overestimate severe stenoses and underestimate less severe lesions.

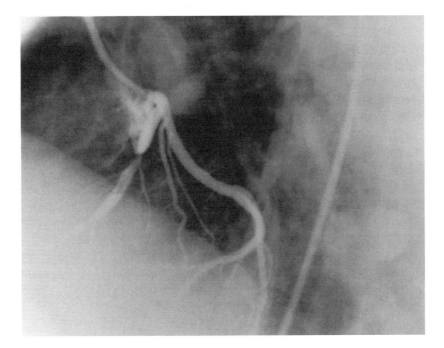

A

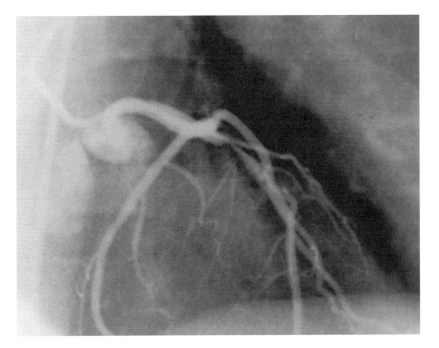

B

Figure 7-16   A thrombus is observed in the proximal LAD distal to a very high grade proximal LAD lesion. The thrombus appears as an ovoid body surrounded by contrast in (**A**) the LAO view and several beads along the inferior surface in (**B**) the cranial RAO view.

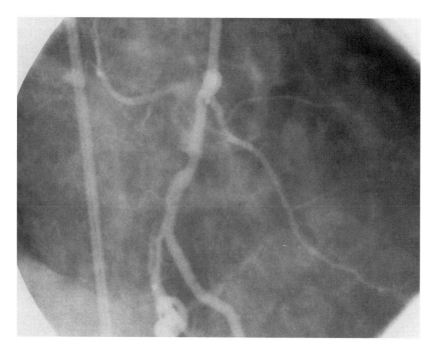

C

Figure 7-16 (**C**) A linear dissection of the mid-RCA following percutaneous transluminal coronary angioplasty (PTCA) is shown in the RAO projection.

Using calipers to compare the diameter of the stenosis with the diameter of the reference segment may be done on the projector or screen or by using tracing paper. The latter method has the advantage of being less of an estimate but the disadvantage of being time consuming. Digital calipers, as part of a computerized program, may be used to measure vessel and lesion size. The physician must place the calipers on the vessel edge to be measured. Thus, high-quality angiography remains necessary to ensure adequate interpretation.

Computer-assisted quantitative coronary angiography (QCA) is the current gold standard for determining the severity of coronary stenosis. It is used routinely in research studies to assess benefits of various interventions, as well as quantify parameters including acute lumen gain and late lumen loss after angioplasty and other interventional procedures. Off-line computer-assisted QCA projects a cine frame onto a TV screen, the image of which is then digitized. A computer program is utilized with either an edge detection or photodensitometry method to measure stenosis severity. The disadvantages of such programs are that they are time consuming, and that significant variability between different QCA systems has been reported. Thus, a particular QCA program may be very reproducible but may have a systematic difference in measurement compared with other QCA systems.

Qualitative Descriptors of Coronary Disease

In the era of interventional cardiology, lesion characteristics have been shown to affect the likelihood of procedural success. Physicians interpreting coronary angiograms should describe coronary lesions both quantitatively and qualitatively. Increasing lesion complexity is associated with decreased success and increasing complication rates in interventional procedures (see Chapter 16).

Flow characteristics of the distal vascular bed subserved by the stenosed vessel also should be described. Standard practice is to define flow according to the Thrombolysis in Myocardial Infarction (TIMI) Trial criteria. TIMI 3 flow is defined as normal flow through the vessel distal to the stenosis, and TIMI 2 flow is present when the dye reaches the distal vessel more slowly than usual. (When viewing a left coronary vessel, the flow is compared with the other vessels concurrently viewed; when viewing the RCA flow, characteristics are compared proximal to and beyond the lesion, or the experienced angiographer bases the decision on what is considered normal.) TIMI 1 flow means the dye goes beyond the lesion but does not reach the terminal portion of the vessel by the end of the cine run, and TIMI 0 flow is present when the angiographic contrast does not traverse the lesion.

It is important to describe the caliber of the vessel distal to the lesion. This finding has implications regarding suitability for bypass surgery and interventional procedures. Collateral blood flow to the distal vessel should be evaluated. The type of collaterals, bridging (from same vessel proximal to stenosis) or via another coronary segment, must be identified. In general, a lesion with bridging collaterals is usually not amenable to interventional techniques. Collateral flow implies a severe stenosis. The presence of collaterals, when a severe stenosis has not been identified, suggests an occluded vessel that must be diligently sought. Collateral flow needs to be observed in both oblique views to be certain of the vascular bed supplied. When distal flow in a vascular segment is not observed and that area of the ventricle moves on ventriculography, there may be an anomalous coronary vessel, or a collateral may have been missed. Collaterals may be overlooked if the injection into the vessel supplying the collateral is not forceful enough, if the vessel supplying the collateral is not injected (i.e., separate ostium conus supplying LAD), and/or if there is inadequate panning. Finally, if the coronary catheter plugs the vessel, forceful injection may push dye into the other coronary via collaterals, even without a significant lesion in the latter vessel (Fig 7-17).

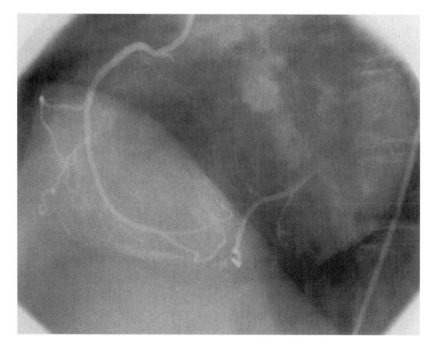

Figure 7-17   In this example, the right coronary catheter is impacted in the RCA without dye overflow into the aorta. Hand pressure forced contrast through collaterals into the left coronary without a lesion in the latter vessel.

Problems in Interpretation

The most frequent problem in interpretation involves vessel overlap. It is imperative that attempts be made to visualize lesions in at least two views, which ideally are perpendicular to each other. During angiography, careful attention to taking all of the views necessary to adequately identify each lesion is mandatory. Frequently, minor adjustments in views (e.g., a steeper RAO caudal or cranial than usual) prove satisfactory. Occasionally, one has to "play around" with different projections until an adequate view is found.

A common problem for the inexperienced angiographer is inadequate opacification. This causes difficulty in defining lesions both quantitatively and qualitatively, and may cause one to "miss" collaterals that are present. Patients with hypertrophied ventricles or increased coronary blood flow require more vigorous injections with more than the usual amount of dye.

Ostial lesions often pose particular difficulties in interpretations. Branch ostial lesions (e.g., LAD and CX) are less of a problem, provided adequate views are taken so that the area is clearly seen. Aorto-ostial lesions can be difficult to detect because the tip of the catheter may obscure the lesion, and streaming of dye from a malaligned catheter may make an area appear abnormal when it in fact is without disease. A clue to significant aorto-ostial disease is the presence of a damped pressure tracing. When this phenomenon occurs in the RCA, administration of nitroglycerin is useful to exclude catheter tip–induced vasospasm. Pressure damping in the left main coronary artery is more troublesome, and great care should be taken in that situation to attempt sinus shots to help identify any ostial lesions. In both the RCA and left main coronary artery, observing for backflow of dye from the orifice is useful, because its absence makes an ostial lesion more likely. In situations in which an ostial lesion is suspected, changing catheters to view the vessel with the catheter sitting differently in or near the ostium may be useful.

Coronary Artery Anomalies

Coronary artery anomalies (Fig 7-18) occur in approximately 1% of patients undergoing catheterization. It is important that these anomalies are understood so that the angiographer recognizes them and performs a safe and complete study. The majority of anomalies are of origin and distribution, with a minority (10%–15%) being coronary artery fistulae. The majority of coronary artery anomalies are found incidentally at the time of coronary angiography and in most cases may be considered benign.

An origin of the LAD and CX separate from the left sinus has an increased incidence in patients with congenital aortic stenosis and left dominant systems. It is often difficult to differentiate separate origins from a short left main. A flush shot in the LAO caudal view with the catheter in the left sinus is helpful in distinguishing these two possibilities. The distribution of the vessels is normal. Failure to recognize this benign anomaly can lead to the erroneous conclusion that a vessel is occluded.

Origin of the CX from the RCA or right sinus of Valsalva is a common anomaly and must be sought in cases in which the CX appears absent (i.e., vessels absent in the lateral wall). Failure to recognize this anomaly leads to an incomplete catheterization. The CX may arise from the proximal RCA and thus will be visualized (with proper panning), provided the right coronary catheter has not intubated the vessel too deeply. When the CX emanates from the right sinus, catheter manipulation to search for this vessel is necessary. The anomalous CX does not cause ischemia in the absence of atherosclerosis.

Other benign anomalous origins of coronary vessels can be discovered. The RCA occasionally originates from the posterior sinus of Valsalva. The left main can also originate from the posterior sinus but does so much less frequently. In both cases, the course of the vessel is normal, and there are no associated symptoms or complications. Occasionally, the coronary arteries arise superiorly

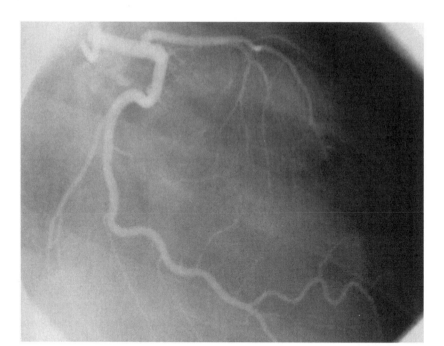

A

Figure 7-18 Examples of a few (of many) coronary anomalies. **(A)** The left coronary artery from the left main consists of only proximal portion and septal perforators.

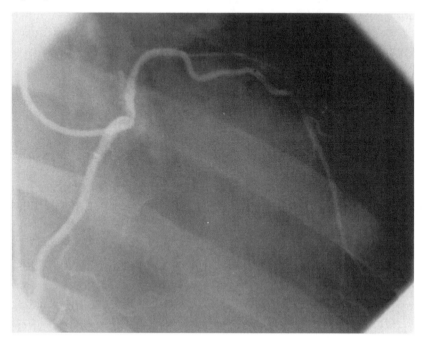

B

Figure 7-18 **(B)** In the RAO, the RCA gives off the LAD, which courses anteriorly.

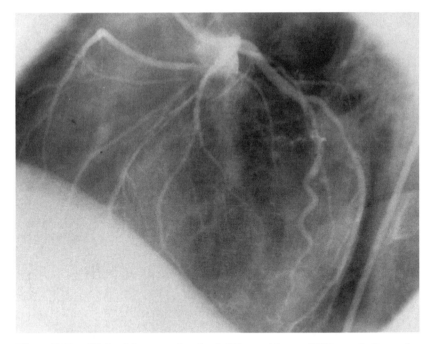

C

Figure 7-18 (**C**) In this example, the LAD provides an RV branch. It can be seen to course to the right heart border.

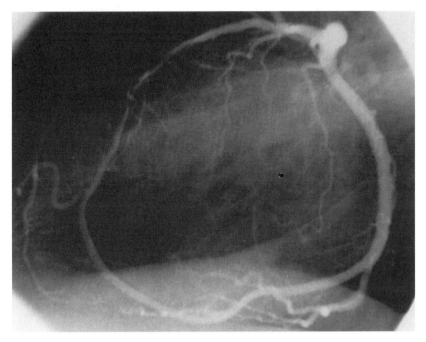

D

Figure 7-18 (**D**) The entire RCA is supplied by a branch from the mid-LAD. The RCA can be seen to course almost parallel with the LAD. (e) A coronary artery fistula from an RV branch of the RCA is shown.

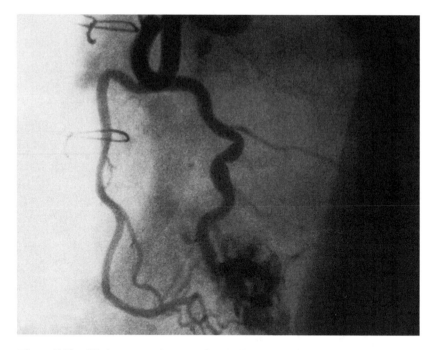

E

Figure 7-18   (E) A coronary artery fistula from an RV branch of the RCA is shown.

above the sinuses of Valsalva. The distribution of these vessels is normal. In circumstances in which the vessel appears to be "missing" and cannot be found, aortography performed in the proximal ascending aorta is helpful.

Potentially serious coronary anomalies comprise approximately 20% of all anomalies. The majority of these lead to signs and symptoms early in life. They include anomalous coronary origin from the pulmonary artery, which usually causes death or profound left dysfunction and heart failure in infancy. Ectopic origin of the RCA from the left sinus is extremely rare and may cause angina with exercise as the aorta expands and squeezes the RCA coursing between the aorta and pulmonary artery. Ectopic origin of the left coronary artery from the right sinus of Valsalva has five subtypes, depending on the relationship of the anomalous artery with the aorta and pulmonary artery. The most serious subtype occurs when the anomalous vessel courses between the aorta and pulmonary artery, which has been reported to provoke ischemia and sudden death. Single coronary arteries also have a number of different patterns, depending on where the vessel originates, its course, and its relationship to the aorta and pulmonary artery.

Small coronary artery fistulae account for approximately 10% to 15% of coronary anomalies. They are usually single and in the majority of cases drain into the pulmonary artery from the RCA. Patients with small AV fistulae do not have signs or symptoms, do not have significant left-to-right shunts, and can be managed without surgical intervention.

Large coronary artery fistulae are rarely seen in adults because they generally are diagnosed and repaired in childhood. Such patients often have continuous murmurs in addition to signs and symptoms of right heart failure.

Complications of Coronary Angiography

The physician performing coronary angiography needs to be aware of complication rates to inform the patient of procedural risks, to take steps to avoid complications, to know how to react when complications occur, and to measure the complication rate for each operator and overall for the catheterization laboratory to determine if its and the operator's complication rates are within the acceptable range.

The mortality risk of coronary arteriography is approximately 0.1% or less. Factors associated with increased risk include age greater than 60 years (doubled mortality), functional class IV, ejection fraction less than 30%, severe aortic stenosis, and left main disease.

The risk of myocardial infarction associated with diagnostic angiography is approximately 0.06%. This rate increases in patients with unstable angina, recent myocardial infarction, left main disease, and insulin-dependent diabetes. Preventing myocardial infarction during catheterization involves adequate anticoagulation, careful catheter manipulation to avoid coronary dissection, adequate flushing of catheters to avoid air embolism or thrombus injection, and prompt management of chest pain, arrhythmias, and hypotension.

Cerebrovascular accidents (CVAs) occur in approximately 0.07% to 0.1% of diagnostic catheterizations. The incidence is increased in patients with prior CVA, ejection fraction less than 30%, and patients more than 60 years old. Most CVAs associated with catheterization are embolic in origin, with atheromatous material dislodged from the aorta by the catheter or a thrombus dislodged from the catheter, wire, or the left ventricle (in patients with a recent myocardial infarction or severe LV dysfunction). Frequently, these embolic neurologic events resolve within days. Attention to catheter manipulation, particularly when the coronary vessel is difficult to cannulate, as well as care in flushing catheters adequately and proper anticoagulation is necessary to minimize risk.

Cardiac arrhythmias requiring treatment occur in approximately 0.5% of cases and include dye-induced bradycardia or asystole, heart block, and sustained ventricular arrhythmias. Risk of serious ventricular arrhythmias is increased in patients with left main coronary disease and patients with depressed LV function. Asystolic episodes (which can precede serious ventricular tachyarrhythmias) can be decreased by minimizing the amount of contrast injected, by ensuring that the patient coughs vigorously when instructed to do so, and by using non-ionic contrast media.

Contrast reactions consist of urticaria in approximately 1% to 2% of patients, angioedema of lips and eyelids and bronchospasm in 0.03%, and anaphylactoid circulatory shock in 0.01%. Patients with "allergic" histories have an increased incidence of mild but not severe reactions. Patients with previous mild reaction to contrast agents have a slightly increased risk on re-exposure to contrast agents, and patients with previous severe reactions are at high risk. Pretreatment for patients at increased risk include use of steroids (e.g., prednisone 40 mg PO two to four times daily in the 24 hours leading to the procedure), H_1-blockers (e.g., diphenhydramine 50 mg on call to the lab), and H_2-blockers (e.g., cimetidine 100 mg IV on call to the laboratory). Non-ionic contrast agents probably should be used in patients with known dye hypersensitivity. When mild contrast reactions occur, IV diphenhydramine (25 mg) may reduce pruritus. When the reaction appears more severe, IV steroids are used. When there is a severe anaphylactoid reaction consisting of bronchospasm and hypotension, the treatment is IV epinephrine (0.2–0.4 mg every 5 min.) associated with volume expansion, as well as treatment with IV diphenhydramine and steroids (hydrocortisone 200 mg intravenously).

The risk of contrast nephropathy is increased in patients with preexisting renal disease (creatinine > 1.5 dL), diabetic renal insufficiency, and multiple myeloma. Serum creatinine rises 24 to 48 hours postprocedure, peaks at approximately day 5, and returns to baseline a few days later in the majority of patients. Less than 2% of patients require dialysis. Limiting the amount of contrast used decreases the risk of contrast nephropathy, as does adequate preprocedure hydration. There are conflicting data regarding the relative nephrotoxicity of non-ionic versus ionic contrast medium (see Chapter 6). In patients at increased risk of contrast nephropathy, it is often advisable to defer left ventriculography and obtain LV function by noninvasive means.

Vascular complications associated with diagnostic coronary angiography occur in approximately 0.6% of patients. With the femoral approach, these are more often localized bleeding, hematoma formation, pseudoaneurysm, or AV fistula development. These complications often occur from excessive or prolonged anticoagulation at the time of sheath removal or reinstitution of anticoagulation shortly thereafter, inadequate compression, inadequate bed rest, and the use of larger Fr sizes of catheters and sheaths. Pseudoaneurysms are often caused by low femoral punctures in association with excessive anticoagulation or inadequate compression. Many pseudoaneurysms can be closed by manual compression using ultrasound guidance. AV fistulae can also be caused by low femoral punctures; small fistulae often close by themselves. Use of the brachial approach is more often associated with arterial thrombosis, the incidence of which can be lessened by adequate anticoagulation, care in manual compression (for percutaneous cases), and closing of the vessel by an experienced operator (for brachial cutdown cases).

This chapter is a beginning for those embarking on a career in invasive cardiology. Acquiring knowledge in the catheterization laboratory is a life-long experience. An open mind, a thirst for knowledge, and concern for patients are required to excel as an angiographer and physician.

SELECTED READINGS

Abrams HL, Adams DF. The coronary arteriogram—structural and functional aspects. N Engl J Med 1969;281:1276–1284, 1336–1344.

Baim DS, Grossman W. Coronary angiography. In: Grossman W, Baim DS, eds. Cardiac catheterization, angiography and intervention. 4th ed. Philadelphia: Lea & Febiger, 1991.

Goss JE, Chambers CE, Heupler FA. Systemic anaphylactoid reactions to iodinated contrast media during cardiac catheterization procedures: guidelines for prevention, diagnosis and treatment. Cathet Cardiovasc Diagn 1995;34:99–104.

Gould KL. Percent coronary stenosis: battered gold standard, pernicious relic or clinical practicality. J Am Coll Cardiol 1988;11:886–888.

Higgins CB. Coronary angiography: a decade of advances. Am J Cardiol 1988;62:7K–10K.

Johnson LW, Lozner EC, Johnson S, et al. Complications of cardiac catheterization: coronary arteriography 1984–1987. A report of the Registry of the Society for Cardiac Angiography and Interventions. I. Results and complications. Cathet Cardiovasc Diagn 1989;17:5–10.

Johnson LW, Krone R. Cardiac catheterization 1991: a report of the Registry of the Society for Cardiac Angiography and Interventions (SCAI). Cathet Cardiovasc Diagn 1993;28:219–220.

Kim D, Orron DE, Skillman JJ, et al. Role of superficial femoral artery puncture in the development of pseudoaneurysm and arteriovenous fistula complicating transfemoral cardiac catheterization. Cathet Cardiovasc Diagn 1992;25:91–97.

King SB, Douglas JS. Coronary arteriography and angioplasty. New York: McGraw-Hill, 1995.

Laskey W, Boyle J, Johnson LW. Multivariable model for prediction of risk of significant complication during diagnostic cardiac catheterization. Cathet Cardiovasc Diagn 1993;30:185–190.

Lozner EC, Johnson LW, Johnson E, et al. Coronary arteriography 1984–1987. A report of the Registry of the Society for Cardiac Angiography and Interventions. II. An analysis of 218 deaths related to coronary arteriography. Cathet Cardiovasc Diagn 1989;17:11–14.

Pepine CJ, Lambert CR, Hill JA. Coronary angiography. In: Pepine CJ, Lambert CR, Hill JA, eds., 2nd ed. Diagnostic and therapeutic cardiac catheterization. Baltimore: Williams & Wilkins, 1994, pp. 211–220.

Sabri N. Complications of cardiac catheterization, coronary angiography and coronary interventions. J Invest Cardiol 1994;6:300–305.

Sos TA, Baltaxe HA. Cranial and caudal angulation for coronary angiography revisited. Circulation 1977;56:119–123.

Tilkian AG, Daily EK. Cardiac catheterization and coronary arteriography. In: Tilkian AG, Daily EK, eds. Cardiovascular procedures. St. Louis: Mosby, 1986.

Wyman RM, Safian RD, Portway V, et al. Current complications of diagnostic and therapeutic cardiac catheterization. J Am Coll Cardiol 1988;12:1400–1406.

Yamanaka O, Hobbs RE. Coronary artery anomalies in 126,595 patients undergoing coronary arteriography. Cathet Cardiovasc Diagn 1990;21:28–40.

8

TRANSSEPTAL LEFT HEART CATHETERIZATION

Igor F. Palacios

TRANSSEPTAL LEFT HEART catheterization was introduced independently in 1959 by Ross and Cope and later modified by Brockenbrough and Mullins.[1-4] The procedure became an agreeable alternative to methods available at that time for directly measuring left atrial and left ventricular pressures, such as the transbronchial and transthoracic approaches.[5] The developments of the flotation pulmonary artery catheter in 1970 by Swan and Ganz[6] and retrograde catheterization of the left ventricle led to a significant decline in utilization of the transseptal technique. Furthermore, with fewer patients with valvular disease and improved echocardiography, a smaller number of cardiologists were adequately trained to perform the procedure.[7,8] With fewer procedures and trained personnel came concern over potentially grave complications and associated mortality; the procedure attained an aura of danger and intrigue.[9] With the introduction of interventional procedures such as percutaneous mitral valvuloplasty, antegrade percutaneous aortic valvuloplasty, and radiofrequency ablation of left-sided bypass tracts, there has been an increased demand for, and rekindled interest in, transseptal catheterization.[10,11] This chapter reviews the technique, indications, and complications of transseptal left heart catheterization.

Technique

The physician performing a transseptal catheterization must be aware of the indications and contraindications of this technique and should be well familiarized with the anatomy of the interatrial septum. Transseptal catheterization is performed using the percutaneous technique only from the right femoral vein. Although the right subclavian and the right jugular veins have been used occasionally, they are not standard techniques. Transseptal catheterization is also possible from the left femoral vein, but it is more painful to the patient due to the sharp angulation between the left iliac vein and the inferior vena cava. Biplane fluoroscopy, if available, is the ideal imaging system. However, a single-plane C-arm fluoroscope, which can be rotated from the anteroposterior to lateral position, may also be used.

There are two different transseptal needles: the Ross and the Brockenbrough. The Ross needle is a 17-gauge needle, has a more pronounced curve, and is typically used with the Brockenbrough catheter. The Brockenbrough needle is more frequently utilized. It is an 18-gauge needle that tapers at the distal tip to a 21-gauge and is typically used with the Mullins sheath.

Prior to attempted puncture of the interatrial septum, full familiarity with the transseptal apparatus (Mullins sheath and dilator and Brockenbrough needle and stylet) is essential (Fig 8-1). The Mullins transseptal introducer (USCI, Billerica, MA) is composed of a 59-cm sheath and a 67-cm dilator. The distance the dilator protrudes from the sheath should be noted prior to the procedure. The Brockenbrough needle is 71 cm in length. The flange of the needle has an arrow that points to the position of the tip of the needle. Before use, the operator should be sure that the needle is straight and that the arrow of

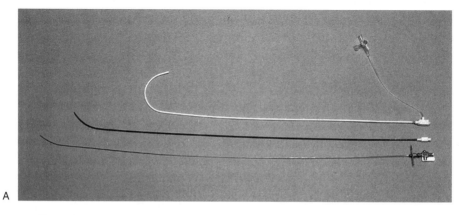

A

Figure 8-1A Brockenbrough needle and Mullins sheath and dilator with the needle within the tip of the dilator.

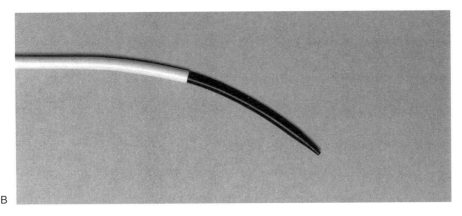

B

Figure 8-1B   The tip of the apparatus.

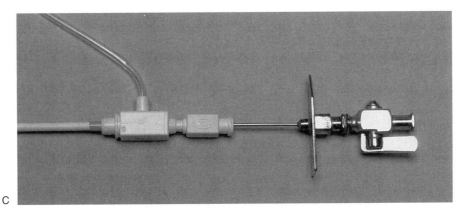

C

Figure 8-1C   The proximal end shows the relationship among the needle, dilator, and sheath. Note the space between sheath/dilator and flange of the needle. The arrow on the flange corresponds to direction of needle tip.

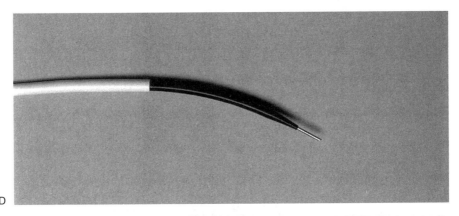

D

Figure 8-1D   With the needle advanced.

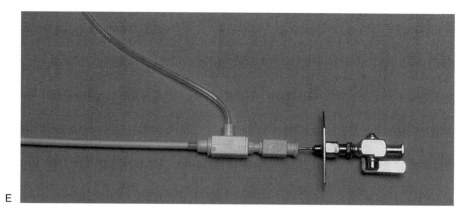

Figure 8-1E the distance between the flange and dilator/sheath is narrowed.

the flange is perfectly aligned with the needle tip. This arrow allows the operator to know exactly where the distal tip of the needle is pointing. When the needle tip lies just within the dilator, there is approximately 1.5 to 2.0 cm distance between the dilator hub and the needle flange. This measurement also should be noted.

Once satisfied with the spatial relationship of the components of the transseptal system, a 0.032″ J-tipped wire is positioned at the junction of the superior vena cava and left innominate vein from the right femoral vein. Venipuncture must be as horizontal as possible to facilitate manipulation of the transseptal system and permit maximal transmission of pulsations. Tactile as well as visual clues are important in properly identifying the puncture site. To ease insertion of the Mullins sheath, predilatation with an 8-Fr dilator is recommended. A pigtail catheter is positioned retrograde at the right coronary sinus. To correctly identify the aorta with the use of the pigtail catheter and biplane fluoroscopy, the spatial relationship of the ascending aorta and its surrounding structures should be known. The pigtail catheter must be flushed with heparinized saline every 3 minutes to prevent clot formation and embolic complications.

Before proceeding, the right and left heart borders and apical pulsations are surveyed under fluoroscopy. Under fluoroscopic guidance, the Mullins sheath and dilator are advanced over the J-wire into the superior vena cava–left innominate vein junction. The sheath must never be advanced without the wire because the stiff dilator can readily perforate the inferior vena cava, superior vena cava, or right atrium. Once the Mullins sheath is properly placed, the wire is removed. The Brockenbrough needle is then advanced to lie just inside the dilator, using the predetermined distance between the needle flange and dilator as a guide. When advancing the needle to this position, it must rotate freely within the dilator, not be forcibly turned, to prevent damage to the needle tip or dilator. Occasionally, there is some resistance to advancing the transseptal needle through the iliac vein or the inferior vena cava, particularly at the pelvic brim. Under these circumstances, the needle should not be forcibly advanced; instead, the needle and the Mullins sheath should be advanced as a unit through the areas of resistance.

Once properly advanced to the tip of the Mullins dilator, the Brockenbrough needle is double-flushed and pressure tubing connected. To avoid confusion, we recommend displaying only this single pressure tracing, and on a 40-mm Hg scale. At this point, proper orientation of the assembly is critical. The side-arm of the sheath and needle flange should always have the same orientation. Initially, they point horizontally and to the patient's left. This directs the tip of the apparatus medially in the anteroposterior fluoroscopic view. The entire system is then rotated clockwise until the needle flange arrow and sheath side-arm is positioned at the 4 o'clock position (with the patient's forehead representing 12 o'clock and the patient's occiput 6 o'clock). This directs the assembly to the left and slightly posterior.

Under anteroposterior fluoroscopy, the entire system is then withdrawn across three sequential landmark "bumps," or leftward movements of the needle. These landmark bumps represent movement of the apparatus (1) as it enters the right atrium–superior vena cava junction, (2) as it moves over the ascending aorta where the tactile sensation of aortic pulsations aids in localization, and (3) as it passes over the limbus to intrude into the fossa ovalis. On a lateral view, the correct position for puncture of the apparatus is posterior and inferior to the aorta (marked by the pigtail catheter) (Figs 8-2 and 8-3).

The system is advanced (needle within the dilator) until further movement is limited by the limbus. In approximately 10% of cases, the foramen ovale is patent and the apparatus directly enters the left atrium. In the remainder, the tip of the Brockenbrough needle is advanced into the left atrium under continuous fluoroscopic and pressure monitoring. Care should be taken to advance only the needle and not the entire apparatus. Successful penetration of the septum is heralded by a change from right atrial to left atrial pressure waveform, accompanied by a small but definite lateral movement of the needle tip on fluoroscopy. A palpable "pop" may occur with septal penetration, confirmed by injecting contrast, which should flow freely into the left atrium. If the pressure tracing is damped, injection of contrast will aid in localizing the puncture site. If there is staining of the interatrial septum, the needle must be advanced further. A stained septum must not be interpreted as failure and, in fact, the tattooed septum may be used as a guide for future attempts. If the left atrium cannot be entered, the entire system must be withdrawn to the inferior vena cava–right atrial junction, the needle removed, and the J-wire advanced through the Mullins system and repositioned in the superior vena cava for a

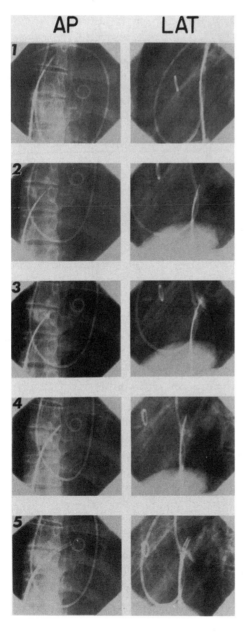

Figure 8-2 Transseptal left heart catheterization as viewed by anteroposterior (left) and lateral fluoroscopy (right). The Mullins sheath and dilator are advanced to the superior vena cava–left innominate vein junction. The J-wire is removed, and the needle and stylet are advanced to lie just inside the dilator (1). After removal of the stylet, the entire system is withdrawn across three sequential "bumps" involving the right atrium, ascending aorta, and fossa ovalis. On a lateral view, the apparatus appears posterior and inferior to the aorta, identified by the pigtail catheter (2). The tip of the needle is advanced into the left atrium, identified by the anticipated change in pressure recordings. This is confirmed by the injection of contrast, which should flow freely into the left atrium. If the pressure tracing is damped, the injection of contrast will stain the interatrial septum (3). Following successful interatrial puncture (4), the Brockenbrough needle and dilator are advanced under fluoroscopic and hemodynamic guidance until the dilator lies within the left atrium. The needle is withdrawn into the dilator and the sheath advanced into the left atrium (5). (Reproduced by permission from Roelke M, Smith AJC, Palacios IF. The technique and safety of transseptal left heart catheterization. The Massachusetts General Hospital experience with 1,279 procedures. Cathet Cardiovasc Diagn 1994;32:332–339.)

second attempt. If there is aortic or pericardial staining, or the presence of an aortic pressure tracing, the tip of the needle must be removed and the patient reevaluated prior to a second attempt. If the procedure is being performed in preparation for percutaneous mitral balloon valvuloplasty (PMV) or antegrade aortic balloon valvuloplasty (PAV), we generally postpone a second attempt for another day, because the patient requires systemic anticoagulation for the

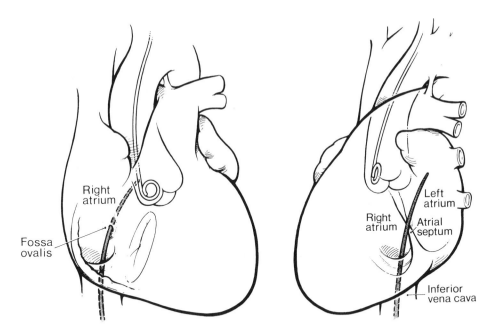

Figure 8-3 The proper orientation of the Mullins sheath/dilator in the left atrium after successful puncture of the interatrial septum. In the antero-posterior view (left), the sheath lies at the midportion of the right atrial silhouette. In the lateral view (right), it is located posterior and inferior to the aortic valve plane (demarcated by the pigtail catheter). (Reproduced by permission from Roelke M, Smith AJC, Palacios IF. The technique and safety of transseptal left heart catheterization. The Massachusetts General Hospital experience with 1,279 procedures. Cathet Cardiovasc Diagn 1994; 32:332–339.

valvuloplasty procedure. If the aorta or pericardium has been entered only with the tip of the needle and the procedure is being performed only in the course of diagnostic catheterization, the procedure may be attempted again.

The proper positioning of the needle after successful puncture is at the midportion of the right atrial silhouette in the anteroposterior view. In the lateral view, it lies posterior and inferior to the aortic valve plane, as demarcated by the pigtail catheter (see Figs 8-2 and 8-3). Slight variations in the technique may be required in the presence of abnormal atrial or aortic anatomy and with different interventional procedures. In patients with left atrial enlargement, the septum lies more horizontally. The site of puncture is more posterior and inferior. In aortic valve disease accompanied by a dilated aorta, the septum is more vertical. The fossa ovalis and the puncture site are therefore more superior and slightly anterior. With right atrial enlargement, the transseptal apparatus may not reach to the septum. A gentle curve placed on the needle 10 to 15 cm from the distal tip may allow engagement of the fossa ovalis. During double-balloon PMV or with antegrade PAV, a low puncture site in the middle posterior third of the septum provides a straight pathway to the mitral orifice and apex of the left ventricle to facilitate manipulation of guidewires and catheters. A slightly higher puncture site is preferred when using a single Inoue balloon (Toray Co., Tokyo, Japan) to allow the straightest course for the flow-directed distal balloon through the mitral valve.

After successful interatrial puncture, the entire system is rotated counterclockwise to 3 o'clock and carefully advanced under fluoroscopic and hemodynamic guidance until it is certain that the dilator lies within the left atrium. The needle is withdrawn into the dilator. The sheath is then advanced into the left atrium, keeping the needle within the sheath to avoid puncturing the left atrium. The needle and dilator are then removed, and the sheath is double-flushed prior to connecting to pressure tubing. If the sheath has entered an inferior pulmonary vein, it must be withdrawn slightly with counterclockwise rotation to position it in the left atrium. Care should be taken after entering the left atrium with the needle. Perforation of the left atrial wall can occur if the system is advanced without careful pressure and fluoroscopic monitoring. If the left atrial pressure becomes damped, the apparatus may be against the left atrial wall and further advancement of the system could result in perforation and tamponade. Heparin, usually 5000 units, is administered after placement of the Mullins sheath has been accomplished.

Indications

In the past, in the majority of cases, transseptal catheterization was performed for diagnostic purposes. Today, however, there is a large group of patients undergoing interventional procedures who require access to the left atrium by the transseptal technique.[10,11]

Transseptal left heart catheterization should be performed whenever direct measurement of left atrial pressure is needed (when accuracy of pulmonary capillary wedge pressure is questionable) or retrograde access to the left ventricle is unobtainable or dangerous (Table 8-1). In patients with mitral stenosis and pulmonary artery hypertension, the true capillary wedge pressure may be unobtainable or inaccurate[5,10–13] and there is a slightly higher incidence of pulmonary artery perforation with balloon flotation in the pulmonary arteries. In patients with prosthetic mitral valves, the pulmonary capillary wedge pressure may overestimate the diastolic gradient across the valve. A false mitral gradient could be the result of either the presence of pulmonary hypertension and/or a phase delay in the pulmonary wedge v waves, resulting in a higher mean diastolic gradient compared with the left atrial pressure obtained by transseptal catheterization (Fig 8-4). This may lead to the calculation of an erroneously small prosthetic mitral valve area and unnecessary repeat mitral valve surgery.[12] In mitral regurgitation, the regurgitant fraction can be quantified by injecting

Table 8-1   Indications for Transseptal Left Heart Catheterization

A. Diagnostic indications
  1. Status postaortic valve replacement
  2. Status postmitral valve replacement and evidence of heart failure with question of prosthesis
      dysfunction
  3. Other
      a. Native severe aortic valve stenosis
      b. Aortic endocarditis/abscess
      c. Mitral stenosis with pulmonary artery hypertension and unreliable pulmonary capillary wedge
          pressure
      d. Hypertrophic cardiomyopathy
      e. Quantitation of mitral regurgitation
      f. Direct measurement of left atrial pressure in patients with unreliable measurement of the
          pulmonary capillary wedge pressure
      g. Cor triatriatum
B. Therapeutic indications
  1. Percutaneous mitral valvuloplasty
  2. Antegrade aortic valvuloplasty
  3. Radiofrequency ablation of left-sided pathways
  4. Atrioseptostomy

indocyanine green dye into the left ventricle and obtaining dye curves by sampling the left atrium and femoral artery.[13]

Aortic valvular disease or aortic valve replacement may preclude safe retrograde left ventricular catheterization. In patients with mechanical aortic valves, retrograde catheterization is not possible. Many cardiologists prefer the transseptal technique in patients with bioprosthetic aortic valves or native aortic stenosis to avoid damaging the valve during catheterization. In critical aortic stenosis, the transaortic gradient is more reliable when left ventricular and aortic pressures are measured simultaneously via transseptal puncture. When the valve area is 0.6 cm^2 or less, the catheter itself may significantly obstruct the orifice and falsely increase the recorded gradient[14] or result in transient hemodynamic deterioration. In heavily calcified valves, transseptal catheterization may avert possible dislodgement and embolization of calcium.[7] Transseptal left heart catheterization should be performed in patients with aortic valve replacements in whom evaluation of the aortic gradient or ventriculography is needed.

Other diagnostic uses for transseptal catheterization include aortic valve endocarditis, in which crossing the valve could be dangerous, and the evaluation of dynamic left ventricular outflow obstruction, both in allowing simultaneous recording of left ventricular and aortic pressures and in distinguishing dynamic outflow obstruction from catheter entrapment. Transseptal catheterization allows direct measurement of left atrial pressure in mitral regurgitation, cor triatriatum, and pulmonary hypertension, and provides access for pulmonary vein angiography in evaluating pulmonary atresia and pulmonary venoocclusive disease.[13]

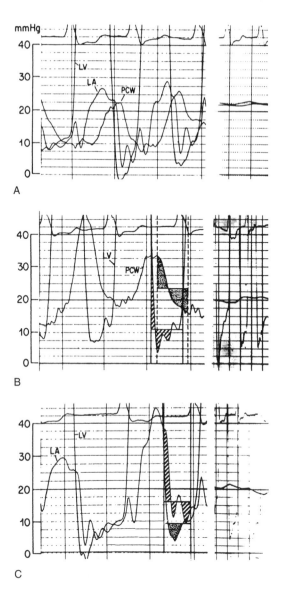

Figure 8-4 **(A)** Simultaneous pulmonary capillary wedge (PCW) and left atrial (LA) recording using the transseptal technique with a phase delay of 0.14 second. **(B)** Simultaneous left ventricular (LV) and PCW recording with a sample gradient measured for one cardiac cycle. Solid vertical lines represent the same diastolic filling period for the left ventricle. Dashed vertical lines represent the same diastolic filling period for the wedge pressure shifted to coincide with the peak of the v wave. **(C)** Simultaneous LV and LA recording using the transseptal technique with a sample gradient measured for one cardiac cycle. Solid vertical lines represent diastolic filling period for both LA and LV tracings. The right side of each panel shows mean LA or mean pulmonary wedge pressure. Reproduced with permission from the American College of Cardiology (Journal of the American College of Cardiology, 1985;5:1387–1392).

The resurgence of interest in transseptal catheterization is a direct result of its role in interventional procedures. Transseptal catheterization is a prerequisite in percutaneous mitral valvuloplasty[15] and antegrade percutaneous aortic valvuloplasty.[16] Likewise, in the pediatric population, balloon atrioseptostomy in the treatment of transposition of the great arteries, pulmonary atresia with intact ventricular septum, total anomalous pulmonary venous return, and tricuspid atresia require transseptal catheterization.[17]

Currently, the vast majority of radiofrequency ablations of left-sided bypass tracts are performed via retrograde left ventricular catheterization. However, successful ablation of left free-wall, posteroseptal, and septal bypass tracts has been reported using a transseptal approach.[18] A transseptal approach may allow for the ablation of otherwise inaccessible pathways and, may facilitate the procedure in some patients, reducing both discomfort and radiation exposure.

Contraindications

Contraindications to transseptal catheterization include the following:

1. Obstruction of the inferior vena cava (e.g., by tumor, thrombus, therapeutic ligation, or filter placement)
2. Systemic anticoagulation
3. Bleeding diathesis
4. Anatomic deformity such as severe kyphoscoliosis, or patients with previous pneumonectomy resulting in severe rotation of the heart
5. Congenital deformities resulting in obscured landmarks of the atrial septum
6. Thrombus in the right or the left atrium documented by echocardiography. Patients with previous clinical emboli can have transseptal catheterization if they have been adequately anticoagulated with coumadin and the left atrium is free of thrombus by transesophageal echocardiography.
7. Presence of atrial myxoma
8. Patients with large right atria, which represent a particular problem, because of the flattening of the septum and the occasional inability of the needle to touch the interatrial septum.

Complications

In part, the decline in the frequency of transseptal catheterization can be ascribed to concern over potentially lethal complications. Penetration of the inferior vena cava, atria, or aorta can occur and may lead to tamponade and/or death.[19–22] Earlier studies utilized a single anteroposterior fluoroscopic view and, in some series, larger-gauge needles than are used today. Lateral fluoroscopy allows the visualization of the needle to place it posterior and inferior to the aortic valve plane, thus avoiding penetration of the aorta and an extreme posterior needle position, which risks left atrial perforation. Today transseptal catheterization can be performed safely with a low incidence of complication,[5,7,10,11,13] which reflects operator experience and perhaps the addition of biplane fluoroscopy. Others, however, have reported low complication rates utilizing single-plane fluoroscopy.[23,24] The transseptal "needle tip only" can inadvertently puncture the atria or the aorta. However, adverse sequelae usually do not develop, provided that this inadvertent puncture is immediately recognized before the apparatus is advanced further. In a series utilizing biplane fluoroscopy, inadvertent pericardial punctures occurred in 3 of 217 patients (1.4%) and none resulted in tamponade.[25] Several series have noted that at operation following uneventful transseptal catheterizations, blood-stained pericardial fluid is not infrequently present, implying unnoticed atrial puncture during the procedure.[3,20,26] Cardiac tamponade occurs with advancement of the larger dilator and not with inadvertent needle puncture. Cardiac tamponade occurs less frequently in patients with prior cardiac surgery, making transseptal catheterization safer in postoperative patients. Tamponade is less likely to occur because of the obliteration of the pericardial space by adhesions.[27]

Two-dimensional transthoracic and transesophageal echocardiography have been used as an adjunct to fluoroscopy to avoid such complications. The interatrial septum and aorta are best visualized in the apical 4-chamber view, and saline contrast allows localization of the needle before and after septal puncture.[28] Needle-tip punctures were not totally eliminated, and occurred in 1 of 13 transseptal catheterizations (with no adverse sequelae).[26] Thus, concomitant echocardiography adds little to biplane fluoroscopy and may be impractical in many catheterization laboratories.

Systemic embolization is another grave complication of transseptal catheterization. Cerebral emboli are most frequently reported, but emboli to coronary, splanchnic, renal, and femoral arteries also have occurred.[20,29,30] We do not routinely perform an echocardiogram prior to diagnostic transseptal catheterization unless the patient is at high risk for an atrial thrombus (e.g., atrial fibrillation, mitral stenosis). As part of the evaluation for percutaneous mitral valvuloplasty, patients obtain an echocardiogram to visualize the atrial appendage and the presence of thrombus, as well as to be ranked by echocardiographic score.[31] Transseptal catheterization in the presence of a non-echogenic atrial myxoma has resulted in embolism.[32] It is also conceivable that not all thrombi are visible by echocardiography. In addition to thrombus, embolization of air to the coronary and cerebral vessels has occurred,[22] as well as embolization of a perforated guide catheter, later discovered in the left popliteal artery.[29] Bleeding and vasovagal reactions occur more frequently but are more easily managed.

Early studies utilized a single anteroposterior view, accounting for higher morbidity and mortality than occur today. Lateral fluoroscopy allows orientation of the catheter posterior and inferior to the aorta and reduces inadvertent penetration of the aorta and left atrium. A high success rate has been reported using modified single-plane fluoroscopy. A right anterior oblique (40- to 50-degree) view provides an end-face view of the atrial septum and defines the inferior, posterior, and superior borders of the right atrium. A pigtail in the aorta demarcates its posterior wall and the level of the aortic valve. The recommended point of puncture lies midway between the posterior borders of the right atrium and aorta and 1 to 3 cm below the aortic valve.[23] Clinical series using this technique have reported atrial perforation in 2 of 118 (1.7%) and cardiac tamponade in 1 of 106 (0.9%), for an overall inadvertent puncture rate of 1.3%.[23,24] This suggests a marked improvement over previous series relying solely on anteroposterior fluoroscopy, but higher numbers are needed before definite conclusions can be drawn. The modified technique offers no advantage over biplane fluoroscopy, although it has been suggested that it may be more appropriate for less experienced, "low-volume" operators because it provides a greater margin of safety in terms of locating the area of septal puncture.[23]

Several authors have suggested that there is a learning curve for transseptal catheterization, and that the majority of complications occur in the first 25 to 50 procedures.[13,33,34] Even at a leading academic catheterization laboratory, the technique had to be "re-learned" for percutaneous mitral valvuloplasty, resulting in a 2 of 61 (3.3%) incidence of tamponade resulting from transseptal catheterization.[35] A higher rate of complications has been noted when the procedure is not regularly performed.[36]

The rate of unsuccessful attempts at transseptal catheterizations also varies with operator experience. Inability to engage the septum in up to 1.4% to 7.0% of attempts has been reported, varying with different patient populations.[25,27,37]

Conclusions

Transseptal left heart catheterization remains an important skill of the invasive cardiologist. Although for diagnostic purposes the technique is less requested than in the past, it remains a necessity in percutaneous mitral valvuloplasty, antegrade percutaneous aortic valvuloplasty, and atrioseptostomy, and may offer advantages in radiofrequency ablation of left-sided pathways. In the proper hands and with the proper equipment, there is little additional risk over routine left heart catheterization. Experienced operators are essential in assuring low morbidity and mortality.

SELECTED READINGS

1. Ross J Jr, Braunwald E, Morrow AG. Transseptal left atrial puncture: new technique for the measurement of left atrial pressure in man. Am J Cardiol 1959;3:653–655.
2. Cope C. Technique for transseptal catheterization of the left atrium: preliminary report. J Thorac Surg 1959;37:482–486.
3. Brockenbrough EC, Braunwald E, Ross J Jr. Transseptal left heart catheterization: a review of 450 studies and description of an improved technic. Circulation 1962; 25:15–21.
4. Mullins CE. Transseptal left heart catheterization: experience with a new technique in 520 pediatric and adult patients. Pediatr Cardiol 1983;4:239–246.
5. Dunn M. Is transseptal catheterization necessary? J Am Coll Cardiol 1985;5: 1393–1394.
6. Swan HJC, Ganz W, Forrester J, et al. Catheterization of the heart in man with use of a flow directed balloon-tipped catheter. N Engl J Med 1970;283:447–451.
7. Schoonmaker FW, Vijay NK, Jantz RD. Left atrial and ventricular transseptal catheterization review: losing skills? Cathet Cardiovasc Diagn 1987;13:233–238.
8. Lundqvist CB, Olsson SB, Varnauskas E. Transseptal left heart catheterization: a review of 278 studies. Clin Cardiol 1986;9:21–26.
9. Baim DS, Grossman W. Percutaneous approach, including transseptal catheterization and apical left ventricular puncture. In: Grossman W, Baim DS, eds., Cardiac catheterization, angiography and intervention. 4th ed. Philadelphia: Lea & Febiger, 1991:62–81.
10. Clugston R, Lau FYK, Ruiz C. Transseptal catheterization update 1992. Cathet Cardiovasc Diagn 1992;26:266–274.
11. Roelke M, Smith AJC, Palacios IF. The technique and safety of transseptal left heart catheterization. The Massachusetts General Hospital experience with 1,279 procedures. Cathet Cardiovasc Diagn 1994;32:332–339.
12. Schoenfield MH, Palacios IF, Jutter AM, et al. Underestimation of prosthetic mitral valve areas: role of transseptal catheterization in avoiding unnecessary repeat mitral valve surgery. J Am Coll Cardiol 1985;5:1387–1392.
13. O'Keefe JH, Vlietstra MB, Hanley PC, Seward JB. Revival of the transseptal aproach for catheterization of the left atrium and ventricle. Mayo Clin Proc 1985;60: 790–795.
14. Carabello BA, Barry WH, Grossman W. Changes in arterial pressure during left heart pullback in patients with aortic stenosis: a sign of severe aortic stenosis. Am J Cardiol 1979;44:424–427.
15. Palacios IF. Techniques of balloon valvotomy for mitral stenosis. In: Robicsek F, ed. Cardiac surgery: state of the art reviews. Philadelphia: Hanley & Belfus, 1991: 229–238.
16. Block PC, Palacios I. Comparison of hemodynamic results of antegrade versus retrograde percutaneous balloon aortic valvuloplasty. Am J Cardiol 1987;60:659–662.
17. Rashkind WJ. Transcatheter treatment of congenital heart disease. Circulation 1983;67:711–716.
18. Saul JP, Hulse JE, Hulse E, et al. Catheter ablation of accessory atrioventricular pathways in young patients: use of long vascular sheaths, the transseptal approach, and a retrograde left posterior parallel approach. J Am Coll Cardiol 1993;21:571–583.
19. Lindeneg O, Hansen AT. Complication in transseptal left heart catheterization. Acta Med Scand 1966;180:395–399.
20. Adrouny AZ, Sutherland DW, Griswold HE, Ritzman LW. Complications with transseptal left heart catheterization. Am Heart J 1963;65:327–333.
21. Braunwald E. Transseptal left heart catheterization. Circulation 1968;37(suppl III): 74–79.
22. Nixon PGF, Ikram H. Left heart catheterization with special reference of the transseptal method. Br Heart J 1965;28:835–841.

23. Croft CH, Lipscomb K. Modified technique of transseptal left heart catheterization. J Am Coll Cardiol 1985;5:904–910.
24. Doorey AJ, Goldenberg EM. Transseptal catheterization in adults: enhanced efficiency and safety by low-volume operators using a 'non-standard' technique. Cathet Cardiovasc Diagn 1991;8:535–542.
25. Ali Khan MA, Mullins CE, Bash SE, et al. Transseptal left heart catheterisation in infants, children, and young adults. Cathet Cardiovasc Diagn 1989;17:198–201.
26. Singleton RT, Scherlis L. Transseptal catheterization of the left heart: observations in 56 patients. Am Heart J 1960;60:879–885.
27. Folland ED, Oprian C, Giancomini J, et al. Complications of cardiac catheterization and angiography in patients with valvular heart disease. Cathet Cardiovasc Diagn 1989;17:15–21.
28. Kronzon I, Glassman E, Cohen M, Weiner H. Use of two-dimensional echocardiography during transseptal cardiac catheterization. J Am Coll Cardiol 1984;4:425–428.
29. Libanoff AJ, Silver AW. Complications of transseptal left heart catheterization. Am J Cardiol 1965;16:390–393.
30. Peckham GB, Chrysohou A, Aldridge H, Wigle ED. Combined percutaneous retrograde aortic and transseptal left heart catheterization. Br Heart J 1964;26:460–468.
31. Wilkins GT, Weyman AE, Abascal VM, et al. Percutaneous mitral valvotomy: an analysis of echocardiographic variables related to outcome and the mechanism of dilatation. Br Heart J 1988;60:299–308.
32. Henderson MA. Transseptal left atrial catheterization. Cathet Cardiovasc Diagn 1990;21:63. Letter.
33. Laskey WK, Kusiak V, Untereker WJ, Hirshfield JW Jr. Transseptal left heart catheterization: utility of a sheath technique. Cathet Cardiovasc Diagn 1982;8:535–542.
34. Weiner RI, Maranhao V. Development and application of transseptal left heart catheterization. Cathet Cardiovasc Diagn 1988;15:112–120.
35. Wyman RM, Safian RD, Portway V, et al. Current complications of diagnostic and therapeutic cardiac catheterization. J Am Coll Cardiol 1988;12:1400–1406.
36. Lew AS, Harper RW, Federman J, et al. Recent experience with transseptal catheterization. Cathet Cardiovasc Diagn 1983;9:601.
37. Gordon JB, Folland ED. Analysis of aortic valve gradients by transseptal technique: implications for noninvasive evaluation. Cathet Cardiovasc Diagn 1989;17:144–151.

9

PRESSURE GRADIENTS

Robert D. Rifkin

A PRIMARY OBJECTIVE of cardiac catheterization is assessment of the hemodynamic significance of obstruction to blood flow due to valvular or vascular stenosis. Almost 50 years ago, Gorlin and Gorlin introduced a simple formula for calculating the cross-sectional area of a valvular stenosis from hemodynamic data. This formula gained rapid acceptance in the catheterization laboratory and became a critical factor in the decision for or against surgical intervention in valvular heart disease.

During the past decade, the use of invasive hemodynamic assessment in a broader spectrum of patients has revealed cases in which the Gorlin formula yields systematically inaccurate results. This finding has led some investigators to question the validity of the simple Gorlin model of flow through a stenotic orifice and to suggest alternative formulas to replace it.

The purposes of this chapter are: (1) to review the basic concepts of fluid flow that underlie the Gorlin formula and to illustrate its application in simple situations, (2) to describe the major limitations of the Gorlin model and how these limitations may be addressed clinically, and (3) to present the current status of some of the controversial issues surrounding use of the Gorlin formula.

Basic Concepts of Fluid Flow

For the purposes of cardiovascular hemodynamics, blood flow can be described in terms of flow velocity, volumetric flow rate, pressure gradient, and certain rheologic properties, such as viscosity. *Hydrostatic pressure* is the force exerted by a fluid per unit area *perpendicular to the direction of fluid flow.* The pressure exerted on a surface facing the direction of flow would be greater, however, because of the additional force of the fluid impacting directly against it. Thus, an end-hole catheter might record a higher apparent pressure, called the *stagnation pressure,* than a side-hole catheter. A *pressure gradient* is a change in hydrostatic pressure over distance within the fluid. Fluids, like all physical objects, possess *inertia,* which is the tendency of mass to continue moving at the same velocity (same speed and direction of motion) unless a force is exerted to alter the motion. Thus, to accelerate fluid to a higher velocity, a pressure gradient in the direction of flow is required to overcome the inertia of the fluid. Similarly, to slow flow to a lower velocity requires a pressure gradient opposite to the direction of flow. *Viscosity* is the tendency for layers of fluid to resist slipping over one another. This is analogous to simple friction experienced when sliding an object over the floor. At the high flow velocities present in valvular stenosis and stenosis of medium-sized arteries, blood is approximately 3 to 5 times as viscous as water. If all elements of a fluid move parallel to each other, the flow is called *laminar.* By contrast, *turbulent* flow is characterized by chaotic or irregular motion of fluid elements, which often move perpendicular to the overall direction of the flow. In a tube such as a blood vessel, viscosity causes the outer layers of fluid to "stick" to the walls and move more slowly than the fluid in the center of the flow. Below a critical velocity, the viscosity also stabilizes the flow by suppressing random mechanical disturbances, thus maintaining a laminar flow pattern consisting of concentric shells moving at different velocities, the fastest shell being in the center.

Turbulence can arise in various ways. In the simple case of flow within a tube of uniform cross-section, when the overall velocity exceeds a critical value, viscous forces are insufficient to suppress local mechanical disturbances. These disturbances spread rapidly throughout the fluid, resulting in turbulent flow. An example of this phenomenon is the peak of systolic flow in the left ventricular outflow tract in aortic stenosis, where Doppler recordings often exhibit spectral broadening. Also, whenever flow is forced to separate from an adjacent surface, turbulence may result. Such separation occurs when fluid flows too rapidly to follow a change in the shape of a tube or a change in the direction of the tube. An extreme example of this phenomenon is a jet emerging from a tube or through an orifice into a large reservoir of stationary fluid, such as in mitral or aortic stenosis. Flow at the carotid bifurcation or the aortic arch is a less extreme example, in which the flow at peak systole may be too fast to negotiate the directional change of the conduit.

Pressure Gradients

It is helpful to think of fluid flowing in a tube as somewhat analogous to a ball rolling down a hill. As the ball rolls down from higher to lower elevation, so the fluid tends to flow from higher pressure toward lower pressure, or "down" the gradient. It is often said that pressure is "lost" in the direction of a falling pressure gradient.

If there is no force opposing the pressure gradient, the fluid accelerates over distance down the gradient, gaining velocity just as a ball would rolling downhill. In this situation, the major effect of the gradient is to overcome the inertia of the fluid, and the existence of the gradient is said to be due to or reflect "inertial effects." By contrast, if a force such as viscosity opposes the fluid motion and exactly balances the gradient, the fluid may move at a constant speed. The main effect of the gradient is to overcome viscous resistance, and the gradient is said to be related to or reflect "viscous effects." Both inertial and viscous effects can be co-existent and the gradients are additive, but in most situations, one of them is dominant.

Pressure Loss Along a Tube Due to Viscosity in the Absence of Stenosis

In steady laminar flow through a tube of uniform cross-section, such as a blood vessel, fluid flows in concentric shells of differing velocity but the velocity in each shell remains the same along the length of the tube (Fig 9-1). Pressure loss

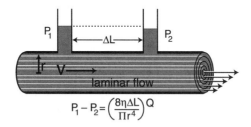

$$P_1 - P_2 = \left(\frac{8\eta\Delta L}{\Pi r^4}\right)Q$$

Figure 9-1 Poiseuille's law of viscous pressure loss for flow in an unobstructed tube with radius r and uniform cross-section. This law is valid only for laminar flow at a steady velocity. The hydrostatic pressure falls from P_1 to P_2 over the distance ΔL according to the formula shown. The arrows at the right end illustrate flow in concentric shells, with fastest flow velocity in the center and slowest flow near the wall. If the average velocity exceeds a critical value given by the Reynold's number, flow becomes turbulent and Poiseuille's law is no longer applicable. Vertical columns depict fluid-filled pressure measuring manometers.

is due exclusively to viscous effects of slippage between adjacent shells. It can be shown that the pressure loss over a length, ΔL, along the tube axis is given by a simple formula called Poiseuille's law:

$$\Delta P = \left(\frac{8\eta\,\Delta L}{\pi\,r^4}\right)\cdot Q$$

where ΔP is the pressure gradient, Q the volume flow rate, η is the viscosity, and r is the radius of the tube.

According to Poiseuille's law, the pressure loss for laminar flow in a tube is proportional to the first power of the volume flow rate, Q. Because the radius r, length ΔL, and viscosity are usually fixed for a given physical situation, the expression in parenthesis is constant and the formula can be rewritten as $\Delta P = K \cdot Q$. The constant, $K = 8\eta\Delta L/\pi r^4 = \Delta P/Q$, has been interpreted as analogous to the resistance, R, in Ohm's law for electrical circuits: $V = I \cdot R$, where the voltage V corresponds to ΔP, and the current, I, corresponds to Q.

Because of the complexity of turbulence, there is no simple formula corresponding to Poiseuille's law to calculate pressure losses over distance with turbulent flow, even for an unobstructed tube of uniform cross-section. Engineers use empirically determined graphs for different types of tubes to assess turbulent pressure losses. In general, pressure losses from turbulence are several times greater than those that would occur if flow were able to remain laminar at the same velocities. This magnified pressure loss is due to the greater viscous resistance imposed by fluid elements moving chaotically, as compared with fluid moving only in the orderly shells that characterize laminar flow.

Figure 9-2 shows the pressure loss per centimeter of length as a function of radius according to Poiseuille's law when flow is 5 liters/min. In a vessel the size of an adult aorta, with a radius of 1 to 2 cm, the pressure drop is less than 0.01 mm Hg/cm. Even at this large flow rate, pressure drop per centimeter would not reach 1 mm Hg unless the tube radius were less than 3 mm. Thus, only tiny pressure losses occur over the physiologic range of flows and lengths of normal-caliber unobstructed large arteries in adults. These tiny viscous losses can therefore be ignored by the cardiologist in the hemodynamic assessment of valvular obstruction. It should be noted that at the assumed flow of 5 liters/ min, this graph of Poiseuille's law is not strictly valid for radii below 0.5 cm, because the critical velocity for development of turbulent flow would be reached within this range of radii. Nevertheless, this fact would not substantially alter the preceding conclusions.

A long stenotic segment of a major epicardial coronary artery could have a length of 1 cm and a radius as small as 0.5 to 1.0 mm, but resting flow through it may be at most only 2.5% of total cardiac output, or 0.1 liter/min. Thus, for

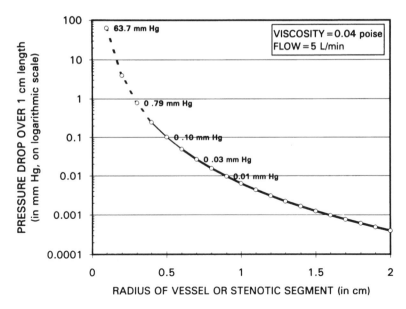

Figure 9-2 Magnitude of viscous pressure loss over a 1-cm length, according to Poiseuille's law for a flow of 5 liters/min as a function of tube radius. Viscosity is that of blood, 0.04 poise. Over this short distance, the pressure loss is very small until the radius falls below 3 mm. The dashed line shows the pressure loss according to Poiseuille's law at these small radii, but is not strictly valid because flow would probably already have become turbulent and pressure losses would have jumped to a value several times greater than that given by Poiseuille's law (see text). The heavy line for radii over 6 mm represents laminar flow where Poiseuille's law is valid. The light line represents the region of transition from laminar to turbulent flow.

a 1-cm segment length and a radius of 1 mm, pressure drop due to laminar viscous effects would be $0.025 \cdot 63.7 = 1.6$ mm Hg (see Fig 9.2). If the flow becomes turbulent, the pressure drop may be several times greater than this figure, reaching perhaps a few millimeters of mercury. This viscous pressure loss would be additive to the pressure drop due to inertial effects, because fluid must accelerate through the stenosis (discussion follows).

The narrowest region of a severely stenotic valve would have a length of only 1 to 2 mm, a radius of perhaps 2 mm, and a flow rate as high as 3 times systemic flow. Flow would be fully turbulent. After adjusting for these factors, viscous pressure losses would amount to a few millimeters of mercury at most. However, the use of Poiseuille's law to analyze this situation is not truly valid because flow is neither laminar nor steady in the region of the orifice, both of which are important assumptions in the use of Poiseuille's law.

Bernoulli's Equation for Pressure Gradient Across a Stenosis

Gorlin and Gorlin recognized that viscous factors are unlikely to explain the large gradients measured across valvular stenoses and that stenotic valves therefore would not behave as simple resistances. They, therefore, focused their attention on the inertial effects of a stenosis, which are described by Bernoulli's law.

When an incompressible fluid such as blood, which is flowing through a rigid tube, enters a narrowed section (Fig 9-3), *conservation of mass* requires that flow velocity in this section be greater than in the preceding wider section, in direct proportion to the ratio of the two cross-sectional areas. The *continuity equation* expresses this principle: $V_2 = V_1 \cdot (A_1/A_2)$ where V_1 and V_2 are the velocities at cross-sections of area A_1 and A_2, respectively. If there is no energy loss due to viscosity or turbulence, the sum of the potential energy, which is represented by the hydrostatic pressure, and the kinetic energy per unit volume is constant at all locations along the axis tube in accordance with *conservation of energy*. Thus, when kinetic energy increases in the narrowed section, hydrostatic pressure falls. This is expressed by Bernoulli's law: $P_1 + KE_1 = P_2 + KE_2$, or

$$P_1 + \frac{1}{2}\rho \cdot V_1^2 = P_2 + \frac{1}{2}\rho \cdot V_2^2$$

where $KE = 1/2\,\rho \cdot V^2$ is the kinetic energy per unit volume and ρ is the density of the fluid. The change in pressure, or pressure gradient between locations 1 and 2, can be found by rearranging this formula to obtain

$$P_1 - P_2 = \Delta P_{12} = \frac{1}{2}(\rho \cdot V_2^2) - \frac{1}{2}(\rho \cdot V_1^2) = \frac{1}{2}\rho \cdot (V_2^2 - V_1^2)$$

This pressure loss is due exclusively to inertial effects.

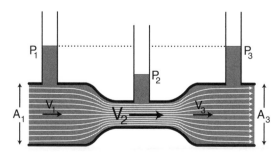

Figure 9-3 Changes in hydrostatic pressure due exclusively to inertial effects when tube cross-section changes gradually. Pressure falls ($P_2 < P_1$) as velocity and kinetic energy rise. Pressure may return to its original value ($P_3 = P_1$) if fluid returns to a tube of the same cross-sectional area ($A_1 = A_3$) and no turbulence develops.

If the flow then returns to a section of the same size as the initial section, the velocity falls and hydrostatic pressure rises back to its original value, *provided that no turbulence develops* (see Fig 9-3). If turbulence develops, however, some of the kinetic energy is lost and hydrostatic pressure will not return to the original value of the initial section. This rise in pressure beyond the stenosis, whether partial or complete, is referred to as *pressure recovery*. Note that in this situation, the fluid flows up the pressure gradient for a short distance by giving up some of its momentum, just as a rolling ball can roll uphill transiently, with slowing.

Bernoulli's Equation Applied to Flow Through a Discrete Stenosis

Gorlin and Gorlin used the preceding equation to obtain the gradient between the region proximal and distal to a discrete stenosis by making several simplifying assumptions (Fig 9-4). First, they assumed that there would be no pressure recovery beyond the stenosis. Thus, the pressure distal to the stenosis, P_d, would equal the pressure in the jet, P_j, and the pressure gradient between the region proximal and distal to the stenosis. $\Delta P_{pd} = P_p - P_d$, which would be measured at catheterization, would equal the pressure gradient between the proximal region and the high-velocity jet at the stenosis, $\Delta P_{pj} = P_p - P_j$. Next, they assumed that the velocity in the jet, V_j, was much higher than the velocity proximal to the stenosis, V_p, so that $V_p^2 \ll V_j^2$. V_p^2 could therefore be removed from the equation for gradient in the preceding section, and the gradient would be approximately correct for a significant stenosis. This is a reasonable assumption for a proximal catheter position in the body of the left ventricle. With these assumptions,

$$\Delta P_{pd} = P_p - P_d = P_p - P_j = \Delta P_{pj} = \frac{1}{2}\rho \cdot (V_j^2 - V_p^2) \approx \frac{1}{2}\rho \cdot V_j^2$$

For flow in a tube, the volume rate of flow, Q, velocity of flow, V, and cross-sectional area, A, are related by the expression $Q = V \cdot A$. Gorlin and Gorlin substituted Q/A_j for V_j, where A_j is the cross-sectional area of the jet, to obtain

$$\Delta P_{pd} = P_p - P_d \approx \frac{1}{2}\rho \cdot V_j^2 = \frac{1}{2}\rho \cdot \left(\frac{Q}{A_j}\right)^2$$

This last equation can be easily solved for the area of the jet, A_j, to yield the Gorlin formula in terms of the difference between two clinically measurable pressures, P_p and P_d, proximal and distal to the stenosis:

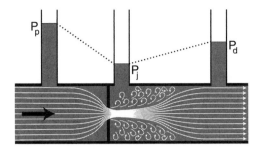

Figure 9-4 Effect of a discrete stenosis. A high-velocity jet develops at the orifice, with a drop in hydrostatic pressure ($P_j < P_p$). The rapidly flowing fluid separates from the walls beyond the stenosis and turbulence develops with energy loss. Pressure recovers when the fluid reattaches to the wall downstream ($P_d > P_j$), but pressure will not return to its original value due to the turbulent losses ($P_d < P_p$). P_p, P_j, and P_d equal the hydrostatic pressures proximal to the stenosis, in the high-velocity jet, and far distal to the stenosis, respectively.

$$A_j \cong \frac{(1/K) \cdot Q}{\sqrt{\Delta P_{pd}}} = \frac{Q}{K \cdot \sqrt{\Delta P_{pd}}}$$

where $1/K = \sqrt{\rho/2}$ and $\rho = 1.05$ g/ml is the density of blood, Q is in units of milliliters per second, pressure is in units of dynes per square centimeter, and A_j is in square centimeters.

$$\text{The constant } K = \frac{1}{\sqrt{\dfrac{\rho}{2}}} = \frac{1}{\sqrt{\dfrac{1}{2} \cdot 1.05}} = 0.72$$

Note that, as initially derived with the original values of all the constants, the Gorlin equation would give the jet area, not the anatomic area of the stenosis. The jet area may be smaller than the anatomic area of the stenosis because the flow can continue to converge for a short distance beyond the stenosis under certain circumstances (discussion follows).

Units

Because 1 mm Hg exerts a pressure of 1330 dyne/cm^2, millimeters of mercury can be used to express the gradient ΔP_{pd} instead of dynes per square centimeter if ΔP_{pd} is multiplied by 1330 in the Gorlin equation. The Gorlin equation then becomes

$$A_j = \frac{Q}{0.72 \cdot \sqrt{1330 \cdot \Delta P}} = \frac{Q}{0.72 \cdot \sqrt{1330} \cdot \sqrt{\Delta P}} = \frac{Q}{50.4 \cdot \sqrt{\Delta P}}$$

Thus, when pressure is expressed in millimeters of mercury, the calculated value of the constant in the Gorlin equation is 50.4. However, this value was adjusted by Gorlin and Gorlin to compensate for various errors to which the equation is subject. The currently accepted values are 37.7 for the mitral valve and 44.4 for the aortic valve (small differences in values seen in the literature are due to the use of different values for the density of blood).

In the clinical use of the Gorlin equation, the measured flow is the systemic cardiac output, F, in liters per minute. Because each valve flow occurs during only a portion of the cardiac cycle, measured systemic cardiac output, F, must be divided by the fraction of time during which blood is actually flowing across the valve to obtain the flow per minute. The period of flow for a single beat, multiplied by the heart rate, gives the number of seconds per minute during which there is flow across the valve: sec/beat · beats/min = sec/min. Dividing this number by 60 sec/min gives the fraction of time, f, occupied by the flow. The actual valve flow per minute is then given as Q = F/f. Also, the units of flow required in the Gorlin equation are in milliliters per second. Flow in liters per minute can be converted to milliliters per second by multiplying by 1000/60 = 16.67.

The Gorlin Constant: A Historical Footnote

In 1951, when Gorlin and Gorlin developed the orifice equation for estimating stenotic valve area, left heart catheterization was not yet being performed routinely. They therefore obtained the diastolic filling period from brachial artery tracings, an approach that yields values that differ from the true diastolic filling period due to pulse wave delay and arterial contour change. Additionally, they were unable to measure the transvalvular mitral gradient; they simply assumed it to be the pulmonary capillary wedge pressure (which they could measure) minus 5 mm Hg ($P_{pcw} - 5$). To correct for errors resulting from this approach, rather than use the calculated value of K, 50.4, the Gorlins determined an empiric value by comparing orifice equation results with the measured areas of 11 excised mitral valve specimens. They recognized that other unknown systematic physical or technical factors affecting accuracy of their equation, such as viscous effects, might also incidentally be corrected by this empiric adjustment of the constant.

The original empiric value of K obtained by the Gorlins for the mitral valve was 31. In 1972, with accurate measurement of the left ventricular diastolic filling period available through left ventricular catheterization, and transvalvular gradient measurable as $P_{pcw} - P_{LV}$, Gorlin recalculated the value of K for the mitral valve to be 37.7.

Because they were not performing left heart catheterization in 1951, the Gorlins were unable to make measurements of transvalvular pressure gradients in patients with aortic stenosis. However, they did compare the orifice equation to an anatomic specimen in one case of pulmonic stenosis, reporting K approximately equal to 44.3. By analogy, they suggested that K = 44.3 was also appropriate for aortic stenosis as well. This value appears to have provided clinically satisfactory estimates of aortic valve area over many years of use and also has furnished reasonable estimates of area in in vitro models of aortic stenosis.

Vascular Stenosis

Vascular stenoses may differ from valvular stenoses in that they may have a greater length, resulting in a contribution of viscous effects to the gradient in addition to the inertial effects. Studies confirm that the viscous contribution to the pressure drop increases with the length and severity of the stenosis. Doppler catheter gradients, calculated as $4 \cdot V^2$, neglect the viscous contribution and may underestimate the gradient obtained by catheter pressure measurements. In most cases, unless the stenosis has a length of greater than 1 to 2 cm, inertial effects are still dominant and the Gorlin equation provides good estimates of the stenosis cross-sectional area.

Major Assumptions in the Gorlin Equation

The Gorlin formula includes several assumptions, many of which are not strictly valid. Fortunately, the net effect on valve area calculation resulting from the inaccuracy of these assumptions tends to produce a systematic error that remains fairly constant under routine conditions. This constancy allows for adequate compensation by a fixed correction factor. As described earlier, Gorlin and Gorlin introduced such a correction factor by adjusting the constant, K, based on empiric measurements. Several of the major assumptions will be reviewed, but this list is not intended to be complete.

A major assumption is that all of the kinetic energy in the high-velocity jet is lost in turbulence beyond the stenosis, allowing pressure at the jet to be equated with distal pressure. This is a good assumption for mitral stenosis where flow stops in the left ventricle. For aortic stenosis, however, flow continues beyond the stenosis and a variable fraction of the kinetic energy is recovered. Downstream hydrostatic pressure may therefore rise slightly above the pressure in the jet at the stenosis. This has been confirmed in both in vitro hydraulic models of valve stenosis and in measurements made in patients. Pressure recovery in patients has been as great as 12 to 15 mm Hg in severe aortic stenosis. It is possible that this effect, on average, is incorporated into the constant 44.4 used for the aortic valve, but occasionally an unusual degree of pressure recovery could distort the Gorlin valve area calculation.

There also is an assumption that viscous forces do not increase the gradient between the region proximal to the stenosis and the outlet region (vena contracta). For most valvular stenoses, this assumption is probably valid at normal flow rates. At low flows, or for some vascular stenoses that have long and very narrow tunnel-like geometries, laminar and turbulent viscous losses at the stenosis may be significant, increasing the gradient beyond that calculated with the Gorlin formula. Nevertheless, for most discrete vascular stenoses, the Gorlin formula is a good first approximation.

It is important to note that A_j in Bernoulli's equation represents the narrowest cross-sectional area of the high-velocity jet, called the vena contracta. For a discrete stenosis, this area may be smaller than the physical orifice area due to continued convergence of flow streamlines for a short distance beyond the jet. Therefore, unless an appropriate correction factor is introduced to account for the difference between anatomic orifice area and vena contracta area, the orifice equation gives the cross-sectional area of the jet at the vena contracta. Because Gorlin and Gorlin determined their corrected value of the constant, K, by comparison with anatomic specimens, their correction presumably includes an average correction for this difference in mitral stenosis, and it is reasonable to assume the Gorlin equation yields anatomic mitral valve area. Because no such systematic comparison was done for the aortic valve, however, it remains unknown whether the Gorlin equation applied to the aortic valve with the constant 44.4 yields a value closer to its anatomic area or to the vena contracta jet area. It is noteworthy, however, that the difference between vena contracta jet area and anatomic area varies with the geometry of the stenosis and may therefore vary from valve to valve, depending, for example, on the degree to which the inlet to the orifice is funnel-shaped, tapered, rounded, or flat. Thus, for a tapering nozzle, the vena contracta jet area is equal to the physical orifice area.

Another major assumption of the Gorlin equation is that valve area is constant throughout the cardiac cycle. This is currently an area of major controversy in the literature. Biologic valves, even when stenotic, are not completely rigid, and some variation in orifice size could be expected to occur during systole.

The Gorlin equation assumes steady-state flow, whereas normal flow is pulsatile. The clinically used flow, which is based on cardiac output measurement is, therefore, actually an average or mean flow, $\bar{Q}$, rather than an instantaneous flow, Q, and the pressure gradient used clinically is actually a mean pressure, $\overline{\Delta P}$. Although the use of mean pressure is valid, for reasons that will not be detailed here, the use of mean flow, $\bar{Q}$, is not. Flow should be calculated as the root mean square of instantaneous valve flow:

$$Q_{rms} = \sqrt{\overline{Q^2}}$$

Although Q, $\bar{Q}$, and Q_{rms} are identical for steady flow, in time-varying flow, Q_{rms} is greater than $\bar{Q}$ by a factor that depends on the temporal shape of the flow profile. For example, if the flow pulse is shaped like a sinusoid, $\bar{Q}$ is 90% of Q_{rms}, potentially causing a 10% underestimation of valve area. For a triangular waveform, $\bar{Q}$ is 86.6% of Q_{rms}, potentially causing a 13% underestimation. For a parabolic flow profile, $\bar{Q}$ is 91% of Q_{rms}. Accordingly, for most commonly encountered flow profiles, use of $\bar{Q}$ tends to cause underestimation of valve area, unless balanced by other corrective factors. As with other assumptions that are not valid, a correction for the use of $\bar{Q}$ instead of Q_{rms} is probably serendipitously incorporated into the modified value of the constant, K, used in the Gorlin equation.

Lastly, in the clinical use of the Gorlin equation, it is assumed that there is no valve regurgitation. Valve regurgitation increases antegrade valve flow above that corresponding to the cardiac output measurement, and this larger flow results in a valve gradient that is greater than it should be for this cardiac output. The numerator of the Gorlin equation is therefore too small when regurgitation is present (not accounting for regurgitant flow), and the calculated area will be smaller than if the regurgitation were absent and all other factors were the same.

Examples of Area Calculation Using the Gorlin Formula

Aortic Stenosis

Assume that in a patient with aortic stenosis in sinus rhythm and no aortic insufficiency, cardiac output is 6 liters/min, transvalvular mean gradient is 45 mm Hg, systolic ejection time is 0.28 sec/beat, and heart rate is 70 beats/min. Antegrade aortic flow occurs for $0.28 \cdot 70 = 19.6$ sec/min, or one-third of the cardiac cycle. Actual valve flow is therefore triple cardiac output or

$3 \cdot 6 = 18$ liters/min. Converting liters per minute to milliliters per second, $(1000/60) \cdot 18 = 16.67 \cdot 18 = 300$ ml/sec. Valve area is thus $300/(44.4 \cdot \sqrt{45})$ $= 300/(44.4 \cdot 6.71) = 1.0$ cm^2.

Mitral Stenosis

Assume that in a patient with mitral stenosis in sinus rhythm and no mitral insufficiency, cardiac output is 5 liters/min, transvalvular mean gradient is 15 mm Hg, diastolic filling time is 0.6 sec/beat, and heart rate is 70 beats/min. Ante-

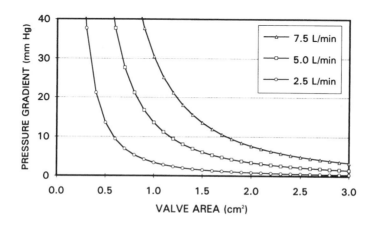

A

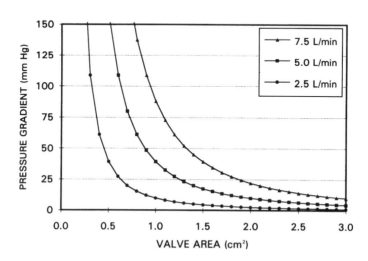

B

Figure 9-5   Pressure gradient as a function of valve area for the (A) mitral and (B) aortic valves, according to the Gorlin equation at three different flow rates. Note that as valve area falls, the rise in pressure becomes increasingly steep. Also, for a given valve area, pressure rises with the square of the flow rate.

grade mitral flow occurs for $0.6 \cdot 70 = 42$ sec/min. Actual valve flow is therefore $5 \cdot (60/42) = 7.14$ liters/min. Converting liters per minute to milliliters per second, $16.67 \cdot 7.14 = 119$ ml/sec. Valve area is thus equal to $119/(37.7 \cdot \sqrt{15}) = 119/(37.7 \cdot 3.87) = 0.82$ cm^2.

These examples illustrate the importance of the flow period in determining the valve gradient. Even at the same systemic cardiac output, if time available for flow per minute falls, valve flow rate increases and the gradient rises. As shown in Figure 9-5, the effect is magnified because the gradient rises with the square of the flow rate. This phenomenon explains the deleterious effect of rapid heart rates in mitral stenosis. Indeed, gradient could rise even though systemic cardiac ouput decreased, because of a reduction in the diastolic filling period per minute, which would result in an increase in net transvalvular flow rate.

Current Controversies Regarding the Gorlin Equation

In recent years, it has been observed by a number of investigators that the valve area calculated using the Gorlin equation, rather than being fixed, may vary with valve flow, showing a tendency toward systematic underestimation in low cardiac output states and overestimation in high flow states. Two competing hypotheses have been offered for these observations. One is that the Gorlin equation is accurate over all flow rates but that anatomic valve area is not fixed with respect to flow as the equation assumes. Thus, stenotic valves open incompletely in low flow states and more fully in high flow states.

The alternative is that valve geometry and orifice area are fixed under changing conditions of flow, but the Gorlin equation is not valid over widely varying flow rates because it does not properly take into account the complete fluid dynamics of flow through a stenosis. In fact, it has been gradually recognized that the Gorlin constant is not truly a constant but varies with flow. However, the magnitude of the variation has been controversial. One group has suggested that under pulsatile flow conditions, the Gorlin constant is proportional to the square root of the mean pressure gradient:

$$K = K' \cdot \sqrt{\Delta P}$$

Substituting this relationship into the Gorlin equation changes the Gorlin equation's dependence on pressure gradient from square root to first power:

$$A_j = \frac{Q}{K \cdot \sqrt{\Delta P}} = \frac{Q}{[K' \cdot \sqrt{\Delta P} \cdot \sqrt{\Delta P}]} = \frac{Q}{K' \cdot \Delta P}$$

This equation can be rearranged as: $\Delta P = Q \cdot [1/(K' \cdot A_j)]$ or $1/(K' \cdot A_j) = \Delta P/Q$. In this form, the relationship between pressure and flow now resembles Poiseuille's law, with the quantity $1/(K' \cdot A_j)$ corresponding to "resistance."

Some investigators have pursued this concept by suggesting that under the pulsatile flow conditions present in biologic circumstances, valve resistance is a more constant and fundamental property of stenotic valves than is the area as defined by the Gorlin equation. Clinically, valve resistance would be calculated simply as $R = \overline{\Delta P}/\overline{Q}$ in much the same way as systemic vascular resistance is calculated. It is worth reiterating the essential difference between this concept and the traditional Gorlin concept. According to the Gorlin viewpoint, the dominant effect of the stenosis is inertial, and the pressure gradient varies with the square of flow rate. The resistance concept implies that the pressure gradient varies with the first power of flow rate. However, recent carefully performed studies with pulsatile flow models failed to confirm the resistance concept as valid. Gorlin valve area, although not absolutely constant within flow variations in these pulsatile models, varied much less than did valve resistance. Moreover, another measure of valve obstruction proposed along with valve resistance, the so-called stroke work loss, also showed more variation with flow rates than the traditional Gorlin valve area.

Many other studies have confirmed that the Gorlin equation provides accurate gradient values over a wide range of flows, both steady and pulsatile, in nearly all situations in which the geometry of the stenotic orifice does not change during the flow cycle. These studies have provided fairly convincing evidence that changes in Gorlin valve area seen in conditions of varying flow, such as low-flow states, most likely represent true changes in the physical orifice size or in some other geometric characteristic of the valve, such as inlet shape, rather than a failure of the Gorlin equation.

Conclusion: Current Status of the Gorlin Equation and Practical Considerations

The Gorlin equation remains the most valid formula for assessing the severity of valvular stenosis. The assumption that valve area does not vary with flow, however, is probably not valid in certain cases. Thus, in low cardiac ouput states, the stiffened valve may not open fully, resulting in a lower valve area than under normal conditions. Conversely, in a high-flow state, the valve may open slightly better, leading to a larger area. This problem is less likely to affect the mitral valve than the aortic valve because the difference between the left atrial–left ventricular gradients seen in low-flow versus normal-flow states with mitral stenosis is probably not as great as the difference in the left ventricular–aortic gradient in these two flow states.

Unfortunately, the degree to which stiffening of the valve affects opening may vary greatly from patient to patient, because it depends on specific structural characteristics. It would be difficult to develop a single equation or correction to the Gorlin equation that would take all possibilities into account. A practical approach to this problem for patients in low-flow states whose valve areas are calculated to be small is to administer an inotropic agent such as dobutamine to increase cardiac output into the normal range. Repeat hemodynamic measurement can then be made and valve area recalculated under these conditions.

Another factor that has been recognized as occasionally affecting assessment of aortic valve hemodynamics is pressure recovery. Generally, pressure recovery is small and may already be accounted for by the modified value of the constant used in the Gorlin equation. However, there may be some difference in the gradients obtained by a catheter just beyond the aortic valve versus one placed more distally. It is probably best to routinely include any pressure recovery in the measured gradient. This approach introduces some standardization to the measurement procedure and more accurately reflects the functional valve area. Because pressure recovery is generally complete by 10 to 15 orifice diameters beyond the stenosis, it is advisable to position the distal measuring catheter in the high ascending aorta or beyond.

SELECTED READINGS

Cannon JD, Zile MR, Crawford FA, Carabello BA. Aortic valve resistance as an adjunct to the Gorlin formula in assessing the severity of aortic stenosis in symptomatic patients. J Am Coll Cardiol 1992;20:1517–1523.

Cohen MV, Gorlin R. Modified orifice equation for the mitral valve area. Am Heart J 1972;84:839–840.

Flachskampf FA, Weyman AE, Guerrero JL, Thomas JD. Influence of orifice geometry and flow rate on effective valve area: an in vitro study. J Am Coll Cardiol 1990;15:1173–1180.

Ford LE, Feldman T, Carroll JD. Valve resistance. Circulation 1994;89:893–894.

Gorlin R, Gorlin SG. Hydraulic formation for calculation of the area of the stenotic mitral valve, other cardiac valves, and central circulatory shunts. Am Heart J 1951;41:1.

Laskey WK, Kussmaul WG. Pressure recovery in aortic valve stenosis. Circulation 1994;89:116–121.

Levine RA, Jimoh A, Cape EG, et al. Pressure recovery distal to a stenosis: potential cause of gradient "overestimation" by Doppler echocardiography. J Am Coll Cardiol 1989;13:706–715.

Teirstein PS, Yock PG, Popp RL. The accuracy of Doppler ultrasound measurement of pressure gradients across irregular, dual, and tunnel-like obstructions to blood flow. Circulation 1985;72:577–584.

Voelker W, Reul H, Nienhaus G, et al. Comparison of valvular resistance, stroke work loss, and Gorlin valve area for quantification of aortic stenosis. Circulation 1995;91:1196–1204.

Voelker W, Reul H, Stelzer T, et al. Pressure recovery in aortic stenosis: an in vitro study in a pulsatile flow model. J Am Coll Cardiol 1992;20:1585–1590.

Yoganathan AP, Cape EG, Sung HW, et al. Review of hydrodynamic principles for the cardiologist: applications to the study of blood flow and jets by imaging techniques. J Am Coll Cardiol 1988;12:1344–1353.

10

SHUNT DETECTION AND MEASUREMENT

Lee Beerman

T HE DETECTION OF intracardiac or great vessel shunts is an essential part of the hemodynamic assessment during a catheterization procedure. Of the numerous methods that have been used to detect and quantitate shunting, oximetry remains the easiest, most commonly utilized, and most consistently reliable technique. This chapter emphasizes the role of oximetric analysis, but other modalities that have been used to assess shunts are mentioned briefly. These include indicator dilution techniques (i.e., indocyanine green, thermodilution, hydrogen gas, ascorbic acid), radionuclide studies, and angiography.

Oximetry

Measuring the level of oxygen saturation in each cardiac chamber and great vessel by direct blood sampling allows both qualitative and quantitative analysis of shunt flows. Because of the ease and accuracy of measurement, oxygen saturation is used rather than content. Using absorption spectrophotometry, a sample of as little as 0.3 to 0.5 ml of blood is sufficient to accurately determine the oxygen saturation at any site in the cardiovascular system. However, to appropriately use oximetry, it is important to be aware of the variability of normal values and numerous limitations and potential pitfalls inherent in the methodology.

Limitations and Pitfalls

One of the most important factors to consider is that this method requires a *steady hemodynamic state,* because subtle changes in ventricular function or cardiac output will render the shunt analysis unreliable. This problem can be overcome to a large degree by obtaining samples from pertinent sites in a rapid and sequential manner. In general, sampling is easily done, except in the setting of complex structural congenital heart disease. Another consideration is that *streaming* of blood flows in various chambers, particularly in the right atrium, can lead to nonrepresentative samples. For instance, superior vena cava (SVC) values are affected by the internal jugular venous saturation, which is lower than the subclavian vein saturation. The inferior vena cava (1VC) saturation is extremely inconsistent because of variable contributions of the highly saturated renal venous flow, lower hepatic venous saturation, and mesenteric venous efflux whose saturation is markedly dependent on the postprandial state. It is therefore easily understood that right atrial saturation may vary widely because of contributions from the cavae as well as the extremely low saturation of blood emptying into the right atrium from the coronary sinus. Streaming is also problematic at the right ventricular and pulmonary artery levels in the presence of left-to-right jets from lesions such as a ventricular septal defect or patent ductus arteriosus. In these circumstances, the site of sampling may be proximal, distal, or directly adjacent to the fully oxygenated jet, leading to a wide discrepancy in the measured saturations. In the normal circulation, saturations may vary as much as 10% within the right atrium, 5% in the right ventricle, and 3% in the pulmonary artery. To counteract the vagaries of streaming, multiple samples from various locations should be obtained and the mean values utilized. Other limitations include the nonlinearity of oxygen saturation determinations by spectrophotometry, with values below 60% and above 95% being less reliable. Increased cardiac output states that lead to a high mixed venous saturation decrease the ability to detect relatively small shunts.

Shunt Run and Normal Values

It is very helpful to plan an orderly process for rapidly and sequentially obtaining blood samples from various locations as close in time to each other as possible to maximize reliability of the oximetric analysis. This is most easily accomplished by advancing an end-hole catheter (either a flow-directed balloon-tipped catheter or one without a balloon) to the pulmonary artery wedge position. A catheter with side and end holes, such as a Goodale-Lubin, is also ac-

Table 10-1 Normal Oxygen Saturations

Site	% O_2 saturation (mean range)
Superior vena cava	70 (65–75)
Inferior vena cava	78 (65–87)
Right atrium	75 (65–85)
Right ventricle	75 (65–85)
Pulmonary artery	75 (65–85)
Coronary sinus	45 (40–50)
Wedge	95 (92–98)
Left atrium	95 (92–98)
Left ventricle	95 (92–98)
Aorta	95 (92–98)

Values are based on a review of values in the medical literature.

ceptable. As the catheter is pulled back to the right atrium and vena cavae, in addition to recording pressures, blood samples for oximetry should be obtained from the following sites: pulmonary artery wedge; branch pulmonary artery; main pulmonary artery; right ventricle; low, mid, and high right atrium; IVC (just below right atrial junction); and SVC (just below the innominate vein insertion). If the catheter passes across the atrial septum, the left atrium and pulmonary veins should be sampled.

Normal values are shown in Table 10-1. In the absence of a left-to-right intracardiac shunt, the most accurate mixed venous saturation is that obtained most distally in the right heart circulation, that is, the average pulmonary artery saturation. This is the value that should be used in calculating systemic arteriovenous oxygen content difference and cardiac output by the Fick technique in the normal circulation.

Shunt Detection and Calculation of Relative Pulmonary and Systemic Blood Flow

A pulmonary artery saturation 3% to 5% greater than that of the SVC strongly suggests the presence of a left-to-right shunt. We recommend using the SVC saturation as representative of the mixed venous saturation in the presence of a suspected shunt. Other authors have suggested using a combination of the IVC and SVC in various proportions, but this does not adequately compensate for the large variation in IVC saturations that may be present independent of the degree of shunting. Oximetry is useful but not definitive in defining the site of the shunt. For instance, a step-up of greater than 7% to 10% going from the SVC to the right atrium suggests an atrial shunt, a step-up greater than 5% between the right atrium and right ventricle would indicate a possible ventricular shunt, and a 3% step-up from the right ventricle to the pulmonary artery is

Table 10-2 Formulas and Abbreviations

O$_2$ capacity	=	Hb (g/100 mL) $\times$ 1.36 mL O$_2$/g Hb
O$_2$ content	=	Saturation $\times$ capacity + dissolved O$_2$
Dissolved O$_2$	=	0.3 mL O$_2$/100 mL/100 mm Hg pO$_2$
O$_2$ consumption	=	Measured O$_2$ consumed (mL/min)*
Flow	=	$\dfrac{\text{O}_2 \text{ consumption (mL/min)}}{\text{Arteriovenous content difference (mL O}_2/\text{liter of blood)}}$

*May be derived from a standard table relating body surface area, age, and heart rate to expected consumption.

suggestive of a great vessel shunt. However, downstream mixing from a more proximal shunt often occurs, compromising this method of shunt localization. Desaturation in either the left atrium, left ventricle, or aorta strongly indicates right-to-left intracardiac shunting when the pulmonary wedge or pulmonary vein positions are fully saturated. Once oxygen consumption is measured and key oxygen saturations are obtained, pulmonary blood flow and its relationship to systemic blood flow can be easily calculated using the Fick principle and a few simple formulas. Table 10-2 shows several of the formulas useful in making such calculations. The central equation is that flow across either the pulmonary or systemic vascular bed is equal to the oxygen consumed (systemic bed) or taken up (pulmonary bed), divided by the difference in arteriovenous oxygen content across that bed. In room air, dissolved oxygen becomes insignificant, and the simplied equation for determining blood flows are as follows:

$$Qp = \frac{O_{2\,consump}}{PV_{SAT \times CAP} - PA_{SAT \times CAP}} \tag{1}$$

$$Qs = \frac{O_{2\,consump}}{AO_{SAT \times CAP} - MV_{SAT \times CAP}} \tag{2}$$

where AO = aortic, CAP = oxygen-carrying capacity, consump = oxygen consumption, MV = mixed venous (typically SVC), PV = pulmonary vein, PA = pulmonary artery, and SAT = saturation.

In the absence of shunting, pulmonary artery saturation should be substituted for mixed venous saturation in determining systemic blood flow, and pulmonary blood flow will be equal to systemic blood flow in this situation. When a shunt is present, SVC saturation should be used for mixed venous saturation.

The physiologic significance of the magnitude of pulmonary blood flow is best understood in its relationship to systemic blood flow. A standard representation of this is expressed as the Qp/Qs ratio. When Equations 1 and 2 are solved for Qp/Qs, several factors cancel out, specifically oxygen consumption and oxygen capacity, and the resultant formula is the easily managable:

$$Qp/Qs = \frac{AO_{SAT} - SVC_{SAT}}{PV_{SAT} - PA_{SAT}} \tag{3}$$

If oxygen is being administered to the patient, the amount of dissolved oxygen may become significant and needs to be included in the calculation of oxygen content. Therefore, the formula for Qp/Qs must be modified to use content rather than saturation.

The concept of effective pulmonary blood flow is infrequently utilized, but provides another way of quantitating shunt flows. Effective pulmonary blood flow (Q_{EP}) can be thought of as the amount of systemic venous return that is effectively oxygenated during its passage through the lungs when there is either a right-to-left or left-to-right intracardiac shunt. When a right-to-left shunt is present, Q_S is made up of the Q_{EP} plus the shunt. Likewise, total Qp (pulmonary flow) consists of Q_{EP} plus the shunt when a left-to-right shunt is present. These values as well as shunt flow expressed as a percent of total flow can be determined by the following formulas:

$$Q_{EP} = \frac{O_{2\,consump}}{PV_{CONTENT} - SVC_{CONTENT}} \tag{4}$$

$$Qs = Q_{EP} + R \rightarrow L \text{ shunt} \tag{5}$$

$$Qp = Q_{EP} + L \rightarrow R \text{ shunt} \tag{6}$$

$$\% \, L \rightarrow R \text{ shunt} = \frac{Qp - Q_{EP}}{Qp} \tag{7}$$

$$\% \, R \rightarrow L \text{ shunt} = \frac{Qs - Q_{EP}}{Qs} \tag{8}$$

Pulmonary and Systemic Resistance

The methods for calculating vascular resistance (R) from flow and pressure relationships are discussed in Chapter 1. In the evaluation of intracardiac shunts associated with elevated pulmonary artery pressure, determination of pulmonary vascular resistance is very important and may have an impact on candidacy for operation intervention. The following formulas are utilized:

$$Rs = \frac{AO_{Pres} - RA_{Pres}}{Qs} \tag{9}$$

$$Rp = \frac{PA_{Pres} - Wedge\ (or\ LA)}{Qp} \tag{10}$$

$$Rp/Rs = \frac{PA_{Pres} - Wedge_{Pres}}{AO_{Pres} - RA_{Pres}} \times \frac{Qs}{Qp} \tag{11}$$

where Pres = mean pressure.

Because of the wide spectrum of body surface areas in the pediatric population, it is important to index systemic and pulmonary flow as well as resistance values (see Example 1 at the end of this chapter). Indexing is not as critical in adults.

The normal range for pulmonary vascular resistance is 1 to 2 index units and a normal Rp/Rs ratio is less than or equal to 0.1. If pulmonary vascular resistance is elevated, oxygen or some other pulmonary vasodilator should be administered to assess pulmonary vascular reactivity.

Other Techniques for Shunt Detection

Alternative methods to oximetry for analysis of shunts have been utilized in the past but are rarely necessary or indicated today. These include indicator dilution techniques using indocyanine green, hydrogen gas, ascorbic acid, and thermodilution. Of these, indocyanine green is the only one available from a practical standpoint and is discussed briefly. Radionuclide studies may allow quantitation of the Qp/Qs but are of questionable reliability unless a laboratory has considerable experience and expertise with this technique. Angiography is very valuable in defining the site of the shunt and anatomic lesions responsible. However, only relatively crude quantitative estimates of the magnitude of the shunt are possible with this methodology.

Green Dye Curves

The injection of indocyanine green into various sites in the circulation allows detection, localization, and quantitation of shunt flows. Because this technique is rarely used in current practice for accurate quantitation of shunts, the reader is referred to other sources for details of the methods utilized. However, it may be of value to have some knowledge of the qualitative analysis of green dye curves.

For left-to-right shunts, dye is injected into the main pulmonary artery and continuous sampling of dye concentration is obtained from an arterial site such as the femoral artery. In the presence of a left-to-right shunt, the peak early concentration is reduced, and the downslope of the curve is less steep because re-

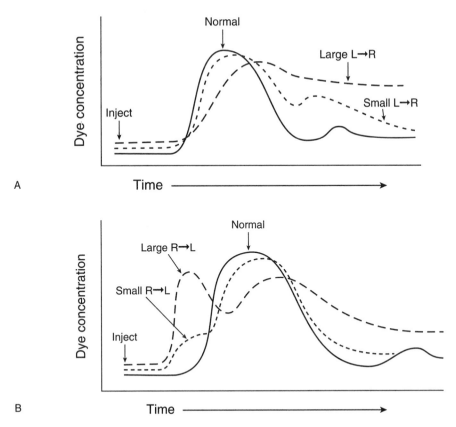

Figure 10-1 **(A)** Idealized normal curve and left-to-right shunt curves utilizing indocyanine green dye indicator injected into the main pulmonary artery. **(B)** Typical tracings associated with right-to-left shunting with injection into SVC. The secondary bump in the normal curve represents recirculation of green dye. Note that in left-to-right shunts the recirculation is earlier than in normal. In right-to-left shunts, the first bump is detected early from dye shunting right to left, and the large second bump is the result of dye traveling by a normal (nonshunted) pathway.

circulation occurs earlier and to a larger degree than in a normal curve. These effects are more pronouced when a larger shunt is present. Figure 10-1 demonstrates idealized green dye curves depicting these situations.

Use of green dye is a very sensitive way to detect even small right-to-left shunts, and the site of shunting can be deduced by injecting into various sites proximal and distal to the defect responsible for the shunt. When the dye is injected proximal to the shunt, the curve will reflect an early appearance time with an early upstroke, followed by a reduced peak concentration. Idealized curves reflecting right-to-left shunts of various magnitudes are also shown in Figure 10-1.

Examples of Left-to-Right Shunts

Common and uncommon lesions resulting in left-to-right shunts, along with the site of initial step-up in oxygen saturation and caveats related to particular lesions, are shown in Table 10-3. Further increases in oxygen saturations frequently occur in the chamber distal to the initial site as more complete mixing occurs. It is important to realize that this does not necessarily reflect a second site of shunting into that distal chamber. Examples of oximetry data and calculations for some common lesions are included in Examples 1 and 2 at the end of this chapter.

If pulmonary hypertension with elevated pulmonary vascular resistance is present, it is common practice to administer 100% oxygen to assess the reactivity of the pulmonary vascular bed to this potent pulmonary vasodilator. If vasodilation occurs, the shunt flow usually increases significantly. When high ambient oxygen is given, sampling from key sites must include pO_2 values in addition to saturations as the amount of dissolved oxygen becomes more important. An example of calculations in a patient with a ventricular septal defect who is given 100% oxygen is shown in Example 3.

Table 10-3   Localization of Left-to-Right Shunts

	Site of initial saturation step-up	Caveat
Common		
Atrial septal defect	RA	Step-up may not occur until RV with ostium primum defect
Ventricular septal defect	RV	Step-up may occur in RA with tricuspid regurgitation or direct LV-RA shunt
Patent ductus arteriosus	PA	Jet enters MPA or LPA (RPA saturation usually lower than LPA); must use distal saturations for Qp/Qs
Uncommon		
Partial anomalous pulmonary venous return	SVC	Very common with sinus venosus defect. Makes Qp/Qs uncertain without reliable MV saturation
Ruptured sinus of Valsalva	RA, RV	Site depends on location of rupture
Coronary artery fistula	RA, RV	Site depends on connection
Aorticopulmonary window	PA	
Anomalous origin of coronary artery from PA	PA	

Abbreviations: RA, right atrium; RV, right ventricle; PA, pulmonary artery; MPA, main pulmonary artery; LPA, left pulmonary artery; RPA, right pulmonary artery; Qp, pulmonary blood flow; Qs, systemic blood flow; SVC, superior vena cava; MV, mixed venous.

Right-to-Left Shunts

The presence of right-to-left shunting should be considered whenever desaturation is noted in the aorta or left heart chambers. In this setting, it is important to rule out pulmonary abnormalities such as ventilation perfusion mismatching or hypoventilation by obtaining pulmonary artery wedge or pulmonary venous samples. These should be fully saturated if the systemic desaturation is due to intracardiac shunting.

Some lesions that would lead to right-to-left atrial shunting include tricuspid atresia, Ebstein's anomaly, and an atrial septal defect with severe pulmonary hypertension. When calculating shunts in the presence of atrial desaturation, pulmonary venous or pulmonary wedge samples must be obtained to be able to assess pulmonary blood flow.

Desaturation that first becomes evident in the left ventricle or aorta may be caused by tetralogy of Fallot, truncus arteriosus, or a ventricular septal defect or patent ductus arteriosus with severe pulmonary hypertension and Eisenmenger's reaction. Example 4 (at the end of this chapter) demonstrates shunt calculations with tetralogy of Fallot.

Summary

Currently available echo and Doppler technology allows accurate and reliable detection and localization of even small intracardiac shunts. Noninvasive quantitation of shunts is also possible with these techniques and to some degree with radionuclide angiography. However, oximetric data obtained by cardiac catheterization remain the most definitive means for quantifying intracardiac shunts. It is important to avoid the pitfalls associated with this technique by obtaining accurate samples from appropriate sites in the circulation close in time to each other during a period of hemodynamic stability.

EXAMPLE 1   Ventricular Septal Defect with Pulmonary Hypertension

This infant had baseline hemodynamics that revealed a Qp/Qs = 2.5 with an Rp/Rs = 0.3 and pulmonary vascular resistance of 6 index units.* FiO_2 of 1.0 was administered for 10 minutes and the following data obtained:

	pO_2	SAT	Pres
SVC	31	58	2
AO	438	98	78
PA	77	95	55
LA	392	98	12

O_2 consumption = 52 ml/min
Hb = 10 g%; body surface area = 0.25 m^2

I. Including dissolved O_2 (using O_2 content)

$$Qp/Qs = \frac{AO_{CONTENT} - SVC_{CONTENT}}{LA_{CONTENT} - PA_{CONTENT}}$$

$$O_{2\,CAPACITY} = 10 \text{ g Hb} /100 \text{ ml} \times 1.36 \text{ ml } O_2/\text{g Hb} \times \frac{1000 \text{ ml}}{\text{liter}} = 136 \text{ ml } O_2/\text{liter}$$

$$O_{2\,CONTENT} = O_{2\,SAT} \times O_{2\,CAP} + \text{dissolved } O_2$$

Dissolved O_2 = 0.3 ml O_2/100 ml/100 mm Hg pO_2

$AO_{CONTENT}$ = 0.98 × 136 ml O_2/liter + 13 ml O_2/liter = 146 ml O_2/liter

$SVC_{CONTENT}$ = 80 ml O_2/liter; $PA_{CONTENT}$ = 132 ml O_2/liter; $LA_{CONTENT}$ = 145 ml O_2/liter

$$Qp/Qs = \frac{146 - 80}{145 - 132} = 5.1$$

$$Qp = \frac{O_{2\,consump}}{LA_{CONTENT} - PA_{CONTENT}} = 4 \text{ liters/min}; \quad Qp \text{ index} = \frac{Qp}{BSA} = 16 \text{ liters/min/m}^2$$

$$Rp = \frac{\overline{PA}\,(mm\,Hg) - \overline{LA}\,(mm\,Hg)}{Qp \text{ index}} = \frac{55 - 12}{16} = 2.7 \text{ index units}$$

$$Rp/Rs = \frac{\overline{PA} - \overline{LA}}{\overline{Ao} - \overline{SVC}} \times \frac{Qs}{Qp} = 0.1$$

II. Ignoring dissolved O_2 (using O_2 saturation rather than O_2 content)

$$Qp/Qs = \frac{AO_{SAT} - SVC_{SAT}}{LA_{SAT} - PA_{SAT}} = \frac{98 - 58}{98 - 95} = 13.3$$

Comments: With the administration of O_2, the Qp/Qs increased substantially and pulmonary vascular resistance fell to near normal levels. If the dissolved O_2 is ignored, the Qp/Qs obtained is nonphysiologic and invalid.

*In the pediatric population, it is critical to use BSA in the equation of

$$R_{index} = \frac{\Delta P}{CO/BSA} = \frac{\Delta P}{CI}$$

where BSA = body surface area, CI = cardiac index, CO = cardiac output.

In the adult population, indexing R is usually unnecessary because there is a smaller range of BSA than in children.

EXAMPLE 2 **Atrial Septal Defect**

Oximetry

Site	Sat%
SVC	75
RA, high	77
RA, mid	82
RA, low	83
RV	84, 87
MPA	88
RPA	86
LA	95
AO	95

$$Qp/Qs = \frac{AO_{SAT} - SVC_{SAT}}{LA_{SAT} - PA_{SAT}}$$

$$Qp/Qs = \frac{95 - 75}{95 - 87} = 2.5/1$$

$$Qp = \frac{O_2 \text{ consumption}}{(LA - PA) \text{ SAT} \times \text{capacity}}$$

Measured O_2 consumption = 240 ml O_2/min

Capacity = g Hb /100 ml $\times$ 1.36 ml O_2/g Hb

Capacity = 14.5 g Hb /100 ml $\times$ 1.36 ml O_2/g Hb $\times$ 1000 ml/liter

Capacity = 197 ml O_2/liter

$$Qp = \frac{240 \text{ ml } O_2/\text{min}}{(0.08) \ 197 \text{ ml } O_2/\text{liter}} = 15.2 \text{ liters/min}$$

Comments: In the absence of a right-to-left shunt, LA, PV, and wedge saturations should be equal. Step-up not complete until RV. Use average PA saturation in calculation.

EXAMPLE 3   **Ventricular Septal Defect**

Oximetry	
Site	*Sat%*
SVC	74, 72
IVC	76
RA, high	75
RA, mid	75
RA, low	77
RV	76, 81
MPA	81
RPA	81
LPA	84
WEDGE	95
AO	97

$$Qp/Qs = \frac{AO_{SAT} - SVC_{SAT}}{PV_{SAT} - PA_{SAT}}$$

$$Qp/Qs = \frac{97 - 73}{97 - 82}$$

$$Qp/Qs = 1.6$$

Comments: Use average SVC saturation and ignore IVC when determining MV saturation. Average all PA saturations. Assume average PV saturation would be equal to aortic saturation if no right-to-left shunt. Note widely divergent saturations in RV.

EXAMPLE 4   **Tetralogy of Fallot**

Oximetry	
Site	*Sat%*
SVC	65
RA	65
LA	95
PV	95
RV	70
LV	90
PA	70
AO	85

$$Qp/Qs = \frac{AO_{SAT} - SVC_{SAT}}{PV_{SAT} - PA_{SAT}}$$

$$Qp/Qs = \frac{85 - 65}{95 - 70}$$

$$Qp/Qs = 0.8$$

Comments: Qp/Qs is calculated in an identical manner to a pure left-to-right shunt. This patient has bidirectional shunting across the VSD with a predominant right-to-left shunt (i.e., Qp/Qs < 1.0). There is no atrial shunting. LV saturation higher than AO because of streaming from LA and sampling proximal to right-to-left shunt.

SELECTED READINGS

1. Antman EM, Marsh JD, Green LH, Brossman W. Blood oxygen measurement in the assessment of intracardiac left to right shunts: a critical appraisal of methodology. Am J Cardiol 1980;46:265–271.
2. Freed MD, Miettinen OS, Nadas AS. Oximetric detection of intracardiac left to right shunts. Br Heart J 1979;42:690–694.
3. Grossman W. Shunt detection and measurement. In: Grossman W, Baim DS, eds. Cardiac catheterization, angiography and intervention. Philadelphia: Lea & Febiger, 1991:167–180.
4. Mathews RA. Shunt detection. In: Neches WH, Park SC, Zuberbuhler JR, eds. Perspectives in pediatric cardiology. Pediatric cardiac catheterization. vol. 3. Mount Kisco, NY: Futura, 1991:71–80.
5. Mayer DC, Artman M. Shunt detection and quantification. In: Pepine CJ, Hill JA, Lambert CR, eds. Diagnostic and therapeutic cardiac catheterization. Baltimore: Williams & Wilkins, 1994:372–393.
6. Vargo TA. Cardiac catheterization—hemodynamic measurements. In: Garson A, Bricker VT, McNamara DG, eds. The science and practice of pediatric cardiology. Philadelphia: Lea & Febiger, 1990:913–945.

11

ENDOMYOCARDIAL BIOPSY

Kenneth Baughman
Edward K. Kasper

C LINICIANS AND INVESTIGATORS have long recognized the non-specific nature of the signs and symptoms of myocardial disease and, therefore, the need to directly examine cardiac tissue to effectively treat disorders of the heart muscle. Biopsy of the heart, compared with that of other organs, is complicated by the fact that the target organ is filled with fluid under high pressure. Bullock et al.[1] established desirable characteristics for the performance of the endomyocardial biopsy procedure, which included "reliability, ease of performance, low morbidity, and essentially no mortality."[2] This chapter reviews the history, current instruments, techniques, complications, uses, and future of endomyocardial biopsy.

Development of Endomyocardial Biopsy

A number of investigators[2,3] first reported the performance of transthoracic biopsy of the left ventricle between 1958 and 1960. Weinberg et al.[2] performed transthoracic open surgical biopsies on five patients through an incision made in the fourth intercostal cartilage in the precordial space. A pericardial patch was resected, and cardiac tissue was removed by surgical incision of an area of the heart through which a suture had been placed. Sutton and Sutton[3] reported 150 biopsy attempts in 54 patients by a percutaneous transthoracic approach using a Terry needle. Two different sites were utilized: (1) the left costosternal angle to biopsy the right ventricle and (2) the apex for the left ventricle. Timmis et al.[4] modified the percutaneous technique, using the tip of the biopsy needle as an exploratory epicardial electrode to ensure recognition of myocardial contact by a transmitted injury current. Shirey et al.[5] reported the largest percutaneous left ventricular biopsy experience when they submitted 198 patients to 254 biopsy procedures with a thin-walled Silverman needle. They acquired adequate tissue for diagnosis in 192 patients, which allowed a specific diagnosis in 27 and documentation of nonspecific abnormalities in 165.

All of the described percutaneous techniques had the potential for significant complications related to the nature of the approach. These included pneumothorax, hemopericardium, postpericardiotomy syndrome, ventricular arrhythmias, and, rarely, death. Additionally, these biopsy procedures rarely demonstrated endocardial tissue, which was felt to be the most likely area to reveal abnormalities. Bullock et al.[1] altered the approach to biopsy in 1965 by attempting percutaneous biopsy of the right ventricular septum through the right internal jugular veins of dogs, utilizing a 50-cm-long, thin-walled, steel tubing through which a cutting needle was inserted.

The modern era of endomyocardial biopsy was introduced by Sakakibara and Konno[6,7] in 1962. They introduced a semirigid bioptome inserted intravascularly for endocardial sampling of the right and left ventricles. The semiflexible forceps were inserted either through the left basilic vein to the right ventricle or through the right axillary artery to the left ventricle. They initially reported that more than 10 biopsies had been performed in five patients without significant complications and with excellent reliability for the acquisition of tissue. The Konno bioptome is relatively large due to its mechanical construction and movable parts. Because of this construction, it is somewhat difficult to sterilize between utilizations and has proved to have somewhat limited durability. Because of the stiffness, it is occasionally difficult to manipulate into the left or right ventricle.

The King myocardial bioptome[8] was introduced as a modified Olympus fiberoptic bronchoscopic bioptome. The bioptome is 105 cm long, is approximately 1.8 mm in diameter, and has no intrinsic shape. The bioptome could be inserted into a vein or an artery and be utilized percutaneously through a sheath. The advantage of the King bioptome relative to the initial Konno instrument was its smaller size and greater flexibility.

In 1974, Caves et al.[9] introduced a modified Konno bioptome. The bioptome has a handle very similar to a surgical instrument with a ratchet mechanism for locking the forceps in the closed position. One jaw of the biopsy cup remains stationary, while the second moves. The biopsy apparatus is either 50 cm or greater than 100 cm in length and can be inserted in the internal jugular or femoral veins. Both have a nearly 90-degree angle bend in the distal portion of the forceps to ease entry across the tricuspid valve into the right ventricle. The biopsy forceps could be appropriately resterilized for repeated use. In Caves' earliest report,[9] the biopsy forceps were used in 19 patients with 100% success in acquiring tissue, were associated with minor complications (one pneumothorax and one episode of atrial fibrillation), and were also associated with shortened procedure times.

Subsequent modifications of the Stanford-Caves bioptome have been made, and disposable systems shaped in the same fashion as the reusable instrument are now available. Most disposable systems have no ratchet handle, but rather a central wire mechanism to control the jaw apparatus like an Olympus fiberoptic bioptome. Biopsy forceps generally come in variable lengths, approximately 50 cm or 105 cm, and can be used for venous or arterial access from the arm, neck, or leg. Bioptome diameter has been decreased over time to accommodate small adults and pediatric patients. Finally, preformed bioptomes have been replaced by bioptomes without any curvature made to be inserted through guiding-sheath systems, which are inserted into the right or left ventricle.[10-13]

Current Biopsy Forceps

Two general bioptome types are available. The first is a preshaped forceps of approximately 50 cm in length for entry from the right internal jugular or subclavian vein; it is inserted through a short entry sheath. The second general category of bioptomes is an unshaped flexible instrument of smaller size that is used through a guiding-sheath system placed in the chamber to be biopsied or that may be shaped by the operator for entry into the heart.

All preshaped 50-cm bioptomes have a greater degree of control due to their shorter length and stiffer shaft. The stiff and preformed nature of the instrument may, however, be a disadvantage, which can make it difficult to reach the interventricular septum of some ventricles. Flexible (or unshaped) disposable systems have the advantage of being guided into almost any chamber with a leading wire or indwelling fluid-filled catheter. The disadvantage of the disposable-sheath system is that the sheath apparatus remains in the ventricle and has much greater potential to cause ventricular arrhythmia between biopsy attempts. Additionally, the disposable system, particularly from the leg, allows less control and a slightly greater risk of perforation due to the tendency of the sheath to partially or completely engage the wall of the ventricle before insertion of the bioptome. Currently available bioptomes and their characteristics are listed in Figure 11-1.

BIOPTOMES

COMPANY	JUGULAR Disposable	Reuseable	Length (cm)	Straight	Pre-Curved	Jaw O.D. (mm)	Vol (mm³)	Diam (French)	FEMORAL Disposable	Reuseable	Length (cm)	Straight	Pre-Curved	Jaw O.D. (mm)	Vol (mm³)	Diam (French)
Argon	√		45	√		2.4	5.4	7.5	√		100	√		2.4	5.4	7.5
	√		45		√	2.4	5.4	7.5	√		100	√		1.8	2.5	7.0
	√		45	√		1.8	2.5	7.0								
	√		45		√	1.8	2.5	7.0								
Cordis	√		50		√	2.4	5.0	7.5	√		104		√	2.4	5.0	7.5
	√		50		√	2.2	5.0	7.0	√		104		√	2.2	5.0	7.0
	√		50	√		2.2	5.0	7.0	√		104	√		2.2	5.0	7.0
	√		50	√		1.8	1.8	5.4	√		104	√		1.8	1.8	5.4
Cook	√		60	√		1.7	4.9	5.2	√		120	√		1.7	4.9	5.2
	√		60	√		1.7	2.3	5.2	√		120	√		1.7	2.3	5.2
	√		60	√		1.1	0.9	3.0	√		120	√		1.1	0.9	3.0
Fehling		√	51	√		2.2	4.9	7.0		√	120	√		2.2	4.9	7.0
	√		51	√		2.2	4.9	7.0	√		120	√		2.2	4.9	7.0
	√		51	√		1.8	3.8	6.0	√		120	√		1.8	3.8	6.0
	√		51	√		1.6	3.2	5.0	√		120	√		1.6	3.2	5.0
	√		80	√		1.8	3.8	6.0	√		100	√		1.8	3.8	6.0
	√		80	√		1.6	3.2	5.0	√		100	√		1.6	3.2	5.0
Mansfield	√		48	√		2.2	4.9	8.0	√		100	√		2.2	4.9	7.0
	√		48	√		2.2	4.9	7.0	√		100	√		1.8	2.4	6.0
	√		48	√		1.8	2.4	6.0								
	√		50	√		1.8	2.4	6.0								
Scholten		√	50	√		2.8	4.5	9.0		√	100	√		2.1		6.5
		√	50	√		2.5	3.4	8.0								
		√	50	√		2.1	2.7	6.5								
		√	40	√		1.6	1.4	5.0								

Figure 11-1 Commercially available bioptomes listed by manufacturer and site of utilization (jugular or femoral).

Technique of Endomyocardial Biopsy

The right ventricular endomyocardium can be easily approached from the right internal jugular, right subclavian, or either of the femoral veins. The left ventricle can be biopsied from the femoral or brachial arteries. Heterotopic heart transplant biopsies may be performed from any of the above venous sites and, in addition, the left subclavian or left internal jugular may occasionally be the most appropriate site for entry.

Certain features are common to endomyocardial biopsy from any site, including informed consent, premedication, monitoring system utilization, preparation, draping, and anesthesia.

Informed Consent

Informed consent allows the physician performing the procedure the opportunity to discuss with the patient the indications for the procedure, the steps involved in the performance of the procedure, potential risks, and management of complications, should they occur.

Premedication

Most endomyocardial biopsy procedures are currently performed on an outpatient basis. Only in rare patients, children or adults with a history of vasovagal reactions, is it necessary to premedicate the patient. Avoidance of complications, particularly perforation of the heart wall, is highly dependent on the ability of the physician to communicate with the patient during the performance of the procedure to ensure that the pain of impending perforation is recognized. Additionally, patients with heart failure may be susceptible to the respiratory depressive effects of usual doses of sedatives. Therefore, anesthesia may, in fact, increase the risk of the most dreaded complications of biopsy, myocardial perforation, and respiratory depression. If necessary, conscious anesthesia with midazolam or other short-acting agents may be used during the procedure itself.

Monitoring Systems

Patients undergoing endomyocardial biopsy are monitored continuously for rhythm disturbances. Additionally, continuous monitoring of BP is appropriate. At Johns Hopkins, we use two methods. The first is an intermittent inflation device measuring and recording BP every 3 minutes. The second device is capable of measuring BP on a beat-to-beat basis through a digital artery. Both techniques are noninvasive and, therefore, advantageous relative to intra-arterial measurement. Continuous BP monitoring is exceedingly important in cardiomyopathy patients, where cardiac perforation can result in dramatic sudden changes in BP. Finally, oxygen saturation should be monitored continuously, particularly in the cardiomyopathy population, to guarantee that the patient's oxygenation remains at an adequate level during the performance of the procedure. Patients are asked how they feel during the procedure to ensure an adequate level of comfort.

Preparation

Standard preparation and draping are performed over the proposed site of venous or arterial access. These techniques are more fully described elsewhere and are similar for all catheterization procedures. In our laboratory, we utilize an iodine solution and alcohol followed by a quadrangular towel draping system, ensuring clear visualization of the site being entered. It is mandatory that a site of adequate size be exposed so that the physician is able to determine appropriate landmarks and cannulate the venous or arterial access systems. Additionally, we place gauze between the edge of the draping system and any exposed portions of the catheterization table.

Anesthesia

The appropriate use of local anesthesia makes general anesthesia or conscious sedation rarely necessary. The most important anesthesia is that which is given with the first needle. Once the upper one-half to three-fourths of an inch of the skin and subcutaneous tissue is anesthetized, only deep visceral structures have large numbers of nerve endings capable of producing significant discomfort.

We use 1% lidocaine without epinephrine. Epinephrine should be avoided in order to prevent sympathetic stimulation of the heart. A 25-gauge needle is utilized to raise a small wheal in the skin, not dissimilar from that produced by a correctly placed PPD. This anesthesic is rubbed gently into the skin for a few seconds. Thereafter, a 25-gauge needle is inserted perpendicular to the skin and advanced by millimeter intervals, aspirating to ensure that no vessel has been entered, and then injecting a very small amount of lidocaine. This is continued to the depth of the small 1.25-inch 25-gauge needle. This lidocaine is then gently massaged into the skin.

For procedures of vascular access, see Chapter 4.

Technique of Biopsy via the Right Internal Jugular Vein

Over 95% of all endomyocardial biopsies are performed through the right internal jugular approach (Figs 11-2 and 11-3). Accessing the right internal jugular vein is described in Chapter 4. It should be emphasized that insertion of the wire or sheath should occur "like a knife through butter." At no time should excessive force be used to advance into any intravascular system. If necessary, fluoroscopy or even dye injection through the lumen of the system being advanced may be necessary to identify its course and resistance.

The preshaped bioptome should be inspected to ensure that it opens and closes appropriately before each insertion into the patient (Fig 11-4). Likewise,

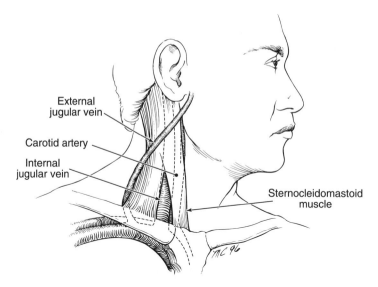

Figure 11-2   The patient is placed flat on the biopsy table, and the head is directed to the left. The lateral head of the sternocleidomastoid muscle, clavicle, and external jugular vein form a triangle within which the internal jugular vein and carotid artery pass. The carotid artery can usually be easily palpated if the internal jugular venous system is not visible. The internal jugular vein should be just lateral to the carotid artery and just beneath the outer border of the sternocleidomastoid muscle. The site of entry should be at least one third of the way from the clavicle to the jaw to ensure that the apex of the lung is avoided and that if the carotid artery is punctured, it can be compressed.

the exterior should be inspected to ensure that there is no debris or clot present on the instrument. The tip is held approximately 5 cm from the end with the right thumb and index finger, and the instrument is cradled in the right arm, with the tip pointed to the right lateral atrial border. The left hand holds the sheath to prohibit motion and irritation while the bioptome is passed through the sheath into the superior vena cava. The bioptome is advanced 5 to 10 cm, and then the left hand is removed from the sheath and placed at the handle end of the bioptome. This allows forward motion to be controlled by the right hand and torque or circular motion to be controlled by the left. The bioptome is advanced to at least the high right atrial lateral border (Fig 11-4A). The biopsy forceps are then turned counterclockwise (anteriorly) 180 degrees, and the handle is pointed towards the patient's head and ear. The plane of the interventricular septum, the desired site for biopsy, is simulated by a 45-degree angle from the tip of the patient's nose to the patient's right shoulder. Therefore, the biopsy handle, which is preshaped to be in the plane of the curvature of the bioptome, is pointed perpendicular to the patient's head or to the floor

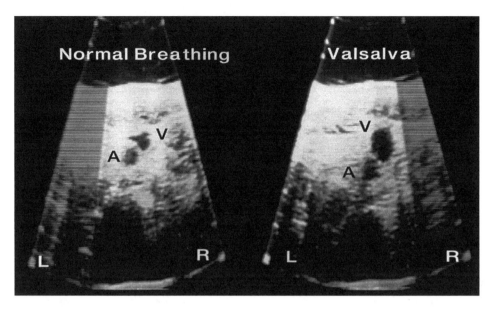

Figure 11-3 Sonographic visualization of the internal jugular vein and carotid artery at baseline and during Valsalva maneuver. The carotid artery is usually smaller in size, thicker walled, medial, and noncompressible relative to the somewhat larger internal jugular vein. Care must be taken not to compress the internal jugular vein with a sonographic apparatus while visualizing or attempting to cannulate the internal jugular vein.

when the biopsy is performed. The tip of the bioptome is visualized under fluoroscopy throughout the entry process and is advanced into the right ventricle. Entry into the right ventricle can usually be confirmed by the greater rocking motion at the distal end of the bioptome and by the appearance of ventricular ectopic beats. The biopsy forceps should be advanced to the right ventricular wall, while assuming a somewhat posterior orientation of the biopsy head, and confirmed by fluoroscopy. To ensure that the biopsy forceps do not become entangled in trabeculae, which could result in their anterior direction, the bioptome is withdrawn 1 to 2 cm from the right ventricular wall once it is engaged and redirected posteriorly to ensure that it points towards the septum.

The biopsy forceps are opened when the bioptome is both withdrawn from the septum and advanced slowly toward the septum. Ventricular ectopic beats will occur when the septum is engaged, and ectopy will continue until firm engagement is established. Therefore, continued ventricular ectopic beats imply that the biopsy head is not well engaged in the septum and that an inadequate piece of tissue will be removed if the bioptome is closed at this time. The septum can usually be palpated by pulsations coming through the rather stiff shaft of the biopsy forceps. Once the right ventricular septum has been engaged,

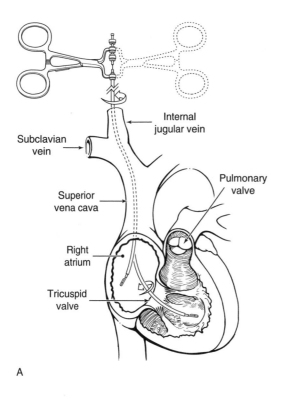

Figure 11-4   Internal jugular reusable right ventricular biopsy technique. **(A)** The bioptome is inserted through the internal jugular on the right side, with the tip pointed to the lateral wall of the right atrium. Excessive stimulation of the atrial wall should be avoided. The bioptome is turned counterclockwise 180 degrees and directed toward the plane of the tricuspid valve. Once right ventricular entry has been confirmed, the bioptome is directed posteriorly to the interventricular septum. **(B)** The presence of premature ventricular contractions implies ventricular contact. The bioptome is retracted 1 cm, the jaws are opened, and the bioptome is advanced to engage the interventricular septum. As the septum is firmly engaged and entrapped in the head of the bioptome, ectopy will stop. The jaws are closed gently, and the ratchet mechanism of the handle is locked. The forceps are then withdrawn. Excessive resistance to withdrawal should be avoided (see text discussion).

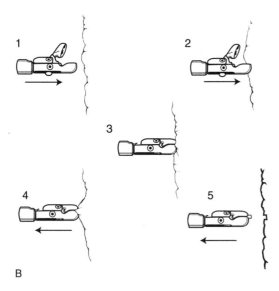

the biopsy forceps are gently closed using the ratchet handle or wire guide system.

The right hand remains on the shaft of the bioptome, while the left is used to hold the venous sheath (Fig 11-4B). Under fluoroscopy, the shaft of the bioptome is pulled. If there is excessive resistance to withdrawal, the forceps should be released and the bioptome repositioned. Usually there will be a slight jerk as the tissue is removed, which may be perceptible to the patient by the myocardial rebound effect. The biopsy forceps are withdrawn quickly through the tricuspid valve to limit ectopy and are removed from the patient while holding onto the sheath with the left hand to ensure that it is not also withdrawn as the bioptome is removed. Fluoroscopy may be stopped once the bioptome "clears" the tricuspid valve.

The forceps are opened and the tissue removed. Tissue removal may be performed with a fine needle with all attempts to minimize tissue trauma and consequent postbiopsy tissue artefact. The bioptome may be rinsed with saline to remove blood while the forceps' jaws are open.

Many disposable unshaped flexible bioptomes may be "shaped" to a curvature appropriate for the angle of entry across the tricuspid valve into the right ventricle. Because most unshaped disposable systems are smaller in diameter than the Stanford Caves bioptome, there is the advantage of selecting a smaller insertion sheath. A disadvantage is that, because the bioptomes are not reusable, procedure costs increase with greater dependence on disposable systems.

Right Internal Jugular Sheath System

In some patients, it is necessary to utilize a right ventricular sheath system from the internal jugular vein (Fig 11-5). Methods of access of the venous system are similar to those described previously. We utilize an entry similar to the technique described previously through which the guiding sheath is inserted. Therefore, a 7-Fr guiding sheath is inserted through an 8-Fr entry sheath. This ensures relatively free motion of the sheath system, which we believe to be advantageous with these fragile guiding sheaths. Alternatively, the ventricular sheath may be inserted primarily into the jugular venous system. The latter approach has the advantage of using a smaller catheter size. This may be critical in some patients, particularly children and smaller adults.

The internal jugular venous sheath and central obturator guiding catheter are pre-shaped to allow more predictable entry into the right ventricle (Fig 11-5A). The obturator and sheath may be inserted in exactly the same fashion that is utilized for the pre-shaped biopsy forceps technique, as described previously. If entry is not gained easily, a 0.038″ flexible J-wire guide may be placed through the obturator catheter, which can be manipulated to identify the proper route to the right ventricle (Fig 11-5B). If successful, the sheath and

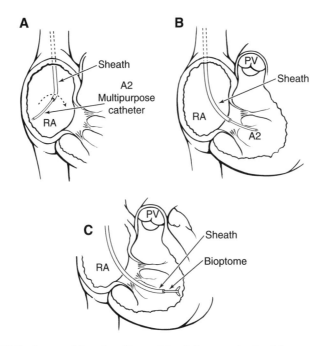

Figure 11-5   Internal jugular disposable right ventricular biopsy technique. **(A)** The preformed sheath is guided into the right atrium (RA) using the A2 multipurpose catheter, Swan-Ganz, or 0.038″ wire guide. As with the reusable bioptome, the sheath is rotated 180 degrees anteriorly and directed toward the tricuspid valve. **(B)** The guiding catheter is advanced across the tricuspid valve into the right ventricle. Occasionally, a guidewire may be necessary to lead the guiding catheter into the appropriate chamber. Once the right ventricle has been entered, the sheath is advanced forward while the guiding catheter and wire are retracted. The sheath is directed posteriorly toward the interventricular septum. The sheath must be free-floating and not engaged in the trabeculae or ventricular septum. **(C)** The bioptome is advanced through the sheath. The jaw handle is manipulated to open the jaws before the bioptome extends from the end of the sheath. This ensures that the bioptome is open as soon as it exits the sheath, reducing the risk of perforation. The technique for removal of biopsy specimens is the same as that performed when using a reusable bioptome system. The flexible and disposable bioptomes, however, do not have a ratchet jaw-locking mechanism, and pressure must be maintained to ensure that the jaws remain closed, retaining the encapsulated specimen, while transporting it out of the interventricular septum and through the guiding sheath. PV, pulmonary valve.

obturator are advanced over the wire guide into the ventricle. If this is unsuccessful, the wire and obturator can be removed and replaced with a balloon-tip device, such as a Swan-Ganz catheter, which eases passage into the outflow system due to its flow-directed characteristics. Once in the right ventricle, the wire, obturator, and/or balloon-tip catheter are withdrawn while the biopsy sheath is advanced, resulting in proper placement of the guiding sheath within the right ventricle. One must ensure that the guiding sheath is advanced adequately over the course of the obturator or guiding balloon catheter so that it remains in the right ventricle once the guiding system is removed, because the guiding systems extend several centimeters beyond the distal end of the biopsy sheath.

The guiding sheath remains in the right ventricle and should be directed medially and inferiorly, as is the case with the disposable or preshaped system. The sheath is attached to a continuous infusion port to ensure that blood does not clot within the sheath due to stasis. The side-arm may also be connected to a pressure transducer to allow for measurement of right ventricular pressure. The unshaped bioptome is inserted into the sheath and advanced to near the tip of the sheath under fluoroscopy. One must ensure that the tip is free-floating and does not become embedded in the myocardium. Dye may be injected to ensure position away from the ventricular wall, and a nondamped ventricular pressure recording guarantees appropriate position. One attempts to open the bioptome before it reaches the end of the sheath so that it will open as soon as it extends beyond the sheath. The open-jaw forceps have a much lesser chance of perforating the ventricular wall when advanced. The biopsy forceps are advanced to the right ventricular wall and, once contact is confirmed by fluoroscopy and ectopy diminished, the bioptome head is closed and the biopsy forceps alone withdrawn and tissue removed (Fig 11-5C).

Biopsy via the Subclavian Vein

Accessing the subclavian vein is described in Chapter 4.

The preshaped bioptome is inserted through the venous sheath pointed toward the right atrial wall. Once there, the bioptome is torqued 180 degrees toward the tricuspid valve and advanced. Again, medial or posterior direction of the biopsy forceps is exceedingly important; however, because of the S-shaped curve of the biopsy forceps, greater reliability on fluoroscopy for this site of biopsy is necessary. This technique relies on great flexibility of the biopsy instrument, and one must ensure that the most flexible of systems is utilized. The guiding-sheath system is not appropriate for the right subclavian site because of the fragility and easy kinking of the sheath.

Biopsy via the Femoral Vein

Accessing the femoral vein is described in Chapter 4.

Although there is a 100-cm Stanford-Caves bioptome that can be used from the leg, this system is used infrequently. Virtually all femoral biopsy procedures are performed using guiding-sheath systems and disposable bioptomes. We prefer to use a "dog-leg" sheath with a 135-degree angle bend, allowing relatively easy access into the right ventricle from the leg (Fig 11-6).

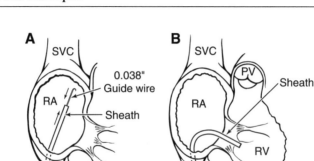

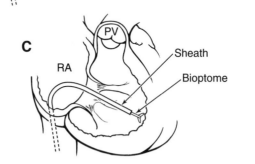

Figure 11-6 Femoral venous disposable right ventricular biopsy technique. **(A)** The sheath is straightened by a central catheter (A2 multipurpose) or guidewire (0.038″). Once in the right atrium (RA), the guidewire may be used to cross the tricuspid valve. Usually, the straightened angulation does not favor this, and the wire is withdrawn as the sheath is advanced. **(B)** The withdrawn stenting wire or catheter allows the femoral venous sheath to assume its normal angulation of approximately 135 degrees. This allows the appropriately shortened sheath (see text discussion) to drop into the right ventricle (RV). As with the disposable internal jugular systems, the sheath must be directed to the interventricular septum and must not engage the right ventricular wall. **(C)** The flexible bioptome is inserted through the guiding sheath into the right ventricular (RV) cavity. The sheath is "straightened," not infrequently, by the advancement of the bioptome itself. Therefore, fluoroscopic assessment of the influence of the bioptome on the dog-leg portion of the catheter must be utilized as soon as resistance is met, implying that the curvature in the sheath has been reached. Because stiffening may be problematic, this aspect of the right ventricular biopsy requires considerable skill. IVC, inferior vena cava; PV, pulmonary valve; SVC, superior vena cava.

Before the long sheath is inserted, the short arm of the sheath must be "sized" to the patient. This is performed by placing the disposable dog-leg angle sheath over the patient's chest under fluoroscopy, with the assumed angle of use mimicked. The right (patient's) portion of the sheath is positioned over the shadow of the right atrial wall, and the length of the shorter dog-leg sheath is assessed relative to the anticipated cavity size of the right ventricle by evaluating the proximity of the sheath to the left ventricular border. All adult sheaths come in one size, whereas all ventricles do not. Therefore, in cases of obvious discrepancy, 1 to several cm of the distal portion of the biopsy sheath must be removed.

The disposable-sheath system may be inserted through an entry sheath (Fig 11-6A). The disposable-sheath system is guided into the right atrium utilizing either a 0.038″ wire guide or balloon-tipped catheter (Swan-Ganz), Mullins, or multipurpose central catheter. The central wire or catheter straightens the sheath angle, allowing passage through the tortuous inferior vena cava.

Once the catheter apparatus is in the right atrium, it is advanced gently into the right ventricle (Fig 11-6B). Unless a central wire apparatus or balloon flotation device is used to guide the sheath into the right ventricle, this usually requires withdrawal of the wire or guiding catheter. Withdrawal of these devices results in the long biopsy sheath attaining its previous dog-leg angulation and dropping into the right ventricle. The right ventricular biopsy sheath should be angled toward the interventricular septum or directed posteriorly. The tip must be free-floating and not embedded in the ventricular wall. If necessary, dye injection or recording undamped ventricular pressure ensures proper positioning.

Once properly placed, the long unshaped disposable biopsy forceps are advanced through the course of the sheath. Once mild resistance is identified, fluoroscopy should be started. The mild resistance is created by the biopsy forceps meeting the sharp angle of the guiding sheath, or may imply a kink in the sheath itself. The biopsy forceps are advanced beyond the resistance to near the end of the sheath. The bioptome handle is opened to ensure that the jaws are open and ready to engage the ventricular wall as soon as the biopsy forceps extend beyond the distal end of the sheath (Fig 11-6C). This reduces the risk of perforation. The sheath remains in a steady position while the forceps are advanced to engage the wall, acquire the tissue, and then withdraw the tissue through the unmoved sheath apparatus.

As with all preshaped sheath systems, the continuous infusion of slightly heparinized solution (1000 units) should be maintained to ensure that clot does not form in the sheath during the biopsy procedure.

Biopsy of the Left Ventricle: Femoral Arterial Approach

Virtually all biopsies of the left ventricle are performed through the femoral arteries. Access into the femoral arteries is described in Chapter 4. Once arterial access is acquired, a high-pressure infusion device must be connected to the sheath to ensure patency and prevent clot formation.

A preshaped guiding biopsy sheath is utilized and manipulated through the short entry sheath. Occasionally, direct insertion of the biopsy sheath into the

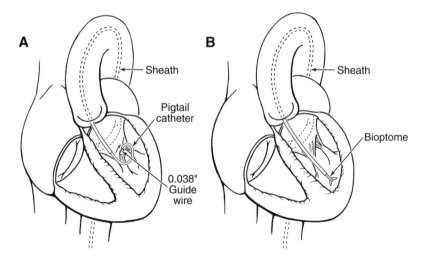

Figure 11-7   Femoral artery left ventricular biopsy technique. **(A)** The bioptome sheath is guided into the left ventricle through the aortic valve, led by a guiding catheter and usually a guiding-wire system. The guidewire is usually a 0.038″ J catheter, and the guiding catheter may be a pigtail, A2 multipurpose, or other catheter appropriate for the aortic arch and aortic valve angulation of the patient. Once in the left ventricle, the guidewire and guiding catheter are withdrawn, while the biopsy sheath is advanced. The biopsy sheath must be free in the interventricular cavity and should not be entrapped in the left ventricular wall. **(B)** The bioptome is inserted through the sheath into the left ventricular cavity. As with the right ventricular approach, the biopsy jaws are opened as soon as the bioptome clears the end of the guiding sheath. The open biopsy forceps are advanced to the left ventricular cavity and the specimen removed. The sheath remains in the left ventricle until the biopsy procedure is completed. The left ventricular sheath, to a much greater extent than the right ventricular disposable systems, must be managed carefully to ensure that there is neither debris nor air forced through the sheath into the left ventricle and systemic circulation.

femoral artery may be advantageous. The preshaped biopsy sheath is led by either a 0.038″ wire guide or a central catheter, which may be a Mullins, multipurpose, or pigtail catheter (Fig 11-7A). The central guiding sheath, with or without a wire guide, is inserted into the left ventricle retrograde through the aortic valve. Once in position, the biopsy sheath is advanced over the guiding catheter into the left ventricle itself, and the guiding wire and central catheter are removed. A constant-infusion device must be attached to the left ventricular catheter to prevent clot formation.

As with the right ventricular biopsy, the bioptome is traversed through the sheath and into the left ventricular cavity using fluoroscopy. The biopsy forceps are opened, the wall engaged, and tissue removed (Fig 11-7B). Because of the greater potential for symptomatic distal embolization, great care must be applied to ensure that no air or clot is allowed to enter the lengthy biopsy sheath.

Heterotopic Heart Biopsy

Some heart transplants are placed in a heterotopic position (piggy-back) as opposed to an orthotopic position (heart replacement). A heterotopic heart shares atrial connections, but the donor right ventricle will characteristically be in a most peculiar location. The right ventricle is usually located in the right chest and pointed toward the armpit. Because heterotopic anatomy may vary somewhat with each recipient, the operator must have a clear understanding from his or her surgical colleague of the exact anatomy created and the anticipated course of venous blood flow.

In virtually all instances, it will be necessary to "experiment" to determine which site of venous access allows successful entry into the ventricular cavity. In our experience, this is usually possible from the left subclavian or femoral venous site, utilizing a Stanford-Caves reusable or arterial sheath disposable system, respectively. Occasionally, contrast studies or echocardiographic analysis may be necessary to identify the most appropriate site.

In all attempts at biopsy procedures, withdrawal of the tissue may result in excessive resistance. Excessive resistance to withdrawal usually implies that either too large a piece has been captured in the jaws, that the annulus as opposed to the septum is being biopsied, that scar tissue is present, or that the patient has an underlying disease characterized by stiff endomyocardial tissue. In all cases except the latter, it is advisable to release the jaws of the forceps and search for a more compliant site to biopsy.

Sonographic Assistance

Two techniques have recently been described to assist in the performance of venous entry and cardiac biopsy: sonographic assessment of the venous access site and echocardiographic assessment of the ventricular biopsy site. A new sonographic instrument has been used to determine the presence, size, and location of the internal jugular vein.[14] This technique uses a small sonographic transducer covered in a sterile wrapper and placed over the site of anticipated venous or arterial entry. The sonogram is calibrated for centimeters in depth. Therefore, the location of the internal jugular vein, its relation to the carotid artery, its size, and its compressibility can be determined. This technique has been demonstrated to improve the frequency of cannulation of the internal jugular vein, decrease the time to acquire access, and decrease complications of venous cannulation.[15] The same device can be utilized for access for almost any venous or arterial system.

The sonographic device is intended to be utilized in conjunction with the venous access needle. This may be cumbersome initially, and the device may inadvertently compress the internal jugular vein. This technique requires modest experience before routine success can be achieved. Others consider this technique to be similar to "fishing with dynamite" and prefer the challenge of a blind approach.

Standard transthoracic echocardiography has been used to visualize the site for ventricular biopsy.[16] Using a subxiphoid or four-chamber view, it is usually possible to identify the tip of the biopsy forceps and define the site of sampling. This should reduce the risk of inadvertent anterior free-wall biopsy with attendant perforation and tamponade. It would also diminish the radiation exposure to patients and operators, because fluoroscopy would be used in a more limited fashion, if at all.

Complications of Endomyocardial Biopsy

To fairly assess the risks of endomyocardial biopsy, one must consider complications of venous access as well as complications related to the performance of the procedure. Most previous studies have concentrated exclusively on the risks of the endomyocardial biopsy without considering the risks of venous or arterial access.

Risks of access include inadvertent arterial puncture, prolonged bleeding, hematoma, vasovagal reaction, Horner's syndrome, brachial plexus injury, pneumothorax, infection, arteriovenous communication, and laceration of the central venous structures. Biopsy complications include arrhythmias (supraventricular and ventricular), conduction abnormalities (bradycardia, bundle branch block, complete heart block), and ventricular perforation resulting in pain, effusion, tamponade, or death. Rarely, allergic reactions to the biopsy forceps or pacemaker dislodgement have been reported, and very rarely a symptomatic embolic event has occurred.

Large series reporting the risk of biopsy alone demonstrate a risk of less than 1% to 1.67%. Stanford reported a 1% or lower risk in 4000 patients, including 0.4% risk of tamponade.[17] A large European survey of 3097 patients reported a risk of 1.55%.[18] A worldwide assessment of 2337 patients reported a risk of 1.67%, with a 0.59% risk of tamponade,[19] whereas a second worldwide series of 6739 patients reported a risk of 1.17%, with a risk of perforation of 0.42%.[20]

Smaller single-site series, which more fully reported risks, included a 4.4% risk to the first 100 patients undergoing biopsy at the Mayo Clinic,[21] an 11% risk to 134 patients undergoing biopsy at Utah,[22] and a 14% risk in the first 50 patients undergoing biopsy at Oregon, followed by a 0.8% risk in the next 250 patients.[23] The risk to pediatric patients is essentially the same, with a 15% risk reported in 53 patients undergoing the procedure.[24]

The risk of venous entry is somewhat diminished in transplantation patients, as is the risk of cardiac complication. Anastasiou-Nana et al.[25] reported 704 transplant-related procedures, compared with 243 cardiomyopathy procedures. An inability to cannulate the site of entry was seen in 0.61% versus 7.0%, and 0 versus 2 patients had a cardiac complication. Two transplant patients had access-site complications: One developed an access-site abscess, and the other suffered laceration of the superior vena cava.

In our published series of 546 consecutive cardiomyopathy and 2454 transplant procedures, we reported an overall procedure risk of 6% in cardiomyopathy patients and 3.1% in transplant patients. The relative risks and nature of the risks are noted in the following data:[26,27]

Entry risks	Cardiomyopathy (%)	Transplant (%)
Overall entry	2.7	2.3
Arterial puncture	2.0	1.8
Prolonged bleeding	0.2	0.4
Vasovagal	0.4	0.1
Horner's syndrome	0.0	0.0
Pneumothorax	0.0	0.0
Infection	0.0	0.0
Laceration of superior vena cava	0.0	0.0
Overall biopsy	3.3	0.77
Arrhythmia	1.1	0.25
Conduction abnormalities	1.0	0.2
Perforation	0.7	0.08
Death	0.4	0.0
Allergic reaction	0.0	0.2
Pacemaker dislodgement	0.0	0.04
Total	6.0	3.1

It is important to note that in both series, a 100% success rate in obtaining tissue was reported. We used the internal jugular approach in 96% and 96.9% of procedures, respectively.

Anderson and Marshall[22] reported that in 12% of cardiomyopathy patients, they could not enter the internal jugular vein; however, there were no failures of access using the femoral venous system. Inadequate tissue was obtained in 6% of patients biopsied using the internal jugular vein versus 0% using the femoral venous system, whereas pericardial effusions were more common in the femoral venous system than through the internal jugular techniques. Although these authors felt that the femoral venous system offered the highest yield with the fewest complications, we consider the femoral venous system to be somewhat more prone to the risk of perforation and to be characterized by less adequate control of the direction of the biopsy sheath and forceps.

Failure to gain access into the internal jugular vein may be related to depleted intravascular volume, lack of neck landmarks due to obesity or previous surgery, or most commonly, bleeding into the carotid sheath or tamponade of the sheath by excessive use of local anesthesia. Problems with inadequate tissue most often relate to use of venous guiding-sheath systems without adequate flushing mechanisms. Without continuous flushing systems, clot may form in the sheath and then be pushed through the sheath by passage of the bioptome. Instead of retrieving myocardial tissue, the bioptome may then mistakenly encapsulate and retrieve clot that has been expelled into the right ventricle. Atrial arrhythmias may be diminished by careful manipulation of the bioptome or sheath through the atrial chambers to avoid wall stimulation, particularly in those patients predisposed by history of previous arrhythmia. Ventricular arrhythmias are virtually impossible to avoid but can be limited by acquiring good contact with the septum with the biopsy forceps and by limiting the time the biopsy forceps are in the ventricle. This may require somewhat more pressure than one is usually comfortable applying to an instrument that may perforate the ventricular wall. Conduction disturbances are likely due to either pressure of the bioptome against the interventricular septum and the right bundle of His, causing a right bundle branch block, or the creation of complete heart block by causing right bundle branch block conduction defects in patients with preexisting left bundle branch block.[28] Occasionally, a conduction problem may be created by an inadvertently high biopsy of the interventricular septum, damaging the conduction system. Pneumothorax can usually be prevented by using an internal jugular approach sufficiently high in the neck to avoid damage to the apex of the lung. The risk of pneumothorax in the subclavian approach can be diminished only by taking a relatively superior approach and ensuring that aspiration occurs during each portion of the procedure. Similarly, any time that the venous system is exposed to air, a finger should be placed over any intravascular cannula to prevent air aspiration through a sheath without a one-way membrane.

The greatest risk of endomyocardial biopsy is that of perforation. One must ensure that the forceps are directed against the interventricular septum. Occasionally, even though directed at the radiographic apex, the forceps will biopsy the anterior free wall when there is marked right ventricular enlargement, resulting in its "wrapping around" and replacing the position of the left ventricular apex. Chest pain experienced during the biopsy must be considered a possible perforation. Respect for any complaint of pain from the patient during the biopsy procedure greatly enhances one's ability to recognize and rapidly treat perforation. Once perforation does occur, the operator must move expeditiously to evacuate the clot if there is hemodynamic compromise. This may be difficult, because rapid bleeding into the pericardial sac may result in clotting.

Indications for Endomyocardial Biopsy

The following diagnoses can be made histologically by endomyocardial biopsy:[4,26,29-54]

Inflammatory/ Immune/Infection	Restrictive heart disease	Malignancy	Vascular	Storage Disease	Other
Cardiac rejection posttransplant	Amyloidosis	Primary cardiac tumors	Ischemia	Glycogen	Hepatolenticular degeneration (Wilson's disease)
Myocarditis	Hemo-chromatosis	Secondary cardiac tumors	Vasculitis	Gaucher	Catecholamine excess
Rheumatic heart disease	Hypertrophy	Anthracycline toxicity	Scleroderma	Fabry	
Löffler's endocarditis	Fibrosis	Radiation toxicity	Thrombotic thrombo-cytopenic purpura		
Kawasaki's syndrome	Sarcoidosis	Carcinoid			
Specific infection (cytomegalo-virus)	Endocardial fibrolastosis Endocardial fibrosis				

To evaluate the usefulness of endomyocardial biopsy, Parillo et al. assessed 100 consecutive patients submitted to endomyocardial biopsy at the Massachusetts General Hospital.[55] The biopsy was considered useful in 54 of 100 patients, including 26 with restrictive heart disease versus pericardial constriction. A specific diagnosis was found in 9 patients, a diagnosis consistent with but not diagnostic of a disorder in 10 patients, and a specific etiology for restrictive hemodynamics in 12 of 26 patients. Nippoldt et al. evaluated 100 consecutive patients undergoing biopsy and separated them into five groups.[21] Of 34 patients with dilated cardiomyopathy, 4 (12%) had myocarditis; of six patients with possible myocarditis, only 1 (17%) had myocarditis, and 2 (33%) had changes compatible with cardiomyopathy. In 27% of patients with arrhythmia and normal heart function, 15% had myocarditis and 30% had changes of cardiomyopathy; in 19 nondilated heart failure patients, 4 (21%) had amyloid; and in 14 patients with some form of systemic disease, 7 (50%) had cardiac findings compatible with that disease. These authors concluded that there was a poor correlation between symptoms compatible with myocarditis and the tissue diagnosis of this disorder. Based on their experience, the authors felt it was reasonable to biopsy patients with dilated cardiomyopathy of unknown etiology, those with suspected myocarditis, patients with arrhythmia and no other identifiable heart disease, and patients with restrictive heart disease. French et al. confirmed the value of biopsy in patients with restrictive or nondilated heart failure.[56] Of 12 patients with normal ejection fractions but congestive heart failure, the biopsy was considered diagnostic in 8 (67%) of the 12 patients, whereas tissue diagnosis was found in only 2 (15%) of 13 patients with depressed ejection fractions. Ferriere et al.[57] evaluated 116 patients submitted to biopsy and found a definitive diagnosis in 14 (12%), two thirds of whom were unsuspected. Olson evaluated 67 patients by endomyocardial biopsy.[58] In 44 (65%) of the patients, the biopsy was helpful in 21 (32%), the suspicion of a specific illness was confirmed; in 22 (33%), suspected diseases were excluded, whereas the biopsy was unhelpful in 19 (28%), and no tissue was demonstrated in 5 (7%). Das et al.[59] evaluated 22 patients, of whom 17 (77%) had tissue obtained. They found unexpected pathology in 1 (4.5%), while confirming a suspected diagnosis in 6 (36%). The diagnosis suspected is somewhat dependent on geographic location, as demonstrated by the histologic identification of endomyocardial fibrosis in 49 (76%) of 64 patients submitted to biopsy by Somers et al.[60] in Uganda.

The usefulness of endomyocardial biopsy has similarly been reported in children. Schmaltz et al.[61] biopsied 60 children, demonstrating a definitive diagnosis in 7 (12%) and determining the biopsy to be helpful in 43 (72%) but of no help in 10 (17%). Leatherbury et al.[62] evaluated 20 children with dilated or hypertrophic cardiomyopathic findings and 2 patients with suspected myocarditis. Of the 16 dilated cardiomyopathy patients, the diagnosis was confirmed in 8 (50%), but 4 (25%) patients had myocarditis, 2 (12.5%) had findings compatible with hypertrophic cardiomyopathy, and 2 (12.5%) had carnitine deficiency. In 2 hypertrophic cardiomyopathy patients, one biopsy confirmed this diagnosis whereas another demonstrated evidence of a cardiac fibroma. Of 2 suspected myocarditis patients, only 1 had the illness, whereas the other had dilated cardiomyopathy. Biopsy was considered helpful in diagnosis or management of 75% of patients and altered the management of 50%.

McKay et al.[63] felt endomyocardial biopsy was of no help in 64 (88%) of 73 patients. Thirteen (18%) of 73 patients had no tissue recovered. These authors categorized biopsies as diagnostic, helpful, of limited help, showing confirmatory findings, of no help, or misleading. The low yield of helpful biopsies was likely due to the case selection, which included 7 patients with rheumatic heart disease and 8 congenital heart patients.

In an early analysis of 610 consecutive patients,[64] we combined histologic diagnoses with strict criteria for nonhistologic diagnoses such as alcohol excess and thyroid disease. Using these criteria, a diagnosis responsible for the dilated cardiomyopathy was found in 366 (60%), with the remaining 244 patients (40%) labeled truly idiopathic dilated cardiomyopathy. The diagnosis was altered by the endomyocardial biopsy in 142 cases (23%). Unsuspected myocarditis was found in 26 patients (4%). A specific diagnosis was identified in 110 patients (18%), whereas nonspecific findings compatible with and supportive of idiopathic dilated cardiomyopathy were found in 244 patients (40%). Therefore, biopsy was considered helpful in 58% (356 of 610 patients).

We feel that patients with malignant ventricular arrhythmias and a structurally normal heart or patients with cancer involving the heart should also be considered for endomyocardial biopsy. Strain et al.[65] submitted 18 patients with ventricular tachycardia or fibrillation without evidence of ventricular dysfunction or coronary artery disease to endomyocardial biopsy. The average ejection fraction was 65%. Despite this, the endomyocardial biopsy was abnormal in 16 (89%) of 18 patients. Nine patients had changes compatible with cardiomyopathy, 3 had unsuspected myocarditis, 2 arteritis, and 2 evidence of right ventricular dysplasia. Those patients without abnormal biopsies (2) had Wolff-Parkinson-White syndrome or mitral valve prolapse. Sugrue et al.[66] similarly submitted 12 patients with normal hearts and malignant ventricular ectopy to biopsy. Eleven (92%) of the 12 were abnormal, demonstrating hypertrophy, fibrosis, endocardial fibrosis, changes of cardiomyopathy, or myocarditis. Vignola et al.[67] evaluated 17 of 65 patients presenting to the Miami Heart Institute without identifiable causes for their ventricular malignant arrhythmias. Twelve of these 17 patients were submitted to biopsy. Six (50%) of those 12 had myocarditis and 3 (25%) had changes compatible with cardiomyopathy, whereas 3 (25%) were normal biopsies. Of note, the 6 patients with myocarditis were treated with immunosuppressive therapy. After 6 months, and without antiarrhythmic medications, 5 (83%) of the 6 did not have inducible ventricular tachycardia at electrophysiologic testing.

Thiene et al.[68] reported the high frequency of right ventricular dysplasia causing sudden death in an Italian population. Right ventricular dysplasia is characterized by lipomatous or fibrin lipomatous transformation of the right ventricular free wall, resulting in the propensity for malignant arrhythmias and sudden death. Endomyocardial biopsy occasionally yields evidence of endocardial fat, which is considered normal. A high proportion of endocardial fat may be considered suggestive of right ventricular dysplasia if combined with a left bundle branch block, ventricular tachycardia and noninvasive evidence by echocardiography and MRI of right ventricular dysfunction, particularly with right ventricular free-wall lipomatous changes.

Malignant disease of the heart is an unusual indication for endomyocardial biopsy. Primary heart tumors occur in less than 0.3% of all autopsies.[45] It is more common for the heart to be affected with metastatic disease, of which bronchogenic carcinoma, breast adenocarcinoma, and malignant melanoma are the most common. The heart may also be infiltrated with diffuse leukemia or metastatic lymphoma. Copeland et al.[69] reported the use of echocardiographic-guided endomyocardial biopsy of mass lesions in the heart.

Biopsy of a mass lesion present in the left ventricle is one of the few indications for a left, as opposed to right, ventricular endomyocardial biopsy. Multiple authors have confirmed the fact that the right ventricular portion of the interventricular septum demonstrates adequately the pathology of the left ventricle, even in cases in which only left ventricular dysfunction is present. The changes in the left ventricular cavity may be somewhat more severe than those in the right, but histologic changes are usually considered more than adequate in the interventricular septum. Similarly, in the few patients who have expired in a time frame close to the performance of endomyocardial biopsy, autopsy has demonstrated confirmatory histopathology.

Histomorphometric Analysis

A multitude of studies have been performed[70–75] to correlate histologic morphology with prognosis. Surprisingly, not all such studies have confirmed the inverse correlation between prognosis and progressive histologic changes. Regardless of the initial insult created, the heart is capable of a limited number of histologic responses. These include development of progressive interstitial fibrosis, cellular hypertrophy, myocyte dropout, and nuclear enlargement. Electron microscopic changes include fiber degeneration or hypertrophy, an increase in mitochondria and stored glycogen, and myofiber loss with an increase in fibrosis.

Most studies[70,71,73–75] have demonstrated the correlation between increased cell size and interstitial fibrosis with poor prognosis. The failure of other studies to demonstrate this effect is likely due to the failure to evaluate patients with idiopathic dilated cardiomyopathy and the disparity in the rate of progression of cardiomyopathies of similar apparent degrees of dysfunction.

Based on these observations, we consider endomyocardial biopsy useful for the following nontransplant indications:

Diagnosis and classification of myocarditis
Diagnosis of the etiology of restrictive heart disease
Establishment of histologic etiology of patients with dilated cardiomyopathy
Understanding of specific cardiomyopathies such as peripartum cardiomyopathy and cardiomyopathy associated with AIDS
Diagnosis of cardiomyopathy
Demonstration of histologic abnormalities in patients with malignant arrhythmia
Provision of tissue for histologic, immunologic, and molecular research

Tissue Management

Tissue obtained from the endomyocardium must be placed in a fixative appropriate for maximizing the information available from the biopsy. The samples from the large-jaw bioptomes may be sectioned with a surgical No. 11 blade into specimens adequate in size for independent analysis. Samples should not be sectioned smaller than 1 μm. Samples may be submitted for analysis in the following ways:

1. *Formalin.* Most tissue is placed in 10% formalin for routine hematoxylin and eosin (H&E) studies. The paraffin-embedded block from which the H&E stains are prepared may be used to perform special stains on histologic tissue as suggested by the initial review of the standard preparation. Special staining may be performed to emphasize fibrosis, glycogen, iron, copper, protein, or immunologic analysis of cellular components.

2. *Glutaraldehyde.* Specimens submitted for electron microscopy are placed immediately in glutaraldehyde. Formalin and glutaraldehyde should be at room temperature when the specimens are inserted. Glutaraldehyde should be placed in iced saline as soon as the tissue is inserted.

3. *Fresh tissue.* Tissue may be submitted in gauze dampened with saline for special studies, such as immunoperoxidase staining.

4. *Liquid nitrogen.* Some analyses, such as genetic markers, require the endomyocardial biopsy tissue to be snap-frozen in liquid nitrogen. This obviously requires special preparation and cooperation with the laboratory to which the specimen will be submitted.

5. *Culture.* Endomyocardial biopsy may be submitted to viral, fungal, or bacterial culture. This approach has produced such a low yield that it has been virtually abandoned in favor of methods capable of identifying these agents by other techniques, including in situ hybridization, polymerase chain reaction, and special stains.

It is the responsibility of the operator to ensure that the endomyocardial biopsy specimens are appropriately placed in fixative and delivered to the laboratory.

Management of the Patient After Biopsy

After the biopsy is performed, the sheaths are removed, and hemostasis is obtained by applying direct pressure. If the patient is biopsied from the internal jugular or subclavian vein, the patient is instructed to sit up to lower the venous pressure and improve the chance for rapid hemostasis. Once the bleeding has stopped, topical antibiotics and a single adhesive strip bandage are placed over the site of entry for 24 hours. If the patient has had the procedure performed through the femoral vein, a 5-lb sandbag is placed over the applied bandage for 2 to 3 hours to ensure that bleeding has stopped. Arterial procedures require that prolonged pressure be applied to ensure that adequate hemostasis is obtained. The patient is laid flat, and a 10-lb sandbag is placed atop the site of entry in the femoral artery for 4 hours. After the 4 hours, 30-degree elevation of the trunk is allowed, and after 6 hours, the patient may ambulate if there is no contraindication.

Complications related to right ventricular endomyocardial biopsy occur during the performance of the biopsy. Therefore, if the patient has no symptoms at the completion of the procedure, one can usually safely assume that there have been no serious complications. Patients are therefore observed for only 30 minutes after routine endomyocardial biopsy from the jugular or subclavian vein and are subsequently discharged. If there is any question that the patient may have suffered perforation, an emergency echocardiogram should be obtained to assess the pericardial fluid status. Patients having left ventricular biopsies may have delayed onset of pericardial accumulation and tamponade and should be observed for at least several hours before being discharged. Fortunately, their hemostasis requirements usually ensure that they are under observation for an adequate length of time. If the patient complains of shortness of breath and there is any question of pneumothorax, an upright chest x-ray should be obtained to assess this potential complication.

The Future of Endomyocardial Biopsy

The indiscriminate use of endomyocardial biopsy with unrealistic expectations for its value will lead to disappointing results. The appropriate use of this procedure can provide invaluable assistance to patients with primary or secondary heart muscle disease, restrictive cardiomyopathy, suspected myocarditis, possible cardiac involvement due to systemic illness, and malignant ventricular arrhythmia and normal heart function.

The potential benefit of endomyocardial biopsy must be weighed against the risk of performance of the procedure. The stated low morbidity and mortality associated with this procedure is a reflection of the expertise present in a limited number of centers around the world. There is likely to be a greater risk of complication at institutions where the procedure is performed infrequently. Similarly, the quality of histologic assessment of the tissue obtained is exceedingly dependent on the experience and interest of the pathologists who interpret the tissue.

The potential of endomyocardial biopsy has never been greater. Endomyocardial biopsy can be used to quantitate the genetic alterations seen in patients with cardiomyopathy and corroborate their correction with treatment of the underlying disorder.[76] Similarly, immunologic techniques, including polymerase chain reaction and in situ hybridization, will allow us to determine whether a patient's ventricular compromise is due to prior myocarditis and whether a viral genome or an immunologic reaction is present. Additionally, molecular techniques are now available that allow assessment of fundamental alterations in patients with heart muscle disease. These techniques, and many others, will allow us to make great strides in the near future to understand and treat a multitude of heart muscle disorders about which we currently know very little.

SELECTED READINGS

1. Bullock RT, Murphy ML, Pearce MB. Intracardiac needle biopsy of the ventricular septum. Am J Cardiol 1965;16:227–233.
2. Weinberg M, Fell EH, Lynfield J. Diagnostic biopsy of the pericardium and myocardium. AMA Arch Surg 1958;76:825–829.
3. Sutton DC, Sutton GC. Needle biopsy of the human ventricular myocardium: review of 54 consecutive cases. Am Heart J 1960;60:364–370.
4. Timmis GC, Gordon S, Baron RH, Brough AJ. Percutaneous myocardial biopsy. Am Heart J 1965;70:499–504.
5. Shirey EK, Hawk WA, Mukerji D, Effler DB. Percutaneous myocardial biopsy of the left ventricle: experience in 198 patients. Circulation 1972;156:112–122.
6. Sakakibara S, Konno S. Endomyocardial biopsy. Jpn Heart J 1962;3:537–543.
7. Konno S, Sekiguchi M, Sakakibara S. Catheter biopsy of the heart. Radiol Clin North Am 1971;9:491–510.
8. Richardson PJ. King's endomyocardial bioptome. Lancet 1974;(i):660–661.
9. Caves PK, Schulz WP, Dong E, et al. New instrument for transvenous cardiac biopsy. Am J Cardiol 1974;33:264–267.
10. Lew BT, Olivari MT, Levine TB. Endomyocardial biopsy with a disposable bioptome: a modified technique. Cathet Cardiovasc Diagn 1987;13:211–213.
11. Brooksby IAB, Swanton RH, Jenkins BS, Webb-Peploe MM. Long sheath technique for introduction of catheter tip manometer or endomyocardial bioptome into left or right heart. Br Heart J 1974;36:908–912.
12. Melvin KR, Mason JW. Endomyocardial biopsy: its history, techniques and current indications. Can Med Assoc J 1982;126:1381–1386.
13. Mason JW. Techniques for right and left ventricular endomyocardial biopsy. Am J Cardiol 1978;41:887–892.
14. Denys BG, Uretsky BF, Reddy PS, et al. An ultrasound method for safe and rapid central venous access. N Engl J Med 1991;324:566.
15. Denys BG, Uretsky BF, Reddy PS. Ultrasound-assisted cannulation of the internal jugular vein. Circulation 1993;87:1557–1562.
16. Piérard L, Allaf DE, D'Orio V, et al. Two-dimensional echocardiographic guiding of endomyocardial biopsy. Chest 1984;85:759–762.
17. Fowles RE, Mason JW. Endomyocardial biopsy. Ann Intern Med 1982;97:885–894.
18. Unpublished data: Olsen EGJ, National Heart Hospital, London.
19. Richardson PJ. Endomyocardial biopsy technique. In: Bolte HD, ed. Myocardial biopsy. Berlin: Springer, 1980:3–7.
20. Przybojewski JZ. Endomyocardial biopsy: a review of the literature. Cathet Cardiovasc Diagn 1985;11:287–330.
21. Nippoldt TB, Edwards WD, Holmes DR, et al. Right ventricular endomyocardial biopsy: clinicopathologic correlates in 100 consecutive patients. Mayo Clin Proc 1982;57:407–418.
22. Anderson JL, Marshall HW. The femoral venous approach to endomyocardial biopsy: comparison with internal jugular and transarterial approaches. Am J Cardiol 1984;53:833–837.
23. Hosenpud JD. Complications of endomyocardial biopsy. In: Kron J, Morton MJ, eds. Complications of cardiac catheterization and angiography: prevention and management. New York: Futura, 1989:135–154.
24. Yoshizato T, Edwards WD, Alboliras ET, et al. Safety and utility of endomyocardial biopsy in infants, children and adolescents: a review of 66 procedures in 53 patients. J Am Coll Cardiol 1990;15:436–442.
25. Anastasiou-Nana MI, O'Connell JB, Nanas JN, et al. Relative efficiency and risk of endomyocardial biopsy: comparisons in heart transplant and nontransplant patients. Cathet Cardiovasc Diagn 1989;18:7–11.
26. Deckers JW, Hare JM, Baughman KL. Complications of transvenous right ventricu-

lar endomyocardial biopsy in adult patients with cardiomyopathy: a seven-year survey of 546 consecutive diagnostic procedures in a tertiary referral center. J Am Coll Cardiol 1992;19:43–47.

27. Baraldi-Junkins C, Levin HR, Kasper EK, et al. Complications of endomyocardial biopsy in heart transplant patients. J Heart Lung Transplant 1993;12:63–67.

28. Castellanos A, Ramirez AV, Mayorga-Cortes A, et al. Left fascicular blocks during right-heart catheterization using the Swan-Ganz catheter. Circulation 1981;64:1271–1276.

29. Caves P, Coltart J, Billingham M, et al. Transvenous endomyocardial biopsy—application of a method for diagnosing heart disease. Postgrad Med J 1975;51:286–290.

30. Billingham ME. Diagnosis of cardiac rejection by endomyocardial biopsy. Heart Transplant 1982;1:25–30.

31. Caves PK, Stinson EB, Billingham ME, Shumway NE. Serial transvenous biopsy of the transplanted human heart—improved management of acute rejection episodes. Lancet 1974;(i):821–826.

32. Mason JW, Billingham ME, Ricci DR. Treatment of acute inflammatory myocarditis assisted by endomyocardial biopsy. Am J Cardiol 1980;45:1037–1044.

33. Rose AG, Uys CJ, Losman JG, Barnard CN. Evaluation of endomyocardial biopsy in the diagnosis of cardic rejection. Transplantation 1978;26:10–13.

34. Yutani C, Go S, Kamiya T, et al. Cardiac biopsy of Kawasaki disease. Arch Pathol Lab Med 1981;105:470–473.

35. Yutani C, Okano K, Kamiya T, et al. Histopathological study on right endomyocardial biopsy of Kawasaki disease. Br Heart J 1980;43:589–592.

36. Marcella JJ, Ursell PC, Goldberger M, et al. Kawasaki syndrome in an adult: endomyocardial histology and ventricular function during acute and recovery phases of illness. J Am Coll Cardiol 1983;2:374–378.

37. Pellikka PA, Holmes DR, Edwards WD, et al. Endomyocardial biopsy in 30 patients with primary amyloidosis and suspected cardiac involvement. Arch Intern Med 1988;148:662–666.

38. Swanton RH, Brooksby IAB, Davies MJ, et al. Systolic and diastolic ventricular function in cardiac amyloidosis. Am J Cardiol 1977;39:658–664.

39. Olson LJ, Gertz MA, Edwards WD, et al. Senile cardiac amyloidosis with myocardial dysfunction. N Engl J Med 1987;317:738–742.

40. Frenzel H, Schwartzkopff B, Kuhn H, et al. Cardiac amyloid deposits in endomyocardial biopsies: light microscopic, ultrastructural, and immunohistochemical studies. Am J Clin Pathol 1986;85:674–680.

41. Short EM, Winkle RA, Billingham ME. Myocardial involvement in idiopathic hemochromatosis: morphologic and clinical improvement following venesection. Am J Med 1981;70:1275–1279.

42. Fitchett DH, Coltart DJ, Littler WA, et al. Cardiac involvement in secondary haemochromatosis: a catheter biopsy study and analysis of myocardium. Cardiovasc Res 1980;14:719–724.

43. Lorell B, Alderman EL, Mason JW. Cardiac sarcoidosis: diagnosis with endomyocardial biopsy and treatment with corticosteroids. Am J Cardiol 1978;42:143–146.

44. Lemery R, McGoon MD, Edwards WD. Cardiac sarcoidosis: a potentially treatable form of myocarditis. Mayo Clin Proc 1985;60:549–554.

45. Flipse TR, Tazelaar HD, Holmes DR. Diagnosis of malignant cardiac disease by endomyocardial biopsy. Mayo Clin Proc 1990;65:1415–1422.

46. Billingham ME, Mason JW, Bristow MR, Daniels JR. Anthracycline cardiomyopathy monitored by morphologic changes. Cancer Treat Rep 1978;62:865–872.

47. Applefeld MM, Wiernik PH. Cardiac disease after radiation therapy for Hodgkin's disease: analysis of 48 patients. Am J Cardiol 1983;51:1679–1681.

48. Nitter-Hauge S, Simonsen S, Langmark F. Myocardial biopsy in diagnosis of endomyocardiopathy in patient with electro- and vectorcardiographic signs of myocardial infarction. Br Heart J 1978;40:1419–1422.

49. Alpert MA, Goldberg SH, Singsen BH, et al. Cardiovascular manifestations of mixed connective tissue disease in adults. Circulation 1983;68:1182–1193.
50. Ridolfi RL, Hutchins GM, Bell WR. The heart and cardiac conduction system in thrombotic thrombocytopenic purpura: a clinicopathologic study of 17 autopsied patients. Ann Intern Med 1979;91:357–363.
51. Edwards WD, Hurdey HP, Partin JR. Cardiac involvement by Gaucher's disease documented by right ventricular endomyocardial biopsy. Am J Cardiol 1983; 52:654.
52. Malcolm AD, Cankovic-Darracott S, Chayen J, et al. Biopsy evidence of left ventricular myocardial abnormality in patients with mitral-leaflet prolapse and chest pain. Lancet 1979;(i):1052–1055.
53. Scully RE, Mark EJ, McNeely WF, McNeely BU. Case 15-1988. N Engl J Med 1988; 318:970–980.
54. Imperato-McGinley J, Gautier T, Ehlers K, et al. Reversibility of catecholamine-induced dilated cardiomyopathy in a child with a pheochromocytoma. N Engl J Med 1987;316:793–797.
55. Parillo JE, Aretz HT, Palacios I, et al. The results of transvenous endomyocardial biopsy can frequently be used to diagnose myocardial diseases in patient with idiopathic heart failure. Circulation 1984;69:93–101.
56. French WJ, Siegel RJ, Cohen AH, Laks HM. Yield of endomyocardial biopsy in patients with biventricular failure: comparison of patients with normal vs reduced left ventricular ejection fraction. Chest 1986;90:181–184.
57. Ferriere M, Donnadio D, Gros B, et al. Biopsie endoventriculaire droite: indications et résultats cent seize observations. Presse Med 1985;14:773–776.
58. Olsen EGJ. Diagnostic value of the endomyocardial bioptome. Lancet 1974; (i): 658–659.
59. Das JP, Rath B, Das S, Sarangi A. Study of endomyocardial biopsies in cardiomyopathy. Indian Heart J 1981;33:18–26.
60. Somers K, Hutt MSR, Patel AK, D'Arbela PG. Endomyocardial biopsy in diagnosis of cardiomyopathies. Br Heart J 1971;33:822–832.
61. Schmaltz AA, Apitz J, Hort W, Maisch B. Endomyocardial biopsy in infants and children: experience in 60 patients. Pediatr Cardiol 1990;11:15–21.
62. Leatherbury L, Chandra RS, Shapiro SR, Perry LW. Value of endomyocardial biopsy in infants, children and adolescents with dilated or hypertrophic cardiomyopathy and myocarditis. J Am Coll Cardiol 1988;12:1547–1554.
63. McKay EH, Littler WA, Sleight P. Critical assessment of diagnostic value of endomyocardial biopsy. Br Heart J 1978;40:69–78.
64. Unpublished data: Kasper EK, The Johns Hopkins Medical Institutions, Baltimore, MD.
65. Strain JE, Grose RM, Factor SM, Fisher JD. Results of endomyocardial biopsy in patients with spontaneous ventricular tachycardia but without apparent structural heart disease. Circulation 1983;68:1171–1181.
66. Sugrue DD, Holmes DR, Gersh BJ, et al. Cardiac histologic findings in patients with life-threatening ventricular arrhythmias of unknown origin. J Am Coll Cardiol 1984;4:952–957.
67. Vignola PA, Aonuma K, Swaye PS, et al. Lymphocytic myocarditis presenting as unexplained ventricular arrhythmias: diagnosis with endomyocardial biopsy and response to immunosuppression. J Am Coll Cardiol 1984;4:812–819.
68. Thiene G, Nava A, Corrado D, et al. Right ventricular cardiomyopathy and sudden death in young people. N Engl J Med 1988;318:129–133.
69. Copeland JG, Valdes-Cruz L, Sahn DJ. Endomyocardial biopsy with fluoroscopic and two-dimensional echocardiographic guidance: case report of a patient suspected of having multiple cardiac tumors. Clin Cardiol 1984;7:449–452.
70. Schwarz F, Mall G, Zebe H, et al. Quantitative morphologic findings of the myocardium in idiopathic dilated cardiomyopathy. Am J Cardiol 1983;51:501–506.

71. Unverferth DV, Fetters JK, Unverferth BJ, et al. Human myocardial histologic characteristics in congestive heart failure. Circulation 1983;68:1194–1200.

72. Baandrup U, Florio RA, Rehahn M, et al. Critical analysis of endomyocardial biopsies from patients suspected of having cardiomyopathy: comparison of histology and clinical/haemodynamic information. Br Heart J 1981;45:487–493.

73. Shirey EK, Proudfit WL, Hawk WA. Primary myocardial disease: correlation with clinical findings, angiographic and biopsy diagnosis. Am Heart J 1980;99:198–207.

74. Noda S. Histopathology of endomyocardial biopsies from patients with idiopathic cardiomyopathy; quantitative evaluation based on multivariate statistical analysis. Jpn Circ J 1980;44:95–116.

75. Baandrup U, Florio RA, Roters F, Olsen EGJ. Electron microscopic investigation of endomyocardial biopsy samples in hypertrophy and cardiomyopathy: a semiquantitative study in 48 patients. Circulation 1981;63:1289–1298.

76. Ladenson PW, Sherman SI, Baughman KL, Feldman AM. Alteration in myocardial gene expression in a hypothyroid man with a reversible dilated cardiomyopathy. Proc Natl Acad Sci U S A 1992;89:5251–5255.

12

MEASURES OF MYOCARDIAL CONTRACTILE AND DIASTOLIC FUNCTION

Michael A. Fifer

ROUTINE CARDIAC CATHETERIZATION provides information regarding overall pump performance of the left ventricle, including left ventricular end-diastolic pressure and volume, cardiac output, stroke volume, and ejection fraction. Understanding of cardiac pathophysiology for clinical and especially for investigative purposes often requires more detailed assessment of the contractile and diastolic function of the myocardium. This chapter summarizes the techniques available in cardiac catheterization for such an evaluation.

Contractile Function

Depression of left ventricular contractile function has long been recognized as both a major cause of symptoms and a predictor of mortality in patients with heart disease. Assessment of myocardial contractility has been hampered by the fact that ventricular performance, although readily measurable, depends not only on contractility, but also on preload and afterload (Fig 12-1). There are four classes of indices that have been advanced for the evaluation of myocardial contractile function: ventricular function curves, isovolumic phase indices, ejection phase indices, and end-systolic indices.

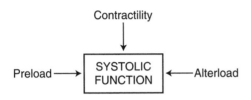

Figure 12-1 Determinants of systolic function.

Ventricular Function Curves

Ventricular function curves relate some measure of systolic performance, such as stroke work, to some measure of preload, such as end-diastolic pressure (Fig 12-2). Ventricular function curves are shifted upward by positive and downward by negative inotropic interventions, but are also shifted upward by decreases in afterload and downward by increases in afterload. Recent reexamination of the relationship between stroke work and end-diastolic volume has led to the so-called preload recruitable stroke work relation, a form of ventricular function curve (Fig 12-3). In the dog heart, this relation is linear, sensitive to inotropic state, and independent of afterload.

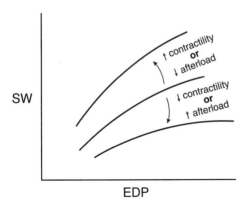

Figure 12-2 Ventricular function curves depicting, in this case, the relationship between stroke work (SW) and end-diastolic pressure (EDP). The position of the curve may be shifted by changes in either contractility or afterload.

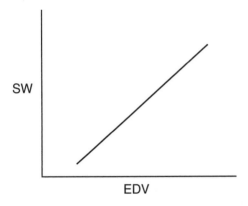

Figure 12-3 The relationship between stroke work (SW) and end-diastolic volume (EDV), termed the preload recruitable stroke work. (Adapted from Glower DD, Spratt JA, Snow ND, et al. Linearity of the Frank-Starling relationship in the intact heart. Circulation 1985;71:994–1009).

Ejection Phase Indices

These, by definition, are measured during ventricular ejection. The most widely used, of course, is *ejection fraction*. Others include percentage fractional shortening (the "one-dimensional" ejection fraction obtained from M-mode echocardiography), mean systolic ejection rate, and mean and peak velocity of circumferential fiber shortening. These measures of ventricular pump performance are sensitive to preload and, in particular, to afterload. At any given level of contractility, these indices vary directly with preload and inversely with afterload. For example, ejection fraction may be low despite normal myocardial contractility in the presence of very high afterload, as in some patients with aortic stenosis. On the other hand, ejection fraction may be normal despite impaired contractility in the presence of high preload and/or low afterload, as in some patients with mitral regurgitation. Thus, because many pathophysiologic conditions alter ventricular preload and afterload, ejection phase indices may not accurately reflect myocardial contractility.

Isovolumic Phase Indices

These indices are derived from measurements made between mitral valve closure and aortic valve opening, during which time (in the absence of mitral regurgitation) blood neither enters nor exits the left ventricle, which is therefore isovolumic. The simplest isovolumic index is the peak rate of left ventricular pressure rise (peak positive dP/dt, Fig 12-4). Although peak positive dP/dt increases when contractility is enhanced, it also increases when preload (left ventricular end-diastolic pressure or volume) increases. Furthermore, dP/dt increases up to the time of aortic valve opening; therefore, the higher the aortic pressure (or afterload), the higher the peak positive dP/dt (a somewhat counterintuitive concept).

In certain instances, application of peak positive dP/dt leads to meaningful conclusions regarding myocardial contractility. For example, when a phosphodiesterase inhibitor such as amrinone is administered to a patient with heart failure, preload and afterload decrease and peak positive dP/dt increases. Because the decreases in preload and afterload would tend to cause peak positive dP/dt to decrease, the fact that it nevertheless increases indicates a positive effect of the drug on myocardial contractility.

In most instances, however, the load sensitivity of peak positive dP/dt renders it less useful as an index of contractility. There have been a number of modifications of peak positive dP/dt that have been made to counter its preload and afterload dependence. The most useful of these is the value of dP/dt at a level of developed pressure (i.e., left ventricular pressure–left ventricular end-diastolic pressure) that occurs at a given level (e.g., at a developed pressure of 40 mm Hg) prior to opening of the aortic valve. The use of developed rather

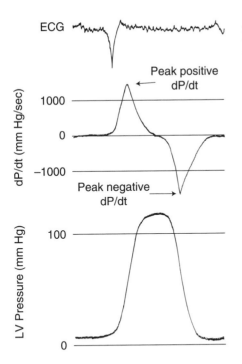

Figure 12-4 The electrocardiogram (ECG), left ventricular (LV) pressure obtained with a micromanometer catheter, and the first time derivative of LV pressure (dP/dt), obtained in this case by electronic differentiation of the pressure signal. Peak positive dP/dt, an index of contractility, occurs at approximately the time of aortic valve opening, whereas peak negative dP/dt, an index of diastolic relaxation, occurs near the time of aortic valve closure.

than absolute pressure obviates much of the preload dependence, whereas the use of a developed pressure that is reached prior to aortic valve opening removes the afterload dependence of dP/dt. Determination of dP/dt requires the acquisition of a high-fidelity ventricular pressure tracing, usually through the use of a micromanometer catheter.

End-Systolic Indices

Three decades ago, it was observed in isolated muscle that the relation between the tension against which the muscle contracts and the length of the muscle at the end of contraction was both linear and independent of the length of the muscle at the beginning of contraction. When this concept was extended to the isolated ventricle, it was seen that (1) the relationship between end-systolic volume and end-systolic pressure (afterload) is linear, (2) this relationship is independent of end-diastolic volume (preload), and (3) this relationship is steeper when contractility is increased with a drug such as epinephrine and decreased with an intervention such as the production of global ischemia (Fig 12-5). These observations indicated that the end-systolic pressure-volume relation (ESPVR) of the ventricle is sensitive to changes in contractility, takes afterload into account, and is independent of changes in preload, suggesting that it would be an ideal index of contractility.

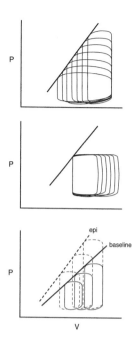

Figure 12-5 Pressure-volume loops depicting the ESPVR. (Top) At a constant inotropic state, the relationship between end-systolic pressure (P) and volume (V) is approximately linear. (Middle) At a constant inotropic state and afterload, the relationship between end-systolic pressure and volume is nearly independent of preload (end-diastolic volume). (Bottom) A positive inotropic intervention, such as administration of epinephrine (epi), shifts the ESPVR upward and leftward, such that end-systolic volume is lower at each end-systolic pressure; a negative inotropic intervention would shift the ESPVR downward and rightward. (Adapted from Suga H, Sagawa K, Shoukas A. Load independence of the instantaneous pressure-volume ratio of the canine left ventricle and effects of epinephrine and heart rate on the ratio. Circ Res 1973;32:314–322.)

In patients undergoing cardiac catheterization, construction of the ESPVR requires manipulation of afterload, high-fidelity ventricular pressure measurement, and multiple determinations of ventricular volume, a time-consuming endeavor attempted only in research studies. Afterload may be increased with a drug such as methoxamine or reduced with a drug such as nitroprusside or a mechanical intervention such as balloon occlusion of the inferior vena cava. In the latter case, a balloon catheter is introduced into the femoral vein, advanced into the right atrium, inflated, and pulled back until it obstructs the junction of the inferior vena cava and the right atrium. This results in a rapid fall in systemic arterial pressure and requires that the technique used to measure left ventricular volume is capable of recording changes on a beat-to-beat basis. Such capability is offered by a "volume" catheter. This catheter is introduced into the left ventricle and measures changes in impedance, which are proportional to the amount of blood within the left ventricle. Alternatively, left ventricular size may be measured by echocardiography, radionuclide techniques, or contrast ventriculography; a disadvantage of the latter method is the large cumulative volume of contrast required.

Pressure and volume measurements throughout the cardiac cycle are combined to form a pressure-volume loop (Fig 12-6). Variation of afterload (end-systolic pressure) generates a series of loops. The line tangent to the upper left-hand corners of the loops is the ESPVR. The slope of this line is the end-systolic elastance (Ees), and is closely related to the maximum elastance (Emax), a measure of the contractile state of the ventricle. If a drug with effects on con-

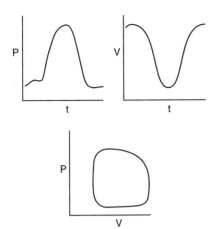

Figure 12-6 Creation of a pressure-volume loop (bottom) from plots of pressure (P) and volume (V) versus time (t) (top left and top right, respectively).

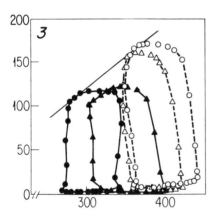

Figure 12-7 Left ventricular pressure-volume loops obtained in a patient with heart failure due to severe systolic dysfunction. A line connecting the loops obtained during a baseline period (open circles), infusion of the vasodilator nitroprusside (closed circles), and another baseline period (open triangles) is the baseline ESPVR. During infusion of the calcium channel blocker nicardipine (closed triangles), the pressure-volume loop is shifted downward and rightward from the baseline ESPVR, indicating a negative inotropic effect of the drug. (Adapted from Aroney CN, Semigran MJ, Dec GW, et al. Inotropic effect of nicardipine in patients with heart failure: assessment by left ventricular end-systolic pressure-volume analysis. J Am Coll Cardiol 1989;14:1331–1338).

tractility is administered and afterload again varied, a new series of loops and a new ESPVR are generated. A slope of the new ESPVR higher than that of the baseline ESPVR indicates a positive inotropic effect, whereas a lower slope indicates a negative inotropic effect. Because generation of the entire ESPVR at baseline and after an intervention may not be practical in the cardiac catheterization laboratory, the position of a single pressure-volume loop after an intervention relative to the ESPVR at baseline may be taken as an indication of the inotropic effect of the intervention (Fig 12-7).

Diastolic Function

In a number of diseases affecting the myocardium, abnormalities of diastolic function may become manifest before those of contractile function, and may

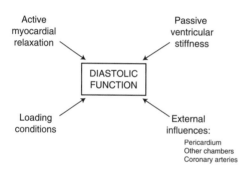

Figure 12-8 Determinants of diastolic function.

predominate even when systolic dysfunction coexists with diastolic dysfunction. Because of this, there has been considerable effort to characterize diastolic function of the left ventricle. Just after ventricular ejection ends with aortic valve closure, ventricular pressure falls precipitously as the myocardium relaxes. Volume remains constant until the mitral valve opens, ending this period of isovolumic relaxation or isovolumic diastole. Ventricular filling ensues, with rapid filling early in diastole, followed by a period of little or no filling, and culminating in filling generated by atrial contraction. Diastolic function is determined by myocardial relaxation, an active, energy-consuming process, by compliance, a passive property of the ventricle, and by factors external to the ventricle, such as the "turgor" of the coronary circulation, compression by the contralateral ventricle, mediated by the pericardium, and loading conditions (Fig 12-8). As is the case for measures of contractility, indices of diastolic function may be conveniently divided into four types: compliance, relaxation, filling, and overall distensibility.

Compliance

Compliance is defined as change in volume divided by change in pressure. To determine compliance, then, one must measure both ventricular volume and ventricular pressure. Volume and pressure measurements are combined to construct the diastolic pressure-volume relation, a portion of the pressure-volume loop for the entire cardiac cycle (Fig 12-9). The slope of this relation is stiffness, and its inverse is compliance. These are measured during mid to late diastole, after active relaxation of the ventricle is completed and before the effects of atrial contraction on left ventricular pressure are evident (i.e., before the a wave). Compliance tends to be decreased in chronic conditions, such as hypertensive left ventricular hypertrophy or restrictive cardiomyopathy, affecting the passive properties of the ventricle.

Relaxation

The simplest measure of the rate of active myocardial relaxation during isovolumic diastole is the maximum rate of fall of left ventricular pressure, which is

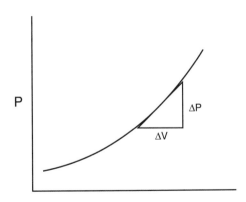

Figure 12-9 Relation between ventricular pressure (P) and volume (V) during diastole, depicting the determination of ventricular compliance ($\Delta V/\Delta P$).

analogous to the maximum rate of rise of pressure, an index of contractility. There is some uncertainty regarding nomenclature (with regard to maximum or minimum), but a useful term is *peak negative dP/dt*, in which case one is considering the absolute value of dP/dt. Like peak positive dP/dt, peak negative dP/dt may be determined from electronic or numerical differentiation of a high-fidelity ventricular pressure recording (see Fig 12-4). Peak negative dP/dt is sensitive to changes in the rate of relaxation, but is also affected by loading conditions. In particular, higher initial (end-systolic) pressure is associated with higher values of peak negative dP/dt.

The afterload dependence of peak negative dP/dt is largely negated by calculation of T, sometimes called τ (tau), the time constant of isovolumic relaxation. Calculation of T is based on the observation that pressure fall during isovolumic diastole is roughly exponential:

$$P = P_0 e^{-t/T}$$

where P_0 is end-systolic pressure. Implicit in this calculation is the assumption that ventricular pressure asymptotically approaches zero. Release of this assumption allows calculation of T and a nonzero asymptote; the reader is referred elsewhere for this derivation.

T is typically approximately 40 msec in a normal human left ventricle. It is chronically prolonged in patients with hypertrophic cardiomyopathy, and acutely and reversibly prolonged during ischemia in patients with coronary artery disease. Interventions that increase the rate of reuptake of calcium into the sarcoplasmic reticulum during diastole, such as the administration of isoproterenol, shorten T.

Filling Indices

Frame-by-frame calculation of left ventricular volume from the contrast ventriculogram allows construction of a plot of volume versus time (Fig 12-10). The

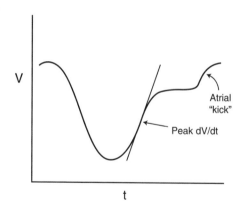

Figure 12-10 Relation between ventricular volume (V) and time (t) throughout the cardiac cycle, showing the derivation of the peak filling rate (dV/dt) as the maximum slope of the curve during early diastolic filling.

maximum slope of this relation (maximum dV/dt) in early diastole is the *peak filling rate* (PFR). The PFR has been determined more recently (and less laboriously) by automated radionuclide techniques and from the transmitral velocity profile determined by Doppler echocardiography. In the latter case, the height (or integrated area) of the early (E) wave is often compared with that of the atrial (A) filling wave, generating the E/A ratio.

Conditions characterized by slow relaxation and diminished ventricular compliance, such as hypertrophic cardiomyopathy, are often associated with a low PFR and a correspondingly greater contribution by filling generated by atrial contraction. The PFR is also depressed when stroke volume is low (as in systolic dysfunction of any cause); this confounding effect may be offset by "normalizing" PFR by dividing it by stroke volume. Unfortunately, in radionuclide studies, PFR is often divided by end-diastolic volume rather than by stroke volume, ensuring that this index of diastolic function will be abnormal in any patient with a high end-diastolic volume due to systolic dysfunction.

A further problem with PFR is that it, too, is load dependent. Increases in left atrial pressure, the "driving" pressure for early left ventricular filling, increase PFR. This leads to the situation wherein a patient with low PFR due to diastolic dysfunction may have an increase (or "pseudonormalization") of PFR when diastolic dysfunction becomes severe enough to bring about an increase in left atrial pressure.

Distensibility

Although compliance and relaxation and filling indices are useful in some clinical and research settings, they have a number of limitations, including load dependence, as indicated in the preceding discussion. Furthermore, they each focus attention on a particular phase of diastole rather than on overall diastolic function, a problem analogous to that of the blind men examining the elephant (Fig 12-11). Overall ventricular distensibility, as defined by the entire diastolic pressure-volume relation, offers a more comprehensive measure of dia-

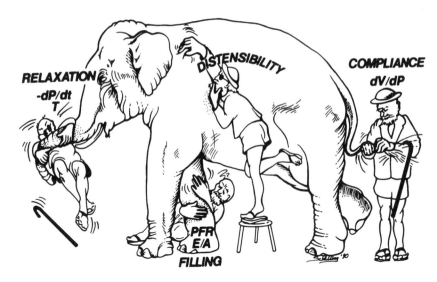

Figure 12-11   Indices used to assess various aspects of diastolic function.

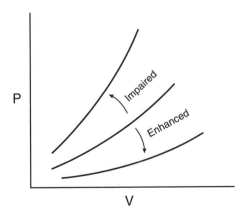

Figure 12-12   Overall distensibility of the ventricle as the relationship between pressure (P) and volume (V). A shift in the position of the curve indicates a change in the distensibility.

stolic performance. If this relationship is shifted upward, so that the ventricular filling requires higher filling pressure, distensibility is impaired; if the relationship is shifted downward, distensibility is enhanced (Fig 12-12). Such shifts may be due to changes in external constraints to ventricular filling as well as to properties of the ventricle itself.

Thus, evaluation of diastolic function is complex. In general, it is best not to draw conclusions based on changes in compliance or in a particular index of relaxation or filling. Instead, one should attempt to assess more than one type of index, including, if possible, overall distensibility. As is the case for the evaluation of contractility, one must also take into account the potentially confounding influences of preload and afterload.

SELECTED READINGS

Fifer MA, Aroney CN, Semigran MJ, et al. Techniques for assessing inotropic effects of drugs in patients with heart failure: application to the evaluation of nicardipine. Am Heart J 1990;19(2 Pt 2):451–456.

Fifer MA, Braunwald E. End-systolic pressure-volume and stress-length relations in the assessment of ventricular function in man. Adv Cardiol 1985;32:36–55.

Grossman W, Lorell BH (eds). Diastolic relaxation of the heart. Boston: Martinus Nijhoff, 1988.

Kass DA, Midei M, Graves W, et al. Use of a conductance (volume) catheter and transient inferior vena cava occlusion for rapid determination of pressure-volume relationships in man. Cathet Cardiovasc Diagn 1988;15:192–202.

II

APPLICATIONS OF CARDIAC CATHETERIZATION IN SPECIFIC DISEASE STATES

13

AORTIC VALVE AND AORTIC ROOT DISEASE

John D. Carroll

Aortic Stenosis

THE GOALS OF cardiac catheterization in patients with aortic stenosis are given in Table 13-1. The explicit definition and prioritization of goals are important because of the elevated risks and the recognized technical difficulties of cardiac catheterization in these patients. Usually, well-tolerated complications such as hematomas, vasovagal reactions, and transient effects of contrast media may lead to cardiovascular collapse in the presence of severe aortic stenosis. In addition, certain complications are unique—tamponade due to left ventricular (LV) perforation from the straight guidewire used to cross the aortic valve. Furthermore, most patients in the current era with severe aortic stenosis are elderly. Prolonged procedures are not likely to be well tolerated, and medication side effects (i.e., lidocaine toxicity from local anesthesia, excessive sedation) are more common in this age group. Technical difficulties should also be anticipated due to the tortuosity of the peripheral circulation, dilated aorta, and the stenotic nature of the valve. Both during and after the procedure, attention to the details of technique, careful intraprocedure decision making, and rapid recognition and correction of problems will yield important clinical data and prevent the vast majority of complications from cardiac catheterization in patients with aortic stenosis.

Table 13-1   Goals of Cardiac Catheterization
in Aortic Valve Disease

1. Assessment of severity of valvular abnormality: obstruction
   and regurgitation
2. Assessment of presence/absence of coronary artery disease
3. Assessment of left ventricular function
4. Assessment of status of thoracic aorta
5. Exclusion of other important cardiac abnormalities

Hemodynamic Assessment: The Valve, the Ventricle, and the Aorta

The properties of not only the aortic valve but also the left ventricle, aorta, and systemic circulation have a major impact on the clinical significance of the aortic stenosis. The valve and these other structures have a functional reserve that eventually becomes exhausted as the stenosis worsens and/or the compensatory mechanisms fail. Understanding these principles aids in performing a useful cardiac catheterization.

The Valve

The normal aortic valve opens to an area of approximately 4 cm^2. At some point when the orifice is reduced to less than 2 cm^2, a pressure overload state is produced and compensatory mechanisms such as myocardial hypertrophy are apparent. Not until the orifice becomes less than 1 cm^2 do symptoms typically emerge.

Valve orifice size is the common way to portray the anatomic basis for hemodynamic obstruction, but other factors are also important. An orifice with an irregular shape versus a round shape increases the surface area over which blood travels, thereby increasing the resistance to flow and the tendency to develop turbulence.[1-3] A more rounded orifice is common in a rheumatically deformed valve, whereas an irregular triangular-shaped orifice is common with degenerative aortic stenosis.

Flow acceleration and deceleration occur upstream and downstream, respectively, in a gradually tapering obstruction. Flow deceleration may be accompanied by a substantial downstream pressure recovery.[2] Aortic stenosis, on the other hand, is characterized by an abrupt, discrete, and severe narrowing with minimal pressure recovery and a substantial net pressure gradient.[4] Slight tapering of the flow field may be present in the hypertrophied outflow tract of the left ventricle. A funnel is also created by the variable degree of residual outward movement of the valve leaflets despite the reduction in orifice area. Downstream of the stenotic aortic orifice there is clearly no tapering, but rather an abrupt expansion of the flow field diameter.

Aortic stenosis has three major effects on blood flow: (1) localized increased transvalvular blood velocity with the formation of jets, (2) a transition from laminar to abnormal turbulent flow, and (3) a reduction in total flow (e.g., cardiac output). Peak LV outflow velocities across the normal aortic valve may reach the 1.5-m/sec level, but in severe aortic stenosis, velocities are often 5 to 6 m/sec. Acceleration of flow may begin below the orifice in a discrete, small anatomic area of the outflow tract. Quantification of stepwise flow acceleration from the left ventricle to the orifice of the valve is routinely noted by Doppler studies. Immediately downstream, the high-velocity laminar jet of blood emerging from the valve orifice peaks (defining the vena contracta) and is then transformed into a turbulent flow field in the ascending aorta.[5] Turbulence causes energy loss and produces a murmur.

The reduction of cardiac output is related to the degree of aortic stenosis, the adaptation of the left ventricle, and secondary circulatory alterations, such as reflex vasoconstriction of the systemic circulation. The reduction in cardiac output may not be present at rest but apparent only during exercise. With advancement in the severity of obstruction, the resting cardiac output is frequently reduced. A discussion of the importance of LV performance differences in patients with aortic stenosis follows.

The net transvalvular pressure gradient is the hallmark of aortic valve obstruction. Using an upstream pressure waveform (LV) and a downstream pressure waveform from the arterial system, the systolic gradient is usually 10 to 20 mm Hg in mild aortic stenosis. Some patients with severe obstruction have small pressure gradients (30–40 mm Hg) due to reduced transvalvular flow, as with severe LV systolic dysfunction and coexistent mitral valve disease. Clinically important aortic stenosis, when flow is not markedly reduced, produces mean systolic gradients often as high as 50 to 100 mm Hg. The highest transaortic mean gradient recorded at rest in our laboratory was 130 mm Hg and occurred in a patient with severe aortic stenosis who had a calculated orifice size of 0.3 cm^2 and an LV ejection fraction of 81%. Substantial transvalvular pressure gradients may occur at rest in mild-to-moderate degrees of obstruction due to unusually high transvalvular flows, as seen in anemia, severe obesity, hyperthyroidism, and coexistent severe aortic regurgitation.

The concept of a transvalvular gradient is a simplification of the complex pressure drop at different locations upstream and downstream from the stenotic orifice (see Chapter 9). Initially, pressure drops upstream of the valve orifice as blood accelerates. It drops further with the onset of turbulence immediately downstream from the orifice. A slight pressure increase or recovery occurs further downstream where laminar flow is reestablished.

A complete hemodynamic description of aortic stenosis must also consider that flow is pulsatile. The transvalvular pressure gradient and blood flow are time dependent (i.e., changing throughout systole), though we frequently speak of mean gradients and mean transvalvular flows. Typically, the pressure gradient, the blood velocity, and the downstream occurrence of turbulence are greatest in early to mid-systole.

Finally, the duration of the systolic ejection period is helpful in the assessment of the degree of aortic stenosis. Aortic stenosis generally increases the duration of ejection.

AORTIC VALVE AREA

The calculated aortic valve area is a standard measurement because it combines three major hemodynamic variables central to the assessment of stenosis severity: the transvalvular pressure gradient, the transvalvular flow, and the duration of flow.[6] Whether obtained invasively or noninvasively, its derivation is theoretically justified and its clinical application has been extensively tested. It also converts a physiologic assessment of stenosis severity into an anatomic representation that is usually semiquantitatively accurate. The term *area* is easily understood by physicians and patients.

The anatomic valve area, such as that derived from planimetry of an image, differs from the effective valve area derived from hemodynamics by the Gorlin equation. The discharge coefficient is an expression of the difference between these two areas. As shown by Flachskampf, the discharge coefficient of the stenotic aortic valve is not constant, as it is portrayed in the Gorlin equation, but varies from patient to patient, and in the same patient before and after

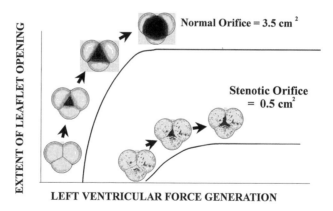

Figure 13-1   The aortic valve leaflets open fully with normal LV force generation and produce a maximum orifice size in the range of 3.5 to 4.0 cm^2. The valve dynamics in aortic stenosis are contrasted to the normal situation in this illustration. The fully opened stenotic valve has an orifice of only 0.5 cm^2 in this example. To open the valve requires more force generation on the part of the left ventricle. If the ventricle becomes myopathic or if the myocardium is acutely depressed, it is apparent that the stenotic valve will be opened even less than when the left ventricle was robust. This emphasizes the importance of LV function on the obstructive physiology of aortic stenosis.

procedures such as valvuloplasty.[3] The formula also contains the controversial assumption that a specific quantitative relationship exists between pressure and flow even in low-flow states.[7] Another controversial assumption is that the valve orifice is fixed. Variations in calculated area with altered flow may be due to true variations in anatomic valve area, as well as to changes in effective valve area, or to incorrect assumptions about the relation between pressure and flow (Fig 13-1).

AORTIC VALVE RESISTANCE

Valve resistance, a measurement of stenosis severity put forward in the 1950s, has been resurrected and studied again in the past several years.[7-11] This physiologic index of stenosis severity is expressed in common terms of opposition to blood flow or resistance units. It therefore lends itself to a variety of useful hemodynamic calculations.[7,8] Valve resistance gives an alternative assessment of stenosis severity in challenging cases, and may yield a more clinically appropriate assessment of stenosis when the gradient and transvalvular flow are low.[11]

The Ventricle

The acute and chronic remodeling of the left ventricle must be considered in assessing the obstructive physiology of aortic stenosis. Chamber properties affect not only the clinical features of aortic stenosis, but also the cardiac output and pressure waveforms used to assess obstructive physiology. The hemodynamic assessment of aortic stenosis takes on a different look when the ventricle is vigorous versus when it is myopathic. When systolic dysfunction sets in, the measured pressure gradient is smaller and the LV ejection time loses its prolonged nature. Furthermore, heart rate is increased when the left ventricle is myopathic, which further reduces the transvalvular pressure gradient and ejection time.

Left ventricular size, including chamber dimensions, geometry, and wall thickness, and LV systolic and diastolic function all reflect a type and degree of adaptation to the pressure overload imposed by the stenotic valve. A spectrum of adaptation of the left ventricle to aortic stenosis has been reported, often related to the patient's gender, and has a significant influence on prognosis.[12]

The Aorta

The poststenotic dilatation of the aorta has been recognized for decades, although the mechanism remains unclarified. Preliminary evidence has shown that reduced aortic compliance significantly influences aortic pressure even in the presence of aortic stenosis.[13,14] The classical abnormalities in the aortic pressure waveform are presented in Figure 13-2. From a clinical standpoint, the status of the ascending aorta also has a significant impact on the type of operation needed and the nature of postoperative complications.

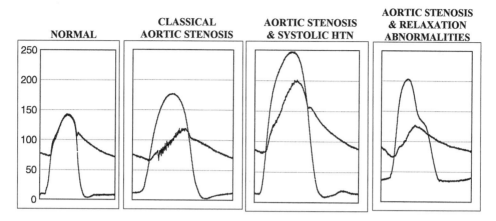

Figure 13-2 High-fidelity aortic and LV pressure waveforms are shown for a patient with a normal aortic valve and three patients with severe aortic stenosis. The patient with classical aortic stenosis demonstrates the large mean gradient and the high-frequency oscillations on the aortic waveform due to turbulence. The patient with systolic hypertension (HTN) has severe aortic stenosis and very elevated aortic *and* LV systolic pressures. Grossly elevated diastolic pressures and abnormal pressure decay are readily apparent in the last patient. Thus, important subsets in aortic stenosis can be determined by an analysis of the pressure waveforms.

The Systemic Circulation

Most patients with severe aortic stenosis have an elevated systemic vascular resistance. The neurohumoral mechanism(s) of this vasoconstriction has not been extensively studied. It is important to realize, however, that either unintentional vasodilation, as in a vasovagal reflex, or intentional pharmacologic manipulation of resistance carries a major risk in aortic stenosis. Not infrequently, the central arterial pressure necessary for cerebral and coronary blood flow is dependent on this high level of systemic resistance. Acute organ ischemia may thus develop, with a lowering of systemic vascular resistance.

Angiographic Assessment

Left ventriculography is routinely performed. The most common indication is to assess systolic function. Echocardiographic studies may be inadequate due to poor image quality and the inability to assess the entire left ventricle, especially the apex. Mitral regurgitation, which often accompanies severe aortic stenosis with depressed systolic function, also must be assessed. Angiography provides a complementary assessment to that of Doppler echocardiography, which may give a misleading categorization of the degree of mitral regurgitation. Additional findings on the left ventriculogram may directly show the presence of aortic stenosis. The degree of valve calcification, leaflet thickening, and leaflet mobility are readily imaged. The degree and location of myocardial hypertrophy can be visualized by the prominence of the papillary muscles, the wall thickness of the anterolateral wall (on the right anterior oblique projection) and the posterior wall (on the left anterior oblique projection), and the prominence and possible encroachment of septal hypertrophy on the LV outflow tract.

Aortography is performed for two major indications: (1) to assess the degree and location of accompanying aortic regurgitation (2) and to assess the aorta itself, including the degree of ascending aorta dilatation. Dissection of the aorta after valve replacement is not a rare complication and is best prevented at the time of valve replacement by replacement or support of the excessively dilated ascending aorta. Also, the size of the aortic annulus is important in planning for homograft replacement of the aortic valve. Furthermore, if the aortic annulus is clearly small and likely to preclude accepting a reasonably sized prosthetic valve, an annular enlargement operation can be anticipated.

Coronary arteriography is performed in the majority of patients with aortic stenosis. Concomitant coronary artery disease is frequently present and impacts on the patient's prognosis and the type of surgical correction needed. The coronary arteriogram may also have a variety of changes that reflect the presence of aortic stenosis. Occasionally, the valvular calcific process will extend up and involve the left and right coronary ostia. The epicardial coronary arteries are often tortuous. The presence of LV hypertrophy magnifies the physiologic importance of any degree of abnormal narrowing of a coronary artery. Major intramyocardial branches (i.e., the septal perforators) may show systolic compression ("milking") from the high intramyocardial compressive pressures.

Catheterization Protocol

Because catheterization of a patient with important aortic stenosis involves some risk and potentially some technical difficulties, the operator must individualize the cardiac catheterization protocol for each patient. In some, for example the 20-year-old with unequivocal severe aortic stenosis by echo/Doppler with no other clinical or noninvasive evidence of co-existing or confounding factors, it can be reasonably argued that cardiac catheterization provides confirmatory information that may or may not be considered important prior to cardiac surgery. In other patients, such as the 80-year-old with a technically limited echocardiographic study, a complete cardiac catheterization is essential. Most adult patients with aortic stenosis come to catheterization for assessment of the presence and degree of concomitant coronary artery disease, the severity of the obstruction, LV function, and the presence or absence of other valvular abnormalities. A consideration also should be given to assessing the ascending aorta, as discussed earlier. A standard protocol is outlined in Table 13-2.

Table 13-2 Standard Cardiac Catheterization Protocol in Aortic Stenosis

Procedure	Technical considerations
1. Vascular access	Femoral versus brachial approach; issues in sizing of catheters; postcatheterization care to minimize groin complications
2. Coronary arteriography	Technical difficulties due to peripheral tortuosity and aortic root dilatation
3. Right heart catheterization	Choice of catheter
4. Temporary pacemaker	Needed when right bundle branch block is present
5. Transvalvular gradient and cardiac output determination	Simultaneous versus pullback method; provocative testing when low gradient; Fick versus thermodilution
6. Left ventricular cineangiography	Safety and technical considerations
7. Aortography	Define the indications and proper projections

Technical Issues and Problems

Vascular Access and Crossing the Stenotic Aortic Valve

Many of today's angiographers were trained that the brachial approach was preferred in the patient with important aortic stenosis. The forward thrusts of the end-hole catheter could be relatively easily controlled in attempting to cross the narrowed orifice. Retrograde catheterization from either femoral artery is now the most widely used technique. Transseptal catheterization from the right femoral vein has the advantage of avoiding the occasionally prolonged time needed to cross the stenotic valve retrogradely.

After insertion of a sheath in the femoral artery, with oversizing relative to the planned catheter, pressure is generally monitored from the side-arm of the sheath. This method not only provides continuous assessment of arterial pressure for safety purposes but also allows a waveform to compare with that from the central aorta and from the left ventricle.

The most common technique (Fig 13-3) for crossing the stenotic aortic valve involves the repetitive forward thrusting of a relatively straight catheter or a catheter with a wire extending out from the catheter tip. An 0.038″ straight wire with a movable core is placed in a standard diagnostic catheter (most commonly a pigtail, but occasionally a right coronary Judkins catheter). By varying the softness of the wire tip and the degree to which it protrudes from the catheter tip, the operator can change the angle of the forward thrust of the catheter-wire assembly. Eventually, the orifice is found and the catheter is gently passed over the wire into the left ventricle. Subsequent removal of the wire and flushing of the catheter gives the sought-after LV waveform. This approach is generally successful but occasionally takes a relatively long period of time to perform (i.e. up to 30 min).

An alternate approach is to employ a catheter with a left Amplatz configuration. The size of the curve is smaller than would be ideal to intubate the left

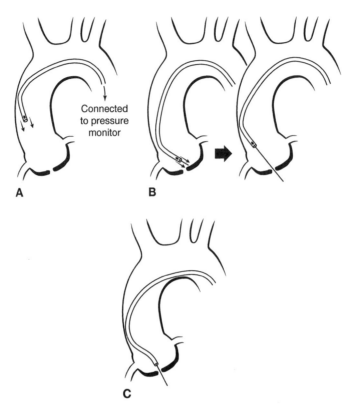

Figure 13-3 Techniques used to cross the stenotic aortic valve. In this example, the valve leaflets are calcified and thickened. The remaining orifice is functionally off-center toward the right. **(A)** A relatively straight catheter (e.g., multipurpose A2), which the operator is thrusting. Success with this technique depends on the amount of valve opening and location of the orifice. **(B)** The approach for placing a 0.035″ to 0.038″ straight-tipped wire, fixing the position of the catheter, and thrusting the wire forward. By changing the position of the tip of the catheter, the thrusting location on the valve changes. In this example, retracting the catheter tip allowed the wire to pass across the stenotic valve. **(C)** The use of an Amplatz-type catheter. The tip is pointed at the presumed residual orifice, and a straight-tipped wire is advanced. The trajectory of the wire can be adjusted by moving the catheter tip (in which case, the wire will point more to the left).

coronary. The catheter tip should be directed in the general vicinity of the remaining orifice. A straight wire is then advanced through the catheter in an attempt to cross the valve. When this maneuver is successful and the patient requires left ventriculography, a 300-cm 0.038″ J-tipped guidewire with a secondary curve is placed to maximize the amount of wire in the left ventricle to minimize the risk of ventricular arrhythmias. Over this wire the Amplatz is removed and typically a pigtail catheter is placed. We have reported on the utility of a series of specially shaped catheters for relatively easy crossing of stenotic aortic valves.[15] The three design variations allow selection of a catheter for different-sized ascending aortas. Using this technique, the aortic valve is routinely crossed in less than 5 minutes by even inexperienced operators.[15]

The thrombogenicity of guidewires and catheters necessitates moderate doses of heparin to reduce the possibility of thrombus formation. A bolus of 5000 units of heparin is standard. In addition, the duration of attempts to cross the valve should be limited to approximately 3 minutes before the wire is removed, wiped, and the catheter lumen aspirated and flushed with clear, heparinized saline.

Measuring the Transvalvular Gradient

The technique used to cross the aortic valve often dictates the method used to assess the transvalvular gradient. The theoretically, hemodynamically ideal method is simultaneous measurement of LV and aortic waveforms with high-fidelity transducers, along with an assessment of the degree of pressure recovery approximately 5 to 10 cm downstream from the valve. The practical methods needed for clinical decision making are less exacting. The degree of accuracy needed is usually that to confirm or disprove the existence of important obstruction. Given this caveat, there are several technical and methodologic considerations of major importance when measuring the transvalvular gradient.

Care must be taken to avoid two pitfalls in LV pressure measurement. The first is the hybrid waveform. Catheters with multiple holes, such as the standard pigtail, may give very misleading waveforms when a few holes sample pressure above and other holes sample pressure below the valve. The result is a waveform that looks ventricular but has a falsely low systolic pressure, which can lead to an important underestimation of the severity of obstruction. The other problem is catheter entrapment in the myocardium. Some patients with severe aortic stenosis have a hypertrophied left ventricle with hyperdynamic shortening characteristics. During systole, the catheter may be entrapped (i.e., compressed by surrounding myocardium). The resultant waveform will have an exaggerated systolic peak, which may lead to an overestimation of the gradient. With a tip transducer catheter (i.e., Millar Instruments, Houston, TX), this peak is easily recognized as a late systolic, spike-like deformity of the waveform. With a fluid-filled catheter, especially one with multiple side holes, the waveform may not suggest entrapment and, in fact, may have a typical LV pressure contour. Thus, when using a fluid-filled catheter to measure LV pressure, it is recommended that a single-lumen catheter be used, or if a multiple-holed catheter is used, be certain the catheter is completely in the chamber but not entrapped.

Care also must be taken to avoid pitfalls in arterial pressure measurement. First, use of arterial pressure from the sideport of the femoral artery sheath requires a sheath size at least one Fr size larger than the catheter being used to measure LV pressure. To ensure that the femoral artery pressure is similar to the central aortic pressure, the two pressures should be recorded together prior to the passing of the central catheter across the aortic valve. Although the waveform and the absolute systolic pressure are different in the central aorta than in the femoral artery, mean arterial pressure should be identical. The modifications of the waveform in aortic stenosis and the properties of the arterial system can be compensated by shifting the pressure during the calculation of the mean gradient.[16]

The measurement of the transvalvular pressure gradient in aortic stenosis can be accomplished with less accuracy using the pullback technique. In brief, a catheter is placed retrogradely in the left ventricle and connected to a pressure transducer. Pressure is recorded in the left ventricle and then, while recording, the catheter is pulled back a few inches to sample pressure in the ascending aorta. The nonsimultaneous pressure waveform from the left ventricle and the aorta are then superimposed, by the computer or by hand. The mean gradient is then determined. It should be noted that in severe aortic stenosis, the catheter across the aortic valve may worsen the degree of obstruction, producing the Carabelli sign—a rise in aortic pressure when the transvalvular catheter is removed.[17]

For the most part, the resting hemodynamic state is used for these measurements. When a relatively low (<30 mm Hg) mean pressure gradient is present, the question arises whether the gradient is low because the transvalvular flow is reduced or because the degree of obstruction is simply not that great. In this situation, exercise and/or pharmacologic manipulation of the cardiac output should be considered. Augmentation of cardiac output increases the pressure gradient to a great degree when severe aortic stenosis is present, but in milder forms of obstruction, the increase is less and occasionally the pressure gradient may decrease due to less obstruction from a greater opening of the thickened cusps from the greater pressure and flow generation of the left ventricle (see Fig 13-1). Dobutamine increases LV pressure and flow generation and is particular useful when reduced LV function is the reason for the small resting gradient. The transaortic pressure gradient increases with dobutamine if the stenosis is severe. Caution is advised, because the hemodynamic effects of dobutamine often remain for up to 30 minutes. These provocative studies should be used in patients who appear to have mild-to-moderate obstruction, with low pressure gradients at rest, and not in patients who clearly have severe stenosis. Furthermore, coronary artery disease should be assessed before considering a provocative test that could induce myocardial ischemia. Nitroprusside can also be used, but great care should be taken to avoid reduction of arterial pressure that compromises coronary blood flow. Exercise-induced symptoms and hemodynamic abnormalities are occasionally used in the assessment of aortic stenosis, but much less often than in mitral stenosis.

Angiography: General

The choice of contrast agents is an important decision. Low-osmolality agents are generally recommended for the patient with severe aortic stenosis. A safe catheterization is frequently made so by minimizing any perturbations in the patient's cardiovascular function.

Left Ventricular Cineangiography

Several important technical issues need to be addressed before performing ventriculography. An appropriate catheter, such as a pigtail, is not likely to have been successfully used to cross the aortic valve because the catheter shape makes crossing the valve difficult. An exchange of catheters can be easily made with a 260-cm 0.038″ exchange wire. First, it is important to create a pigtail configuration of the distal wire, as in making a ribbon curl, which more easily remains in the left ventricle without important ventricular ectopy during the exchange procedure. If an end-hole catheter is used instead of a pigtail catheter, the performance of ventriculography must be done with the standard precautions. A lower injection rate and, generally, volume are used, and the position of the catheter must be verified with a test injection. This enhances the chance of a high-quality ventriculogram with sinus beats, and reduces the chance of an LV perforation from the high-velocity injection.

Aortography

No unusual technical problems are specific to aortography in patients with aortic stenosis. A well-placed catheter and a standard injection protocol of 40 to 60 ml at 20 ml/sec through a pigtail catheter will delineate the degree of valve regurgitation, the size and shape of the ascending aorta, and the patency of the proximal coronary arteries. The additional dye load may impact on the decision to use low-osmotic nonionic contrast agents.

Coronary Arteriography

Performing selective coronary arteriography in patients with aortic stenosis may be difficult, not so much due to the valve abnormality, but rather to peripheral vessel tortuosity, which in turn is related to aging and the frequent presence of atherosclerosis. Dilation of the ascending aorta should be anticipated and the selection of left Judkins catheters should be modified. The routine shape should be a 5 left Judkins, but when marked aortic dilatation is expected, a 6 left Judkins catheter is usually successful. In extremely tortuous and difficult cases, engagement of both coronary arteries may be most expeditiously performed by engaging the coronary ostia with the 0.038″ wire (possibly an extra-support variety) within the coronary catheter. The wire serves to stiffen and lengthen the catheter such that it may reach and engage the coronary artery.

This should be followed by slow aspiration to ensure an air-free system and limited flushing of the catheter and immediate verification that the coronary ostia have been successfully engaged and the pressure waveform does not exhibit dampening. The use of non-preformed catheter shapes is problematic in the patient with vascular tortuosity because of limitations in catheter control in the ascending aorta. Finally, the number of coronary injections may be modified not only by the stability of the patient and tolerance to angiography, but also by the degree of vessel tortuosity and overlap, which may demand additional injections in oblique projections.

Right Heart Catheterization

Measurement of right heart pressures and sampling of blood for the determination of cardiac output and the exclusion of shunts are the usual factors dictating the choice of right heart catheter design. A balloon-tipped catheter is preferred to the classical Cournand design because less ventricular ectopy occurs during catheter passage through the right ventricle. In addition, the presence of conduction system disease, which is common in aortic stenosis, may dictate temporary pacing capabilities.

Intravascular Ultrasound

Direct visualization of the orifice of the stenotic valve is an additional means under development to better characterize the obstruction in patients with stenosis of unclear severity. Intravascular ultrasound is currently being used to directly visualize valve area and shape.[18,19] Combined with a pharmacologic manipulation of transvalvular flow, it should be possible to assess valvular reserve in cases with poor baseline LV systolic function.

Postcatheterization Observation

The postcatheterization protocol should receive a major emphasis in the patient with severe aortic stenosis. Dehydration and hematomas are to be vigorously avoided because they may be lethal in this setting. The osmotic diuresis from contrast medium should be counterbalanced by intravenous hydration. Sheath removal should occur only after the majority of the heparin effect has worn off. A closely monitored setting, in which recognition and treatment of complications can be performed quickly by skilled personnel, is mandatory. The cardiac catheterization–related risk of death in aortic stenosis is in part related to the quality of surveillance in the postcatheterization period.

Important Clinical Subsets

High Output/High Gradient

Conditions such as obesity, anemia, systemic infection, thyrotoxicosis, and pregnancy increase cardiac output. It may be difficult to distinguish whether the symptoms are due to progression of the valvular disease or to the condition increasing cardiac output. The acutely reversible conditions of anemia, infection, and thyroid disease should be treated prior to cardiac catheterization. Unlike mitral stenosis, aortic stenosis is usually better tolerated during pregnancy, allowing postponement of cardiac catheterization and therapy. The obese individual with aortic stenosis may have a higher than average cardiac output but physiologically needs a greater absolute valve orifice than other patients. A large mean pressure gradient (over 40 mm Hg) across an anatomically abnormal valve with a calculated valve area and resistance suggesting at least moderate obstruction are usually adequate catheterization information to proceed with a valve replacement in the symptomatic patient.

Combined Valvular and Subvalvular Obstruction

Obstruction in some patients with aortic stenosis exists not only at the orifice level, but also in the subvalvular region of the LV outflow tract. Some degree of anatomic narrowing at this location may be present in patients with valvular obstruction and echocardiographic evidence of severe hypertrophy of the interventricular septum. The precatheterization echocardiogram may show a variant of systolic anterior motion of the anterior leaflet of the mitral valve and considerable flow acceleration in the outflow tract. These patients are often women with small, markedly hypertrophied left ventricles with normal to supernormal ejection performance. At cardiac catheterization, a subvalvular pressure gradient may be recorded in the outflow tract, with meticulous attention to pressure recording using high-fidelity tip transducers. Ventriculography may show a narrowed outflow tract in systole. It is important that these patients be identified pre-operatively. Postoperative hypotension may occur from worsening of the outflow tract obstruction—now a true obstruction versus an oddity of the pre-operative hemodynamic assessment. Prophylactic septal myectomy is often recommended along with careful medical management in the early postoperative period.[20]

Systolic Hypertension

In the past, systolic hypertension and severe aortic stenosis were thought to only rarely coexist. Today, perhaps with a greater number of elderly patients, more than 27% have important systolic hypertension (systolic pressure > 160 mm Hg).[13,14] Cardiac catheterization in these patients requires certain caveats. First, do not casually exclude critical aortic stenosis when finding a markedly elevated arterial systolic pressure. The transvalvular gradient may appear smaller, because absolute pressure in the ventricle may be almost 300 mm Hg, with aortic pressures in the 200s (see Fig 13-2). Second, do not be cavalier in acutely reducing these elevated systolic pressures. Myocardial ischemia due to relative coronary hypoperfusion can occur after a standard dose of antihypertensive medications.

Elderly Women with Severe Aortic Stenosis

In our experience, we continue to be impressed by the substantial percentage of elderly women with aortic stenosis who have small, hypertrophied left ventricles with hyperdynamic shortening and elevated diastolic pressures.[12] These patients are frequently included in the subsets described earlier with systolic hypertension and subvalvular obstruction. Despite normal systolic chamber function, many have markedly elevated diastolic pressures and abnormal pressure decay (see Fig 13-2). Contrast ventriculography may be suboptimal due to the induction of frequent extrasystoles. Concomitant pulmonary hypertension is common.

Aortic Regurgitation

The goals of cardiac catheterization in patients with aortic regurgitation are similar to those for aortic stenosis (see Table 13-1). There are several special considerations, however, in the patient with aortic regurgitation. A major defining characteristic is the difference between acute and chronic aortic regurgitation. Another relates to the mechanism of regurgitation; an increasing number of patients in the current era have aortic root disease with secondary valvular regurgitation, as compared with a disease destructive of the aortic cusps themselves. Technical difficulties are not infrequent and usually relate to performing coronary arteriography in a patient with a very dilated aortic root. Finally, vascular access complications can be more frequent due to the wide pulse pressure disrupting vascular hemostasis after sheath removal.

Hemodynamic Assessment: The Valve, the Aorta, and the Ventricle

The structural integrity of the normal aortic valve is noteworthy. In the vast majority of individuals, the valve opens and closes 100,000 times each day for 80 years. Closure occurs with no important backward movement of blood into the left ventricle. The three cusps, and also the design of the sinus of Valsalva and the entire aortic root, maintain hemodynamic competence despite wide variations in the cardiac output, aortic pressure, and body movement and position.

The development of aortic regurgitation represents an additional workload for the left ventricle. To achieve the same forward cardiac output, the left ventricle must pump more blood; that is, it has a volume overload. In addition, a greater systolic pressure is typically achieved that imposes a pressure component to the abnormal workload.

The Valve

The aortic valve in aortic regurgitation may appear fairly normal in the patient with root disease or may appear severely deformed, as in the patient with endocarditis, rheumatic heart disease, isolated perforation of a cusp, or a bicuspid valve. The regurgitant jet will vary in its direction and width, depending on the cause of the regurgitation.

Although it is logical to envision a regurgitant orifice when there is a perforation in a cusp, it is important to consider the degree of regurgitation as a somewhat dynamic process. First, the size of the regurgitant orifice may be modified by the distending pressure of the ascending aorta. An acute increase in central aortic pressure may increase the space between poorly coaptating aortic cusps. Second, the volume of regurgitant flow is dependent on the driving pressure across the regurgitant orifice. An excellent example of this is the diminishing volume of regurgitant flow from early to late diastole. With severe aortic regurgitation, retrograde flow frequently stops due to the equilibration of LV and aortic pressure from the torrential early diastolic regurgitation. Finally, the ability to pharmacologically reduce the regurgitant volume is currently being used to prolong the time to aortic valve replacement.

The Aorta

Annuloaortic ectasia, either in isolation or as part of Marfan's syndrome, has emerged as an important etiology of aortic regurgitation.[21] Lesser degrees of regurgitation are not uncommonly seen in systemic hypertension with ascending aortic dilatation. Therefore, the competence of the aortic valve can be disrupted by processes that primarily affect the ascending aorta. On the other hand, patients with severe aortic valve disease usually have a secondary enlargement of the ascending aorta.

The Ventricle

The hemodynamic load of aortic regurgitation elicits a complex remodeling of the left ventricle. Chamber size increases, often enormously, demonstrating the cor bovinum described in classical pathology textbooks. Chamber and myocardial properties are altered to allow the chamber to become more compliant, thus maintaining relatively normal filling pressures despite the massive chamber enlargement. Hypertrophy with increase in wall thickness may maintain wall stress in a range where normal systolic chamber function is maintained. Eventually one or more of these compensatory mechanisms fail. Either directly or through activation of neurohumoral systems, hemodynamic deterioration becomes manifest either at rest or during exercise. The development of systolic dysfunction in aortic regurgitation has important clinical consequences, even if the patient is initially asymptomatic. Recognized early, valve replacement can be hemodynamically and clinically successful, but if discovered late or ignored, systolic dysfunction can lead to irreversible myocardial failure. The results of valve replacement then become suboptimal and occasionally have no benefit. Therefore, assessment of LV function is an important component of cardiac catheterization in the patient with aortic regurgitation.

Angiographic Assessment

Aortography

The grading of aortic regurgitation from an aortogram is based on the degree and rapidity with which the left ventricle opacifies from contrast regurgitating from an injection in the ascending aorta (Fig 13-4). The aortogram also provides other important information. The left ventricle often opacifies adequately to assess LV regional and global systolic function. Furthermore, the presence and, to some extent, degree of mitral regurgitation can be determined in many patients. Therefore, a high-quality aortogram can replace a left ventriculogram in many patients with severe regurgitation.

Aortography also shows the degree of aortic dilatation, some morphologic characteristics of the aortic valve, and the character of the regurgitant jet. In the United States, an increasing proportion of patients with severe aortic regurgitation have aortic root problems as the bases of their aortic valve incompetence. With aortography, the very dilated aortic root and arch can be well visualized, along with the frequent effacing of the sinotubular junction. Primary

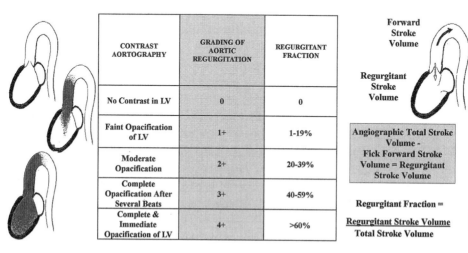

Figure 13-4 Angiographic assessment of the degree of aortic regurgitation is compared with the calculation of regurgitant fraction. Contrast aortography grades the degree of regurgitation in a 1 to 4+ scale, which corresponds roughly to a regurgitant fraction that varies from 1% to more than 60%.

abnormalities of the aortic valve leaflets also can be defined. Cusp prolapse, sinus of Valsalva aneurysm, rheumatic deformities, and a congenitally bicuspid valve can often be identified and characterized by aortography.

Ventriculography

When the degree of regurgitation is mild or the degree of mitral regurgitation needs to be accurately assessed, a separate ventriculogram should be performed.

Coronary Arteriography

Unlike aortic stenosis, coronary artery disease does not frequently accompany aortic regurgitation. Important coronary artery disease must be defined, however, and may be found increasingly frequently as the predominant demographics of isolated aortic regurgitation evolve from the young to middle-aged patient to the more elderly patient with aortic root disease.

Catheterization Protocol

Catheterization of a patient with important aortic regurgitation requires some planning. The protocol should reflect the prioritization of data needed. Most adult patients with aortic regurgitation come to catheterization for the assessment of the presence and degree of concomitant coronary artery disease. Many also come for a second type of assessment of the degree of regurgitation.

Technical Issues and Problems

Aortography

Optimal visualization of the aorta, aortic valve, and degree of regurgitation is achieved when a large volume of contrast is rapidly delivered to the ascending aorta. A high-flow pigtail catheter is typically used. Recoil from a small Fr size catheter may invalidate the usefulness of an injection. This problem can be minimized by first pushing the catheter so that it touches the valve and then pulling it back to a position immediately above the sinotubular junction. An injection protocol of 40 to 60 ml delivered at 18 to 20 ml/sec is completed at this location. No test injection is usually needed unless catheter position is uncertain.

Coronary Arteriography

The dilated ascending aorta, the torrential coronary flow, and the frequently unobstructed coronary artery system in aortic regurgitation all present technical challenges for the performance of coronary arteriography. The ascending aorta is often markedly dilated in aortic regurgitation, such that catheter shape should be chosen accordingly. A large bolus of dye is frequently needed to adequately visualize the coronary arteries. Occasionally, there is reversal of proximal epicardial coronary blood flow due to the regurgitation into the left ventricle. In general, although smaller Fr-sized catheters may be selected initially to reduce vascular problems, larger sizes should be considered when poor visualization is preventing the acquisition of important data on the status of the coronary arteries.

Groin Complications

To achieve hemostasis at the femoral entry sites, compression techniques may take a prolonged period in patients with severe aortic regurgitation. The major explanation is that the marked pulsatility of the circulation disrupts the hemostatic process in the arterial wall. Large hematomas develop rapidly. For this reason, the level of heparinization may be reduced, with attention to careful and frequent flushing of catheters on the systemic arterial side.

Important Clinical Subsets

Aortic Regurgitation from Infective Endocarditis

There are a variety of special considerations in this group, the timing of cardiac catheterization being one. The second is the potential danger of crossing into the left ventricle with a catheter and dislodging material that embolizes peripherally.

Combined Aortic Regurgitation and Stenosis

Although the hemodynamic, angiographic, and clinical findings of these patients fall in a spectrum between the two pure hemodynamic lesions, several special considerations should be noted when the valvular lesion is truly combined regurgitation-stenosis. The first is the transvalvular flow used to assess the degree of stenosis. The total flow across the valve is the sum of both the net forward cardiac output and the regurgitant volume. Thus, gradients of 30 to 50 mm Hg often indicate a mild stenotic component in the patient with severe regurgitation.

Prosthetic Valve Assessment in the Aortic Position

There are diverse prosthetic valves used in the aortic position. The assessment of an aortic prosthesis starts with identification of the type of valve. Hemodynamic abnormalities are present when there is malfunction, and the cardiac catheterization assessment is similar to that previously discussed for native valve stenosis and regurgitation. The unique problems relative to prosthetic valves are covered in this section.

Fluoroscopic and Angiographic Assessment

The majority of prosthetic valves used in the aortic patient are radiopaque, homografts being the major exception. The identification of the type of prosthetic valve is made by its appearance at fluoroscopy or on plain chest x-ray.[22,23] By recent count, 32 types of mechanical prostheses have been implanted in patients in the United States.[24]

Cinefluoroscopic assessment of prosthetic valves allows an accurate measurement of function for most mechanical valves in current use. Isolated frames from several examples are shown in Figure 13-5. The major goals of cinefluoroscopy are listed in Table 13-3.

Aortography is typically used to assess regurgitation. Pathologic regurgitation may be from a perivalvular leak, a thrombus or tissue ingrowth limiting closure, or a missing leaflet or ball.

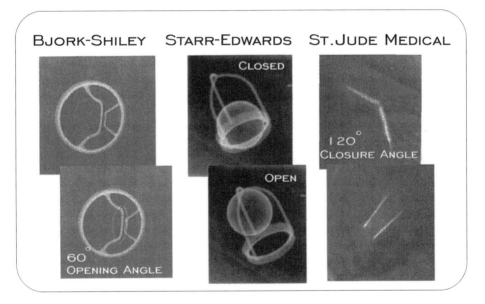

Figure 13-5 Several types of prosthetic valves, with demonstration of the radiographic assessment of function. The Bjork-Shiley (Pfizer, Irvine, CA) valve disk opens to 60 degrees and is best measured in a view (not shown here) that is perpendicular to the plane of the sewing ring and in-line to the plane of the disk. The Starr-Edwards (Baxter Edwards, Irvine, CA) ball should move the entire length of the cage. The St. Jude Medical valve (St. Jude Corp., Minneapolis, MN) opens to reveal two parallel leaflets (lower panel) and closes completely with a 120-degree angle between the two leaflets (upper panel).

Table 13-3 Goals of Cinefluoroscopy
of Aortic Valve Prosthesis

1. Identification of model and assessment of structural integrity
2. Assessment of rocking motion
3. Assessment of leaflet or poppet excursion
4. Assessment of closure of leaflet(s) or poppet

This pathologic regurgitation must be distinguished from normal degrees of regurgitation that are dynamic (i.e., that occur immediately before the prosthetic valve closes) and static (i.e., in diastole through the mechanical structure of certain types of valves).

Hemodynamic Assessment

The homograft is the first valve substitute that is truly nonobstructive. Mechanical and tissue valves with struts all produce a transvalvular pressure gradient. The use of certain models (e.g., Starr-Edwards [Baxter Edwards, Irvine, CA]), increased cardiac output states, and relatively small sizes of prosthetic valves are three situations in which there may be significant obstructive findings, such as a moderate to large pressure gradient (20–40 mm Hg) across the valve.

Technical Issues

Retrograde crossing of a mechanical valve is relatively contraindicated. Catheter entrapment may occur in the minor orifice of the Bjork-Shiley valve. More commonly, the catheter causes the prosthetic valve to acutely malfunction with severe regurgitation. Within seconds, hemodynamic deterioration is apparent. Thus, limited information is obtainable by this technique.

If the left ventricle must be entered for pressure measurement or angiography, the transseptal approach is recommended. If a mechanical valve is also in the mitral position, LV access may be obtained by an apical transthoracic puncture. With the availability of echocardiography, it is rare that such an approach is necessary.

Aortic Dissection

Emergency cardiac catheterization for aortic dissection is performed in most institutions, especially in patients in whom the ascending aorta is thought to be involved with the dissection. There are generally three goals in the cardiac catheterization of the patient with aortic dissection: (1) define the extent of dissection, especially whether it involves the ascending aorta and arch; (2) define complications of dissection, including pericardial hemorrhage, aortic regurgitation, and coronary occlusion; and (3) define any co-existent coronary artery disease.

Performing cardiac catheterization in this patient group has multiple caveats. The operator must work fast and get the information needed despite the frequent difficulty in staying within the true lumen. An inordinate delay in the patient's transfer to the operating room can result in death from rupture. The invasive cardiologist must also be extremely careful with catheter movement in the vicinity of a dissection. A frequent operating room observation is that of an extremely thin-walled dissected aorta in which extensive catheter manipulation had been performed minutes before. Not all patients with acute aortic dissection can or need to undergo cardiac catheterization. The hemodynamically unstable patient with solid evidence for dissection on transesophageal echocardiographic study or computerized tomography needs an immediate operation despite the incomplete diagnostic evaluation.

Finally, communication with the surgeon is essential. Institution-to-institution and physician-to-physician differences pervade the diagnosis and management of patients with aortic dissection. An agreement of what information is needed, the time available to obtain it, and any special procedural concerns (i.e., leaving a femoral arterial sheath in place for initial cardiopulmonary bypass) will optimize the chances of a successful outcome in a life-threatening situation with high surgical mortality.

Technical Issues and Problems

Vascular Access

The site of vascular entry in acute aortic dissection is dependent on the dissection itself. Lack of a pulse at an entry site precludes its use. A strong pulse does not preclude the local extension of the dissection. Usually, the femoral and brachial entry sites are not involved. Rather, the false lumen is frequently entered when the catheter is making its retrograde journey to the heart.

True Versus False Lumen

The major problem in cardiac catheterization of the patient with aortic dissection is maintaining the catheter in the true lumen for aortography, selective coronary arteriography, and LV pressure measurement and ventriculography. The pressure waveform in the false lumen is indistinguishable from the true lumen. Retrograde catheter movement in the false lumen usually offers no resistance until the base of the aortic root is reached, and generally no alteration in the patient's symptomatic status occurs during this retrograde journey. Therefore, the retrograde movement of the catheter from, for example, the femoral artery should be accompanied by frequent, small, hand injections ("puffs") of contrast to verify a location in the true lumen. Verification is by the downstream pulsatile movement of the contrast dye. When the false lumen is encountered, the contrast dye appears static, and occasionally the rough borders of the dissected aorta are visualized. At this point, the catheter position relative to the last true lumen position is studied, the catheter is withdrawn to this point, and with a leading 0.038″ guidewire, the catheter is steered away from the false lumen location. Confidence of a true lumen pathway is generally assured when the catheter can freely enter the left ventricle or when the coronary arteries can be visualized by selective or nonselective injection. A catheter or a guidewire should not be aggressively pushed in an attempt to enter the left ventricle from the ascending aorta without confidence that the catheter is in the true lumen. Otherwise, entry into the pericardial or other extravascular location will occur, with immediate and fatal hemodynamic collapse.

Once the true lumen of the ascending aorta is achieved, the operator should not leave this position until all information is obtained. Catheter exchanges should be performed with a long guidewire (250–300 cm) curled in the base of the aorta or even the left ventricle.

Successful entry into the left ventricle and completion of coronary arteriography can be achieved in approximately 90% cases of acute dissection involving the ascending aorta. In others, the problem is usually inability to stay in the true lumen. Occasionally, the deformation of the true lumen of the ascending aorta makes selective engagement of the coronary ostia extremely difficult.

Aortography

Aortography establishes the diagnosis and often documents the location of the proximal and distal extent of dissection.[25] Ascending aortic injection of 40 to 60 ml at a 18- to 20-ml/sec rate will show (1) the degree of any aortic regurgitation; (2) the proximal coronary arteries; (3) the "flap" of the false lumen, often waving back and forth in the middle of the ascending aorta; and (4) the deformed true lumen of the ascending aorta (Fig 13-6). Most cardiac catheterization laboratories have small image intensifiers that preclude visualizing the entire thoracic aorta in the field of view. Instead, the table is moved during the cineangiogram of the ascending aorta to show the arch vessels and the descending thoracic aorta. Additional injections in the arch or descending aorta are often needed but usually not absolutely necessary for the surgeon.

Biplane aortography is generally preferred with a straight anteroposterior projection and a left anterior oblique or lateral projection. Flaps not visible in one plane are usually apparent in another projection. If only the false lumen can be reached, it is important to document this on film. Caution must be exercised in considering a power injection in the false lumen. Extensive thrombus can be dislodged, and perforation of a thin-walled, dissected aorta is often a worry. Nonetheless, dye injected into the false lumen often spills over into the true lumen via the tear. Sometimes this is adequate to verify the patency of

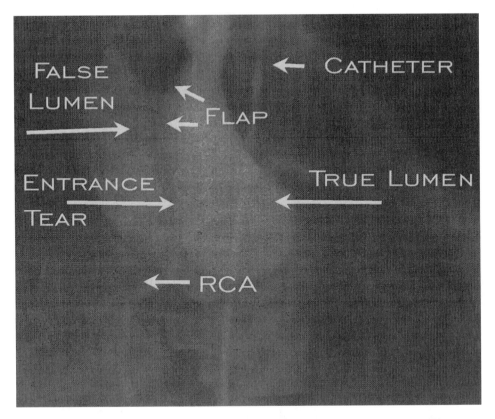

Figure 13-6 Contrast aortographic findings in acute aortic dissection. The dissection is characterized by a true and false lumen with a thin, movable flap between the two. Aortography should be performed in the true lumen and often shows the coronary ostia and whether the aortic valve is competent.

the proximal coronary arteries and the presence or absence of important aortic regurgitation.

Anticoagulation

Heparin is not given because of the greater risk of hemorrhage or rupture than with catheter-based thrombosis or embolism. Rather frequent flushing of the catheter system is mandatory.

Coarctation of the Aorta

Cardiac catheterization of the adult with coarctation of the aorta is generally performed to confirm the diagnosis and assess associated anomalies. It is uncommon that coarctation be first suspected in an older adult; most adult cases present themselves in the 20- to 30-year age bracket. While measurement of the pressure gradient is performed, the robust collateral circulation often maintains distal pressure and blood flow. Exercise is an excellent method for assessing the severity of obstruction. Even with extensive collateralization, the gradient during exercise is substantial. In addition, exercise is useful in assessing the residual or recurrent obstruction after prior corrective surgery or balloon dilatation. Visualization of the obstruction is performed with aortography and complements the assessment of the pressure gradient. Angiography will localize the obstruction (pre- or postductal) and determine the severity of the narrowing in terms of absolute diameter reduction and the length of the narrowing. The major associated cardiac anomaly is bicuspid aortic valve. Other complications include LV failure and aortic dissection. Brachial artery catheterization is usually necessary if coronary arteriography is needed.

Discrete Subaortic Stenosis

This subvalvular obstruction is typically from a discrete fibromuscular ring of tissue if the patient is first presenting as a young adult. The obstructive physiology usually resembles more that of valvular aortic stenosis than hypertrophic cardiomyopathy.[26] Catheterization is done to localize and quantify the obstruction with ventriculography, pressure measurement, and cardiac output determination. Aortic regurgitation is a complication that occurs in many cases and should be assessed with aortography.

Thoracic Aortic Aneurysms

Aortography is the major procedure performed during cardiac catheterization of patients with thoracic aortic aneurysms. These occur generally as a consequence of severe systemic atherosclerosis. Therefore, coronary arteriography is frequently performed, anticipating the technical difficulty often accompanying a very large aorta.

S E L E C T E D   R E A D I N G S

1. Krabill KA, Sung HW, Tamura T, et al. Factors influencing the structure and shape of stenotic and regurgitant jets: an in vitro investigation using Doppler color flow mapping and optical flow visualization. J Am Coll Cardiol 1989;13:1672–1681.
2. Yoganathan AP, Edward GC, Sung HW, et al. Review of hydrodynamic principles for the cardiologist: applications to the study of blood flow and jets by imaging techniques. J Am Coll Cardiol 1988;12:1344–1353.
3. Flachskampf FA, Weyman AE, Guerrero JL, Thomas JD. Influence of orifice geometry and flow rate on effective valve area: an in vitro study. J Am Coll Cardiol 1990; 15:1173–1180.
4. Carroll JD, Carroll EP, Chiu YC, Feldman T. Effect of turbulence and downstream pressure recovery on quantification of the severity of aortic stenosis. Circulation 1988;78:II-213. Abstract.
5. O'Toole MF, Carroll JD, Feldman T. Turbulence intensity in aortic stenosis: frequency characteristics and effects of alterations in left ventricular function. J Heart Valve Dis 1993;2:94–102.
6. Carabello BA, Grossman W. Calculation of stenotic valve orifice area. In: Grossman W, ed. Cardiac catheterization and angiography. 4th ed. Philadelphia: Lea & Febiger, 1990:152–165.
7. Ford L, Feldman T, Carroll JD. Valve resistance. Circulation 1994;89:893–895.
8. Ford LE, Feldman T, Chiu YC, Carroll JD. Hemodynamic resistance as a measure of functional impairment in aortic valvular stenosis. Circ Res 1990;66:1–7.
9. Beyer RW, Olmos A, Bermudez RF, Noll HE. Mitral valve resistance as a hemodynamic indicator in mitral stenosis. Am J Cardiol 1992;69:775–779.
10. Feldman T, Ford LE, Chiu YC, Carroll JD. Changes in valvular resistance, power dissipation, and myocardial reserve with aortic valvuloplasty. J Heart Valve Dis 1992; 1:55–64.
11. Cannon JD, Zile MR, Crawford FA, Carabello BA. Aortic valve resistance as an adjunct to the Gorlin formula in assessing the severity of aortic stenosis in symptomatic patients. J Am Coll Cardiol 1992;20:1517–1523.
12. Carroll JD, Carroll EP, Feldman T, et al. Sex associated differences in left ventricular function in aortic stenosis of the elderly. Circulation 1992;86:1099–1107.
13. Carroll JD, Hellman K, Feldman T. Systolic hypertension complicating aortic stenosis. Circulation 1993;88:I-102 (abstract).
14. Carroll JD, Hellman K, Feldman T, Levin TN. Systolic hypertension in aortic stenosis: a dynamic ventricle or a noncompliant arterial system? Circulation 1994;90: I-52 (abstract).
15. Feldman T, Carroll JD, Chiu YC. An improved catheter design for assessing stenosed aortic valves. Cathet Cardiovasc Diagn 1989;16:279–283.
16. Folland ED, Parisi AF, Carbone C. Is peripheral arterial pressure a reliable substitute for ascending aortic pressure when measuring aortic valve gradients? J Am Coll Cardiol 1984;4:1207–1214.
17. Carabello BA, Barry WH, Grossman W. Changes in arterial pressure during left heart pullback in patients with aortic stenosis: a sign of severe aortic stenosis. Am J Cardiol 1979;44:424–430.
18. Follman DF, Levin TN, Lang RM, et al. Low frequency intracardiac ultrasonographic imaging before and after balloon pulmonary valvuloplasty. Am Heart J 1993;125:259–262.
19. Jiang L, dePrada JV, He J, et al. Quantitative assessment of stenotic aortic valve area using intravascular echocardiography: in vitro validation. Circulation 1993;88:541. Abstract.
20. Turina M. Asymmetric septal hypertrophy should be resected during aortic valve replacement. Z Kardiol 1986;75:198–200.

21. Guiney TE, Davies MJ, Parker DJ, et al. The aetiology and course of isolated severe aortic regurgitation: a clinical, pathological, and echocardiographic study. Br Heart J 1987;58:358–368.
22. Mehlman DJ. A guide to the radiographic identification of prosthetic heart valve: an addendum. Circulation 1984;69:102.
23. Steiner RM, Mintz G, Morse D, et al. Radiology of cardiac valve prosthesis. Radiographics 1988;8:277.
24. Atkius CW. Mechanical valvular prosthesis. Ann Thorac Surg 1991;52:161–172.
25. Lindsay J Jr. Aortic dissections. In: Lindsay J Jr, ed. Diseases of the aorta. Malvern PA: Lea & Febiger, 1994:127–143.
26. Feldman T, Chiu C, Carroll JD. Catheter balloon dilatation for discrete subaortic stenosis in the adult. Am J Cardiol 1987;60:403–405.

14

MITRAL, PULMONIC, TRICUSPID, AND PROSTHETIC VALVE DISEASE

Howard C. Herrmann

T HE PURPOSE OF this chapter is to describe the major issues confronting the cardiologist in the cardiac catheterization laboratory in the assessment of the patient with mitral, tricuspid, pulmonic, and prosthetic valvular heart disease. For each of the valvular lesions, the role of catheterization, both hemodynamic approach and angiographic assessment, will be discussed. It should be remembered, however, that the history, physical examination, and especially noninvasive imaging techniques are essential for the full evaluation of patients with valvular heart disease. In some cases, catheterization may be unnecessary or serve only a confirmatory role, whereas in other cases it is diagnostic and/or therapeutic. The integration and proper use of catheterization in the evaluation of valvular heart disease is a critical skill for the practicing cardiologist.

Mitral Valve Stenosis

Role of Catheterization

Mitral stenosis is rarely an unsuspected diagnosis in a patient undergoing cardiac catheterization. The apical diastolic rumble is pathognomonic, and the echocardiographic features are not subtle. Therefore, the role of cardiac catheterization is often confirmatory. The mitral valve area can be calculated using the Gorlin formula (see next section), but the result may be only a little more accurate than carefully performed echocardiographic valve area determinations using planimetry or the pressure half-time formula. During catheterization, pulmonary artery and pulmonary capillary wedge pressure can be directly measured, which may be useful in assessing the need and risk of surgery or valvuloplasty. These pressures may provide important data on other potential causes of dyspnea. Left ventriculography or other angiography may be performed to assess the degree of frequently co-existing mitral regurgitation and other valvular lesions. Finally, coronary angiography is necessary in selected patients prior to percutaneous therapeutic intervention or surgery.

Thus, cardiac catheterization is indicated in patients prior to cardiac surgery or other therapeutic interventions to confirm the diagnosis and to assess co-existing cardiac conditions, including coronary artery disease. The goals of the procedure should include hemodynamic measurements to calculate the mitral valve area, level of pulmonary artery pressure, determination of the existence of other valve lesions, and assessment of the degree of valve calcification and mitral regurgitation, which could influence suitability for percutaneous balloon valvuloplasty and surgical repair.

Hemodynamic Assessment

The hemodynamic assessment of mitral stenosis requires an understanding of both the pathophysiology of this disease and the limitations of the catheterization techniques used in its assessment. Mitral stenosis is usually a late (10- to 40-yr) sequela of rheumatic fever and often (>75%) co-exists with other valvular lesions, particularly mitral and aortic regurgitation. Rare causes of mitral stenosis include congenital malformations and severe annular calcification. Differentiation of the etiology is best accomplished with two-dimensional echocardiography.

The normal mitral valve apparatus is a complex structure including the annulus, the larger C-shaped anterior leaflet that divides the left ventricular inflow and outflow tracts, the small posterior leaflets, the two papillary muscles, and the attaching chordae tendinae. From a hemodynamic standpoint, all of these structures contribute to the pattern of blood flow from the left atrium to the left ventricle. It is simplistic, but useful, to think of the mitral valve opening as a circular area. However, it should not be forgotten that this area is an approximation of a more complex funnel-like three-dimensional structure. Normal mitral valve dimensions include an open area of 4 to 5 cm^2 that varies throughout diastole by as much as 20% to 40%.

In patients with rheumatic mitral stenosis, pathologic changes include commissural fusion, leaflet thickening, chordal thickening and shortening, and cal-

cification. Most patients with rheumatic mitral stenosis will not develop symptomatic dyspnea until the valve area narrows to less than 1.5 cm^2; critical mitral
stenosis is often defined as a valve area less than 1.0 cm^2. In the catheterization laboratory, the mitral valve area (MVA) is calculated using the modified
Gorlin formula (discussion below), which is derived from standard fluid dynamic principles:

$$MVA\ (cm^2) = \frac{Cardiac\ output\ (ml/min)/diastolic\ filling\ period\ (sec/min)}{37.9\ \sqrt{Mean\ diastolic\ gradient\ (mm\ Hg)}}$$

Each of the factors in this equation requires careful measurement, and potential errors or pitfalls of measurement may be compounded in the final calculation.

The cardiac output determination is critical and can be obtained by the
thermodilution technique in the absence of significant tricuspid regurgitation.
Alternatively, the cardiac output also can be determined in the patient with
multivalvular disease by the indicator dilution technique or the Fick principle.
The Fick principle relates the patient's oxygen consumption to the arteriovenous oxygen difference and the cardiac output (CO) as follows:

$$CO\ (ml/min) = \frac{Oxygen\ consumption\ (ml/min)}{10 \times [Arterial-mixed\ venous\ oxygen\ content\ (vol\ \%)]}$$

The patient's oxygen consumption can either be measured, using a metabolic
cart or Douglas collection bag, or assumed, using nomograms based on the patient's body surface area. In our laboratory, we have found variability in both
thermodilution and direct oxygen consumption measurements and therefore
use the assumed Fick technique to determine cardiac output (total oxygen consumption ~ 110–120 ml/min × body surface area).

The diastolic filling period is the mean time that the valve is open during
a cardiac cycle, and it must be used to correct the total cardiac output to the
portion flowing across the stenotic valve during diastole. The time in seconds is
measured on the pressure tracing obtained at fast paper speeds (100 mm/sec)
from mitral valve opening (when left ventricular pressure falls below left atrial
or pulmonary capillary wedge pressure) to valve closure (when the rising left
ventricular pressure during systole exceeds left atrial pressure) (Fig 14-1). The
time per beat is multiplied by the heart rate to derive the total diastolic filling
period in seconds per minute.

The mean transmitral gradient is derived from simultaneous measurements of left atrial and left ventricular pressures. Usually, the more easily obtained pulmonary capillary wedge pressure is substituted for a direct left atrial

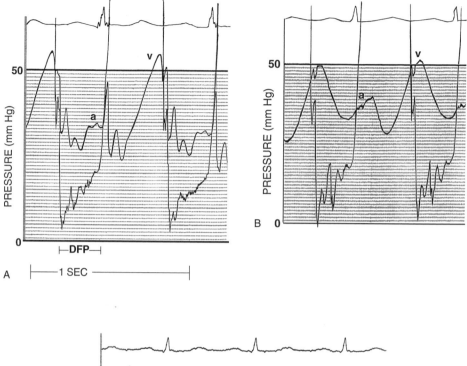

Figure 14-1 **(A)** Simultaneous left atrial and left ventricular pressure recordings from a 56-year-old woman with rheumatic mitral stenosis. Note the diastolic pressure gradient and diastolic filling period (DFP). The mean transmitral gradient was 19 mm Hg and the calculated mitral valve area was 1.0 cm^2 (cardiac output = 4.8 liters/min). **(B)** Simultaneous pulmonary capillary wedge and left ventricular pressure recordings in the same patient. Note the rightward displacement (delay) in the a and v waves on the wedge tracing. **(C)** Simultaneous pulmonary capillary wedge and left atrial pressure recordings in the same patient. The wedge pressure is delayed approximately 75 msec relative to the left atrial pressure. Note the slower (attenuated) y descent after the v wave on the wedge pressure recording.

pressure measurement, and is a frequent potential source of error in the mitral valve area calculation (see Fig 14-1b). The pulmonary capillary wedge pressure should be measured through a large-caliber rigid catheter to avoid pressure damping with a blunting (attenuation) of the wave peaks. The entire pressure tubing must be well flushed and free of air, and the position of the catheter in wedge position must be confirmed by recording a characteristic pressure wave form with a and v waves, the fluoroscopic position in a peripheral lung field, and/or by obtaining a fully saturated blood sample from the tip. A Swan-Ganz thermodilution catheter is usually *not* adequate for pressure measurement due to the small lumen caliber of the distal port, resulting in attenuation of the rate of pressure descent. Seven Fr Cournand, Goodale-Lubin, Lehman, or balloon-tipped catheters with a single large lumen are preferred. Left ventricular pressure is most commonly recorded by retrograde catheterization.

One source of error in gradient measurement involves the correction of the wedge pressure measurement for time delay. The wedge pressure measurement is delayed relative to left atrial pressure, because the waveforms have to be transmitted back through the pulmonary venous circulation. This delay (see Fig 14-1c) varies between 55 and 100 msec. The pressure tracing must be moved back this amount in time (using tracing paper) before it is used to measure the difference from the left ventricular pressure. This difference is graphically averaged over the time the mitral valve is open, utilizing a planimeter or simple computer program to calculate the mean gradient during diastole. An alternate practical method of correction is to move the wedge pressure tracing back until the v wave is bisected by the decreasing left ventricular pressure waveform. Despite this correction, as shown in Figure 14-1, the wedge pressure falls more slowly than the true left atrial pressure and tends to overestimate the gradient (and underestimate the valve area) by a small, and not usually clinically relevant, amount.

Another common potential source of error in mitral valve area determination can arise when the right (wedge pressure) and left (ventricular) heart transducers are not carefully calibrated to each other. In our laboratory, this is checked before each pressure measurement by simultaneously recording from the same intravenous (IV) tubing of a solution bag hung on an IV pole at about 50 cm above the transducers. Alternatively, the gradient can be remeasured after switching the transducers to ensure that it is unchanged.

It should be recognized that the gradient measured is in part dependent on the flow across the valve. Although most patients with severe and symptomatic mitral stenosis will have cardiac outputs between 3 and 3.5 liters/min, transmitral gradients between 12 and 18 mm Hg, and valve areas between 0.9 and 1.2 cm^2, a wide range of potential combinations of these parameters is theoretically possible (Fig 14-2). The maximum tolerable left atrial/pulmonary capillary wedge pressure is approximately 30 mm Hg. At a mitral valve area of 1.5 cm^2, a pressure gradient of about 7 mm Hg (mean left atrial pressure

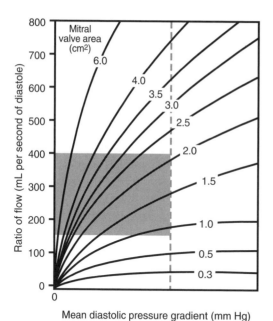

Figure 14-2 Hemodynamics of mitral stenosis. These curves illustrate the quadratic relationship between the mitral valve flow and gradient during diastole at varying severity of valve obstruction. The dotted lines show the physiologic limits of left atrial pressure and cardiac output. (From Wallace AG, Pathophysiology of cardiovascular disease. In: Smith LH, Thier SO, eds. Pathophysiology. The biological principles of disease. Philadelphia: Saunders, 1981:1192).

of about 15 mm Hg) is needed to provide the normal resting blood flow of 150 ml/sec of diastole. If the valve area is reduced to 1.0 cm^2, a 16-mm Hg gradient is required to provide the same flow. However, at this valve area, the gradient can be increased only a small amount before the maximum tolerated left atrial pressure is achieved, thereby effectively limiting the transvalvular flow to a small range, hence the term *critical mitral stenosis* (see Fig 14-2). Measurements should be recorded over several beats and averaged for the final valve area calculation; at least 5 beats should be utilized for the patient in normal sinus rhythm, and 10 beats during atrial fibrillation. Finally, the cardiac output, pressure gradient, and diastolic filling time must be measured simultaneously.

Angiographic Assessment

The angiographic assessment of mitral valve stenosis does not usually add much information to noninvasive imaging techniques. Fluoroscopic valve calcification may be present and has been shown to be an important predictor of both acute and chronic outcomes of percutaneous balloon valvuloplasty. Left ventriculography in the right anterior oblique projection can be used to assess left ventricular systolic function and mitral regurgitation. Sufficient angulation (usually about 45 degrees) should be chosen to separate the left atrium from the spine and descending aorta so that contrast entering the atrium can be visualized easily. The mitral valve leaflets may be seen with this negative contrast and the immobility (of the posterior leaflet) or prolapse of either leaflet assessed. The left ventricle often appears somewhat flattened or "pancaked" due to increased right ventricular pressure and volume, which displaces the left ventricle, particularly the septum. Left ventricular dysfunction may also occur due to abnormal papillary muscle function or associated cardiomyopathy. Cardiomyopathy may be due to chronic underfilling, rheumatic carditis, or concomitant conditions, but systolic dysfunction, if present and ascribed to rheumatic heart disease, is usually mild.

The size of the left atrium may be determined if even mild mitral regurgitation is present. Greater opacification of the left atrium can be obtained either by direct injection or by cineangiography of the late phase of a pulmonary artery injection; however, these techniques are rarely needed.

Special Issues in Mitral Stenosis

Several special issues may arise during the catheterization of a patient with mitral stenosis. Patients with very severe mitral stenosis and pulmonary hypertension may have a low cardiac output and/or a low gradient. In such patients, the valve area calculation is highly dependent on the gradient, and extra care should be taken in its determination. The administration of saline to raise the flow and gradient if the left atrial pressure is not already too high may improve the accuracy of the calculations. The use of two or more methods of cardiac output determination also may be necessary in this setting.

A low transmitral gradient (4–8 mm Hg) may also be due to only *mild* mitral stenosis (e.g., valve areas between 1.4 and 1.7 cm^2). Symptomatic patients with mild mitral stenosis can be difficult to assess, particularly if they have another potential cause for dyspnea, such as mild or moderate obstructive lung disease. Exercise can be performed in the catheterization laboratory with either repetitive single-leg raising or with arm raising using hand weights. After 3 minutes of exercise, measurement of the pulmonary capillary wedge pressure, gradient, and cardiac output can be helpful in determining whether a patient's dyspnea is due to mitral stenosis or another cause. Occasionally, in a patient with cardiomyopathy, the left ventricular pressure will rise substantially with the small gradient, suggesting that left ventricular dysfunction rather than mitral stenosis is the major pathology. In patients with mild-to-moderate mitral stenosis and no other cause for symptoms, relief of the obstruction with percutaneous balloon valvuloplasty has been shown to result in immediate and sustained clinical improvement. In some of these patients, the valve area may be elevated due to other conditions that increase the cardiac output (e.g., pregnancy, thyrotoxicosis), whereas in others, the valve area normalized for body surface area will be relatively small.

Transseptal left heart catheterization may be necessary to fully assess the transmitral gradient in some patients. When a satisfactory wedge recording cannot be obtained or when the recorded pressure is discrepant with other assessments of the expected pressure, direct left atrial pressure recording is warranted. The Gorlin formula constant should be increased slightly (to 40) when utilizing direct left atrial pressure.

With the use of multiple catheters and attempts to wedge them in multiple positions, a satisfactory wedge pressure can be obtained in the great majority of patients. However, one needs to be constantly vigilant for false measurements, such as a large gradient in a patient with few symptoms, mild stenosis by echo, and low pulmonary artery pressure, in whom the wedge pressure is inaccurately reflecting left atrial pressure due to catheter malposition, transducer error, or the presence of pulmonary veno-occlusive disease. When a transseptal technique is utilized, the left ventricular pressure can be recorded in an antegrade fashion.

Mitral Valve Regurgitation

Mitral regurgitation is one of the most difficult valvular lesions to assess due to the lack of easily measured quantitative parameters, the myriad causes of this disorder, and its effects on left ventricular function. Mitral valve incompetence may result from conditions affecting any of the complex parts of the mitral valve apparatus: the annulus, leaflets, chordae tendinae, or papillary muscles. In addition, disorders of the left ventricle may distort the anatomic relationships of the valve parts or stretch the annulus, resulting in functional regurgitation.

Following the development of mitral regurgitation, the left ventricle initially compensates by enlarging to take advantage of Starling's law relating end-diastolic volume to stroke volume. This allows the patient to increase total left ventricular stroke volume and maintain forward stroke volume despite the "backward" regurgitant volume. Chronically, the left ventricle undergoes eccentric hypertrophy in response to the excess volume load. This ventricular remodeling creates a more compliant chamber. Increased compliance allows the ventricle to accommodate the larger left ventricular volume at lower diastolic pressures. Chronic remodeling may eventually produce myocardial dysfunction. At this point, left ventricular function will deteriorate, and surgical correction of the valvular lesion may no longer restore normal function.

Patients develop symptoms due to the increased left atrial pressure, the development of pulmonary artery hypertension, and/or left ventricular systolic failure. Symptoms tend to be more pronounced when the regurgitant lesion develops acutely due to the greater rise in left atrial pressure as the regurgitant volume enters the normal, relatively noncompliant left atrium. Chronically, the atrium dilates and becomes more compliant, allowing the regurgitant volume to be accommodated with a smaller increase in pressure.

Role of Catheterization

In young patients (age < 40 years), physical examination and noninvasive imaging are often sufficient to establish the diagnosis, assess severity, and guide management. In older patients and those with chest pain, coronary angiography is necessary. Catheterization may be useful in many patients to provide an additional measure of severity by left ventriculographic visual assessment, and to measure the hemodynamic consequences. This approach is particularly important in cases in which the estimated valve lesion severity and symptoms do not correlate well.

Hemodynamic Assessment

The hemodynamic assessment of mitral regurgitation requires right and left heart catheterization. The left atrial v wave may be measured on pulmonary capillary wedge pressure or direct left atrial pressure recordings (Fig 14-3). The size of the v wave depends on a number of factors, including the regurgitant volume, the position on the atrial pressure-volume relationship (volume status of the patient), and the actual pressure-volume relation (compliance). In general, large v waves (more than twice the mean left atrial pressure or > 10 mm Hg above the mean pressure) correlate with severe regurgitation. However, other conditions that increase left atrial pressure (e.g., left-to-right shunts, congestive heart failure) also may cause large v waves, and large v waves may be absent even in the presence of severe regurgitation if the left atrium is very compliant (chronic mitral regurgitation) or the patient has been diuresed to a "flatter" portion of their atrial diastolic pressure-volume relation (Fig 14-4). In clinical studies, both the sensitivity and specificity of v waves for diagnosing mitral regurgitation have been 60% to 70%.

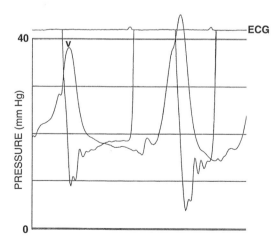

Figure 14-3 Simultaneous pulmonary capillary wedge (PCW) and left ventricular (LV) pressure recordings in a 68-year-old man with severe (3+) mitral regurgitation. Note the large v wave on the wedge recording to 40 mm Hg. The mean wedge pressure is 28 mm Hg and there is only a small a wave present.

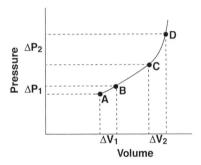

Figure 14-4 Hypothetical left atrial pressure-volume relationship demonstrating the dependence of the v wave on the amount of mitral regurgitation, the shape of this relationship, and the position on the relation. In the normal patient at point A, a regurgitant volume (ΔV) generates a small pressure change (B minus A). If the same patient has increased left atrial volume (due to heart failure or a ventricular septal defect) and moves up to a steeper portion of the curve, the same regurgitant volume results in a larger pressure wave (D minus C). Similarly, an increase in left atrial compliance (due to enlargement with chronic mitral regurgitation) will shift the curve rightward so that pressure changes are decreased at any given volume. (Adapted from Fuchs RM, Heuser RR, Yin FCP, Brinker JA. Limitations of pulmonary wedge V waves in diagnosing mitral regurgitation. Am J Cardiol 1982;49:849–854.)

Other hemodynamic parameters that are assessed include pulmonary pressure and cardiac output. Pulmonary artery pressure elevation is less common in patients with mitral regurgitation than in those with mitral stenosis. Early diastolic v waves exceeding systolic pressure may be seen on the pulmonary artery pressure recording correlating with the left atrial v waves in patients with severe regurgitation, noncompliant left atria, or low pulmonary vascular resistance, all characteristic of recent-onset regurgitation. In some patients, this finding may result in early closure of the pulmonic valve. Cardiac output tends to be below normal and decreases further as left ventricular dysfunction develops. The failure of forward cardiac output to increase with exercise in the catheterization laboratory may be another useful parameter to judge the severity of mitral regurgitation in relation to patient symptoms.

Angiographic Assessment

The severity of mitral regurgitation can be assessed angiographically (see Chapter 6). Left ventriculography is performed in the right anterior oblique (RAO) projection, usually at a steeper angle (e.g., 45 degrees) than for assessment of contractile function, to displace the left atrium to the right of the spine. Care must be taken to fully opacify the ventricle and to avoid ectopic beats. Approximately 40 to 60 ml of dye should be injected at a rate of 14 to 20 ml/sec through a minimum 6-Fr catheter with multiple side holes (pigtail). In biplane laboratories, the 40-degree left anterior oblique (LAO) projection may provide complementary information.

The grading of the severity of regurgitation is subjective and depends on the degree of opacification of the left atrium (Fig 14-5). Sellers first described this qualitative grading system on a scale of 1 (mild) to 4 (severe) in 1964, and it remains the current standard (Table 14-1).

A more quantitative assessment of the severity of regurgitation can be obtained by measuring total left ventricular stroke volume and subtracting forward stroke volume to obtain the regurgitant volume. The regurgitant volume

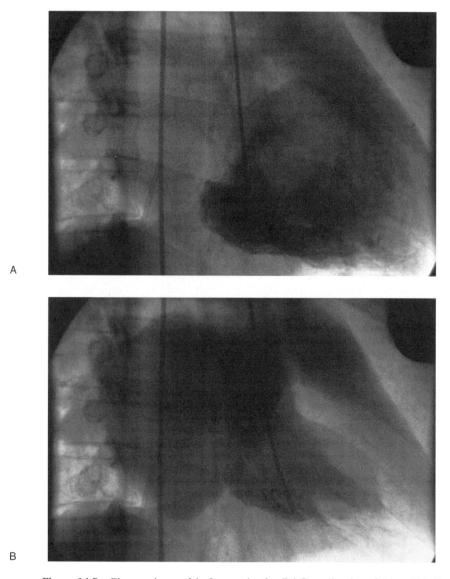

Figure 14-5   Cineangiographic frames in the RAO projection during (**A**) diastole and (**B**) systole in a patient with severe mitral regurgitation. Note the complete and equal opacification of the enlarged left atrium with reflux into the superior pulmonary veins.

Table 14-1   Angiographic Assessment of Mitral Regurgitation

1+	Mild	Dye clears from LA with each beat and does not opacify the entire atrium.
2+	Moderate	Dye does not clear with each beat and faintly opacifies entire atrium after several beats.
3+	Moderately severe	LA is completely opacified and equals density of left ventricle.
4+	Severe	LA opacifies completely with one beat, becomes progressively more dense, and refluxes into pulmonary veins.

Abbreviation: LA, left atrium.

can be normalized for body surface area and may exceed 3 liters/min/m^2 in patients with severe regurgitation. Total left ventricular stroke volume can be determined angiographically using the Sandler and Dodge area-length method to calculate left ventricular end-diastolic and end-systolic volumes. Forward stroke volume can be measured using the Fick or thermodilution methods. The regurgitant fraction is then derived by dividing the regurgitant volume by the total stroke volume. In severe mitral regurgitation, the regurgitant fraction may exceed 0.60.

Unfortunately, the correlation between quantitative and angiographic measures of mitral regurgitation is not precise. This disparity is especially marked for the higher grades of angiographic regurgitation. Larger left atria and ventricles are particularly prone to underestimation of the severity of regurgitation angiographically. Finally, the quantitative measurement of regurgitant fraction and volume in the catheterization laboratory is often difficult due to inaccuracies in the measurement of each of the required variables. Accuracy depends on the quality of chamber opacification, normality of chamber dimensions assumed in the calculation, and exact correlation for magnification.

Thus, a more precise and reproducible assessment of mitral regurgitation severity is needed. Decisions for surgery are based on symptoms, the severity of regurgitation, and evidence of left ventricular dysfunction (including deterioration on serial examinations). Echocardiography provides the simplest method to serially follow left ventricular dimensions and function. Furthermore, an echocardiographic method utilizing the proximal flow convergence method to calculate regurgitant stroke volume, flow rate, and effective orifice area has recently been introduced and validated. Its clinical value will be determined during the next few years.

Tricuspid Valve Disease

Tricuspid valve disease may be primary or secondary to right ventricular dysfunction. The trileaflet normal valve has the largest annular circumference (~10 cm) and orifice area (~7 cm^2) of the four cardiac valves. The subvalvular apparatus includes approximately 25 chordae arising from one to three papillary muscles on the right ventricular posterior and septal walls.

A large series of 363 abnormal tricuspid valves removed surgically at the Mayo Clinic over a 25-year period demonstrated rheumatic heart disease in 192 (53%), congenital heart disease in 94 (26%) (most frequently Ebstein's anomaly), pulmonary venous hypertension in 55 (15%), and infective endocarditis in 11 (3%). The relative frequency of a rheumatic etiology decreased over the 25 years of study, whereas the proportion due to congenital abnormalities increased. All of the patients with rheumatic tricuspid valve disease had associated mitral valve pathology. Finally, the incidence of pure regurgitation greatly exceeded the occurrence of mixed disease and pure stenosis (74% versus 23% and 2%, respectively).

Tricuspid Stenosis

Tricuspid stenosis is rare, usually results from rheumatic fever, and is almost always associated with mitral stenosis. The clinical diagnosis may be masked by the symptoms of mitral stenosis and is often first discovered echocardiographically. Diastolic doming, commissural fusion, and thickening are very sensitive markers of tricuspid valve disease, and hemodynamically significant stenosis will be present only in a minority of patients with these echocardiographic signs.

Hemodynamic assessment of tricuspid stenosis requires simultaneous recording of right atrial and ventricular pressures with two identical catheters due to the small gradient and frequent occurrence of atrial fibrillation. The catheters should be calibrated together in the right atrium to confirm identical zero positions and transducer gain before passing one into the right ventricle. The mean transvalvular gradient may be quite small (e.g., 2–4 mm Hg), even in severe tricuspid stenosis (Fig 14-6). The a wave on the right atrial pressure recording is large and frequently exceeds the maximum systolic pressure by more than 5 mm Hg. The y descent will be slow, consistent with impairment of rapid right ventricular filling. The mean right atrial pressure may be normal or only slightly elevated, reflecting the low cardiac output, which also fails to rise more than twofold with exercise. Exercise (or atropine administration) to increase the heart rate and volume administration may be helpful to increase the transvalvular gradient and confirm the diagnosis. The Gorlin formula may be used to calculate the tricuspid valve area, but often underestimates the valve area due to frequently associated regurgitation. Clinically important stenosis usually occurs at valve areas less than 1.5 cm^2.

Angiographic study of tricuspid stenosis should include right atrial angiography in a shallow RAO projection (10 to 15 degrees). This minimizes overlap of the right atrium and ventricle and often allows visualization of the leaflet thickening and doming.

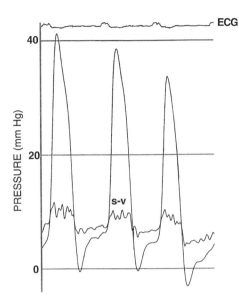

Figure 14-6 Hemodynamic tracings in a 54-year-old woman with mixed rheumatic tricuspid valve disease. Simultaneous right ventricular (RV) and right atrial (RA) pressure recordings demonstrate a small diastolic gradient (mean = 3 mm Hg); the calculated minimum effective valve area is 1.2 cm^2 with a low cardiac output of 2.9 liters/min. Note the systolic (s-v) wave on the right atrial pressure recording due to tricuspid regurgitation.

Patients with symptoms of low cardiac output or peripheral edema and hepatomegaly may benefit from relief of their obstruction. Percutaneous balloon valvuloplasty has resulted in hemodynamic and symptomatic improvement in patients with rheumatic tricuspid stenosis that is similar to surgical commissurotomy and valve replacement.

Tricuspid Regurgitation

As with tricuspid stenosis, mitral valve pathology is frequently present in patients with tricuspid regurgitation. The hemodynamic hallmarks of this condition are increased right atrial pressure and decreased cardiac output.

The mean right atrial pressure is high and exhibits large systolic waves (see Fig 14-6). The y descent is rapid and increases with inspiration. The size of the systolic wave correlates with the severity of regurgitation and may be indistinguishable from the right ventricular pressure (ventricularization) in the most severe cases. The right atrial pressure wave due to regurgitation is called the s wave and occurs slightly earlier than the v wave. It may form a single systolic wave with the normal ventricular filling v wave in severe regurgitation.

Right ventricular angiography is essential to evaluate the severity of tricuspid regurgitation, although careful catheter placement to avoid interfering with the leaflet closure and inducing premature contractions is essential. A specially preshaped catheter may be helpful in this regard. Quantification of the severity of regurgitation is qualitative, utilizing a scale similar to the Sellers criteria for mitral regurgitation. The best projection is RAO with a pigtail or Berman catheter positioned in the mid-right ventricle. Care should be taken to insert the catheter sufficiently to place all of the side holes in the ventricle. Injection rates of 12 to 14 ml/sec for 45 to 60 ml are most often utilized.

Pulmonic Valve Disease

Pulmonic Stenosis

One of the most common congenital valve defects is pulmonic valve stenosis, occurring in approximately 10% of children with congenital heart disease. It is usually diagnosed and treated, often with balloon dilation, in infancy or childhood. Most adults with congenital pulmonic stenosis were either corrected as children or have hemodynamically insignificant stenosis with a benign course. A minority of adults, however, will develop symptoms of dyspnea, fatigue, and chest pain requiring assessment and treatment. The efficacy and safety of balloon valvuloplasty in this condition may also warrant treatment for asymptomatic patients with severe right ventricular pressure elevation.

The role of catheterization includes a careful hemodynamic and angiographic assessment of both the severity and location of obstruction, as well as identification of other congenital abnormalities. In most cases, obstruction is at the level of the valve itself; however, obstruction also may be present in the subvalvular region due to infundibular stenosis, supravalvular, or in the peripheral pulmonary artery branches.

Hemodynamic assessment is performed with an end-hole catheter pulled slowly back from the branch pulmonary artery to the right ventricle. Advancing the catheter through the obstruction can be accomplished with a J-tipped wire. The pulmonary artery pressure is low to normal with a step-up as the catheter enters the right ventricle (Fig 14-7). Right ventricular systolic pressure reflects the severity of obstruction and will exceed 50 mm Hg in moderate pulmonic stenosis, and is greater than 75 mm Hg in severe stenosis. The right atrial pressure may be normal in mild pulmonic stenosis, but may be elevated (with a large a wave) in more severe obstructions. A separate gradient may be detected across the infundibulum, reflecting anomalous muscle bundles or severe hypertrophy. The use of two catheters, one for pullback and a second in the right ventricular body, may facilitate the determination of an intraventricular gradient. The infundibular gradient may worsen following successful balloon dilation of valvular stenosis and the consequent reduction in right ventricular systolic pressure. In patients with severe pulmonic stenosis, a right-to-left shunt through either a patent foramen ovale or atrial septal defect may explain the finding of cyanosis. A full saturation run is also important to check for an occasionally associated ventricular septal defect.

The valvular obstruction is best visualized angiographically by anteroposterior (or 10-degree RAO) and lateral biplane right ventriculography through a

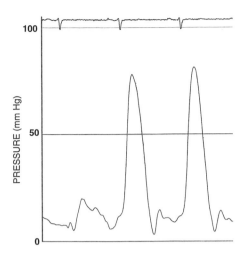

Figure 14-7 Pullback pressure recording with an end-hole catheter from the pulmonary artery (lower pressure left-side pressure tracing) to the right ventricle (higher pressure, right-sided pressure tracing) in a 27-year-old woman with congenital pulmonic stenosis and prior surgical commissurotomy. Note the step-up from the pulmonary artery systolic pressure of 20 mm Hg to the right ventricular systolic pressure of 80 to 85 mm Hg.

pigtail or Berman catheter using 40 to 60 ml of contrast at 12 to 18 ml/sec). Ten to 20 degrees of cranial angulation in the anteroposterior or RAO view places the proximal pulmonary artery and bifurcation in a less foreshortened position. The valve will appear domed and thickened with a central jet that opacifies a dilated poststenotic pulmonary artery (Fig 14-8A). The infundibular narrowing is most apparent during systole and in the lateral projection (Fig 14-8B). If the valve annulus is small or the leaflets large, a dysplastic valve should be suspected. The results of balloon valvuloplasty have been excellent in both children and adults with valvular pulmonic stenosis, but less successful in dysplastic valves. Finally, branch stenoses may be better visualized with cranial or other compound views.

Pulmonic Regurgitation

Pulmonic regurgitation results in a wide pulse pressure on the pulmonary artery recording, but it may be difficult to confirm solely on this basis. Angiographic assessment with main pulmonary artery injection of contrast at a fast rate (20–25 ml/sec) may allow a visual determination of the severity,

Prosthetic Valve Disease

Mechanical valves were first developed and implanted by Harken, Edwards, and Starr in 1960. Subsequently, homograft and porcine xenografts were pioneered by Ross, Carpentier, and Barratt-Boyes. The assessment of function of prosthetic heart valves begins with an understanding of the various prostheses. Mechanical valves include the caged-ball (Starr-Edwards, Baxter-Edwards, Irvine,

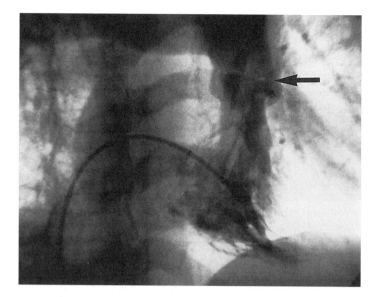

A

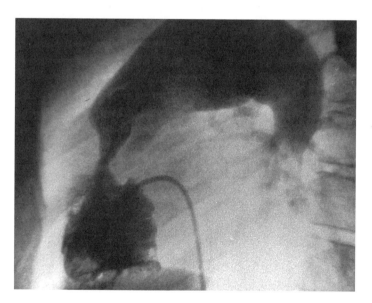

B

Figure 14-8   Right ventricular cineangiograms from two patients with congenital pulmonic valve stenosis. **(A)** The RAO projection demonstrates right ventricular function and shows the thickened and doming pulmonic valve (arrow) during systole. **(B)** The lateral projection demonstrates stenosis of the right ventricular outflow tract (infundibulum) after balloon valvuloplasty.

CA), tilting-disk (Medtronic-Hall, Medtronic Corp., Minneapolis, MN; Bjork-Shiley, Pfizer, Inc., Irvine, CA), and bileaflet (St. Jude, St. Jude Corp., Minneapolis, MN; CarboMedics, Austin, TX) designs. These valves all require chronic anticoagulation and have rates of thromboembolism of 1.5% to 4.0% per year. Tissue valves (bioprostheses) include the porcine xenograft (Carpentier-Edwards [Baxter-Edwards, Irvine, CA], Hancock [Medtronic, Minneapolis, MN]), which is glutaraldehyde fixed, and bovine pericardial valves (Edwards, Baxter-Edwards, Irvine, CA). The bovine valve offers an improved orifice-to-annulus ratio, but its durability compared with other bioprostheses is not yet clear. The bioprosthetic valves do not require long-term anticoagulation to avoid thromboembolic events, but degenerate over time, particularly in young patients and in the mitral position. Recently, cryopreserved "viable" cadaver homograft prostheses have become popular, based on the absence of need for anticoagulation and a probably improved durability compared with other bioprostheses.

Valvular dysfunction may result from structural failure (which is rare for current mechanical prostheses but not uncommon for porcine and pericardial valves after 7 to 10 years) and valve thrombosis, from development of valvular or paravalvular regurgitation due to infection, or from tissue ingrowth. Successful catheterization laboratory assessment of prosthetic heart valves requires a thorough understanding of the specific size, type, and normal function of the specific prosthesis.

Hemodynamic Assessment

The hemodynamic assessment of valvular prostheses requires measurement of the gradient by measuring pressure in the cardiac chamber or vascular structure on either side of the valve, determination of the cardiac output, and calculation of the effective orifice area. Mechanical valves should never be crossed with a catheter in either the antegrade or the retrograde direction. Although retrograde catheterization of mechanical valves has been reported, the catheter may disrupt or dislodge moving parts or become entrapped in the valve. Furthermore, even a small catheter will often disrupt valve function sufficiently to render useless any pressures that are recorded.

In contrast, bioprostheses are frequently crossed with catheters. However, the risk of damaging a friable leaflet in an old or dysfunctional prosthesis should make one cautious. When the valve can be assessed without crossing it (e.g., transseptal approach for aortic prosthesis), this is a preferable approach (Fig 14-9). If a prosthetic valve must be crossed, a nontraumatic catheter (such as a balloon-tipped one for antegrade crossings) is preferred. Similarly, crossing valves with suspected thrombosis, recent embolism, or mobile vegetations should be avoided. Direct left ventricular puncture has occasionally been utilized to assess valve function in the patient with mechanical aortic and mitral

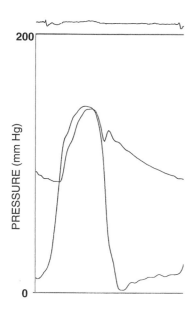

200

PRESSURE (mm Hg)

0

Figure 14-9 Normal hemodynamics of a Starr-Edwards aortic valve prosthesis. Simultaneous left ventricular pressure (catheter inserted transseptally) and ascending aortic pressure were recorded, demonstrating a small early systolic gradient (mean = 10 mm Hg). The peak instantaneous and mean gradients obtained by echocardiographic Doppler evaluation were 38 and 21 mm Hg, respectively.

Table 14-2 Prosthetic Valve Gradients and Effective Valve Areas Assessed by Cardiac Catheterization

Valve (size)	Diastolic gradient (mm Hg)	Valve area (cm²)
Standard St. Jude (No. 29)	2.3±0.6	3.1±0.8
Starr-Edwards (No. 30)	6.3±2.0	1.8±0.4
Bjork-Shiley (No. 29)	4.5±1.6	2.2±0.5
Standard St. Jude (No. 23)	—	2.2±0.3
Starr-Edwards (No. 24)	—	1.4±0.2
Bjork-Shiley (No. 23)	—	1.5±0.3
Hancock	5.2±3.3	1.9±0.5

Source: Data from Horstkotte D, Haerten K, Seipel L. Central hemodynamics at rest and during exercise after mitral valve replacement with different prostheses. Circulation 1983;68(II):161–168.

prostheses. However, complications of this procedure are not uncommon and include death; in most situations, noninvasive assessments can be substituted.

Table 14-2 lists the effective valve areas (Gorlin formula) of a number of mechanical prosthesis in the mitral and aortic positions assessed by catheterization 1 year after implantation. More comprehensive assessments of normal hemodynamic values for prosthetic values have come from echocardiographic studies. Doppler echocardiographic measurement of prosthetic valve hemodynamics have important limitations, including localized high-flow velocities and underestimation of the recovery of pressure loss. These limitations tend to result in overestimation of the mean pressure gradient and underestimation of the effective orifice area (see Fig 14-9).

Angiographic Assessment

The assessment of prosthetic heart valves involves direct inspection of the valve for normal operation as well as angiography to assess valvular and paravalvular regurgitation. Angiography should be performed in standard views (RAO for mitral valves; LAO or biplane for aortic valves). The exact angle should be fine-tuned to place the annulus of the prosthesis perpendicular to the imaging plane. Fluoroscopic evaluation should include inspection for evidence of structural deterioration or fracture evidence of excessive "rocking" of the annulus and determining any abnormality of opening and closing parameters. For example, the Bjork-Shiley 60-degree convex-concave model valve has had the problem of strut fracture, which may be assessed fluoroscopically. Similarly, opening (10- to 13-degree) and closing (120- to 127-degree) angles for various sizes of normally functioning St. Jude valves are published and can be measured on a cineangiogram to assess leaflet thrombus or impedance to closure due to tissue ingrowth (Fig 14-10).

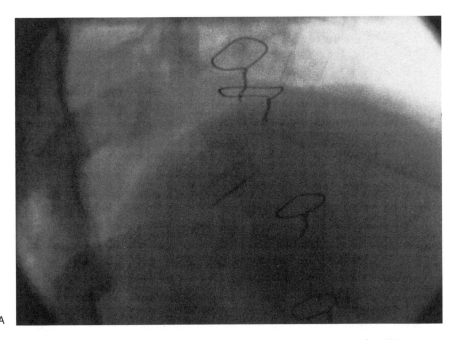

A

Figure 14-10   Cineangiograms of a St. Jude aortic prosthesis in the (**A**) open and (**B**) closed positions. The opening and closing angles can be measured to assess normal or abnormal function.

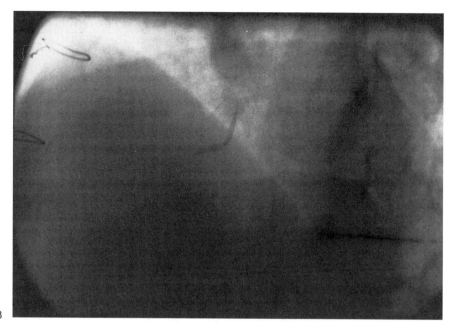

B

SELECTED READINGS

Cha SD, Desai RS, Gooch AS, et al. Diagnosis of severe tricuspid regurgitation. Chest 1982;82:726–731.

Cohn LH, Collins JJ, DiSesa VJ, et al. Fifteen-year experience with 1678 Hancock porcine bioprosthetic heart valve replacements. Ann Surg 1989;210:435–443.

Croft CH, Lipscomb K, Mathis K, et al. Limitations of qualitative angiographic grading in aortic or mitral regurgitation. Am J Cardiol 1984;53:1593–1598.

Czer LS, Weiss M, Bateman TM, et al. Fibrinolytic therapy of St. Jude valve thrombosis under guidance of digital cinefluoroscopy. J Am Coll Cardiol 1985;5:1244–1249.

Fuchs RM, Heuser RR, Yin FCP, Brinker JA. Limitations of pulmonary wedge V waves in diagnosing mitral regurgitation. Am J Cardiol 1982;49:849–854.

Gorlin R, Gorlin SG. Modified orifice equation for the calculation of mitral valve area. Am Heart J 1972;84:839–840.

Grose R, Strain J, Cohen MV: Pulmonary arterial V waves in mitral regurgitation: clinical and experimental observations. Circulation 1984;9:214–222.

Hammermeister KE, Murray JA, Blackmon JR. Revision of Gorlin constant for calculation of mitral valve area from left heart pressures. Br Heart J 1973;35:392–396.

Hauck AJ, Freeman DP, Ackermann DM, et al.: Surgical pathology of the tricuspid valve: A study of 363 cases spanning 25 years. Mayo Clin Proc 1988;63:851–863.

Henneke KH, Pongratz G, Bachmann K. Limitations of doppler echocardiography in the assessment of prosthetic valve hemodynamics. J Heart Valve Dis 1995;4:18–25.

Herrmann HC. Acute and chronic efficacy of percutaneous transvenous mitral commissurotomy. Implications for patient selection. Cathet Cardiovasc Diagn 1994;Suppl 2:61–68.

Herrmann HC, Feldman T, Isner JM, et al. Comparison of results of percutaneous balloon valvuloplasty in patients with mild and moderate mitral stenosis to those with severe mitral stenosis. Am J Cardiol 1993;71:1300–1303.

Herrmann HC, Hill JA, Krol J, et al. Effectiveness of percutaneous balloon valvuloplasty in adults with pulmonic valve stenosis. Am J Cardiol 1991;61:1111–1113.

Horstkotte D, Haerten K, Seipel L, et al. Central hemodynamics at rest and during exercise after mitral valve replacement with different prostheses. Circulation 1983;68(II):161–168.

Johnson LW, Grossman W, Dalen JE, Dexter L: Pulmonic stenosis in the adult. N Engl J Med 1972;287:1159–1163.

Khan SS. Assessment of prosthetic valve hemodynamics by doppler: lessons from in vitro studies of the St. Jude valve. J Heart Valve Dis 1993;2:183–193.

Kitchin A, Turner R. Diagnosis and treatment of tricuspid stenosis. Br Heart J 1964;26:354–379.

Lange RA, Moore DM, Cigarroa RG, Hillis LD. Use of pulmonary capillary wedge pressure to assess severity of mitral stenosis: is true left atrial pressure needed in this condition? J Am Coll Cardiol 1989;13:825–829.

Ribeiro PA, Zaibag MA, Kasab SA, et al. Percutaneous double balloon valvotomy for rheumatic tricuspid stenosis. Am J Cardiol 1988;61:660–662.

Sandler H, Dodge HT, Hay RE, Rackley CE. Quantitation of valvular insufficiency in man by angiocardiography. Am Heart J 1963;65:501–513.

Sellers RD, Levy NJ, Amplatz K, Lillehei CW. Left retrograde cardioangiography in acquired cardiac disease. Am J Cardiol 1964;14:437–447.

Vandervoort PM, Rivera M, Mele D, et al. Application of color doppler flow mapping to calculate effective regurgitant orifice area. Circulation 1993;88:1150–1156.

15

PERICARDIAL DISEASE

Andrew A. Ziskind

The Normal and Abnormal Pericardium

THE NORMAL FUNCTION of the pericardium is to help maintain the anatomic position of the heart, reduce friction, and provide a barrier against the spread of infection from adjacent structures. In addition, the pericardium may assist in the diastolic function of the heart by preventing overdistension and facilitating ventricular coupling.[1-4] Pericardial pressure is normally the same as intrapleural pressure, varying from 0 to −2 mm Hg with the respiratory cycle. The normal pericardial space contains approximately 20 to 30 ml of serous fluid.

Pericardial disease processes include pericarditis (with or without accompanying effusion), cardiac tamponade, pericardial constriction, and subacute effusive-constrictive disease. Symptoms may be due to the inflammatory process itself or the hemodynamic consequences of inflammation. When an effusion, constriction, or effusive-constrictive disease develops, diastolic function can be affected. As biventricular filling becomes impaired, stroke volume decreases, leading to decreased cardiac output.

Pericardial Effusion and Cardiac Tamponade

Hemodynamics

The pericardium is a relatively inelastic fibrous structure. Thus, the hemodynamic consequences of a pericardial effusion depend on the quantity of fluid in the pericardial space and the rate at which that fluid has accumulated. The rapid accumulation of as little as 150 ml into the pericardial space can produce marked elevations in intrapericardial pressure, yet 1 to 2 liters of fluid may accumulate slowly before pericardial pressure rises. In comparison to constriction, the hemodynamic effect of cardiac tamponade occurs throughout the entire cardiac cycle. As fluid accumulates and the pericardial pressure rises, transmural distending pressures fall, leading to impaired ventricular filling. The impairment of rapid diastolic filling of the right ventricle leads to loss of the Y descent in the right atrial waveform. Negative intrapleural pressure can still be transmitted to the pericardial space. This permits right atrial pressure to fall with inspiration and explains the absence of Kussmaul's sign. Pulsus paradoxus, an exaggeration of the normal inspiratory fall in systolic BP, may be seen due to inspiratory augmentation of right ventricular filling at the expense of left ventricular filling. Although compensatory tachycardia can initially maintain cardiac output, as ventricular filling is further compromised, hemodynamic collapse can develop. To further aid in the differentiation of tamponade from constriction, tamponade is characterized by lack of an early dip-and-plateau pattern in the ventricular waveform and absent early Y descent in the right atrial waveform. For some patients, vasoconstriction can be a prominent part of the hemodynamic response, so BP may be normal or elevated despite hemodynamics consistent with cardiac tamponade.[5]

Low-pressure tamponade may be seen when volume depletion is present. These patients demonstrate equalization of pericardial pressures, impaired cardiac output, and tenuous hemodynamics at pericardial pressures less than 15 mm Hg.[6]

It is prudent to perform right heart catheterization at the time of pericardiocentesis. Right heart catheterization can confirm the hemodynamic significance of the pericardial effusion, but it is also clinically important to remeasure pressures after withdrawal of pericardial fluid. It is worth noting that up to 40% of patients with cardiac tamponade have other cardiac or pulmonary disease that is contributing to their dyspnea.[7] When cardiac tamponade is present, there is elevation and equalization of diastolic pressures (Fig 15-1). As fluid is withdrawn, the pericardial pressure should return to intrapleural pressure, oscillating around zero. The right atrial waveform should normalize with reappearance of the diastolic Y descent (Fig 15-2). If right atrial pressure remains elevated, but a prominent Y descent appears, the diagnosis of effusive-constrictive disease must be considered.

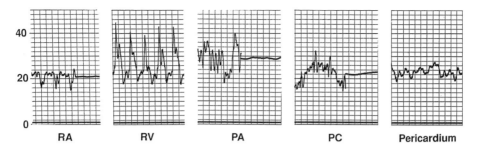

Figure 15-1 Pressure tracings from right heart catheterization demonstrating elevation and equalization of diastolic pressures due to cardiac tamponade. PA = pulmonary artery; PC = pulmonary capillary wedge; RA = right atrium; RV = right ventricle.

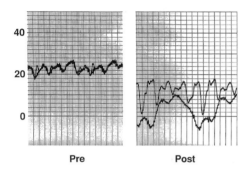

Figure 15-2 With cardiac tamponade, right atrial and pericardial pressures are elevated and equal to each other. Following withdrawal of pericardial fluid, they separate, with a return to the normal contour.

Etiologies of Effusive Pericardial Disease

On a medical service, malignant disease is the most common cause for pericardial effusion. Other etiologies include autoimmune disease, infectious processes (viral, bacterial, fungal), uremia, postmyocardial infarction (particularly patients on anticoagulation), trauma, such as following invasive procedures (pacemaker placement), or idiopathic.[8]

Symptoms and Physical Findings

Patients with acute development of tamponade are often in extremis with clinical shock. When cardiac tamponade develops gradually, exertional dyspnea, malaise, and other constitutional symptoms are often seen. These complaints, accompanied by prominent neck veins, tachycardia, and pulsus paradoxus, usually lead to an echocardiogram that confirms cardiac tamponade (Fig 15-3).

The ECG may reveal electrical alternans, beat-to-beat alteration in the amplitude, or polarity of the P, QRS, or T waves (Fig 15-4). The mechanism is felt to be pendulum-like swinging of the heart within the fluid-filled pericardial space.

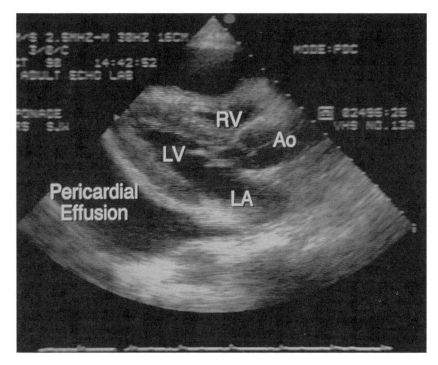

Figure 15-3   Echocardiogram (parasternal long axis view) revealing a large pericardial effusion with diastolic collapse of the right atrium and right ventricle consistent with tamponade. LV, left ventricle; RV, right ventricle; LA, left atrium; Ao, aorta.

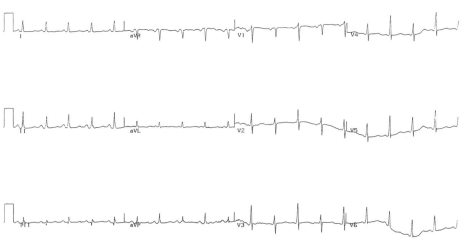

Figure 15-4   Electrocardiogram tracing demonstrating electrical alternans, suggesting the presence of a large pericardial effusion/tamponade.

Unless critical hemodynamic compromise is present, echocardiography is usually performed to identify the presence of pericardial fluid and confirm its location and quantity. Caution must be exercised when evaluating acute hemorrhagic tamponade because clotted blood may be echodense.

Radiographic Findings

When pericardial fluid accumulates slowly, the cardiac silhouette is typically enlarged, with a water bottle configuration on chest x-ray (Fig 15-5). However, when the volume of fluid is small, particularly when its development is acute, the cardiac silhouette can be normal. It may be helpful to identify the epicardial fat stripe, which can be seen separated from the pericardial silhouette. In the catheterization laboratory, the fluoroscopic appearance is remarkable for

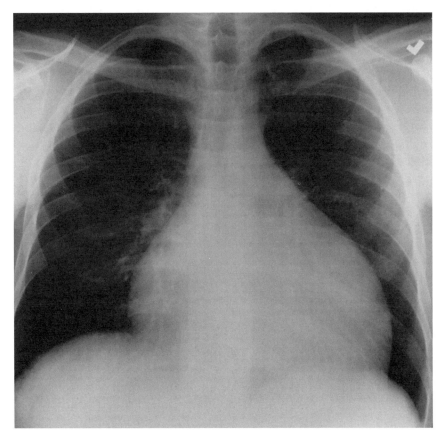

Figure 15-5 Posteroanterior chest x-ray of a patient cardiac tamponade: The cardiac silhouette is markedly enlarged with a "water bottle" configuration.

an immobile cardiac silhouette, within which can be seen motion of the epicardial fat stripe.

Treatment

Pericardiocentesis

The technical approach and difficulty of pericardiocentesis may vary according to the amount and location of the fluid. The risks decrease and the likelihood of successful pericardiocentesis increases with increasing size of the effusion.[7] A variety of techniques have been used to guide appropriate needle placement to reduce the possiblity of injury to the heart and surrounding structures. Pericardiocentesis may be performed "blindly," or with ECG, echocardiographic, or fluoroscopic guidance. Often a combination of these techniques is used. The degree of hemodynamic compromise may influence the approach, particularly when immediate removal of fluid is warranted to restore hemodynamic stability. Rapid intravenous administration of volume may provide transient hemodynamic improvement by raising right atrial pressure above pericardial, thereby improving ventricular filling and cardiac output.[9] Although vasodilators may improve cardiac output, they may be risky in hypotensive patients and are unlikely to improve organ perfusion.[9] If the patient is acutely ill, hypotensive, and in severe distress, pericardiocentesis should be attempted without delay for further diagnostic studies. If the situation is more stable, an expedient approach to drainage should be undertaken. It must be recognized that there is no single best way to approach pericardial drainage. The preferred approach is frequently dictated by institutional preferences based on their patient population and the availability of cardiology and surgery resources.

Pericardiocentesis is most commonly performed via a subxiphoid approach. After administration of local anesthesia to the skin and deeper tissues, the pericardial needle is connected to an ECG V lead. The most common needle orientation is from the left subxiphoid skin entry site toward the posterior aspect of the left shoulder (Fig 15-6). A discrete "pop" may be felt as the needle enters the pericardial space. If the needle contacts the epicardial surface, ST segment elevation will be seen on the V lead tracing (Fig 15-7). This may be accompanied by premature ventricular contractions. The needle should then be retracted slightly until ST elevation disappears. Once the pericardial space has been entered, a guidewire is introduced through the pericardial needle. The needle is removed, and a catheter is inserted over the guidewire. The catheter is frequently left in place for a period of time to ensure effective drainage and if necessary provide a route for instillation of sclerosing or chemotherapeutic agents. Alternative approaches to simple ECG-guided pericardiocentesis include monitoring pressure through the pericardial needle or using fluoroscopic or echocardiographic guidance.

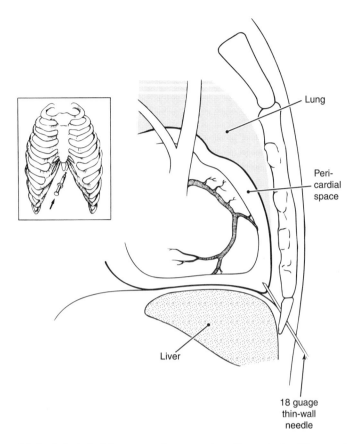

Figure 15-6 Subxiphoid approach to pericardiocentesis. The pericardial needle is advanced from the left costoxiphoid junction directed toward the posterior aspect of the left shoulder. Reprinted with permission from Tilkian AG, Daily EK. Cardiovascular Procedures. St. Louis: CV Mosby & Co. 1986:242.

Echocardiography is useful in directing the approach of the needle toward the most readily accessible portion of the pericardial space. Institutions that rely heavily on echocardiographically guided pericardiocentesis frequently utilize less conventional apical and parasternal approaches.[10] Echocardiographic guidance for pericardiocentesis may also help identify the amount and location of pericardial fluid. This is particularly important when fluid is localized, or small in quantity (e.g., diagnostic pericardiocentesis), or when the thoracic configuration is abnormal.[10–12] For selected patients with hepatomegaly due to metastatic disease, the use of echocardiographic guidance may help prevent inadvertent liver injury during a subxiphoid approach.

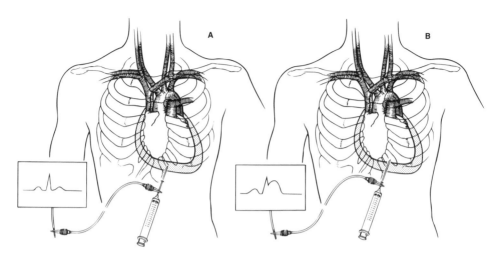

Figure 15-7   Electrocardiogram recording from pericardial needle. If contact is made with the epicardial surface, ST segment elevation is seen. Reprinted with permission from Tilkian AG, Daily EK. Cardiovascular Procedures. St. Louis: CV Mosby & Co. 1986:248.

Pericardial Fluid Analysis

At the time of pericardiocentesis, pericardial fluid should be sent for analysis. When the diagnosis is unclear, the following studies should be considered: protein, amylase, glucose, cholesterol, hematocrit, white blood cell count and differential, culture (aerobic, anaerobic, tuberculosis, fungal), special stains (including Gram's, fungal, and acid-fast), and cytology. In cases of suspected autoimmune disease, immunologic studies are occasionally useful (complement levels, ANA).

Adjunctive Therapeutic Approaches

Therapeutic approaches for the managment of pericardial effusion may be divided into catheter-based strategies and surgical strategies. The first step is to identify, if possible, the etiology of the effusion and determine the appropriate diagnostic and therapeutic level relative to the patient's underlying disease process. Recurrences following simple catheter drainage have been reported in 14% to 50% of patients with pericardial effusion and tamponade.[13-16] Leaving the pericardial catheter in place for 24 to 72 hours may allow the visceral and parietal pericardial surfaces to maintain apposition, thereby allowing autosclerosis to occur. The pericardial catheter itself may also contribute to inflammatory obliteration of the pericardial space.[10,17,18] Prophylactic antibiotics may be used during the time that the catheter is in place to prevent secondary infection of the pericardial space.

For many patients, initial treatment consists of catheter drainage, with removal of the catheter when drainage is less than 75 to 100 ml/day. A more aggressive approach is then undertaken if pericardial drainage continues or if fluid recurs after catheter removal.

Sclerotherapy

Instillation of sclerosing agents may obliterate the pericardial space. Tetracycline,[19-21] doxycycline, and bleomycin[22] are most commonly used. The use of bleomycin is growing because the parenteral form of tetracycline is no longer manufactured.

The technique for use of sclerosing agents is varied, but usually involves delivering the sclerosing agent in 30 to 50 ml of saline, allowing it to remain in the pericardial space for 1 to 2 hours, then draining the pericardial space to maintain apposition of the visceral and parietal pericardial surfaces.[19] This is repeated until drainage is less than 50 to 75 ml/24 hr. When discomfort accompanies sclerotherapy, the instillation of 5 ml of lidocaine into the pericardial space may help.

Percutaneous Balloon Pericardiotomy

For patients with advanced malignancy and limited life expectancy, it is desirable to minimize surgical procedures. In 1991 Palacios et al. first reported the technique of percutaneous balloon pericardiotomy (PBP) via the subxiphoid approach as an alternative to subxiphoid surgical windowing.[23] Since that initial report on eight patients, the multicenter PBP registry has reported data on a larger number of patients.[24,25]

Percutaneous balloon pericardiotomy uses a balloon-dilating catheter to create a pericardial window (Fig 15-8). It is performed in the catheterization laboratory with local anesthesia and mild sedation with intravenous narcotics and a short-acting benzodiazepine. After administration of local anesthesia to the skin and deeper tissues, the pericardium is entered via a standard subxiphoid approach and a catheter is inserted.

After measuring pericardial pressure, most of the pericardial fluid should be withdrawn to limit the volume left to pass into the pleural space once the window is created. A 0.038″ J-tipped extra-stiff guidewire is advanced into the pericardial space and its location confirmed fluoroscopically by looping in the pericardial space. After predilation along the track of the wire with a 10-Fr dilator, a 20-mm diameter by 3-cm-long balloon dilating catheter (Mansfield, Watertown, MA) is advanced over the guidewire and positioned to straddle the parietal pericardium. Precise localization of the balloon is confirmed by gentle inflation to identify a waist at the pericardial margin (Fig 15-9A). The balloon is inflated manually until the waist produced by the parietal pericardium disappears (Fig 15-9B).

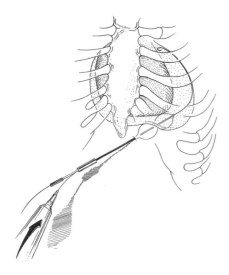

Figure 15-8 Schematic representation of PBP technique via the subxiphoid approach. Reprinted with permission from the American College of Cardiology (Ziskind AA, Pearce AC, Lemmon CC, et al. Journal of the American College of Cardiology, 1993, 21: 1–5).

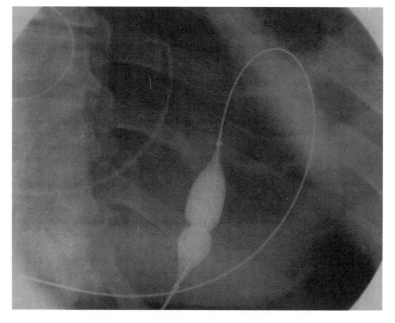

A

Figure 15-9 Anteroposterior fluoroscopic images (20 mL radiographic contrast has been instilled for illustrative purposes): (A) As the balloon is inflated manually, a waist is seen at the pericardial margin. (B) The waist disappears with full inflation of the balloon as the pericardial window is created.

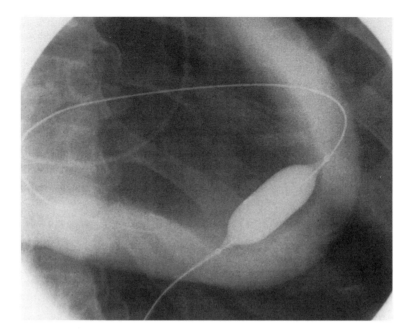

B

If the pericardium is apposed to the chest wall, as indicated by failure of the proximal portion of the balloon to expand, a countertraction technique can be used in which the catheter is gently advanced while the skin is pulled in the opposite direction to isolate the pericardium for dilatation (Fig 15-10).[26] The balloon-dilating catheter is then removed, leaving the 0.038" guidewire in the pericardial space. The pigtail catheter is then advanced over this guidewire and placed into the pericardial space.

The risk of cardiac injury during PBP is minimal because it requires successful pericardiocentesis before the dilating balloon is advanced. If the right ventricle were inadvertently entered and the balloon advanced, the results would be disastrous. For this reason, PBP should be performed only by operators who have extensive experience with pericardiocentesis.

After PBP, the pericardial catheter should be aspirated every 6 hours and flushed with heparin (5 ml, 100 u/ml). Pericardial drainage volumes should be recorded and the catheter removed when the volume is less than 100 ml/24 hr. Follow-up echocardiography and chest x-rays are performed within 24 to 48 hours after removal of the pericardial catheter and monthly to monitor for reaccumulation of pericardial fluid or development of a pleural effusion.

Patients with malignancy may be candidates for PBP if they have undergone prior pericardiocentesis and have either persistent drainage from the pericardial catheter (after 3 days continue to drain greater than 100 ml/24 hr) or

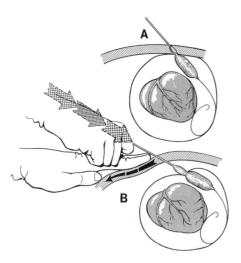

Figure 15-10 The countertraction technique to separate the pericardium from the adjacent chest wall (transverse view from below): **(A)** Initial trial inflation of the balloon demonstrates trapping of the proximal portion of the balloon within the chest wall structures. **(B)** Simultaneous traction on the skin and pushing of the balloon catheter results in displacement of the pericardium away from the chest wall, allowing proper inflation to occur. (Modified from Ziskind AA, Burstein S. Echocardiography vs. fluoroscopic imaging. Cathet Cardiovasc Diagn 1992; 27:86–88.)

have recurrent pericardial effusion after catheter removal. In addition, PBP may be offered as primary treatement at the time of initial pericardiocentesis when the clinical diagnosis of malignancy is clear. It remains unresolved whether PBP should be used for the treatment of nonmalignant pericardial disease.

Patients with uncorrectable platelet or coagulation abnormalities should be excluded. For this reason, PBP is not recommended for the treatment of uremic pericardial effusions or when coagulation parameters cannot be normalized (refractory coagulopathy, thrombocytopenia, or irreversible platelet dysfunction). Echocardiography must be performed prior to PBP to exclude the presence of loculated pericardial fluid. If pericardial fluid is not free-flowing, a surgical approach is preferable. Patients with marginal pulmonary reserve (e.g., after pneumonectomy or with a preexisting large pleural effusion) should be evaluated with caution, because most patients develop a left pleural effusion after PBP. If a left effusion is moderate or large before PBP, the chance of needing subsequent thoracentesis is increased. Patients with suspected bacterial or fungal pericardial infection should not undergo PBP due to the risk of spreading the infection.

The precise mechanism by which PBP works is not clear. Balloon inflation results in localized tearing of the parietal pericardial tissues, leading to a communication of the pericardial space with the pleural space and possibly the abdominal cavity. The use of a flexible fiberoptic pericardioscope introduced over a guidewire after PBP has revealed that the pericardial window freely communicates with the left pleural space (Fig 15-11).[27] Although a communication between the pericardial and pleural spaces is created, it is unlikely that this remains open indefinitely. It is possible that the early communication between pericardial and pleural spaces allows more complete internal drainage of the

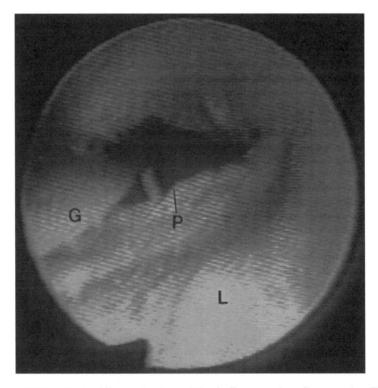

Figure 15-11   Pericardioscopic view of the balloon pericardiotomy site. The fiberoptic endoscope has been withdrawn over a guidewire to visualize the external pericardial surface. This figure demonstrates direct communication of the pericardial window with the left pleural space. G, guidewire; P, pericardial window created by balloon dilatation; L, lung in left pleural space immediately outside the pericardium.

pericardium than can be obtained with simple catheter drainage. By keeping the parietal and visceral pericardial surfaces apposed, autosclerosis can occur. Alternatively, PBP may trigger an inflammatory response that leads to sclerosis of the pericardial space.

Multicenter Percutaneous Balloon Pericardiotomy Registry

The technique of PBP has been studied in a multicenter registry to systematically evaluate the therapeutic efficacy and risks. Data on 130 patients undergoing PBP from 1987 to 1994 in 16 centers have been presented.[24,28] Clinical characteristics of the 130 patients are shown in Table 15-1.

Percutaneous balloon pericardiotomy was defined as successful if there was no recurrence of pericardial effusion on echocardiographic follow-up and if no complications occurred that required a surgical pericardial window. It was successful in 75 (87%) of 86 patients with no recurrences of pericardial effusion/tamponade during a mean follow-up of 5.1 months + 5.3 months.

Table 15-1 Clinical Characteristics of
130 PBP Registry Patients

Age (years, mean + SD)	58 + 13 (range 25–87)
Male/Female	68/62
Tamponade present	90 (69%)
Prior pericardiocentesis	75 (58%)
Clinical history	
Known malignancy	110 (85%)
Lung	55
Breast	21
Other malignancies	34
Nonmalignant	20 (15%)
Idiopathic	5
HIV disease	4
Postoperative trauma	4
Uremia	2
Renal transplant	1
Hypothyroidism	1
Congestive heart failure	1
Viral	1
Autoimmune	1

Three patients were considered failures due to pericardial bleeding and underwent surgical windowing. Eight patients had recurrence of pericardial effusion (mean time to recurrence 54 ± 65 days). Seven of those underwent surgical windowing, but four again recurred. Minor complications occurred in 11 (13%), the most frequent being fever. No patient had documented bacteremia or positive pericardial fluid cultures. Following PBP, thoracentesis or chest tube placement was required in 10 patients, seven of whom had preexisting pleural effusions.

Sixty-two (83%) of the 75 patients with a history of malignancy died, compared with 2 (13%) of 16 with nonmalignant disease. The mean survival for patients with a history of malignancy was 3.8 ± 3.3 months. No procedure-related variables were found to influence either survival or freedom from recurrence (e.g., number of sites dilated, visualization of free fluid exit, duration of catheter placement). There was no significant difference in recurrence rate whether PBP was performed as primary treatment (4 [11%] of 38) or after failed pericardiocentesis (7 [15%] of 48).

Surgical Therapies

When the etiology of the pericardial effusion is unclear based on pericardial fluid analysis and the patient has a projected survival that merits a more invasive approach, a surgical drainage procedure with sampling of the pericardium may be appropriate. Surgical procedures range from a simple subxiphoid pericardial window under local anesthesia, to a partial pericardiectomy, to a full pericardiectomy.[29-33]

Treatment Strategies

Studies comparing all the different treatment strategies for effusive pericardial disease are not only unavailable, but also virtually impossible to do, due to the relatively infrequent nature of the disease. Vaitkus et al. did a meta-analysis of prior studies in which treatment of malignant pericardial effusions was defined as successful if the patient survived the procedure, the symptoms did not recur, and no other interventions directed at the pericardium were required, regardless of the length of survival.[34] Success rates for the various treatments are shown in Figure 15-12. To a large extent, the treatment of recurrent pericardial effusions should be guided by institutional strengths and preferences.

Whether to perform PBP versus pericardiocentesis with or without sclerotherapy may also depend on both patient and institutional variables. Percutaneous balloon pericardiotomy should be considered when pericardial fluid recurs after primary pericardiocentesis. In those institutions with an aggressive approach toward malignant pericardial disease, this "less invasive" alternative to a surgical pericardial window may be considered for the primary treatment of malignant pericardial tamponade. In contrast, pericardiocentesis alone, without PBP at that time, is preferred first-line management when the etiology of pericardial fluid is unknown. Simple pericardiocentesis is also preferred when uremic platelet dysfunction or other coagulation abnormalities are present and

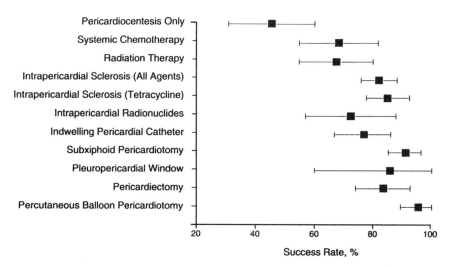

Figure 15-12 Success rates with 95% confidence intervals (indicated by bars) for different treatment modalities of malignant pericardial effusions. (From Vaitkus PT, Herrmann HC, LeWinter MM. Treatment of malignant pericardial effusion. JAMA 1994;272:63. Copyright 1994, American Medical Association.)

when there is the possibility of bacterial or fungal infection that could spread to the pleural space.

Constrictive Pericarditis

Constrictive pericardial disease is characterized by fibrosis of the pericardium. Although tuberculosis was the most frequent cause in the past, in the United States, the most frequent etiologies *now* are other inflammatory processes, particularly those with recurrent episodes. These include renal failure, recurrent idiopathic or viral pericarditis, malignant pericardial disease (especially after radiation therapy), autoimmune diseases, and following cardiac surgery or trauma when a hemorrhagic pericardial effusion has occurred.

In constrictive pericarditis, symptoms result from chronic elevation of biventricular filling pressures and impaired cardiac output. These include fatigue, exercise intolerance, poor appetite, dyspnea, and orthopnea. Marked jugular venous distension, hepatic engorgement, and peripheral edema are usual signs of full-blown pericardial constriction. Tachycardia may compensate initially for the decreased stroke volume; however, lethargy and cachexia are

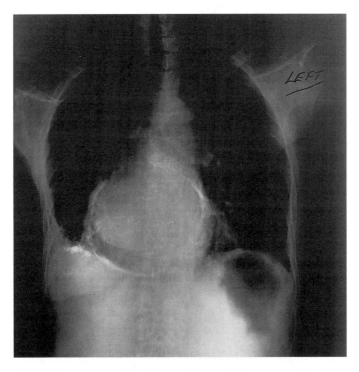

Figure 15-13 Anteroposterior chest radiograph demonstrating thick curvilinear calcification in a patient with a history of tuberculosis.

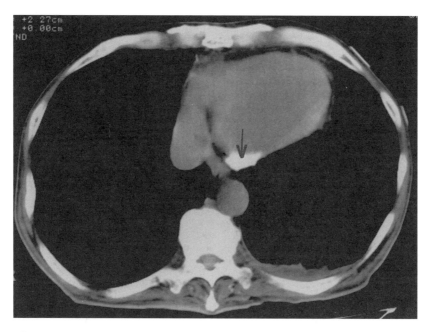

Figure 15-14   Computed tomography scan demonstrating pericardial thickening and calcification (arrow) around posterior margin of left ventricular free wall.

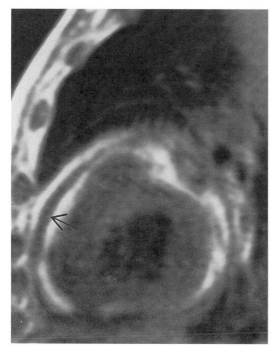

Figure 15-15   T1-weighted spin echo magnetic resonance image (sagittal section) demonstrating diffuse pericardial thickening (arrow).

observed as stroke volume declines to the point that increased heart rate cannot adequately compensate. Atrial fibrillation may be seen not uncommonly with chronic constriction.

Radiographically, calcification of the pericardium may be seen, particularly when the etiology is tuberculosis (Fig 15-13); however, the cardiac silhouette is not typically larger than normal. Echocardiography may show a thickened pericardium and an abrupt end to diastolic filling. Computed tomography (CT) and magnetic resonance imaging (MRI) may be helpful in demonstrating pericardial thickening (Figs 15-14 and 15-15).

Patients with suspected constrictive pericardial disease should undergo right and left heart catheterization to confirm the diagnosis, differentiate constrictive from restrictive disease, and exclude other or co-existing causes of elevated right atrial pressure.

Hemodynamic Findings

Although constrictive pericardial disease may occasionally be a focal process, it more often involves all cardiac chambers. The diagnosis is made by simultaneously recording right and left ventricular pressures, optimally with identical catheters to ensure similar damping and resonance. Severe pulmonary hypertension is uncommon with constrictive disease. The tracings reveal elevation and equalization (within 5 mm Hg) of right and left ventricular mid-diastolic pressures (Fig 15-16). Inducing premature ventricular contractions usually uncouples the diastolic pressures of the right and left ventricles. If uncoupling does not occur, constriction should be considered. Diastolic pressures are usually greater than one third of right ventricular systolic pressure.[35] Because the constrictive process limits expansion of ventricular volume, most of the filling occurs in early diastole. Ventricular filling is rapid due to elevation of atrial pressure, but stops abruptly, leading to the characteristic dip and plateau or square root sign. The rapid filling results in a prominent y descent in the right atrial waveform. As atrial systole occurs against a ventricle with limited capacity, a prominent a wave is present. This is followed by a prominent x descent. The prominent x and y descents lead to the characteristic M configuration (Fig 15-17).

As constriction becomes more severe, the negative intrapleural pressure during inspiration is not transmitted to the ventricular chambers. This results in loss of respiratory variation in right atrial pressure. Kussmaul's sign, a rise in right atrial and central venous pressures with inspiration, can be seen when constriction is severe.[35]

Occasional constriction patients who have undergone rigorous diuresis may have low or normal filling pressures. Hemodynamics suggestive of constrictive physiology may be evoked by the rapid infusion of 1.0 to 1.5 liters of saline.[36]

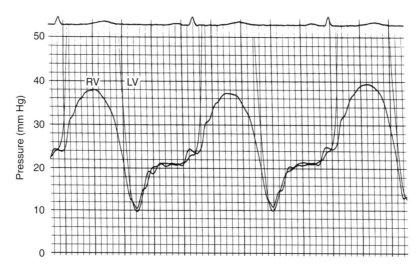

Figure 15-16   Pericardial constriction. Simultaneous right (RV) and left ventricular (LV) pressure measurement demonstrates elevation and equalization of diastolic pressures.

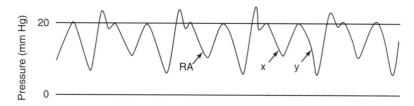

Figure 15-17   Pericardial constriction. Right atrial waveform reveals prominent x and y descents with a characteristic M configuration.

Angiographic Findings

With pericardial constriction, systolic function is typically preserved, but left ventriculography demonstrates a marked reduction in end-diastolic volume and an abrupt diastolic relaxation pattern. Although it is rare for constrictive processes to impinge on the coronary arteries,[37] older patients should undergo coronary angiography if surgical pericardiectomy is anticipated so that simultaneous treatment of coronary disease can be performed, if appropriate.

Differentiation of Constriction from Restrictive Cardiomyopathy

It is important to distinguish constrictive states from restrictive disease in which a myocardial process interferes with diastolic filling. Restrictive processes due to, for example, amyloidosis or hemochromatosis may present with similar clinical findings.

Obtaining simultaneous right and left ventricular pressures may help to distinguish constrictive from restrictive processes. Because restriction involves a myocardial process, and the left ventricle may have a larger myocardial mass involvement, left ventricular diastolic pressures are usually greater than the right. Rarely, an infiltrating process involves the right ventricle more than the left, with a consequently higher right than left ventricular diastolic pressure. This finding is in contrast to constriction in which the constrictive process is transmitted equally to all chambers regardless of muscle mass, leading to equally elevated biventricular filling pressures.[38] Maneuvers such as fluid loading, exercise, or unloading with nitroglycerin or nitroprusside may increase the separation of right and left ventricular diastolic pressures. Pulmonary hypertension is more common in restrictive disease than in constriction. Typically, the stroke volume is relatively *decreased* due to the inability of the ventricle to dilate. In the early phases of constriction, an increase in heart rate will maintain the cardiac output. As the disease progresses, stroke volume will fall further and the cardiac output will not be *maintained,* despite sinus tachycardia.

When hemodynamic measurements are not helpful in distinguishing constrictive from restrictive processes, myocardial biopsy should be considered as a means to identify an *infiltrative* process. Newer imaging modalities, such as gated MRI or cine-CT, may identify pericardial thickening that would suggest a constrictive process. In occasional patients, thoracotomy may be necessary to evaluate the pericardium, with stripping performed at that time if the pericardium is abnormal.

Effusive-Constrictive Pericarditis

Successful pericardiocentesis for effusive pericardial disease should restore intrapericardial pressure to zero. When pericardial and right atrial pressures remain elevated, the diagnosis of effusive-constrictive disease must be considered. These patients typically demonstrate a mixed picture, with components of effusion under pressure as well as constriction.[39] To make the diagnosis, hemodynamic measurements before and after pericardiocentesis are essential.

Typically, initial hemodynamics suggest tamponade with elevation and equalization of pericardial, atrial, and ventricular end-diastolic pressures. The right atrial waveform demonstrates loss of Y descent. Following withdrawal of pericardial fluid, intrapericardial pressure becomes zero, but right atrial pressure remains elevated and assumes a pattern suggestive of constriction with a prominent Y descent. The right ventricular waveform may assume a dip-and-plateau configuration.

Adjunctive Techniques for the Diagnosis of Pericardial Disease

Although patients may have a history of malignancy, it has been shown that only 50% of such patients have malignancy as the etiology of their pericardial effusion.[7,40,41] Although pericardial fluid cytology may aid in the diagnosis, PBP suffers from the limitation that pericardial tissue is not obtained for pathologic analysis as it would be if a surgical pericardial window were performed. To address this need, a percutaneously introduced pericardial bioptome has been successful in providing diagnostic quality tissue.[42] At the present time, this technique is considered investigational.

Percutaneous pericardial biopsy is performed after successful placement of a pericardial catheter. The catheter is then withdrawn over the 0.035-in guidewire and an 8-Fr 23-cm-long percutaneous vascular introducer is inserted into the pericardial space. The distal tip of the sheath is positioned 5 to 7 cm within the pericardial margin. Under fluoroscopic guidance, a bioptome is inserted so that the jaws protrude 1 cm beyond the tip of the sheath. The jaws are

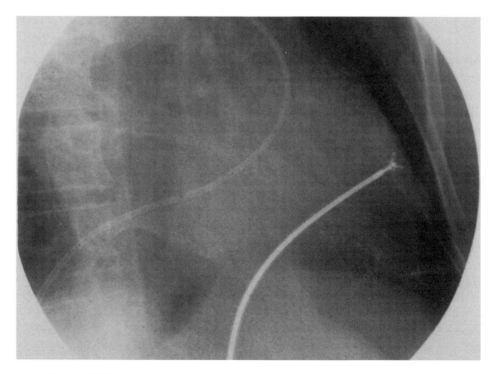

Figure 15-18 Anteroposterior fluoroscopic image of the pericardial bioptome being directed toward the posterolateral surface of the parietal pericardium.

Figure 15-19 The pericardial bioptome with center needle and aggressive serrated jaw configuration.

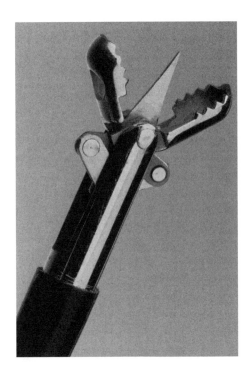

opened and the bioptome is withdrawn until resistance is felt, indicating contact with the distal tip of the sheath. Then the sheath and bioptome are advanced as a unit to biopsy the posterolateral portion of the parietal pericardium (Fig 15-18). Samples are best obtained with a bioptome consisting of an 8-Fr system with center needle and aggressive serrated jaws mounted on a stiff 80-cm shaft (Fig 15-19) (Mansfield/Boston Scientific Corporation, Watertown, MA).

Summary

The evaluation and treatment of pericardial disease require an integrated clinical approach that involves a high index of suspicion for its presence, good noninvasive imaging, and careful hemodynamic assessment before and after treatment.

SELECTED READINGS

1. Hoit B, Dalton N, Bhargava V, Shabetai R. Pericardial influences on right and left ventricular filling dynamics. Circ Res 1991;68:197–208.
2. Gilbert JC, Glantz SA. Determinants of ventricular filling and of the diastolic pressure-volume relation. Circ Res 1989;64:827–852.
3. Ringertz HG, Misbach GA, Tyberg JV. Effect of the normal pericardium on the left ventricular diastolic pressure-volume relationship. Acta Radiol 1981;22:529–534.
4. Ross JJ. Acute displacement of the diastolic pressure-volume curve of the left ventricle: role of the pericardium and the right ventricle. Circulation 1979;59:32–37.
5. Brown J, MacKinnon D, King A, Vanderbush E. Elevated arterial blood pressure in cardiac tamponade. N Engl J Med 1992;327:463–466.
6. Antman E, Cargill V, Grossman W. Low-pressure cardiac tamponade. Ann Intern Med 1979;91:403–406.
7. Krikorian JG, Hancock EW. Pericardiocentesis. Am J Med 1978;65:808–814.
8. Guberman B, Fowler N, Engel P, et al. Cardiac tamponade in medical patients. Circulation 1981;64:633–640.
9. Gascho JA, Martins JB, Marcus ML, Kerber RE. Effects of volume expansion and vasodilators in acute pericardial tamponade. Report: The American Physiological Society, The Cardiovascular Center, University of Iowa Hospital, 1981.
10. Callahan JA, Seward JB, Nishimura RA, et al. Two-dimensional echocardiographically guided pericardiocentesis: experience in 117 consecutive patients. Am J Cardiol 1985;55:476–479.
11. Gatenby RA, Hartz WH, Kessler HB. Percutaneous catheter drainage for malignant pericardial effusion. J Vasc Interv Radiol 1991;2:151–155.
12. Pandian NG, Brockway B, Simonetti J, et al. Pericardiocentesis under two-dimensional echocardiographic guidance in loculated pericardial effusion. Ann Thorac Surg 1988;45:99–100.
13. Markiewicz W, Borovik R, Ecker S. Cardiac tamponade in medical patients: treatment and prognosis in the echocardiographic era. Am Heart J 1986;111:1138–1142.
14. Flannery EP, Gregoratos G, Corder MP. Pericardial effusions in patients with malignant diseases. Arch Intern Med 1975;135:976–977.
15. Kopecky SL, Callahan JA, Tajik AJ, Seward JB. Percutaneous pericardial catheter drainage: report of 42 consecutive cases. Am J Cardiol 1986;58:633–635.
16. Patel AK, Kosolcharoen PK, Nallasivan M, et al. Catheter drainage of the pericardium. Practical method to maintain long-term patency. Chest 1987;92:1018–1021.
17. Lock JE, Bass JL, Kulik TJ, Fuhrman BP. Chronic percutaneous pericardial drainage with modified pigtail catheters in children. Am J Cardiol 1984;53:1179–1182.
18. Erdman S, Levinsky L, Deviri E, Levy MJ. Closed pericardial drainage for relief of pericardial tamponade. Thorac Cardiovasc Surg 1986;34:66–67.
19. Shepherd FA, Morgan C, Evans WK, et al. Medical management of malignant pericardial effusion by tetracycline sclerosis. Am J Cardiol 1987;60:1161–1166.
20. Davis S, Sharma SM, Blumberg ED, Kim CS. Intrapericardial tetracycline for the management of cardiac tamponade secondary to malignant pericardial effusion. N Engl J Med 1978;299:1113–1114.
21. Abubakar S, Malik I, Ali SM, Khan A. Management of malignant pericardial effusion with tetracycline induced pericardiodesis. Jpma J Pak Med Assoc 1991;41:20–22.
22. Van Belle SJP, Volckaert A, Taeymans Y, et al. Treatment of malignant pericardial tamponade with sclerosis induced by instillation of bleomycin. Int J Cardiol 1987;16:155–160.
23. Palacios IF, Tuzcu EM, Ziskind AA, et al. Percutaneous balloon pericardial window for patients with malignant pericardial effusion and tamponade. Cathet Cardiovasc Diagn 1991;22:244–249.

24. Ziskind AA, Pearce AC, Lemmon CC, et al. Percutaneous balloon pericardiotomy for the treatment of cardiac tamponade and large pericardial effusions: description of technique and report of the first 50 cases. J Am Coll Cardiol 1993;21:1–5.

25. Ziskind AA, Rodriguez S, Lemmon CC, et al. Percutaneous balloon pericardiotomy for the treatment of effusive pericardial disease—104 patient follow-up. J Am Coll Cardiol 1994;23:274A.

26. Ziskind AA, Burstein S. Echocardiography vs. fluoroscopic imaging. Cathet Cardiovasc Diagn 1992;27:86–88.

27. Ziskind AA, Pearce AC, Lemmon CC, et al. Feasibility of percutaneous pericardial biopsy and pericardioscopy as an adjunct to balloon pericardiotomy for the diagnosis and treatment of pericardial disease. J Am Coll Cardiol 1992;19:267A.

28. Ziskind A, Lemmon C, Rodriguez S, et al. Final report of the percutaneous balloon pericardiotomy registry for the treatment of effusive pericardial disease. Circulation 1994;90:I-121.

29. Fontanelle LJ, Cuello L, Dooley BN. Subxyphoid pericardial window: a simple and safe method for diagnosing and treating acute and chronic pericardial effusions. J Thorac Cardiovasc Surg 1971;62:95–97.

30. Santos GH, Frater RWM. The subxiphoid approach in the treatment of pericardial effusion. Ann Thorac Surg 1977;23:467–470.

31. Palatianos GM, Thurer RJ, Kaiser GA. Comparison of effectiveness and safety of operations on the pericardium. Chest 1985;88:30–33.

32. Palatianos GM, Thurer RJ, Pompeo MQ, Kaiser GA. Clinical experience with subxiphoid drainage of pericardial effusions. Ann Thorac Surg 1989;48:381–385.

33. Little AG, Kremser PC, Wade JL, et al. Operation for diagnosis and treatment of pericardial effusions. Surgery 1984;96:738–744.

34. Vaitkus PT, Herrmann HC, LeWinter MM. Treatment of malignant pericardial effusion. JAMA 1994;272:59–64.

35. Shabetai R, Fowler N, Guntheroth WG. The hemodynamics of cardiac tamponade and constrictive pericarditis. Am J Cardiol 1970;26:480–489.

36. Bush CA, Stang JM, Wooley CF, Kilman JW. Occult constrictive pericardial disease: diagnosis by rapid volume expansion and correction by pericardiectomy. Circulation 1977;56:924–930.

37. Goldberg E, Stein J, Berger M, Berdoff R. Diastolic segmental coronary artery obliteration in constrictive pericarditis. Cathet Cardiovasc Diagn 1981;7:197–202.

38. Shabetai R, Fowler N, Fenton J. Restrictive cardiac disease. Pericarditis and the myocardiopathies. Am Heart J 1965;69:271–286.

39. Hancock E. Subacute effusive-constrictive pericarditis. Circulation 1971;43:183–192.

40. Mills SA, Julian S, Holliday RH, et al. Subxiphoid pericardial window for pericardial disease. J Cardiovasc Surg 1989;30:768–773.

41. Goudie RB. Secondary tumors of the heart and pericardium. Br Heart J 1955;17:183–188.

42. Ziskind AA, Rodriguez S, Lemmon CC, Burstein S. Percutaneous pericardial biopsy as an adjunctive technique for the diagnosis of pericardial disease. Am J Cardiol 1994;74:288–291.

16

INVASIVE EVALUATION OF CORONARY ARTERY DISEASE

Andrew P. Chodos
Alice K. Jacobs

T
HE MOST IMPORTANT reason to confirm the diagnosis and characterize the extent of coronary artery disease is our increasing ability to modify its natural history by decreasing morbid events and death through medical, interventional, and surgical approaches. Coronary artery disease exacts heavy psychological and financial costs. The chronic and often progressive nature of the disease results in life-long treatment with all of its implications. Failure to adequately secure the diagnosis may lead to unwarranted patient morbidity, inefficient care, and patient dissatisfaction. This chapter reviews current approaches, particularly invasive strategies, to characterize coronary disease.

Evaluation of the Patient with Chest Pain

Outpatient Evaluation of Chest Pain and Other Symptoms of Myocardial Ischemia

Chest "pain" or "pressure" is the most common presenting symptom of myocardial ischemia. It may be classified as "typical" for myocardial ischemia (i.e., angina pectoris) if it is provoked by stress, either physical or emotional, is visceral in quality, is of short (<15 min) but definite (>30 sec) duration, and is relieved by sublingual nitroglycerin or removal of the provoking stimulus. The great majority (~90%) of patients with typical angina pectoris have significant obstructive coronary disease (>50%–70% diameter stenosis of at least one epicardial coronary vessel by coronary arteriography). Patients who have "atypical" angina pectoris, but in whom the treating physician concludes it is cardiac in origin, have an intermediate probability (~50%) of having significant coronary disease at catheterization. Examples of atypical presentations include dyspnea on exertion (not felt to be pulmonary in origin) that is promptly relieved by rest or visceral chest pain primarily at rest. Patients who have atypical chest pain

Table 16-1   Conditions to Consider in the Differential Diagnosis of Chest Pain

Syndrome	*Distinguishing characteristics*
Myocardial ischemia	Visceral chest pain, ST-T changes usual
Aortic dissection	Frequently sudden onset; severe, tearing chest pain, radiates to back; hypertensive patient
Pulmonary embolism	Dyspnea prominent, frequently sudden onset, often pleuritic chest pain, tachycardia, oxygen desaturation
Spontaneous pneumothorax	Pleuritic chest pain, absent breath sounds over affected area
Chest wall syndrome	Pain reproduced by palpation of chest or upper body parts
Chest wall twinge syndrome	Very common, brief (seconds), nonexertional pain, dramatically worse with deep inspiration, better with shallow breaths, relieved with popping sensation
Costochondritis (Tietze's syndrome)	Tenderness in junction of rib and sternum
Pneumonia with pleuritis	Pain usually varies with respiration, tubular breath sounds
Epidemic pleurodynia (Bornholm's disease, devil's grip)	Frequently severe pain similar to myocardial infarction, sometimes associated with upper respiratory symptoms, headache common, friction rub in 25%
Pericarditis	Frequently associated with pleuritic pain and viral syndrome, may improve by sitting forward, characteristic evolving electrocardiographic pattern
Esophagitis	"Heart burn," history of reflux may be exacerbated by swallowing or some foods
Pneumonia	Cough, leukocytosis, fever, auscultatory/chest x-ray findings
Abdominal conditions	For all abdominal conditions, look for associated symptoms and physical exam important
Peptic ulcer	Pain on empty stomach, relieved by food
Gastritis	Clinical setting important
Acute cholecysitis	Pain radiates to back, fatty foods precipitate
Pancreatitis	Clinical setting, abnormal abdominal exam, elevated amylase and/or bilirubin

that is believed by the physician not to be angina have a low probability (10%–20%) of having angiographic coronary disease.

Coronary angiography is performed in the high-probability group primarily to define the coronary anatomy, in the intermediate-probability group to diagnose the presence of coronary disease as well as determine its extent, and in the low-probability group to rule out coronary disease in patients in whom noninvasive tests are equivocal. The refinement of several noninvasive tests to determine myocardial ischemia (e.g., exercise, adenosine, dipyridamole, or dobutamine thallium scintigraphy, or echocardiography) allows patients to be further characterized as to the significance of the coronary lesions.

The evaluation of chest pain in the ambulatory patient may include diagnostic evaluation of all or some of the conditions listed in Table 16-1. A discussion of the workup of these conditions is beyond the scope of this chapter. The order of the workup (i.e., cardiac or noncardiac) is usually determined by the physician's level of suspicion of significant coronary disease.

Emergency Room Evaluation of Chest Pain

The emergency room evaluation for cardiac chest pain must exclude all major life-threatening conditions (see Table 16-1). These include pulmonary embolism, aortic dissection, and spontaneous tension pneumothorax as well as myocardial ischemia. These diagnoses should be considered in all patients presenting to the emergency room with chest pain, particularly if the pain is severe, persistent, or associated with hemodynamic compromise. A normal ECG should alert the clinician to the possibility of alternate life-threatening conditions rather than myocardial ischemia. However, a normal ECG does not exclude the diagnosis of ischemia. Patients with a critical stenosis in the posterior coronary circulation (left circumflex) may present without diagnostic electrocardiographic changes due to the relatively "electrically silent" nature of posterior ischemia. Patients with intermittent chest pain without diagnostic ST changes between attacks should have a 12-lead ECG recorded during pain because of the dynamic nature of ST segment changes from ischemia.

The pain associated with pulmonary embolism is quite variable, ranging from mild to severe, and may be confused with ischemic pain. Patients usually have the sudden onset of dyspnea or pain that can be located anywhere within the chest. The pain ranges from mild to severe and is often pleuritic in nature. The most common physical findings in pulmonary embolism are tachycardia and tachypnea. Cardiac examination may reveal a prominent pulmonic valve closure sound or a right ventricular heave. Pulmonary examination may reveal wheezing or rales, but is frequently unremarkable. Massive embolism and pulmonary infarction may present with acute right heart failure and shock due to the acute afterload mismatch. Arterial pO_2 is typically decreased. The ECG usually shows a sinus tachycardia and not uncommonly, new right axis deviation manifesting an S1, Q3, and T3 pattern. If the etiology of the chest pain in the patient in the emergency room remains uncertain and pulmonary embolism is a consideration, a ventilation/perfusion scan should be performed.

Aortic dissection should be considered in all patients who present with the sudden onset of severe, tearing back or retrosternal pain. Other than severe distress and diaphoresis, the physical examination may be unremarkable, as may be the ECG. Physical findings, when present, may reflect either proximal or distal extension of the dissection. Proximal extension can result in the disruption of a coronary ostium, most commonly the right coronary artery, resulting in the electrocardiographic appearance of acute inferior myocardial infarction (MI). In this situation, the aortic dissection may be difficult to diagnose because the symptoms of MI predominate and the chest pain from dissection is mistaken for that of acute MI. For this reason, it is imperative that all patients presenting to the emergency room with unexplained chest pain have BP checked in both arms and pulses documented in all distributions. Proximal propagation of aortic dissection can also lead to acute aortic insufficiency or hemopericardium. A diastolic murmur should alert the clinician to this diagnostic possibility. Distal extension of an aortic dissection may present with asymmetric limb BP measurements or unilateral loss of pulses. Focal neurologic findings may also occur due to ischemia in an affected region of the CNS. Aortic dissection may be diagnosed by transesophageal echocardiography, computerized tomographic angiography, or magnetic resonance angiography, which has largely supplanted contrast angiography. The diagnostic modality of choice is often determined by the study with the shortest time delay and the level of local institutional clinical expertise in one study or the other. Coronary arteriography may be useful preoperatively to elucidate coronary anatomy. However, the emergent nature of this problem often requires expeditious definitive surgical therapy.

Patients presenting with a spontaneous pneumothorax often have the sudden onset of sharp, pleuritic chest pain and may develop severe dyspnea and/or shock if there is a tension pneumothorax. The diagnosis is made by auscultation of unilaterally absent breath sounds in the setting of a chest x-ray showing absent lung markings and a mediastinal shift.

The Physical Examination in Coronary Artery Disease

The physical examination is usually unimpressive in patients with chest pain from coronary disease. Physical examination is most useful in diagnosing other conditions causing pain (as previously noted) or in findings related to the effect of ischemia or infarction (e.g., ischemically mediated mitral regurgitation). Patients presenting to the emergency room with acute, severe chest pain should have a rapid directed examination. The examination should include BP measurement in both arms, characterization of pulses (radial, brachial, carotid, femoral, dorsalis pedis, and posterior tibialis), the presence of bruits in the carotid and femoral locations, carotid and jugular venous waveform analysis, heart sounds including systolic murmurs (ischemic mitral regurgitation, aortic stenosis), diastolic murmur (e.g., from aortic dissection), and second heart sound. Pulmonary examination should evaluate the presence of alveolar congestion (rales) and exclude important pulmonary causes for chest pain (see Table 16-1). Likewise, the abdominal examination should exclude any acute conditions that might account for the symptoms of chest pain. Signs of an acute abdomen or abdominal aneurysm should be specifically evaluated. Lower extremity examination should assess the presence of edema, signs of phlebitis or peripheral vascular disease, and the relative state of systemic perfusion.

Laboratory Examination of Ischemic Heart Disease

The ECG and chest x-ray are the primary tests to assess the patient with acute and severe chest pain. The electrocardiographic findings of ischemia (focal ST-T changes), pericarditis (diffuse ST-T changes), or acute right heart strain consistent with pulmonary embolism are useful findings. Noncardiac causes of chest pain may be diagnosed radiographically. Unilateral absence of lung markings (pneumothorax) and a wide mediastinum (aortic dissection) are useful x-ray findings. Other laboratory studies that may be useful include a WBC count with a shift to the left (bacterial pneumonia) or arterial desaturation (pulmonary embolism, pneumonia). In most emergency rooms, creatinine phosphokinase isoenzymes are of limited value in the diagnosis of infarction either because of the short duration of symptoms or ischemia without necrosis. Newer tests (e.g., CK-MB isoenzymes) may allow for earlier detection of myocardial necrosis in the emergency room diagnosis of acute MI.[1]

Provocative Noninvasive Testing in the Evaluation of Chest Pain

Stress testing to provoke evidence of regional myocardial ischemia is an important aspect of evaluation in determining the presence and severity of myocardial ischemia. It is particularly important in defining the probability of significant coronary disease in stable outpatients and in inpatients with a recent MI or "stabilized" unstable angina pectoris. Recently, provocative studies have been utilized within the first 24 hours in "low-risk" patients in an outpatient emergency room setting. The most commonly utilized stress test employs exercise to increase myocardial oxygen demand. Evidence of ischemia may be diagnosed by the development of chest pain, electrocardiographic ST-T changes, radionuclide redistribution (sestamibi, thallium), or left ventricular (LV) echocardiographic wall motion abnormalities. The method used to document ischemia depends in part on the status of the ST-T configuration on the resting

ECG, the type of information being sought, and the expertise of a given institution in performing the study. Patients with abnormal baseline ST-T wave segments, such as those with LV hypertrophy or patients taking digoxin, will frequently have nondiagnostic electrocardiographic changes with exercise and should therefore have some form of myocardial imaging performed with exercise. Myocardial imaging also may be employed if ischemia in a specific vascular territory is sought, for example, when trying to identify a "culprit" vessel in the setting of multivessel disease.

Pharmacologic agents may be employed to create supply-demand imbalance. These tests can be divided into those that increase myocardial oxygen demand (dobutamine) and those that act to increase the relative discrepancies in supply that exist between areas supplied by normal and stenosed coronary arteries (dipyridamole, adenosine). Regardless of the agent used, all pharmacologic provocations utilize an imaging modality in addition to standard electrocardiographic recording. These tests are most frequently employed in patients who are unable to exercise and who require some objective assessment of ischemia or as a second study to rule in or out coronary disease when the first study has equivocal results.

The most common indication for stress testing is to secure the diagnosis of coronary artery disease. The utility and accuracy of these tests is strongly related to the pre-test likelihood that coronary artery disease is present. Bayes' theorem suggests that patients with a very low or very high pre-test likelihood of coronary artery disease will have little additional diagnostic benefit from the stress test results. In such patients, a result opposite of that expected is more likely to be either a false-positive or a false-negative finding. For this reason, the diagnostic utility of stress testing is greatest in those patients with an intermediate pre-test suspicion of coronary artery disease.

Stress testing is particularly useful in estimating prognosis in patients with known or suspected coronary artery disease. Patients with coronary artery disease have a very wide range of probabilities of adverse outcomes. Stress test parameters including the duration of exercise, maximum rate-pressure product, and the extent and duration of ischemia are all used to identify high- and low-risk subgroups. High-risk stress test results include ischemia at a low workload (occurring ≤ stage 2 of the Bruce protocol), widespread ischemia (multiple leads with ST depression or abnormal thallium redistribution in two or more perfusion regions), severe ischemia (> than 2 mm of ST depression), hypotension during the stress test, prolonged ischemia (chest pain or ST changes lasting > 6 min into recovery), transmural ischemia (ST elevation in the absence of Q waves), or signs of LV dysfunction (increased thallium pulmonary uptake in the absence of severely reduced LV function at rest). Patients manifesting any of these findings after exercise are at higher risk for left main and multivessel disease. A patient exercising for 12 minutes who develops chest pain late in the protocol with only 1 mm of ST depression in two leads has an excellent long-term prognosis. Conversely, the patient who develops chest pain early in the protocol at a low rate-pressure product with electrocardiographic evidence of widespread ischemia has a much less favorable prognosis. This type of information then can be used to tailor therapy.

A third major indication for stress testing is to aid in the decision to perform revascularization. Angiography provides a coronary "road map" but does not provide information regarding the functional significance of a given lesion. In situations in which the angiogram and clinical presentation are not congruent (e.g., minimal symptoms, high-grade proximal lesion), a stress test may be employed to provide objective evidence of ischemia or myocardial viability. Other examples of this application of stress testing are in determining the significance of borderline angiographic lesions and myocardial viability in regions of abnormal dysfunction. This information then facilitates selection of the most appropriate treatment strategy.

Finally, a stress test *after* a revascularization procedure, either coronary bypass or percutaneous intervention, may be used as a baseline for long-term noninvasive follow-up.

Coronary Angiography in the Evaluation of Coronary Disease

Coronary angiography is the gold standard for diagnosing coronary disease, estimating long-term prognosis, and determining the preferred treatment strategy.[2] The most effective use of coronary angiography requires an understanding of its limitations and strengths. Studies evaluating coronary arteries with intravascular ultrasound (see Chapter 19), angioscopy (see Chapter 21), and functional angiometry (see Chapter 20) have emphasized that the angiogram is a *luminogram*. It is inadequate to characterize the vessel wall (as is possible with intravascular ultrasound), the endoluminal surface (as may be observed with angioscopy), and any blood flow limitation (which may be determined by angiometry). Older pathologic studies and more recent intravascular ultrasound studies have demonstrated that many angiographically normal or "reference" segments have atherosclerotic disease.[3,4] As such, areas of angiographic luminal narrowing are often underestimated.

Coronary angiography is a two-dimensional representation of a three-dimensional structure (see Chapter 7). Vessel foreshortening and misrepresentation of eccentric lesions are two angiographic manifestations of this problem.[5,6] These problems are partially overcome by obtaining orthogonal projections of each vessel. Vessel tortuosity and overlap can limit the accurate interpretation of coronary angiograms. Percent stenosis measured angiographically continues to guide most clinical decisions regarding coronary disease, but this measurement does not always predict the physiologic significance of a lesion.[6] Dynamic coronary vasomotion plays an important role in many clinical syndromes, but is poorly studied during routine angiography.

Despite the invasive nature of cardiac catheterization, the procedure is relatively safe in the hands of a skilled operator (see Chapters 6 and 7). Patient subgroups with multiple risk factors for catheterization-related complications must have this information factored into the decision of whether to perform the procedure. Unfortunately, patients deemed to be at greatest risk for angiography-related complications are frequently the very same patients who most require the collection of catheterization data to be properly managed. For example, patients who have left main disease diagnosed at catheterization have a 10- to 20-fold increase in procedural risk.[7-9] At the same time, they are the subgroup that has the greatest benefit from bypass surgery. In general, if a patient is an acceptable revascularization candidate (either with bypass surgery or a percutaneous procedure), the risk of catheterization, even if substantial, should not preclude the procedure.

The strengths and limitations of coronary angiography are reflected in the American College of Cardiology/American Heart Association guidelines for cardiac angiography. The indications for cardiac catheterization designated as class I, II, or III conform to the most recently published version of these guidelines (Table 16-2).

Several specific patient subgroups in which coronary angiography is especially useful in diagnosing coronary artery disease include the following: (1) patients with recurrent symptoms of chest pain with a nondiagnostic stress test result; (2) patients with frequent hospital admissions or disabling symptoms despite a negative stress test; (3) patients with rest pain without electrocardiographic changes, in whom stress testing is considered unsafe and contraindicated;, and (4) young patients (< 35 years old) recovering from an acute MI in whom confirmation of the diagnosis and exclusion of unusual causes of infarction are important.

Determining prognosis and communicating it to the patient are central to good medical practice. Angiographic data, particularly LV systolic function and

Table 16-2   American College of Cardiology/American Heart Association Indications for Coronary Angiography

Class I	Conditions for which there is general agreement that coronary angiography is justified
Class II	Conditions for which coronary angiography is frequently performed, but there is a divergence of opinion with respect to its justification in terms of value and appropriateness
Class III	Conditions for which there is general agreement that coronary angiography is not ordinarily justified

extent of coronary artery disease, are important in delineating low- and high-risk patient subgroups in patients with stable coronary disease. Patients with single-vessel coronary artery disease or normal LV systolic function, as a group, have a favorable prognosis compared with those patients with multivessel disease and/or reduced LV function.[10]

The prognostic value of angiography also has been demonstrated in stable postinfarction patients. In one study, stable postinfarction patients who underwent angiography soon after their event revealed that LV function and extent of disease were predictors of 5-year event-free survival (Fig 16-1).[11] The prognostic value of other data obtained at catheterization, such as lesion morphology and percent stenosis, has also been evaluated. Although certain morphologies have been associated with acute coronary syndromes,[12] the ability to predict future events from this knowledge remains uncertain.

Although lesion morphology has an uncertain prognostic role, it clearly impacts on revascularization decision making. The American College of Cardiology/American Heart Association Committee on Percutaneous Transluminal Coronary Angioplasty (PTCA) has published guidelines for the performance of coronary angioplasty. Lesions are divided into three groups, depending on expected success and complication rates (Table 16-3).[13] Although these guidelines are imperfect and have been challenged, they provide a basis for procedural risk assessment and consequently patient selection for percutaneous revascularization. Additionally, the choice of revascularization method (angioplasty vs. coronary bypass grafting) is dependent on the quality of the distal vessels (e.g., diffuseness of disease, quality of the run-off) and the extent and complexity of the coronary lesions. In general, in patients with extensive disease and greater lesion complexity, bypass surgery is often the procedure of choice. Revascularization strategy continues to evolve as newer percutaneous devices that successfully treat more extensive and complex coronary anatomy become available and experience with them grows.

The number of vessels with a significant (>50% diameter narrowing) lesion has proven to be a durable predictor of prognosis. Several clinical trials have demonstrated that with increasing numbers of vessels with significant disease there is a concomitant worsening of survival. The location of the most severe stenosis, which has an intuitive appeal as a predictor of future ischemic events, has not been helpful in pinpointing the location of subsequent occlusion.[14] In one study, moderate stenoses, often less than 60% diameter narrowing, were more commonly the site of eventual acute occlusion than were more severe stenoses. Plaque rupture, the presumed mechanism leading to MI, is probably more closely related to lesion composition and geometry rather than the severity of stenosis. Angiography does not provide information on lesion composition, which may explain its inability to predict the location of future occlusions.

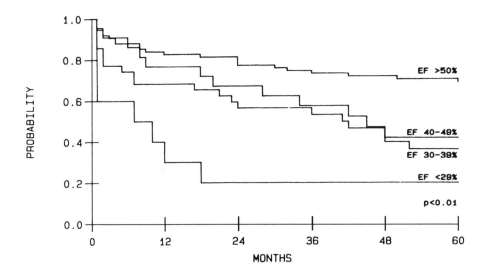

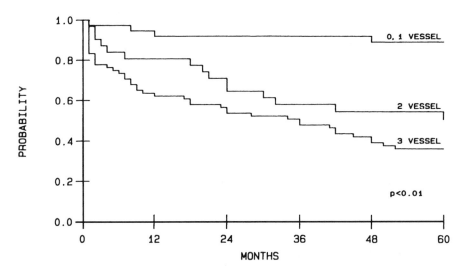

Figure 16-1 Relationship between LV ejection fraction or number of diseased vessels and event-free survival in postinfarction patients. Nonfatal MI and coronary artery bypass surgery are considered events. (Top panel) Patients with a depressed ejection fraction had the lowest probability of an event-free survival. (Lower panel) Patients with two- and three-vessel disease had a lower probability of an event-free survival than patients with single-vessel disease. (Reproduced with permission from the American College of Cardiology [Schulman ST, Achuf SC, Griffith LS, et al. Journal of the American College of Cardiology, 1988, 11, 1164–1172].)

Table 16-3   Lesion-Specific Characteristics of Type A, B, and C Lesions

Type A lesions (minimally complex)
   Discrete (length < 10 mm)
   Concentric
   Readily accessible
   Nonangulated segment (<45 degrees)
   Smooth contour
   Little or no calcification
   Less than totally occlusive
   Not ostial in location
   No major side branch involvement
   Absence of thrombus
Type B lesions (moderately complex) *
   Tubular (length 10–20 mm)
   Eccentric
   Moderate tortuosity of proximal segment
   Moderately angulated segment (>45 degrees, <90 degrees)
   Irregular contour
   Moderate or heavy calcification
   Total occlusions < 3 mo old
   Ostial in location
   Bifurcation lesions requiring double guidewires
   Some thrombus present
Type C lesions (severely complex)
   Diffuse (length > 2 cm)
   Excessive tortuosity of proximal segment
   Extremely angulated segments (> 90 degrees)
   Total occlusions > 3 mo old and/or bridging collaterals
   Inability to protect major side branches
   Degenerated vein grafts with friable lesions

*Although the risk of abrupt vessel closure *with PTCA* may be moderately high with Type B lesions, the likelihood of a major complication may be low in certain instances, such as in the dilation of total occlusions < 3 mo old or when abundant collateral channels supply the distal vessel. Type B lesions may be further classified into those with only one type B characteristic (B1) and greater than one (B2).
Reprinted with permission from the American College of Cardiology. Ryan TJ, Bauman WB, Kennedy JW, et al. Guidelines for percutaneous transluminal coronary angioplasty. A report of the American College of Cardiology/American Heart Association Task Force on assessment of diagnostic and therapeutic cardiovascular procedures (Committee on Percutaneous Transluminal Coronary Angioplasty). Journal of the American College of Cardiology, 1993;22:2033–2054.

Invasive Evaluation for Specific Coronary Syndromes

Asymptomatic Patients

The indication to perform cardiac catheterization in truly asymptomatic individuals is to prevent future events (death, MI) and/or to provide prognostic information. Three asymptomatic patient groups in which cardiac catheterization should be considered are those patients with reduced LV function, certain patients with silent ischemia, and those surviving sudden cardiac death. Most patients with LV dysfunction and survivors of sudden death are not truly asymptomatic, but may not have chest pain from ischemia as part of the clinical picture.

The majority of patients with reduced LV systolic function should undergo stress testing. Patients with an equivocal or positive test for ischemia should be considered for catheterization. This recommendation is based in part on the proven survival advantage achieved by coronary artery bypass surgery as compared with medical therapy in patients with multivessel disease, particularly in the setting of reduced LV function (Figs 16-2, 16-3).[10,15-17] Chronic ischemia may cause a reversible reduction in LV systolic function, termed *hibernating myocardium*. Several studies have demonstrated that revascularization in patients with poor LV function in the setting of viable myocardium may improve both regional wall motion and overall ejection fraction.[18,19] Refinement of noninvasive techniques such as thallium or deoxyglucose imaging, stress echocardiography, or PET imaging should improve predicting which myocardial regions will be expected to improve function after revascularization.

The management and evaluation of patients with silent ischemia remain controversial. Studies have suggested that prognosis in patients with silent ischemia is governed by the same angiographic variables that affect patients with symptomatic coronary artery disease.[20,21] Therefore, most clinicians agree that patients with silent ischemia and findings on exercise testing consistent with high risk should be considered for catheterization. This recommendation is based on the higher frequency of left main or three-vessel disease seen in patients with these stress test results, even if unaccompanied by angina. Data from the Coronary Artery Surgery Study (CASS) registry have shown that patients with minimal or no symptoms with triple-vessel disease demonstrated a mortality advantage with bypass surgery.[22] Revascularization of asymptomatic patients

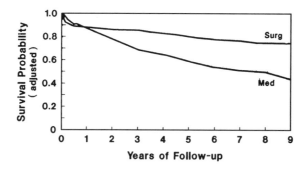

Figure 16-2 Kaplan-Meier survival estimates during 9 years of follow-up, adjusted for known prognostic factors in patients with LV ejection fraction less than or equal to 40%, treated with medical therapy or coronary artery bypass surgery. In comparison to patients treated with surgical therapy, patients treated medically had a lower probability of survival. Med, medical therapy; Surg, coronary artery bypass surgery. (Reproduced with permission from the American Heart Association, Inc, from Bounous EP, Mark DB, Pollack BG, et al. Surgical survival benefits for coronary disease in patients with left ventricular dysfunction. Circulation 1988;78[suppl I]:I-151–I-157.)

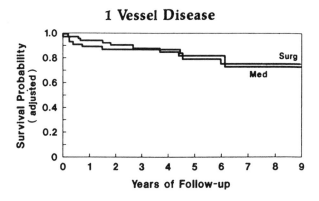

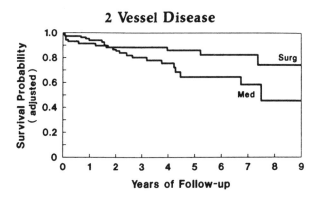

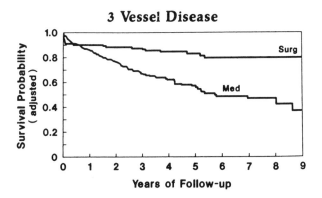

Figure 16-3 Kaplan-Meier survival estimates during 9 years of follow-up, adjusted for known prognostic factors in patients treated with medical therapy or coronary artery bypass surgery. (Top panel) Patients with one-vessel disease; (middle panel) patients with two-vessel disease; (bottom panel) patients with three-vessel disease. Patients with single-vessel disease had a similar probability of survival when treated with medical or surgical therapy. Patients with multivessel disease appeared to have a survival advantage when treated with surgical therapy compared with medical therapy. Surg, coronary artery bypass surgery; Med, medical therapy. (Reproduced with permission from the American Heart Association, Inc, from Bounous EP, Mark DB, Pollack BG, et al. Surgical survival benefits for coronary disease in patients with left ventricular dysfunction. Circulation 1988;78[suppl I]:I-151–I-157.)

with silent ischemia has not been validated by prospective studies and should be considered an attractive but unproven strategy.

In asymptomatic patients who have evidence of ischemia on stress testing and whose occupation involves the safety of others (e.g., pilots) or whose work may require a burst of activity (police officers, fire fighters, athletes), cardiac catheterization may be considered a class I indication. In asymptomatic patients with known or suspected coronary disease, there are several American College of Cardiology/American Heart Association class II indications for angiography. In all cases, some evidence of ischemia by stress testing is required. Examples of such patients are those with documented silent ischemia following MI, angioplasty or bypass surgery, or peripheral vascular surgery. In the latter group, cardiac catheterization is part of a pre-operative evaluation when ischemia is documented during stress testing. This recommendation is based on data that show these patients to be at higher than average risk for infarction and death during surgical procedures.[23]

Patients who do not have angina and have survived sudden cardiac death should usually undergo cardiac catheterization. If coronary artery disease is documented at catheterization, its relative contribution to the sudden cardiac death must be assessed. The sequence of coronary angiography relative to the time of electrophysiologic testing is not standardized, but frequently catheterization precedes electrophysiologic study to provide the eletrophysiologist with maximal information.

Chronic Stable Angina

Chronic stable angina is defined as angina that is not progressive, not prolonged (>20 min), or not occurring at rest unless in an unchanged pattern. The most recent American College of Cardiology/American Heart Association guidelines list four class I indications for cardiac catheterization in patients with chronic stable angina: (1) angina inadequately responsive to medical therapy, (2) angina associated with high-risk stress test characteristics, (3) angina in patients undergoing major vascular surgery, and (4) resuscitation from sudden cardiac death in the absence of acute MI.[2]

Angina that is "inadequately responsive" to medical therapy may be interpreted broadly to include dissatisfaction by the patient and/or the treating physician with the current medical regimen. Dissatisfaction may be due to side effects from the medical regimen but more commonly is related to persistent symptoms interfering with a patient's occupation or ability to participate in routine daily activities (Canadian Cardiovascular Society class III and IV angina), or the patient's desire not to take medicines and be revascularized. These indications are quite subjective and are directly dependent on the patient's and physician's expectations.

The strategy of angioplasty as an alternative to medical therapy in patients with single-vessel disease for angina has been validated. In a study of single-vessel disease, relief of angina was shown to be superior with PTCA, as compared with medical therapy.[24] Multicenter studies comparing angioplasty with bypass surgery in selected patients with multivessel disease who were candidates for both procedures have documented the effectiveness of angioplasty for the treatment of anginal symptoms.[25,26] It must be communicated to patients that whereas angioplasty is an acceptable treatment for chronic stable angina, it is associated with the risk of serious short-term morbidity, an angiographic restenosis of 40% to 60%, and a clinical restenosis rate of 25% to 40%. Serious immediate complications of angioplasty include abrupt closure requiring stent placement or bypass surgery (2%–8%), non-Q-wave MI (2%–8%) Q-wave MI (1%–5%), emergency bypass surgery (0.1%–0.5%), and death (0.1%–0.5%). Because of these risks, some clinicians prefer advising medical therapy for patients with stable symptoms, reserving angioplasty for patients with refractory symptoms, those intolerant of medical therapy, or those felt to be at higher risk on medical management.

Major vascular surgery in patients unable to perform an exercise stress test is also a class I indication for cardiac catheterization. Recent data suggest that not all of these patients require catheterization and that further risk stratification on the basis of clinical features and pharmacologic stress testing results is possible. In a study of 200 patients scheduled for vascular surgery, five prospective variables, including pathologic ECG Q waves, ventricular ectopy, diabetes mellitus, advanced age as well as angina pectoris, were able to identify patients at low risk (no variables present) and high risk (> three variables), with expected adverse cardiac event rates at surgery of 3.1% and 5.0%, respectively.[27] Patients with one or two risk variables represent a group with an intermediate prognosis, which was further stratified using dipyridamole thallium stress testing. Patients manifesting no redistribution had a very low event rate (3.2%) during their vascular surgery, whereas patients with redistribution present had nearly a 30% event rate.[27] This study suggests that high-risk groups consisting of patients with three or more variables or those with one or two variables present and a positive dipyridamole thallium stress test should be considered for preoperative catheterization. This study also suggests that patients with no clinical risk factors present may proceed to their vascular surgery without either stress testing or cardiac catheterization being performed. The usefulness of dipyridamole thallium testing in patients with peripheral vascular disease has been suggested by some but not all investigators.[28,29] There are no prospective studies at this time demonstrating that mechanical revascularization in this patient group will prevent peri-operative death or MI. In a retrospective study, patients scheduled for peripheral vascular surgery underwent pre-operative elective angioplasty[30] with a very low cardiac event rate during and after vascular surgery that was quite favorable when compared with historical controls. It is our practice to pursue pre-operative revascularization in patients with peripheral vascular disease only if the revascularization procedure is indicated in the absence of upcoming noncardiac surgery. This approach is based on the appreciation that the theoretic gains from pre-operative mechanical revascularization of the coronary circulation may indeed be offset by the added morbidity associated with the prophylactic procedure.

Specific Procedural Aspects of Catheterization in Patients with Stable Angina

Both echocardiography and radionuclide ventriculography can evaluate systolic LV function. The unique diagnostic aspect of cardiac catheterization is defining the coronary anatomy. If the clinical suspicion of severe coronary disease (e.g., significant left main disease) is high, coronary angiography should be considered for the first use of dye. Performing coronary arteriography first should also be performed in patients with a history of contrast reaction, even if prophylaxis has been given. Utilizing a right coronary catheter first and passing it into the ventricle prior to coronary arteriography allow baseline measurement of LV pressure. Because dye injection transiently depresses LV function and vasodilates the peripheral vasculature, performing left ventriculography first provides the most accurate assessment of ventricular function. Right heart catheterization with measurement of right-sided pressures, cardiac output, and pulmonary artery saturation should be performed in patients with LV dysfunction and evidence of heart failure.

Unstable Angina

Patients with unstable angina are a heterogeneous group. The unifying feature is an intensification of the anginal pattern or recent onset of angina. Plaque rupture and superimposed thrombosis is often the mechanism, as it is in acute MI by which the clinical syndrome develops. Unlike patients with acute infarction, however, these patients undergo no tissue necrosis and therefore do not release creatine phosphokinase into the systemic circulation. There is no objective test to confirm the diagnosis; thus, unstable angina remains a clinical diagnosis. The Agency for Health Care Planning and Research has developed criteria for diagnosis and risk stratification in this patient group.[31]

The prognosis of patients with unstable angina is worse than for patients with chronic stable angina. Adverse risk is related in turn to the severity of significant coronary artery disease and to factors affecting the likelihood of a large infarction or death if an ischemic event occurs. The wide range of event rates reported for the unstable angina patient groups reflects, in part, the inclusion in many studies of patients with noncardiac causes of their symptoms. Therefore, an important goal when assessing a patient with unstable angina is

Table 16-4   Short-term Risk of Death or Nonfatal Myocardial Infarction
in Patients with Unstable Angina

High risk	Intermediate risk	Low risk
At least one of the following features must be present:	No high-risk feature but must have any of the following:	No high- or intermediate-risk feature but may have any of the following features:
Prolonged, ongoing (>20 min) rest pain	Prolonged (>20 min) rest angina, now resolved, with moderate or high likelihood of CAD	Increased angina frequency, severity, or duration
Pulmonary edema, most likely related to ischemia	Rest angina (>20 min or relieved with rest or sublingual nitroglycerin)	Angina provoked at a lower threshold
Angina at rest with dynamic ST changes (>1 mm)	Noctural angina	New-onset angina with onset 2 weeks to 2 mo prior to presentation
Angina with new or worsening MR murmur	Angina with dynamic T-wave changes	Normal or unchanged ECG
Angina with S3 or new/worsening rales	New onset CCSC III or IV angina in the past 2 weeks with moderate or high likelihood of CAD	
Angina with hypotension	Pathologic Q waves or resting ST depression < 1 mm in multiple-lead groups (anterior, inferior, lateral)	
	Age > 65 yr	

Note: Estimation of the short-term risks of death and nonfatal MI in unstable angina is a complex multivariable problem that cannot be fully specified in a table such as this. Therefore, this table is meant to offer general guidance and illustration rather than rigid algorithms.
Abbreviations: CAD, coronary artery disease; MR, mitral regurgitation, CCSC, Canadian Cardiovascular Society Classification.
Reprinted with permission from the American College of Cardiology (Journal of the American College of Cardiology, 1991, 17: 1053–1057).

to determine the likelihood that the symptoms are ischemic in origin. Known prior coronary artery disease, classic angina in an older patient, and hemodynamic or electrocardiographic changes with chest pain are all consistent with a high likelihood of an ischemic etiology of the symptoms. Conversely, the absence of such findings or a younger patient with more atypical symptoms or a normal or nondiagnostic ECG makes the diagnosis of coronary artery disease less likely. After determining the probability that the presenting symptoms are related to coronary artery disease, the clinician should estimate the patient's risk for an adverse outcome. High-risk patients for an adverse outcome include those who have prolonged rest pain (>20 min), pain accompanied by acute pulmonary edema, hypotension, ST changes or worsened mitral regurgitation with pain, or known moderate to severe LV dysfunction.[31]

Conversely, at somewhat lower risk for an adverse event are those patients in whom the tempo of presentation has been slower. Chronic angina that occurs at a lower threshold and angina that is more frequent and severe but slowly progressing over an extended period are examples. Table 16-4 summarizes the characteristics of these risk types. For patients in the high-risk group or patients whose symptoms persist despite intensive medical therapy including intravenous heparin and aspirin, early catheterization and revascularization are indicated. For stabilized patients deemed not to be at high risk, the diagnostic evaluation is more flexible.

Noninvasive Evaluation of "Stabilized" Unstable Angina

Prior to the utilization of antithrombotics as front-line therapy for patients with unstable angina, subsequent MI and death occurred relatively frequently. The appropriate use of aspirin and heparin has led to a 50% reduction in the event rate in patients with stable angina.[32,33] With aggressive use of medical therapy, less than 10% of patients are truly refractory to maximal multidrug therapy.[34] The natural history of "stabilized" unstable angina, however, is not well documented. The approach to these patients consists of further stratification by stress testing (noninvasive approach) or early cardiac catheterization (invasive approach).

Multiple studies have documented the safety of early stress testing following a presentation of unstable angina.[35,36] The primary goal of noninvasive testing is to identify high-risk patients in whom further invasive testing may be indicated. The clinical practice guidelines from the Agency for Health Policy and Research for the diagnosis and management of unstable angina suggest two patient groups as appropriate for the noninvasive strategy.[32] These are low-risk patients with unstable angina who are to be managed as outpatients and non-high-risk stabilized inpatients (no chest pain or congestive heart failure for >48 hr). In the noninvasive strategy, stress testing should be carried out in a timely fashion, probably within 48 to 72 hours. These guidelines suggest that the type of stress test performed should, in large part, depend on the status of the resting ECG and on the local expertise available to perform the study. In general, patients with normal ECGs should undergo standard treadmill exercise testing. The addition of an imaging modality is appropriate in patients with an abnormal baseline ECG, such as those manifesting digoxin effect, LV hypertrophy, or baseline ST abnormalities. In patients unable to exercise, there are limited data suggesting that pharmacologic stress testing provides useful prognostic information.

Invasive Evaluation of Unstable Angina

Although advances have been made in the medical management of unstable angina, many clinicians still prefer to perform cardiac catheterization in this patient group. There are four conceptual approaches that govern the decision to perform cardiac catheterization in unstable angina. Cardiac catheterization can be pursued: (1) as a pre-revascularization procedure in patients refractory to medical management, (2) in all stabilized patients as a pre-revascularization test, (3) in all stabilized patients as a prognostic test and (4) in selected patients deemed to be at high risk with medical management.

Unstable angina that is refractory to medical therapy is considered a class I indication for catheterization. Patients with refractory symptoms on medical therapy have a poor prognosis, with high infarction and mortality rates. This group includes patients with unstable angina that develop either spontaneous or provoked ischemia after an initial stabilization with medical therapy.

More controversial is the strategy to catheterize all patients with unstable angina, with the goal being revascularization of all appropriate vessels. This strategy has been evaluated in the Thrombolysis in Myocardial Infarction (TIMI) IIIB investigation.[37] This study compared an invasive strategy consisting of early catheterization and revascularization with a conservative approach applying catheterization and intervention only for provoked or spontaneous ischemia in patients with acute coronary insufficiency (unstable angina or non-Q-wave MI [NQMI]). The early invasive strategy did not lead to an improvement in any primary endpoints that consisted of death, MI, or positive stress test at 42 days when compared with outcomes in patients treated with the conservative strategy. Earlier studies evaluating the role of angioplasty in patients presenting with unstable angina have consistently shown that angioplasty in these patients is associated with a higher risk of acute complications and late restenosis compared with patients with stable angina.[38,39] At present, the early invasive and conservative strategies in patients presenting with unstable angina should be considered equivalent in terms of important clinical endpoints. Which approach is selected for any given patient should depend on the patient's clinical risk, the availability of a skilled interventional team, and the patient's informed preference. The early invasive strategy is attractive to some because of the potential to decrease hospital length of stay. It is still unclear whether the reduction in anti-anginal medication and rehospitalization seen with the early invasive approach in the TIMI IIIB study outweighs the increased number of interventions associated with that strategy.

The strategy of performing cardiac catheterization for prognostic purposes in all patients presenting with unstable angina is supported by many clinicians. This information may allow for a more patient-specific application of medical or invasive resources. It has been estimated that of all patients with unstable angina undergoing catheterization, between 10% and 20% will have normal coronaries and another 30% will have insignificant epicardial disease.[31] These patient groups have an excellent prognosis and may be candidates for early discharge and further evaluation as outpatients. Approximately 15% of patients will be found to have left main disease or three-vessel disease with reduced LV function and would be expected to have a survival benefit with revascularization. Other patients may have findings at catheterization that allow for the institution of more patient-specific therapies. For example, patients found to have akinetic or dyskinetic walls could be placed on afterload therapy, and those patients with angiographic evidence for intracoronary thrombus might be treated with thrombolytics or prolonged antithrombotic therapy. A final rationale for performing a prognostic catheterization in these patients is to determine "lesion risk" and suitability for intervention, which can be determined only by coronary angiography. A disadvantage of this routine application of catheterization is that "reperfusion momentum" may lead to overusage of revascularization procedures.

A fourth invasive strategy is to perform angiography only in patients at high risk with medical management. This approach would include patients who fulfill the high-risk criteria seen in Table 16-4. This strategy has the advantage of intervening in patients at high risk, and thus expediting care, while reserving stress tests for patients thought to be at lower risk.

Invasive Evaluation of Non-Q-Wave Myocardial Infarction

Clinical Presentation and Prognosis

Non-Q-wave myocardial infarction is defined by a characteristic rise and fall in cardiac enzymes in patients who fail to develop pathologic ECG Q waves. The clinical presentation may be characteristic of MI (e.g., chest pain, nausea and/or vomiting, etc.), or may be similar to the patient's angina. The ECG may demonstrate ischemic ST-T changes, but such changes are not required to make the diagnosis. The chest pain of NQMI is generally more severe and of greater duration than that seen in chronic or unstable angina. However, the quality and duration of pain is quite variable.

In the present era of thrombolytic therapy, ST elevation may be the presenting ECG finding in up to 40% of patients with an NQMI.[37] Because the ECG changes in the other 60% are so nonspecific, the diagnosis requires enzyme evidence of myocardial necrosis.

The diagnostic evaluation of patients with NQMI requires an understanding of both short- and long-term prognosis in these patients. Non-Q-wave myocardial infarction is thought to represent an incomplete infarction. Many studies have shown that patients with NQMI have smaller infarctions and better preserved LV systolic function than that seen in patients with Q-wave infarctions.[40,41] NQMI has a favorable early prognosis with early mortality of about half that seen with Q-wave infarcts. Additionally, approximately 60% of these patients will have a patent infarct-related artery. Again, this is much higher than seen in Q-wave infarctions (in the absence of thrombolytic therapy).[41,42] Several investigators have shown that those patients with NQMI more frequently have myocardium at risk in the infarct zone.[43] The combination of a patent infarct-related artery and myocardium at risk may explain the high rates of recurrent angina and reinfarction seen in these patients. Ultimately, despite this early favorable prognosis, the 1-year mortality rates for these patients reach and may actually surpass that seen in patients with Q-wave infarctions.[40-44]

Catheterization and Revascularization in Non-Q-Wave Myocardial Infarction

Because of the high rates of recurrent angina, reinfarction, and late mortality demonstrated in NQMI, many clinicians favor an aggressive diagnostic evaluation in these patients, including early catheterization and revascularization. The TIMI IIIB study,[37] which included patients with NQMI, is the only large, randomized, prospectively designed study that has compared invasive and "conservative" approaches in NQMI. There was no difference in the primary endpoints of 42-day death, reinfarction, or positive stress test between patients treated with early catheterization and revascularization and those patients treated medically who underwent revascularization only for spontaneous or provoked ischemia. Further analysis of prospectively defined subgroups has shown that only older patients (> 65 years) benefited from the invasive strategy. Interestingly, the TIMI IIIB has been used to support both the invasive and noninvasive approaches to patients with NQMI. Although primary endpoints were not different between these two strategies, patients treated in the invasive arm had shorter hospital stays, 50% less readmission, significantly fewer days of rehospitalization, and fewer antianginal drug requirements. There was a very high crossover rate to cardiac catheterization, with nearly 60% of patients in the noninvasive arm undergoing angiography by day 42. Hence, the similar primary endpoints between these two strategies came at a cost of more hospitalizations and frequent crossover to catheterization and revascularization in the noninvasive arm. The argument for the noninvasive approach is that the conservative approach avoided "unnecessary" catheterization in one third of the patients.

Central to the therapeutic approach to all patients with coronary artery disease is the concept of risk stratification. Dividing patients into low- and high-risk populations allows us to identify high-risk patients who are most likely to derive benefit from an intervention while avoiding the morbidity associated with any intervention in patients whose prognosis is already favorable. Patients with NQMI as a group are at high risk for late events. Several studies suggest that ST depression on presenting ECG, particularly if persistent, congestive heart failure, older age, and prior infarction or reinfarction are all independent predictors of poor outcome following NQMI.

Using the TIMI IIIB study and prognostic data, an overall strategy for revascularization in NQMI is proposed (Fig 16-4). Application of this risk stratification allows identification of those low-risk patients who could be considered appropriate for early triage based on stress-testing data. Those patients identified at higher risk based on the clinical data would proceed directly to

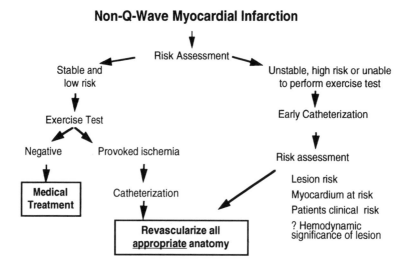

Figure 16-4 Strategy for management of patients following non-Q-wave myocardial infarction.

catheterization and revascularization. This evaluation would promote the excellent outcomes seen in the recent TIMI IIIB study while potentially avoiding some of the "unnecessary" procedures that result when using an unselective invasive approach.

Procedural Approach in Patients with Non-Q-Wave Myocardial Infarction or Unstable Stable Angina

The catheterization protocol in patients with NQMI or unstable stable angina is modified from that performed in patients with chronic stable angina, reflecting the acuity and higher risk of these patients. It is our usual practice to place an 8-Fr venous sheath in the femoral vein in addition to the usual arterial access. This permits rapid right heart pressure monitoring or pacing if necessary. It also facilitates performing on-line intervention if this strategy is pursued. Unlike the strategy in patients with stable ischemic syndromes, in patients with recent or acute coronary insufficiency, we perform coronary angiography before ventriculography. This approach allows the early collection of the important coronary angiographic data and also limits the contrast load in these patients who may undergo same-sitting coronary intervention. In patients with persistent instability (angina within 24 hr), a non-ionic contrast agent is used. Right heart catheterization is undertaken if the patient has primarily symptoms of dyspnea, recurrent pulmonary edema, or prior knowledge that significant LV dysfunction exists or symptoms of congestive heart failure are present.

Acute Myocardial Infarction

The strategies governing patient selection for catheterization following MI may be divided into three broad categories: (1) immediate emergent, (2) unplanned urgent, and (3) elective. Immediate coronary angiography is performed with the goal of mechanical revascularization to achieve patency of the infarct-related artery (Fig 16-5). The major proven strategy is the application of direct (or primary) angioplasty in lieu of thrombolytic therapy. The Primary Angioplasty in Myocardial Infarction (PAMI) study analyzed outcomes in 395 patients presenting within 12 hours of the onset of MI who were randomized to primary angioplasty or treatment with t-PA.[45] Primary angioplasty was associated with a high initial successful revascularization rate of 97% with no patients requiring emergency bypass surgery. The inhospital mortality rates in the angioplasty- and t-PA–treated groups were 2.6% and 6.5%, respectively. Six-month follow-up showed significantly lower reinfarction or death rate in the angioplasty-treated group compared with the t-PA group (8.5% vs. 16.8%, respectively). Smaller studies have generally confirmed the excellent outcomes seen in the PAMI study.[46,47] The feasibility of routine primary angioplasty as a reperfusion ther-apy in acute MI is dependent on the proximity of a hospital that has both cardiac catheterization facilities and a skilled interventional team committed to 24-hour coverage. These requirements have generally limited the widespread use of this approach, although defining the outer limits of PTCA in this setting continues to evolve.

The strategy of angioplasty after thrombolytic therapy has been tested in the Thrombolysis and Angioplasty in Myocardial Infarction (TAMI-1) trial,[48] the European Cooperative Study Group (ECGS),[49] and the TIMI-IIA study.[50] All three studies showed similar mortality rates without benefit in LV function or reinfarction in patients undergoing infarct-related ("culprit") vessel angioplasty after intravenous thrombolysis, compared with those patients receiving thrombolysis alone. Based on these data, PTCA after thrombolysis should not be performed routinely, except for certain specific indications. The primary circumstances are evidence of persistent ischemia after thrombolysis or impending or present cardiogenic shock. Clinically failed thrombolysis, severe postinfarction angina, evidence of infarct vessel reocclusion, and hemodynamic instability are examples of such indications. Some clinicians have suggested that failed thrombolysis should be treated with "rescue" angioplasty. Rescue angioplasty refers to angioplasty performed in the early hours after thrombolysis in patients with persistent symptoms and presumed failure of thrombolysis to achieve reperfusion of the culprit vessel. In a meta-analysis of 12 studies of rescue angioplasty, Ellis et al. reported a procedural success rate of 80% and an overall mortality of 10.6%.[51] In this meta-analysis, successful reperfusion of the infarct-related artery resulted in a relatively favorable mortality rate. Unfortunately, leaving the catheterization laboratory with a closed vessel following a failed angioplasty

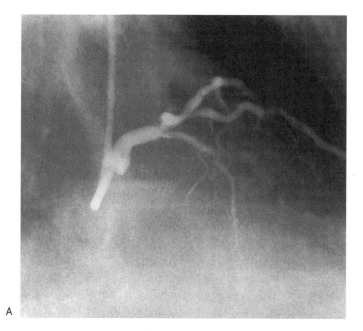

A

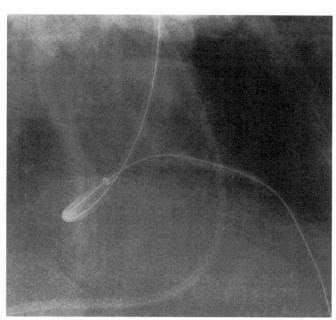

B

Figure 16-5 Single-frame cineangiograms of the left coronary artery in a shallow right anterior oblique projection with cranial angulation. (**A**) Total occlusion of the left anterior descending artery after the first septal perforator artery. (**B**) Inflated balloon catheter positioned over intracoronary wire at site of lesion.

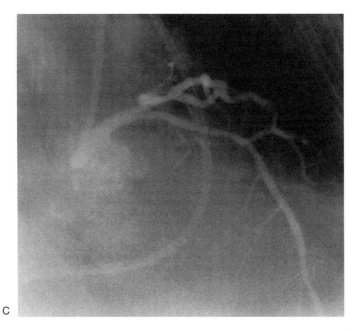

Figure 16-5 (**C**) Patent left anterior descending artery with minimal residual stenosis at site of inital total occlusion.

translated into a mortality rate approaching 40%. This is notable, given the somewhat high failure rate (20%) of angioplasty in this setting. In a smaller study of 151 patients, the same author showed no difference in resting ejection fraction, only a slight improvement in exercise ejection fraction, and a borderline decrease in the combined endpoint of death or severe heart failure in patients undergoing rescue angioplasty, compared with those undergoing no rescue angioplasty.[52] Proponents of rescue angioplasty point to the overall low mortality rate and improved patency obtained by this strategy. Opponents of this approach argue that new lytic agents and dosing protocols are improving patency rates, that clinical markers of reperfusion are unreliable and will therefore result in many patients undergoing catheterization who already have a patent infarct vessel, and that extremely poor outcomes occur in patients with failed angioplasty in this setting.

Recurrent angina following MI identifies a group of patients at high risk for reinfarction and/or death. Patients with recurrent inhospital symptoms, especially if associated with electrocardiographic changes or in those with multiple or prolonged episodes of chest pain, are at higher risk for reinfarction and should undergo urgent catheterization and revascularization. Special note should be made of patients presenting with recurrent chest pain associated with recurrent ST elevation following thrombolysis. These patients usually have reocclusion of the culprit vessel and require urgent attention. Our approach to these patients follows the outline in Figure 16-6. In summary, it is our approach

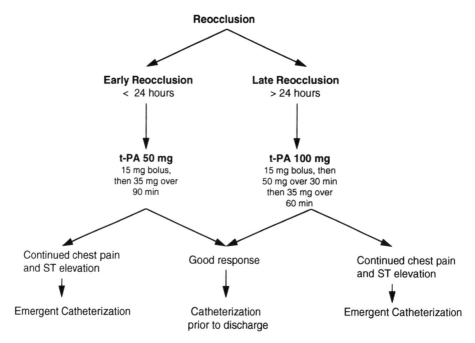

Figure 16-6 Strategy for management of patients following reocclusion of the infarct-related coronary artery. If reocclusion occurs at an institution where a cardiac catheterization laboratory is available, urgent coronary angiography is performed.

to recommend catheterization and, when appropriate, rescue PTCA in patients with ongoing chest pain, particularly if the ECG shows preservation of R waves in the infarct territory.

Urgent to emergent catheterization following MI is often required in patients presenting with impending cardiogenic shock following MI. Cardiogenic shock has been reported to have an extremely high mortality rate of 50%–100%. Several small, nonrandomized series using PTCA have shown that producing patency of the infarct-related artery was associated with improved survival (60%–75%).[53,54] Patients taken to the catheterization laboratory tended to be younger and had better LV function than patients in whom no revascularization was undertaken; as such, these data are biased in favor of PTCA. The appropriateness of emergent catheterization and revascularization in this high-risk population is being evaluated. Placement of a right heart catheter to titrate fluid requirements is often helpful, as is intra-aortic balloon placement, which often may stabilize these patients (see Chapter 22).

Patients with acute MI complicated by mechanical defects such as ventricular septal defect or papillary chordal rupture and acute mitral regurgitation represent a very high risk subgroup and should undergo emergent catheterization. A new murmur, often holosystolic, at the left sternal border, with profound elevation of venous pressure and relatively clear lungs, should alert the clinician to the possibility of an acquired ventricular septal defect. Swan-Ganz catheterization with sampling of oxygen saturations in the superior vena cava, right atrium, right ventricle, pulmonary artery, and systemic artery can estimate the size of the shunt. If the patient is not in frank shock, a two-dimensional echocardiogram will usually localize the septal lesion. Because these patients are typically hemodynamically unstable, contrast dye injection should be minimized wherever possible and limited to coronary arteriography. Non-ionic or low-osmolar ionic contrast agents are preferred. The proper timing of surgery remains controversial, but consensus at present is to perform surgery as early as is feasible.[55] Even more ominous is rupture of the tip of one of the heads of one of the papillary muscles. The result is torrential mitral regurgitation, typically acute pulmonary edema, and severe hypotension. Emergency placement of an intra-aortic balloon pump, characterization of the coronaries, and emergency surgery is the recommended approach.[56] Even if all of these procedures are expeditiously performed and surgery is undertaken, mortality remains high (>75%).

Catheterization in acute MI may also be performed as a planned, elective procedure prior to discharge. Postinfarction patients with spontaneous angina that is not progressive and patients with provoked ischemia at predischarge stress testing should be considered for catheterization. Patients who are stable postinfarction without chest pain or congestive heart failure may benefit from cardiac catheterization to obtain further prognostic information. In the pre-thrombolytic era, one study described risks for outcome based on catheterization data and concluded that multivessel disease (defined as disease in the left anterior descending and at least one other vessel), ejection fraction, and the presence of other risk segments were significant predictors of outcome (see Fig 16-1). Angiographic variables added significantly to clinical variables in predicting cardiac events during the follow-up period. Two studies from the thrombolytic era, Should We Intervene Following Thrombolysis (SWIFT) and TIMI IIB, compared the usefulness of early elective catheterization and a strategy employing catheterization only for spontaneous or provoked ischemia following MI. These studies showed no difference in major endpoints of death, reinfarction, or ejection fraction over the short-term between patients receiving an early elective catheterization compared with those with a "watchful waiting" strategy.[57,58] Both approaches resulted in excellent short-term mortality of less than 10%. Our practice is not to perform catheterization in patients who are stable following thrombolysis, instead using a modified Bruce stress test prior to discharge and a symptom-limited stress test at 4 to 6 weeks to further risk stratify these patients. Patients who have either spontaneous ischemia or a positive stress test undergo elective catheterization and revascularization as appropriate. With this watchful waiting approach, nearly 60% of patients will undergo catheterization by 1 year.[59]

Procedural Approach in Acute Myocardial Infarction

Cardiac catheterization in the first few hours of an acute MI is performed with the expectation of proceeding to immediate culprit vessel angioplasty. Because these patients are in the midst of a MI, the diagnostic catheterization must be performed rapidly by experienced operators. Our practice is to initially place an 8-Fr sheath in a femoral artery and femoral vein. If the patient has recently received thrombolytics, a single wall arterial puncture should be attempted to minimize bleeding complications. Next, we float a pacing-capable, right heart catheter into the pulmonary artery to assess LV filling pressures and to permit cardiac pacing if the need arises during the ensuing angioplasty procedure. If not already heparinized, a heparin bolus is given and a constant infusion is started to achieve an activated clotting time of greater than 300 seconds. Coronary angiography is performed of both coronary vessels using non-ionic contrast. If the anatomy is appropriate, an 8-Fr guiding catheter is placed into the appropriate ostium, and angioplasty of the culprit vessel is carried out.

Chest Pain with Normal or Near-Normal Coronaries

A significant minority (10%–30%) of patients presenting with chest pain will have normal or nearly normal coronary arteries at cardiac catheterization.[60,61] As a group, the prognosis in patients with completely normal coronaries is favorable. In a CASS registry study of 3136 patients with normal coronary arteries, the 7-year survival rate was 96%.[62] In a second large study of nearly 20,000 patients undergoing cardiac catheterization, 1491 patients had normal coronaries and had an excellent survival rate of 98% at 10 years.[63] Patients having abnormal yet insignificant coronary disease (defined as having epicardial obstructions of less than 60%) generally have an excellent survival rate, but are more likely to develop a nonfatal MI in the future than are those patients with completely normal coronaries.[64] The pathophysiology of chest pain in patients with normal coronary arteries can be divided into cardiac and noncardiac etiologies. The common nonatherosclerotic, nonobstructive cardiac causes of chest pain are reviewed in the following sections.

Coronary Artery Spasm

Anginal pain from coronary artery spasm at the site of a preexisting fixed epicardial stenosis was described by Prinzmetal et al. in 1959.[65] Coronary artery spasm may also occur at angiographically normal sites.[66–68] Bertrand et al. administered methergine to 1089 consecutive patients undergoing cardiac catheterization for standard indications. They found that 131 patients (12%) developed coronary spasm.[69] The majority of these patients had nonexertional rest pain as the presenting symptom, and spasm occurred predominantly at atherosclerotic sites.

Use of a direct vasoconstricting agent such as ergonovine to provoke coronary artery spasm in patients presenting with chest pain and insignificant coronary artery disease has been described. Unfortunately, the lack of a gold standard for this diagnosis means the sensitivity and specificity of this test are difficult to determine. Additionally, logistics that require holding calcium channel blockers and nitrates for 24 hours prior to catheterization in patients presenting with rest symptoms, the time-consuming in-lab protocol, and finally the ambiguous significance of the test results have discouraged many clinicians from using this test. Ergonovine has recently been withdrawn from the market. Experience with a substitute agent, ergometrine, is limited in the United States.[68] In many catheterization laboratories, however, infusion of acetylcholine (normally an endothelium-dependent vasodilator) is being used to evaluate coronary artery vasospasm[70] and abnormal coronary artery endothelial function. Several studies have reported a paradoxic coronary vasoconstriction in response to acetylcholine in patients with early atherosclerosis as well as in patients with traditional risk factors for coronary artery disease such as hypertension.[71–73] In our laboratory, in the presence of a pacing catheter positioned in the right heart and an intracoronary flow wire (FloWire, Cardiometrics, Inc., Mountain View, CA), acetylcholine (15–30 μg/min) is infused via a subselective 3-Fr intracoronary catheter. Coronary cineangiography is performed before and after each 3-minute infusion, and coronary flow velocity is recorded. Next, nitroglycerin (200 μg), an endothelium-independent vasodilator, is given as a bolus injection via the guiding catheter, and repeat coronary angiography and measurement of coronary flow velocity are performed.

Syndrome X

Syndrome X describes a syndrome in which patients have typical exertional angina, normal epicardial coronaries, and no other clear cardiac etiology such as coronary spasm or LV hypertrophy to explain the symptoms. Cannon et al.[74] have suggested the term *microvascular angina* to describe these patients, believing that an abnormality of coronary artery reserve secondary to structural or functional abnormalities of the microcirculation is the underlying pathophysiology. The same group has also argued that ischemia may not be the pathologic mechanism in these patients but rather an enhanced visceral nociception.[74] Because the pathologic mechanism for this proposed syndrome is unproven, because there is no gold standard for diagnosis, and because the ability to test for abnormalities of the microvascular circulation is limited in most catheterization laboratories, the diagnosis of syndrome X remains one of exclusion.

Other Ischemic Causes of Chest Pain

There are several other ischemic causes of pain that are not due to obstruction of major epicardial vessels. Patients with LV hypertrophy (from hypertension, aortic stenosis, or hypertrophic cardiomyopathy) may develop angina presumed to be caused by an abnormal supply-demand ratio. Several studies have suggested an abnormality in coronary flow reserve in patients with hypertension, both with and without associated LV hypertrophy.[75,76] Patients with LV hypertrophy, in general, have a higher myocardial oxygen demand; as such, limitations in myocardial oxygen supply could result in exertional angina.

An interesting nonatheromatous abnormality of the macrocirculation that may cause angina is myocardial bridging. Normally, conduit coronary vessels lie on the epicardial surface of the heart. *Myocardial bridging* refers to a segment of a vessel that is intramyocardial and is obliterated during systole. At angiography, systolic compression of the vessel is observed. Because the great majority of blood flow occurs during diastole, it is unlikely that myocardial ischemia occurs in most cases. Occasionally, the intramyocardial vessel is partially occluded during diastole; as such, it may provoke ischemia. This condition is reported in 2% to 12% of patients undergoing catheterization; its incidence is dependent to some extent on the diligence with which the diagnosis is sought. In general, the prognosis is excellent.

Mitral Valve Prolapse

Patients with mitral valve prolapse frequently present with atypical chest pain. The association between chest pain and mitral valve prolapse has been suggested in many studies. Because of design flaws and inherent bias found in many of these studies,[77] the finding of mitral valve prolapse in patients with chest pain and normal coronary vessels does not prove cause and effect.

Evaluation of Borderline Angiographic Stenoses

The clinical significance of chest pain in the setting of a borderline angiographic lesion represents a common and difficult problem. As previously reviewed, provocative stress testing is often used to determine the clinical and hemodynamic significance of such lesions. Recent advances in percutaneous technologies has lead to on-line assessment of such lesions using intracoronary techniques. Initial attempts at intracoronary interrogation of lesions utilized the measurement of a pressure gradient across a stenosis. This was accomplished by crossing a stenosis with a very small catheter (2–3 Fr in diameter) using standard angioplasty techniques and then measuring the gradient across the lesion. This measurement may be confirmed by recording a pullback gradient across the stenosis. Gradients of more than 20 to 25 mm Hg have been considered to be hemodynamically significant, particularly when very small catheters are utilized.[78] In instances in which the measured gradient has been considered borderline, vasoactive substances (e.g., adenosine) have been infused to maximize flow, and hence the gradient, across a given stenosis.

More recently, intracoronary ultrasound[79] (see Chapter 19) and intracoronary Doppler flow wires[80,81] (see Chapter 20) have been used to assess the significance of borderline angiographic lesions. These techniques may become more common diagnostic modalities in the future.

Special Considerations in Women

Cardiovascular disease is the leading cause of death in women, accounting for nearly 500,000 deaths annually in the United States. In fact, twice as many women die of cardiovascular disease than of cancer, with the majority of deaths due to MI and stroke.[82] Although it is true that more men have MIs than do women, and men have them earlier in life, several studies have shown that women sustaining an acute MI have a higher inhospital mortality rate, are more likely to experience recurrent infarction, and have a higher long-term relative risk of death than do men, even when thrombolytic therapy is used.[83–85]

The concept that cardiovascular disease is an affliction of men and not of women is based on the fact that very few women develop the manifestations of the disease before menopause. In addition, in any given decade, the incidence of coronary heart disease and MI is higher in men than in women. Of note, however, is that women develop coronary heart disease at the same rate as men but approximately 10 years later.[85]

Noninvasive Diagnosis

Whereas almost two thirds of men with coronary artery disease present with MI or sudden death as the initial manifestation of the disease, just over one half of women have angina pectoris as their first symptom.[86] Yet, establishing the diagnosis of coronary heart disease in women is more problematic than in men. This is due, in part, to the relatively high prevalence of chest pain syndromes among women who do not have significant coronary artery disease. In general, noninvasive tests to diagnose coronary heart disease are less sensitive and specific in women than in men. The prevalence of coronary heart disease, especially multivessel disease, is generally lower in premenopausal women than in men with comparable chest pain syndromes; the lower pre-test likelihood of a positive exercise response limits the diagnostic yield of the test.[86] The higher prevalence of hypertension and LV hypertrophy, particularly in older women, tends to confound interpretation of the electrocardiographic findings. In addition, many elderly women are unable to exercise to a sufficient degree to yield definitive diagnostic information. It is important to note, however, that correction for factors contributing to false-positive exercise tests and the prevalence of disease in women results in comparable diagnostic accuracy of exercise tests in both women and men.[87]

As in men, chest pain compatible with angina pectoris in women warrants evaluation for coronary artery disease. Electrocardiographic exercise testing is recommended for women if the resting ECG is normal. When the resting ECG is abnormal, thallium or other perfusion imaging improves the specificity of exercise testing in women.[88-90] Dipyridamole and exercise echocardiography, which have been reported to retain predictive accuracy in the setting of single-vessel disease, may be useful in women, and pharmacologic stress testing may be helpful in women who are unable to exercise.[91,92]

When the results of exercise testing reveal evidence of myocardial ischemia, particularly in combination with a history of typical angina, referral for diagnostic coronary angiography should be considered. However, several studies have suggested that women are referred less often or later in the course of their disease than are men, even when the results of noninvasive testing suggest the presence of coronary artery disease.[93,94] These observations have fueled debate about a possible *gender bias*, a term that must be interpreted with caution. First, it is unclear whether the difference in referral pattern for diagnostic cardiac catheterization is appropriate in women, based on other risk parameters such as age, LV function, and comorbid disease. Second, numerous studies have shown that women undergoing coronary revascularization with coronary angioplasty or coronary artery bypass surgery have a higher inhospital mortality than do men.[95,96] Third, when women present for diagnostic cardiac catheterization, despite the fact that they are older with more risk factors and unstable angina than men, they have a similar (or lesser) extent of epicardial coronary artery disease and better LV function.[97] Last, and perhaps most important and certainly most difficult to study, it is unclear whether the decision to undergo coronary angiography is made *for* women by the physician or *by* women who may opt to pursue medical therapy.

Invasive Diagnosis

As discussed, the indications for diagnostic cardiac catheterization in women are similar to those in men. From a procedural standpoint, the approach is similar in women and men. Women have smaller coronary arteries and a higher incidence of coronary artery spasm. Therefore, catheter engagement of the coronary ostia should be undertaken after injecting contrast into the sinus to exclude ostial disease. Catheter damping should be anticipated when the arteries are small. In this setting, it may be helpful to use 5- or 6-Fr diagnostic catheters. Catheter-induced spasm should be treated with nitroglycerin, and angiography should be repeated. If coronary spasm or the small size of an artery precludes reflux of contrast into the sinus, a sinus injection just under the coronary ostium should be performed. Non–catheter-induced coronary spasm may be evaluated with provocative testing, as noted previously.

It is noteworthy that for a given extent of epicardial coronary artery disease, women are more symptomatic (with more CCS class III–IV angina and unstable angina) than men. This is nicely demonstrated in the CASS Registry wherein the severity of angina among 2385 women and 12,938 men was stratified according to the number of vessels diseased.[96] Perhaps the more intense angina that occurs in women is due to more extensive myocardial ischemia based on an impaired vasodilator response at the level of the resistance vessels that remain unvisualized at the time of coronary angiography. This may be due to more prevalent endothelial vasomotor dysfunction in women, which may correlate with their estrogen levels, their lipid profiles, or simply their higher prevalence of hypertension and diabetes.

Myocardial ischemia with angiographically normal coronary arteries may represent microvascular angina in women.[98] In this setting, diagnostic testing for abnormal endothelial function using intracoronary infusions of acetylcholine and nitroglycerin may be useful.[71]

Management

Once the diagnosis of coronary heart disease is made, therapy for women is similar to that for men. Information on the results of pharmacotherapy for MI suggests that women and men fare equally well. The beta-blocker timolol has been shown to reduce fatal and nonfatal reinfarction in both women and men following MI.[99] Thrombolytic therapy also appears to be equally beneficial to both women and men in that reperfusion rates are similar and mortality is reduced, although the absolute reduction in mortality may be less in women.[100] However, a greater incidence of bleeding complications has been noted in women. It is unclear whether this phenomenon reflects an intrinsic gender effect or that the fixed dose of thrombolytic agent administered may be relatively greater for the average woman's smaller body size.

Despite the fact that women may be referred less often for diagnostic coronary angiography, once the diagnosis of coronary artery disease is established, referral patterns for coronary revascularization, particularly coronary angioplasty, tend to be similar to those for men.[101,102] However, the acute and long-term outcome of women undergoing revascularization procedures differs from that of men. Women in whom coronary bypass surgery is performed experience a higher surgical mortality, a higher incidence of incomplete revascularization, a higher incidence of recurrent symptoms, and a higher incidence of early and late graft occlusion, but a similar long-term mortality in comparison with men.[102–106] These differences may be due, in part, to the smaller body size of women and with smaller vessel diameter, or baseline differences in that women are older and have a higher risk profile.[106] A higher incidence of congestive heart failure in the setting of LV hypertrophy and diastolic LV dysfunction has also been implicated.[107]

Similarly, women undergoing coronary angioplasty are older and have more unstable angina, congestive heart failure, hypertension, and diabetes mellitus than do men.[95,108] Although current acute success rates are equal to those in men,[108-110] inhospital mortality is significantly higher in women undergoing coronary angioplasty.[95] In fact, female gender is an independent predictor of early mortality. In addition, inhospital complications, particularly vascular problems, are increased in women.[93] It is noteworthy, however, that women undergoing coronary angioplasty in 1993–1994, in comparison with 1985–1986, within the NHLBI PTCA Registries had a lower incidence of nonfatal MI and emergency coronary bypass surgery and a higher clinical success rate despite the fact that they were older and had more diabetes, congestive heart failure, and comorbid disease.[111] This study suggests that coronary angioplasty has been extended to women with more advanced disease with favorable results.

SELECTED READINGS

1. Puleo PR, Meyer D, Wathens C. Use of a rapid assay of subforms of creatine kinase MB to diagnose or rule out acute myocardial infarction. N Engl J Med 1994;331: 561–566.

2. Ross J, Brandenburg RO, Dinsmore RE, et al. Guidelines for coronary angiography: a report of the American College of Cardiology/American Heart Association Task Force on Assessment of Diagnostic and Therapeutic Cardiovascular Procedures (Subcommittee on Coronary Angiography). J Am Coll Cardiol 1987;4: 935–950.

3. Grondin C, Dyrda I, Paternac A, et al. Discrepancies between cineangiographic and postmortem findings in patients with coronary artery disease and recent myocardial revascularization. Circulation 1974;49:703–708.

4. Arnett R, Isner J, Redwood D, et al. Coronary artery narrowing in coronary heart disease: comparison of cineangiographic and necropsy findings. Ann Intern Med 1979; 91:350–356.

5. DeRouen T, Murray J, Owen W. Variability in the analysis of coronary arteriograms. Circulation 1976;55:324–328.

6. White C, Wright C, Doty D, et al. Does visual interpretation of the coronary arteriogram predict the physiologic importance of a coronary stenosis? N Engl J Med 1984;310:819–824.

7. Kennedy JW. The Registry Committee of the Society of Cardiac Angiography, Symposium on Catheterization Complications: Complications associated with cardiac catheterization and angiography. Cathet Cardiovasc Diagn 1982;8:5–11.

8. Bourassa MG, Noble J. Complication rate of coronary arteriography. A review of 5250 cases studied by percutaneous femoral technique. Circulation 1976;53: 106–114.

9. Johnson W, Lozner EC, Johnson S. Coronary angiography 1984–1987: a report of the Registry of the Society for Cardiac Angiography and Interventions. I. Results and complications. Cathet Cardiovasc Diagn 1989;17:5.

10. Bounous EP, Mark DB, Pollock BG, et al. Surgical survival benefits for coronary disease patients with left ventricular dysfunction. Circulation 1988;78(suppl I): I-151–I-157.

11. Schulman ST, Achuf SC, Griffith LS, et al. Prognostic cardiac catheterization variables in survivors of acute myocardial infarction: a five year prospective study. J Am Coll Cardiol 1988;11:1164–1172.

12. Ambrose JA, Winters SL, Arora RR, et al. Angiographic evolution of coronary artery morphology in unstable angina. J Am Coll Cardiol 1986;7:472–481.

13. Ryan TJ, Bauman WB, Kennedy JW, et al. Guidelines for percutaneous transluminal coronary angioplasty. A report of the American College of Cardiology/American Heart Association Task Force on assessment of diagnostic and therapeutic cardiovascular procedures (Committee on Percutaneous Transluminal Coronary Angioplasty). J Am Coll Cardiol 1993;22:2033–2054.

14. Little WC, Constantinescu M, Applegate RJ, et al. Can coronary angiography predict the site of a subsequent myocardial infarction in patients with mild-to-moderate coronary artery disease? Circulation 1988;78:1157–1166.

15. The Veterans Administration Coronary Bypass Surgery Cooperative Study Group. Eleven-year survival in the Veterans Administration randomized trial of coronary artery bypass surgery for stable angina. N Engl J Med 1984;311:1333–1339.

16. European Coronary Surgery Study Group. Prospective randomized study of coronary artery bypass surgery in stable angina pectoris. Lancet 1980;2:491–495.

17. CASS Principal Investigators and their associates. Coronary Artery Surgery Study (CASS). A randomized trial of coronary artery bypass surgery: survival data. Circulation 1983;68:939–950.

18. Cigarroa CG, deFilippi CR, Brickner ME, et al. Dobutamine stress echocardiography identifies hibernating myocardium and predicts recovery of left ventricular function after coronary revascularization. Circulation 1993;88:430–436.

19. Ragosta M, Beller GA, Watson DD, et al. Quantitative planar rest-redistribution 201TI imaging in detection of myocardial viability and prediction of improvement in left ventricular function after coronary bypass surgery in patients with severely depressed left ventricular function. Circulation 1993;87:1630–1641.

20. Weiner DA, Ryan TJ, McCabe CH, et al. Risk of developing an acute myocardial infarction or sudden coronary death in patients with exercise-induced silent mycardial ischemia. A report from the Coronary Artery Surgery Study (CASS) Registry. Am J Cardiol 1988;62:1155–1158.

21. Weiner DA, Ryan TJ, McCabe CH, et al. Significance of silent myocardial ischemia during exercise testing in patients with coronary artery disease. Am J Cardiol 1987;59:725–729.

22. Weiner DA, Ryan TJ, McCabe CH, et al. Comparision of coronary artery bypass surgery and medical therapy in patients with exercised-induced silent myocardial ischemia: a report from the Coronary Artery Surgery Study (CASS) Registry. J Am Coll Cardiol 1988;12:598–599.

23. Leppo J, Plaja J, Gionet M, et al. Noninvasive evaluation of cardiac risk factors before elective vascular surgery. J Am Coll Cardiol 1987;9:269–276.

24. Parisi A, Folland ED, Hartigan P, et al. A comparison of angioplasty with medical therapy in the treatment of single-vessel coronary artery disease. N Engl J Med 1992;326:10–16.

25. Hamm CW, Reimers J, Ischinger T, et al. A randomized study of coronary angioplasty compared with bypass surgery in patients with symptomatic multivessel coronary disease. N Engl J Med 1994;331:1037–1043.

26. King SB, Lembo NJ, Weintraub WS, et al. A randomized trial comparing angioplasty with coronary bypass surgery. N Engl J Med 1994;331:1044–1050.

27. Eagle KA, Coley CM, Newell JB, et al. Combining clinical and thallium data optimizes preoperative assessment of cardiac risk before major vascular surgery. Ann Intern Med 1989;110:859–866.

28. Baron JF, Mundler O, Bertrand M, et al. Dipyridamole-thallium scintigraphy and gated radionuclide angiography to assess cardiac risk before abdominal aortic surgery. N Engl J Med 1994;330:663–709.

29. Wong T, Detsky AS. Preoperative cardiac risk assessment for patients having peripheral vascular surgery. Ann Intern Med 1992;116:743–753.

30. Huber KC, Evans MA, Bresnahan JF, et al. Outcome of noncardiac operations in patients with severe coronary artery disease successfully treated preoperatively with coronary angioplasty. Mayo Clinic Proc 1992;67:15–21.

31. US Department of Health and Human Services. Unstable angina: diagnosis and management. Clin Pract Guidel Number 10;1994:22.

32. Lewis HD, Davis JW, Archibald DG. Protective effects of aspirin against acute myocardial infarction and death in men with unstable angina. Results of a Veterans Administration Cooperative Study. N Engl J Med 1983;309:396–403.

33. Theroux P, Ouimet H, McCans J, et al. Aspirin, heparin or both to treat acute unstable angina. N Engl J Med 1988;319:1105–1111.

34. Grambow DW, Topol EJ. Effect of maximal medical therapy on refractoriness of unstable angina pectoris. Am J Cardiol 1992;70:577–581.

35. Wilcox I, Freedman SB, Allman KC, et al. Prognostic significance of a predischarge exercise test in risk stratification after unstable angina pectoris. J Am Coll Cardiol 1991;18:677–683.

36. Brown K. Prognostic value of thallium-201 myocardial perfusion imaging in patients with unstable angina who respond to medical treatment. J Am Coll Cardiol 1991;17:1053–1057.

37. The TIMI IIIB Investigators. Effects of tissue plasminogen activator and a comparison of early invasive and conservative strategies in unstable angina and non-Q-wave myocardial infarction. Circulation 1994;89:1545–1556.
38. Myler RK, Shaw RE, Stertzer SH, et al. Unstable angina and coronary angioplasty. Circulation 1990;82(suppl II):II-88–II-95.
39. DeFeyter PJ, Suryapranata H, Serruys PW, et al. Coronary angioplasty for unstable angina: immediate and late results in 200 consecutive patients with identification of risk factors for unfavorable early and late outcome. J Am Coll Cardiol 1988; 12:324–333.
40. Nicod P, Gilpin E, Dittrich H, et al. Short- and long-term clinical outcome after Q-wave and non-Q-wave myocardial infarction in a large patient population. Circulation 1989;79:528–536.
41. Gibson RS. Non-Q-wave myocardial infarction: diagnosis, prognosis, and management. Curr Probl Cardiol 1988;13:9–72.
42. Theroux P, Kouz S, Bosch X, et al. Clinical and angiographic features of non-Q-wave and Q-wave myocardial infarction (MI). Circulation 1986;4(suppl II):303.
43. Gibson RS, Beller GA, Gheorghiade M, et al. The prevalence and clinical significance of residual myocardial ischemia two weeks after uncomplicated non-Q-wave infarction. Circulation 1986;73:1186–1198.
44. Schechtman KB, Capone RJ, Kleiger RE, et al. Risk stratification of patients with non-Q-wave myocardial infarction. The critical role of ST segment depression. Circulation 1989;80:1148–1158.
45. Grines CL, Browne KF, Marco J, et al. A comparison of immediate angioplasty with thrombolytic therapy for acute myocardial infarction. N Engl J Med 1993; 328:673–679.
46. Zijlstra F, Jan de Boer M, Hoorntje JCA, et al. A comparison of immediate angioplasty with intravenous streptokinase in acute myocardial infarction. N Engl J Med 1993;328:680–684.
47. Gibbons RJ, Holmes DR, Reeder GS, et al. Immediate angioplasty compared with the administration of a thrombolytic agent followed by conservative treatment for myocardial infarction. N Engl J Med 1993;328:685–691.
48. Topol EJ, Califf RM, George BS, et al. A randomized trial of immediate versus delayed elective angioplasty after intravenous tissue plasminogen activator in acute myocardial infarction. N Engl J Med 1987;317:581–585.
49. Simoons ML, Betriu A, Col J, et al. Thrombolysis with tissue plasminogen activator in acute myocardial infarction: no additional benefit from immediate percutaneous coronary angioplasty. Lancet 1988;(i):197–202.
50. The TIMI Research Group. Immediate vs delayed catheterization and angioplasty following thrombolytic therapy for acute myocardial infarction: TIMI II A results. JAMA 1988;260:2849–2858.
51. Ellis SG, Van DeWerf F, Ribeiro-DaSilva E, et al. Present status of rescue coronary angioplasty: current polarization of opinion and randomized trials. J Am Coll Cardiol 1992;19:681–686.
52. Ellis SG, Ribeiro-DaSilva E, Heyndrickx G, et al. Randomized comparison of rescue angioplasty with conservative management of patients with early failure of thrombolysis for acute anterior myocardial infarction. Circulation 1994;90:2280–2284.
53. Bengtson JR, Kaplan AJ, Pieper KS, et al. Prognosis in cardiogenic shock after acute myocardial infarction in the interventional era. J Am Coll Cardiol 1992; 20:1482–1489.
54. Hibbard MD, Holmes DR. Can angioplasty improve survival when cardiogenic shock complicates myocardial infarction? Coronary Artery Dis 1993;10:34–42.
55. Jones MT, Schofield PM, Dark JR, et al. Surgical repair of acquired ventricular septal defects: determinants of early and late outcome. J Thorac Cardiovasc Surg 1987; 93:670–687.

56. Miller DC, Stinson EB. Surgical management of acute mechanical defects secondary to myocardial infarction. Am J Surg 1988;116:1330–1341.
57. The TIMI Study Group. Comparison of invasive and conservative strategies after treatment with intravenous tissue plasminogen activator in acute myocardial infarction. N Engl J Med 1989;320:618–627.
58. de Bono DP, Pocock SJ, the SWIFT Investigators Group. The SWIFT study of intervention versus conservative management after anistreplase thrombolysis. Br Med J 1991;302:555–560.
59. Rogers WJ, Babb JD, Baim DS, et al. Selective versus routine predischarge coronary arteriography after therapy with recombinant tissue-type plasminogen activator, heparin and aspirin for acute myocardial infarction. J Am Coll Cardiol 1991; 17:1007–1016.
60. Proudfit WL, Shirey EK, Sones FM. Selective cine coronary arteriography: correlation with clinical findings in 1,000 patients. Circulation 1966;33:901–910.
61. CASS Principal Investigators. Coronary artery surgery study (CASS): a randomized trial of coronary artery bypass surgery. J Am Coll Cardiol 1984;3:114–128.
62. Kemp HG, Kronmal RA, Vlietstra RE, et al. Seven year surival of patients with normal or near normal coronary arteriograms: a CASS Registry study. J Am Coll Cardiol 1986;7:479–483.
63. Papanicolaou MN, Califf RM, Hlatky MA, et al. Prognostic implications of angiographically normal and insignificantly narrowed coronary arteries. Am J Cardiol 1986;58:1181–1187.
64. Proudfit WL, Bruschke AVG, Sones FM. Natural history of obstructive coronary artery disease: ten-year study of 601 nonsurgical cases. Prog Cardiovasc Dis 1978; 21:53–78.
65. Prinzmetal M, Kennamer R, Merliss R, et al. Angina pectoris. I. A variant form of angina pectoris. Am J Med 1959;27:375–388.
66. Oliva PB, Potts DE. Coronary arterial spasm in Prinzmetal angina. N Engl J Med 1973;288:745–751.
67. Schroeder JS, Bolen JL, Quint RA, et al. Provocation of coronary spasm with ergonovine maleate. New test with results in 57 patients undergoing coronary arteriography. Am J Cardiol 1977;40:487–491.
68. Conti CR. Coronary artery spasm: provocative testing. Clin Cardiol 1994;17:353.
69. Bertrand ME, LaBlanche JM, Tilmant PY, et al. Frequency of provoked coronary arterial spasm in 1089 consecutive patients undergoing coronary arteriography. Circulation 1982;65:1299–1306.
70. Yasue H, Horio Y, Nakamura N, et al. Induction of coronary artery spasm by acetylcholine in patients with variant angina: possible role of the parasympathetic nervous systems in the pathogenesis of coronary artery spasm. Circulation 1986;74: 955–963.
71. Ludmer PL, Selwyn AP, Shook TL, et al. Paradoxical vasoconstriction induced by acetylcholine in atherosclerotic coronary arteries. N Engl J Med 1986;315: 1046–1051.
72. Vita JA, Treasure CB, Mabel EG, et al. Coronary vasomotor response to acetylcholine relates to risk factors for coronary artery disease. Circulation 1990;81:491–497.
73. Brush JE, Faxon DP, Salmon S, et al. Abnormal endothelium-dependent coronary vasomotion in hypertensive patients. J Am Coll Cardiol 1992;19:809–815.
74. Cannon RO, Quyyumi AA, Schenke WH, et al. Abnormal cardiac sensitivity in patients with chest pain and normal coronary arteries. J Am Coll Cardiol 1990;16: 1359–1366.
75. Strauer BE. Ventricular function and coronary hemodynamics in hypertensive heart disease. Am J Cardiol 1979;44:999–1006.
76. Opherk D, Mall G, Zebe H, et al. Reduction of coronary reserve: a mechanism for angina pectoris in patients with arterial hypertension and normal coronary arteries. Circulation 1984;69:1–7.

77. Devereux RB, Kramer-Fox R, Brown WT, et al. Relation between clinical features of the mitral prolapse syndrome and echocardiographically documented mitral valve prolapse. J Am Coll Cardiol 1986;8:763–772.

78. Anderson HV, Roubin GS, Leimgruber PP, et al. Measurement of transstenotic pressure gradient during percutaneous transluminal coronary angioplasty. Circulation 1986;73:1223–1230.

79. Nissen SE, Gurley JC, Booth DC, DeMaria AN. Intravascular ultrasound of the coronary arteries: current applications and future directions. Am J Cardiol 1992; 69:18H–29H.

80. Kern MJ, Donohue TJ, Bach RG, et al. Clinical applications of the doppler flow velocity guidewire for interventional procedures. J Intervent Cardiol 1993;6: 345–363.

81. Joye JD, Schulman DS, Lasorda D, et al. Intracoronary doppler guide wire versus stress single-photon emission computed tomographic thallium-201 imaging in assessment of intermediate coronary stenoses. J Am Coll Cardiol 1994;24:940–947.

82. Tofler GH, Stone PH, Muller JE, et al. Effects of gender and race on prognosis after myocardial infarction: adverse prognosis for women, particularly black women. J Am Coll Cardiol 1987;9:473–482.

83. Greenland P, Reicher-Reiss H, Goldbourt U, Behar S. In-hospital and 1-year mortality in 1,523 women after myocardial infarction: comparison with 4,315 men. Circulation 1991;83:484–491.

84. Gruppo Italiano per lo Studio della Streptochinasi nell'Infarto Miocardico (GISSI). Long-term effects of intravenous thrombolysis in acute myocardial infarction: final report of the GISSI study. Lancet 1987;2:871–874.

85. Lerner DJ, Kannel WB. Patterns of coronary heart disease morbidity and mortality in the sexes: a 26-year follow-up of the Framingham population. Am Heart J 1986;111:383–390.

86. Weiner, DA, Ryan TJ, McCabe CH, et al. Correlations among history of angina, ST-segment response and prevalence of coronary artery disease in the Coronary Artery Surgery Study (CASS). N Engl J Med 1979;301:230–235.

87. Melin JA, Wijns W, Vanbutsele RJ, et al. Alternative diagnostic strategies for coronary artery disease in women: demonstration of the usefulness and efficiency of probability analysis. Circulation 1985;71:535–542.

88. Hung J, Chaitman BR, Lam J, et al. Noninvasive diagnostic test choices for the evaluation of coronary artery disease in women: a multivariate comparison of cardiac fluoroscopy, exercise electrocardiography and exercise thallium myocardial perfusion scintigraphy. J Am Coll Cardiol 1984;4:8–16.

89. Goodgold HM, Rehder JG, Samuels LD, et al. Improved interpretation of exercise T1-201 myocardial perfusion scintigraphy in women: characterization of breast attenuation artifacts. Radiology 1987;165:361–366.

90. Friedman TD, Greene AC, Iskandrian AS, et al. Exercise thallium-201 myocardial scintigraphy in women: correlation with coronary arteriography. Am J Cardiol 1982;49:1632–1637.

91. Sawada SG, Ryan T, Fineberg NS, et al. Exercise echocardiographic detection of coronary artery disease in women. J Am Coll Cardiol 1989;14:1440–1447.

92. Masini M, Picano E, Lattanzi F, et al. High dose dipyridamole-echocardiography test in women: correlation with exercise-electrocardiography test and coronary arteriography. J Am Coll Cardiol 1988;12:682–685.

93. Steingart RM, Packer M, Hamm P, et al. Sex differences in the management of coronary artery disease. N Engl J Med 1991;325:226–230.

94. Ayanian JZ, Epstein AM. Differences in the use of procedures between women and men hospitalized for coronary heart disease. N Engl J Med 1991;325:221–225.

95. Kelsey SF, James M, Holubkov AL, et al. Results of percutaneous transluminal coronary angioplasty in women: 1985–1986 National Heart, Lung and Blood Institute's Coronary Angioplasty Registry. Circulation 1993;87:720–727.

96. Philippides GJ, Jacobs AK. Coronary angioplasty in women: is there an increased risk? Cardiol Rev 1994;2:189–198.

97. Davis KB, Chaitman B, Ryan T, et al. Comparison of 15-year survival for men and women after initial medical or surgical treatment in coronary artery disease: a CASS Registry Study. J Am Coll Cardiol 1995;25:1000–1009.

98. Cannon RO III, Camici PG, Epstein SE. Pathophysiological dilemma of syndrome X. Circulation 1992;85:883–892.

99. Pedersen TR. Six-year follow-up of the Norwegian Multicenter Study on timolol after acute myocardial infarction. N Engl J Med 1985;313:1055–1058.

100. Gruppo Italiano per lo studio della Streptochinasi nell'Infarto Miocardico (GISSI). Effectiveness of intravenous thrombolytic treatment in acute myocardial infarction. Lancet 1986;1:397–402.

101. Bell MR, Berger PB, Holmes DR, et al. Referral for coronary artery revascularization procedures after diagnostic coronary angiography: evidence for gender bias? J Am Coll Cardiol 1995;25:1650–1655.

102. Loop FD, Golding LR, MacMillan JP, et al. Coronary artery surgery in women compared with men: analysis of risks and long-term results. J Am Coll Cardiol 1983; 1:383–390.

103. Tyras DH, Barner HB, Kaiser GC, et al. Myocardial revascularization in women. Ann Thorac Surg 1978;25:449–453.

104. Douglas JS, King SB III, Jones EL, et al. Reduced efficacy of coronary bypass surgery in women. Circulation 1981;64(suppl II):11–16.

105. Eaker EP, Kronmal R, Kennedy JW, et al. Comparison of the long-term, postsurgical survival of women and men in the Coronary Artery Surgery Study (CASS). Am Heart J 1989;117:71–81.

106. O'Connor GT, Morton JR, Diehl MJ, et al. Differences between men and women in hospital mortality associated with coronary artery bypass graft surgery. Circulation 1993;88(part 1):2104–2110.

107. Fisher LD, Kennedy JW, Davis KB, et al. Association of sex, physical size, and operative mortality after coronary artery bypass in the Coronary Artery Surgery Study (CASS). J Thorac Cardiovasc Surg 1982;84:334–341.

108. Judge KW, Pawitan Y, Caldwell J, et al. Congestive heart failure symptoms in patients with preserved left ventricular systolic function: analysis of the CASS registry. J Am Coll Cardiol 1991;18:377–382.

109. Cowley MJ, Mullin SM, Kelsey SF, et al. Sex differences in early and long-term results of coronary angioplasty in the NHLBI PTCA Registry. Circulation 1985; 71:90–97.

110. Welty FK, Mittleman MA, Healy RW, et al. Similar results of percutaneous transluminal coronary angioplasty for women and men with postmyocardial infarction ischemia. J Am Coll Cardiol 1994;23:35–39.

111. Jacobs AK, Kelsey SF, Yeh W, et al. A documented decline in morbidity and mortality for women undergoing angioplasty: the 1993–94 NHLBI PTCA Registry. Circulation 1995;92:I-75, 0359A.

17

PULMONARY HYPERTENSION, CARDIAC TRANSPLANTATION, AND THE CARDIOMYOPATHIES

Srinivas Murali

Pulmonary Hypertension

THE HUMAN PULMONARY circulation, unlike the systemic circulation, is a very low resistance vascular bed. The normal pulmonary artery peak systolic pressure is 15 to 30 mm Hg, end-diastolic pressure is 4 to 12 mm Hg, and mean pressure is 9 to 18 mm Hg. *Pulmonary hypertension* is defined as pulmonary artery peak systolic pressure in excess of 30 mm Hg and a mean pressure in excess of 20 mm Hg. According to the hydrodynamic equation, which draws an analogy from Ohm's law, the resistance to flow (R) varies directly with the pressure drop (ΔP) and inversely with the rate of flow (Q) across the vascular bed such that $R = \Delta P/Q$. The normal pressure drop across the pulmonary vascular bed (transpulmonary gradient [TPG]), that is, the difference between mean pulmonary artery pressure and mean pulmonary venous (left atrial, pulmonary capillary wedge) pressure, ranges from 2 to 10 mm Hg. Thus, the normal pulmonary vascular resistance (PVR), as calculated by the preceding equation, ranges from 0.25 to 1.60 mm Hg/liters/min (also referred to as Wood units). This calculated resistance, however, does not represent the true resistance to blood flow through the pulmonary circulation because it does not take into account determinants such as

461

blood viscosity, inertia to flow, vascular compliance, lung compliance, and extramural forces such as alveolar pressure. The transpulmonary gradient is directly measured. It may be more representative of vascular resistance across the pulmonary bed because it is not affected by flow across the pulmonary circulation. Increases in pulmonary flow will distend the vessels by increasing transmural pressure, thereby diminishing vascular resistance without altering TPG. In addition, augmentation of flow may also recruit parallel pulmonary vascular channels, which may further decrease resistance without affecting TPG. A TPG in excess of 12 mm Hg is consistent with pulmonary hypertension.

Classification of Pulmonary Hypertension

The causes of pulmonary hypertension can be classified in four categories (Table 17-1). Increased resistance to flow across the pulmonary circulation may develop because of decreased cross-sectional area of the vascular bed or increased resistance to flow through the large pulmonary arteries. In primary pulmonary hypertension or pulmonary hypertension of unknown cause, medium and large pulmonary arteries typically demonstrate intimal proliferation, medial hypertrophy, concentric laminar intimal fibrinoid necrosis with or without arteritis, and plexiform lesions. Eisenmenger's syndrome refers to patients who have congenital cardiac disease with severe pulmonary hypertension in whom a reversal of a left-to-right shunt has occurred. The augmented pulmonary blood flow is initially associated with a passive reduction in PVR with consequent minimal elevation of pulmonary pressures. However, chronic augmentation of blood flow results in pulmonary arterial vasoconstriction stimulated by distention of muscular pulmonary arteries and arterioles. This vasoconstriction leads to intimal fibrosis, medial hypertrophy, and reduction in cross-sectional area. Pulmonary thromboembolism results in obstruction of major pulmonary arteries and their branches, with the resultant decrease in vascular cross-sectional area and increase in resistance to blood flow. Pulmonary hypertension may also result from a decrease in vascular cross-sectional area at the capillary level. In chronic obstructive lung disease, destruction of alveoli and the subsequent reduction of the cross-sectional area of the pulmonary capillary bed result in pulmonary hypertension. Restrictive lung disease, such as interstitial pulmonary fibrosis, leads to a major reduction in pulmonary vascular cross-sectional area with the destruction and obliteration of many small arteries and arterioles. In collagen vascular disease, such as the CREST syndrome, lupus erythematosus, and rheumatoid arthritis, vasculitis with fibrous obliteration of the pulmonary vascular bed may occur.[1,2] Peripheral pulmonic stenosis is a congenital disease seen in association with supravalvular aortic stenosis. Depending on the extent, location, and severity of pulmonary stenoses, significant pulmonary hypertension may develop.

Table 17-1 Classification of Pulmonary Hypertension

1. Increased resistance to flow across pulmonary circulation
   a. Decreased cross-sectional area of pulmonary arterial bed
      - Primary pulmonary hypertension
      - Eisenmenger's syndrome
      - Chronic obstructive lung disease
      - Restrictive lung disease
      - Collagen vascular disease
   b. Increased resistance to flow through large pulmonary arteries
      - Pulmonary thromboembolism
      - Peripheral pulmonic stenosis
2. Increased resistance to pulmonary venous drainage
   a. Elevated left ventricular end-diastolic pressure
      - Left ventricular failure
      - Constrictive pericarditis
   b. Left atrial hypertension
      - Mitral valve disease
      - Left atrial myxoma
   c. Pulmonary veno-occlusive disease
3. Increased resistance from vasoconstriction secondary to hypoxia and/or hypoventilation
   a. Obesity
   b. Neuromuscular disorders
   c. Disorders of chest wall
4. Miscellaneous causes
   a. High altitude
   b. Intravenous drug abuse
   c. Hepatic cirrhosis and/or portal hypertension

A frequent cause of increased resistance causing pulmonary hypertension is pulmonary venous outflow obstruction from left heart pathology. Left ventricular systolic and/or diastolic failure from primary cardiomyopathy or ischemic heart disease may result in an elevated left atrial pressure with consequent pulmonary venous and pulmonary arterial pressures. Pulmonary hypertension is often seen in constrictive pericarditis because of an increase in the resistance to pulmonary venous return to the left atrium. Mechanical obstruction to mitral outflow, as seen in mitral stenosis and left atrial myxoma, can cause left atrial hypertension and consequent pulmonary hypertension. Likewise, pulmonary veno-occlusive disease results in pulmonary hypertension because of mechanical obstruction to pulmonary venous drainage. Acute elevation of pulmonary venous pressure to greater than or equal to 25 mm Hg results in pulmonary edema. Chronic gradual elevation, however, to pressures as high as 30 to 35 mm Hg may not result in pulmonary edema because of marked augmentation of lymph drainage in the pulmonary interstitium, diminished permeability of the alveolar capillary membrane, and reactive constriction of small pulmonary arteries and arterioles. These adaptive mechanisms explain the lack of clinical and radiographic findings of pulmonary edema in patients who have chronic elevations of left ventricular end-diastolic pressure in excess of 25 mm Hg.

Pulmonary hypoventilation due to obesity hypoventilation syndrome, neuromuscular disorders such as myasthenia gravis and poliomyelitis, and disorders of the chest wall can all result in pulmonary hypertension. Hypoxia, which is common to all of these conditions, causes pulmonary vasoconstriction.[3] High-altitude pulmonary edema is often associated with reversible pulmonary hypertension. Intravenous (IV) drug abuse can result in pulmonary vascular occlusion and pulmonary vasoconstriction. Hepatic cirrhosis with or without portal hypertension may result in pulmonary hypertension. The proposed mechanism is the inability of the damaged liver to catabolize endogenous circulating catecholamines, resulting in vasoconstriction of the pulmonary arterioles.[4]

Indications for Cardiac Catheterization

Cardiac catheterization is indicated in pulmonary hypertension, both for diagnosis and for therapy (Table 17-2). Although the presence of pulmonary hypertension can be detected with a high level of accuracy by noninvasive Doppler echocardiography, cardiac catheterization is often needed to confirm the severity and to ascertain the cause. A peak pulmonary artery systolic pressure of 30 to 45 mm Hg and a mean pressure of 20 to 30 mm Hg are considered mild pulmonary hypertension. Moderate pulmonary hypertension is defined as a pulmonary artery peak systolic pressure of 46 to 60 mm Hg and a mean pressure of 31 to 40 mm Hg. Pressures in excess of this level define severe pulmonary hypertension.

The precise cause of pulmonary hypertension can often be detected during cardiac catheterization. For instance, an oximetry run (see Chapter 10), with blood samples from the pulmonary artery, right ventricle, right atrium, superior vena cava, inferior vena cava, and a systemic artery, may detect the presence of an intracardiac shunt, its anatomic location, and its size. Intracardiac shunting should be suspected when there is an unexplained desaturation of the

Table 17-2 Indications for Cardiac
Catheterization in Pulmonary Hypertension

A. For diagnosis
   - Determination of cause
   - Assessment of severity
   - Localization of intracardiac shunt
   - Quantification of shunt
B. Pulmonary angiography
C. For therapy
   - Primary pulmonary hypertension
   - Left ventricular failure
   - Intracardiac shunt
   - Mitral valve disease

arterial blood (right-to-left shunt) or when the pulmonary artery oxygen saturation is greater than 80% (left to right). Generally, an oxygen step-up of 7% or greater at the atrial level and 5% or greater at ventricular level is considered significant. The location of the shunt may be determined by the site of the abnormal step-up. Shunt quantification requires the calculation of both pulmonary and systemic blood flow using the standard Fick equation. The ratio of pulmonary to systemic blood flow then gives the size of the shunt (for method to calculate shunt, see Chapter 10). Bidirectional shunts can be calculated by using separate formulae for left-to-right and right-to-left shunts.

The oximetry method of shunt calculation has certain limitations. It is important to ensure that a steady state is present when the serial blood samples are collected. Because the method is not very sensitive, small intracardiac shunts may be missed when utilizing this technique. Large shunts that need surgical repair, however, are detected by this method.

Pulmonary angiography is indicated for the diagnosis of suspected pulmonary embolism, pulmonary artery stenosis, pulmonary arteriovenous malformations, and intrapulmonary shunts. Pulmonary embolism often can be diagnosed on clinical grounds along with a positive ventilation-perfusion lung scan. Pulmonary angiography is indicated when the lung scan is inconclusive and the clinical suspicion is high. When multiple pulmonary thromboemboli are present, a ventilation-perfusion lung scan may not show a mismatch, and angiography is required to make the diagnosis. Pulmonary angiography is generally safe, even in those patients who are critically ill. It may, however, cause profound bradycardia, hypotension, and right ventricular failure (see Chapter 6).

Primary pulmonary hypertension remains a diagnosis of exclusion. There is no known cure. According to the National Institutes of Health registry on primary pulmonary hypertension, the median survival is 2.8 years from the time of diagnosis.[5] A number of hemodynamic variables have been shown to correlate strongly with survival in primary pulmonary hypertension.[5] A mean right atrial pressure greater than or equal to 20 mm Hg, a mean pulmonary artery pressure greater than or equal to 85 mm Hg, and a mean cardiac index less than or equal to 2 liters/min/m^2 are all associated with a poor outcome. In fact, a decrease in pulmonary pressures with vasodilator therapy in itself is an indicator of a better prognosis.[6] This fact arises because there is a vasoreactive component as well as a fixed component in most patients with pulmonary hypertension. Initially, most if not all of the pulmonary vasculature is vasoreactive. Toward the latter stages of the disease, most of the vasculature has irreversible histologic changes and the pulmonary hypertension is fixed. The response to vasodilator therapy in a given patient, therefore, depends on the proportion of the fixed and reversible components.

Significant spontaneous fluctuations occur over time in pulmonary artery pressure and PVR in patients with primary pulmonary hypertension. This spontaneous variability may be as high as 25% to 36%.[7] This fact has to be borne in mind whenever vasodilator response is quantified and target hemodynamic endpoints for effectiveness of vasodilator therapy are defined. Routine vasodilator therapy usually requires higher than conventional doses to elicit a hemodynamic response, and many patients are intolerant to such doses.[8] Patients must therefore undergo vasodilator drug testing under hemodynamic monitoring so that the appropriate dosage (i.e., that which results in a targeted hemodynamic response) may be determined.

High doses of calcium channel blockers (nifedipine or diltiazem) cause both acute and sustained reductions in pulmonary artery pressure and PVR.[6] In uncontrolled trials during long-term therapy with these agents, patients have demonstrated improvement in symptoms, reduction in right ventricular size, reduction in the QRS voltage in the right ventricular leads, and improved survival. To determine the precise dosage of calcium channel blocker necessary to produce these desirable effects, a gradual up-titration of dose (e.g., nifedipine 10 mg every hour or diltiazem 30 mg every hour) under continuous hemodynamic monitoring is recommended.

Prostacyclin (PGI$_2$ or epoprostenol) is a potent short-acting vasodilator produced by the vascular endothelium. In pharmacologic doses, it lowers PVR and pulmonary artery pressure and inhibits platelet aggregation. Acute administration of prostacyclin in patients with primary pulmonary hypertension lowers PVR and pulmonary artery pressure while improving cardiac output and systemic venous oxygen saturation.[9] Continuous administration of prostacyclin for 12 weeks has been shown to improve hemodynamics, symptoms, submaximal exercise, tolerance, and survival.[10] This drug was approved in 1994 by the Food and Drug Administration for treatment of primary pulmonary hypertension. Hemodynamic monitoring may be necessary to determine the precise dosage of prostacyclin needed to begin chronic therapy.

Another short-acting IV pulmonary vasodilator is adenosine. It may be used in an individual patient to test whether there is a component of pulmonary vasoreactivity.[11] If desirable hemodynamic effects are seen with IV adenosine (70–140 μg/kg/min for 10 min), it has been hypothesized that long-term oral therapy with other vasodilators such as calcium channel blockers or prostacyclin may be beneficial. On the other hand, if there is no response to IV adenosine, one may assume that the pulmonary hypertension is mostly fixed and therefore unresponsive to chronic vasodilator therapy. This approach requires empiric testing.

Nitric oxide is a product of the vascular endothelium involved in a number of complex biochemical reactions that elicit a variety of important biologic effects. In the endothelial cell, nitric oxide is produced by nitric oxide synthase and is an important, perhaps one of the most important, determinants of resting vascular tone.[12] Recent evidence suggests the possibility that pulmonary hypertension may be associated with a diminished expression of endothelial nitric oxide synthase.[13] Exogenous nitric oxide administration may therefore have a role in the treatment of pulmonary hypertension. Acute inhalation of nitric oxide reduces pulmonary arterial pressure and PVR without affecting cardiac output. Long-term therapy with this compound is being investigated.

Endothelin is a powerful endogenous vasoconstrictor produced by the vascular endothelium.[14] In primary pulmonary hypertension and pulmonary hypertension secondary to liver disease, increased plasma levels of endothelin and reduced clearance of endothelin have been observed.[15] In addition, increased expression of vascular endothelin RNA has been observed in explanted lungs in patients with primary pulmonary hypertension.[16] These data suggest the possibility of endothelin's involvement in the pathogenesis of pulmonary hypertension. Specific endothelin inhibitors are being tested to determine their value in this disorder.

Cardiac Transplantation

Cardiac transplantation is recommended for certain patients with end-stage heart failure whose symptoms are refractory to all available therapy. As a therapeutic strategy, transplantation is seriously limited by the relative unavailability of suitable donor hearts. Currently, approximately 3200 cardiac transplant procedures are performed annually in the United States.[17] This figure contrasts starkly with the approximately 25,000 patients with end-stage heart failure who could potentially benefit from transplantation. Because of this mismatch between supply and demand, transplantation is offered only to select patients who meet specific criteria.[18] According to the International Society for Heart and Lung Transplantation, the 1-year survival rate after cardiac transplantation is 90%, 5-year survival is 70%, and 10-year survival is 45%.[17] As the experience with cardiac transplantation has grown over the past 15 years, patient groups that have less than optimal outcome with this procedure have been identified.[18]

Orthotopic heart transplantation in patients with chronic congestive heart failure who have significant pulmonary hypertension can result in intraoperative and early postoperative right ventricular failure of the donor heart. The donor right ventricle, which is accustomed to normal PVR, may acutely fail when called on to pump into a higher-resistance pulmonary vasculature. The failing right ventricle will initially dilate and eventually become unable to maintain adequate pulmonary blood flow and left ventricular filling pressure, leading to a markedly reduced left ventricular stroke volume and cardiac output. Operative mortality with cardiac transplantation ranges from 2% to 5%, and is four- to fivefold higher if the patient has significant pulmonary hypertension.[19] The precise level of pulmonary hypertension beyond which the risk of posttransplantation donor right ventricular failure is excessive has not been completely clarified. A pre-operative calculated PVR greater than 5 Wood units or a TPG greater than 15 mm Hg have been used clinically to arbitrarily define significant pulmonary hypertension in heart transplantation candidates.[20,21] Of these two parameters, the directly measured TPG is perhaps a more accurate measure of the total pulmonary resistance than the calculated PVR, because it is flow-independent and takes into account other factors that provide resistance to flow across the pulmonary vasculature. Potential mechanisms for the development of pulmonary hypertension in chronic end-stage heart failure include the need for a high left ventricular end-diastolic pressure to fill the dilated non-compliant left ventricle, neurohormonal activation with increased circulating levels of vasoconstricting substances, structural changes in the pulmonary vasculature, and pulmonary parenchymal factors such as alveolar hypoventilation and interstitial edema. Depending on the severity and duration of congestive heart failure, pulmonary hypertension may be reactive and easily reversible with vasodilating drugs or relatively fixed as a result of medial hypertrophy, intimal thickening, and adventitial fibrosis in the pulmonary vessels.

Vasodilator Drug Testing of Pulmonary Hypertension During Pretransplantation Evaluation

A number of vasodilator drugs have been utilized to evaluate pulmonary vascular reactivity during pretransplantation evaluation. Acute administration of IV nitroglycerin can cause significant reduction in pulmonary artery pressures, pulmonary artery wedge pressure, and PVR, which are accompanied by a reduction in systemic arterial pressure and a small increase in cardiac output. Both the pulmonary artery wedge and the pulmonary artery pressures decline similarly without affecting the TPG. Therefore, the calculated PVR declines but there is no change in the TPG.

Acute administration of sodium nitroprusside also reduces both right and left heart filling pressures, systemic arterial pressure, and the calculated PVR. The cardiac output increases and a small reduction in TPG is observed. If the calculated PVR decreases to less than 3 Wood units without the systolic arterial pressure dropping to less than 85 mm Hg, it is considered an adequate vasodilator response to sodium nitroprusside.[22]

Prostaglandin E-1, which is a linoleic acid derivative, is a potent pulmonary vasodilator (arterial and venous). It has been utilized in the postoperative management of pulmonary hypertension following mitral valve surgery and for the maintenance of ductal patency in the treatment of certain cyanotic congenital heart diseases. Acute administration of IV prostaglandin E-1 usually results in a reduction in pulmonary artery pressure, pulmonary artery wedge pressure, and PVR.[23] This is accompanied by a reduction in systemic arterial pressure and an increase in cardiac output. Unlike the effect of sodium nitroprusside and nitroglycerin, the reduction in pulmonary artery pressure is of a substantially greater magnitude than the reduction in pulmonary artery wedge pressure. Therefore, the TPG declines significantly. A reduction in TPG to less than 15 mm Hg

Table 17-3 Pulmonary Vasodilator Testing During Pretransplantation Evaluation

A. Sodium nitroprusside
- Administer in incremental doses (0.5, 1.0, 1.5 μg/kg/min) at 10-min intervals

B. Prostaglandin E-1
- Administer in incremental doses (0.05, 0.1, 0.2, 0.3 μg/kg/min) at 10-min intervals

C. Adenosine
- 100 μg/kg delivered over 10 min

D. Nitric oxide
- 80 ppm inhaled over 10 min

Reduction of TPG to less than 15 mm Hg and/or PVR less than 3 Woods without reduction of systemic arterial pressure to less than 85 mm Hg systolic indicates acceptable vasoreactive response.

accompanied by a reduction in PVR to less than 5 Wood units following prostaglandin E-1 administration is considered evidence for pulmonary vasoreactivity[24] (Table 17-3).

Intravenous adenosine and inhaled nitric oxide have also been utilized for pulmonary vasodilatory testing during pretransplantation evaluation.[25,26] Both of these drugs are potent pulmonary vasodilators and reduce pulmonary arterial pressures without significant change in pulmonary artery wedge pressure, and may prove to be useful in pretransplantation evaluation.

Inotropic agents such as dobutamine, milrinone, and amrinone can also acutely lower calculated PVR by augmenting cardiac output. Little or no change in pulmonary arterial pressures is noted with dobutamine, but both amrinone and milrinone can reduce systemic and pulmonary arterial pressures and the pulmonary artery wedge pressure. However, the TPG tends to remain the same.[23]

The comparative effects of all of these drugs on pulmonary vasoreactivity are shown in Figure 17-1. The relationship of the TPG to calculated PVR is evaluated over a wide range of cardiac output. In normal subjects, the TPG is 10 mm Hg and the cardiac output 5 liters/min; calculated PVR is 2 Wood units. When the cardiac output decreases to 2 liters/min and the TPG is maintained at 10 mm Hg, the PVR increases to 5 Wood units. When the acute effects of nitroglycerin, nitroprusside, prostaglandin E-1, dobutamine, and amrinone are examined in a group of severe heart failure patients with pulmonary hypertension, heterogeneous responses are observed. All drugs increase cardiac output and decrease PVR, but only nitroglycerin, nitroprusside, and prostaglandin E-1 also lower the TPG. Prostaglandin E-1 is the most effective in lowering the TPG and PVR. There is a significant correlation between baseline TPG and the magnitude of reduction observed following acute prostaglandin E-1 infusion.

The pharmacologic agent that is used to demonstrate pulmonary vasoreactivity may then be used both intra-operatively and early postoperatively to prevent acute donor right ventricular failure after transplantation. Early mortality following cardiac transplantation is high in patients with severe pulmonary hypertension, irrespective of whether TPG or PVR is utilized to define

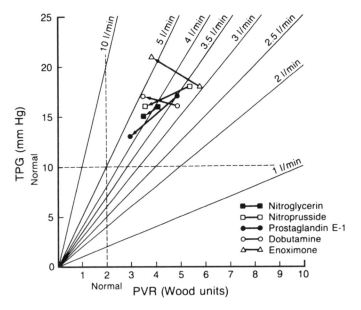

Figure 17-1   Effects of different drugs on the TPG, PVR, and cardiac output. The observed values of TPG, PVR, and cardiac output at baseline and after each drug intervention are plotted against a background of theoretical pressure-resistance lines representing different rates of flow or cardiac output as predicted by the hydrodynamic equation for streamlined flow. Note: dotted lines represent normal values for TPG and PVR and they intersect at normal cardiac output. Enoximone is a phosphodiesterase inhibitor like amrinone and milrinone. Prostaglandin E-1 is most effective in lowering both TPG and PVR. (Reprinted with permission from Murali S, Uretsky BF, Reddy PS, et al. Reversibility of pulmonary hypertension in congestive heart failure patients evaluated for cardiac transplantation: comparative effects of various pharmacologic agents. Am Heart J 1991;122:1375.)

severe pulmonary hypertension (Fig 17-2A). The mortality in the first 2 days following transplant surgery is three- to fourfold higher in patients with TPG greater than or equal to 15 mm Hg or those with calculated PVR greater than or equal to 5 Wood units. Later mortality rates (3- to 7-day, 8- to 30-day) are similar in patients with and without pulmonary hypertension. The donor right ventricle can dilate and hypertrophy to compensate for the pulmonary hypertension. This remodeling process normally begins by 48 hours following transplant surgery. Thirty-day mortality in patients undergoing cardiac transplantation who are arbitrarily grouped into four hemodynamic subsets based on their pulmonary hemodynamics is shown in Figure 17-2B. Transplant recipients who have a TPG greater than or equal to 15 mm Hg and PVR greater than or equal to 5 Wood units have the highest mortality, whereas those with a TPG less than 15 mm Hg and PVR less than 5 Wood units have the lowest 30-day mortality. It is of interest to note that mortality in patients who have a TPG greater than or equal to 15 mm Hg and PVR less than 5 Wood units is higher than those who have a TPG less than 15 mm Hg and PVR greater than or equal to 5 Wood units. These data suggest that the directly measured TPG may better predict operative risk than calculated PVR in patients undergoing cardiac transplantation.

In addition to the assessment of pulmonary hypertension, cardiac catheterization also provides important hemodynamic data to develop strategies for management of these patients while they await cardiac transplantation. The waiting period for cardiac transplantation is often long and approximately 25% to 33% of patients die on the waiting list before a suitable organ can be identified.[27] Therapies tailored to meet specific hemodynamic targets often are necessary to provide optimal care to these patients.[28] For example, if the patient has normal filling pressures and a markedly reduced cardiac output, then inotropic therapy with a beta-agonist or a phosphodiesterase inhibitor is most appropriate. On the other hand, if the filling pressures are markedly increased and the cardiac output markedly reduced, either vasodilator therapy to reduce both preload and afterload or a combination of vasodilators and inotropes may be necessary. Assessment of hemodynamics is also helpful in deciding the need for mechanical circulatory support, either with an intra-aortic balloon pump or a ventricular assist device.

Generally, a cardiac index of less than 2 liters/min/m^2 and a pulmonary artery wedge pressure greater than or equal to 20 mm Hg on maximal medical

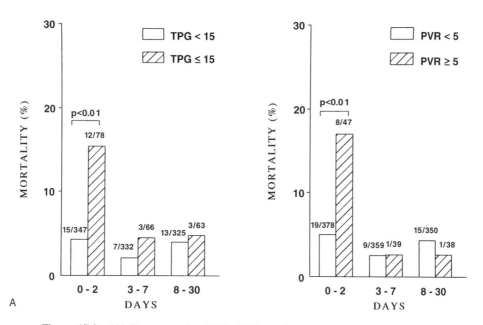

Figure 17-2 (**A**) Pre-operative TPG, PVR, and posttransplant mortality. Patients with pre-operative TPG greater than or equal to 15 mm Hg or PVR greater than or equal to 5 Wood units had a significantly higher 0- to 2-day posttransplant mortality rate.

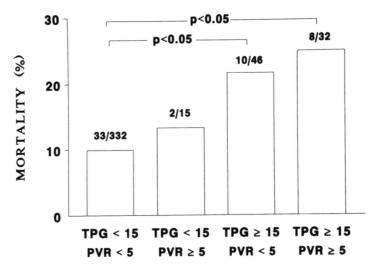

Figure 17-2 **(B)** Thirty-day posttransplant mortality in patients arbitrarily grouped into four hemodynamic subsets. The subset with a TPG greater than or equal to 15 mm Hg and PVR greater than or equal to 5 Wood units has the highest mortality rate, and the subset with a TPG less than 15 mm Hg and PVR less than 5 Wood units had the lowest mortality rate. (Reprinted with permission from Murali S, Kormos RL, Uretsky BF, et al. Preoperative pulmonary hemodynamics and early mortality after orthotopic heart transplantation: the Pittsburgh experience. Am Heart J 1993;126:896.)

therapy are considered indications for mechanical circulatory support. Intra-aortic balloon counterpulsation augments cardiac performance by diastolic augmentation of coronary blood flow and systolic reduction of cardiac afterload. It is a safe and effective "bridge" to transplantation in patients with end-stage heart failure irrespective of whether the etiology is ischemic or non-ischemic heart disease. Both univentricular and biventricular assist devices have also been successfully used in severe heart failure as a bridge to transplantation. Precise measurement of right atrial and right ventricular pressures along with assessment of the severity of pulmonary hypertension is necessary for proper selection of the type of ventricular assist device.

Posttransplant Hemodynamic Assessment

Following cardiac transplantation, relatively normal hemodynamics are restored rapidly. Cardiac output and left ventricular end-diastolic pressure return to normal within the first posttransplant month, whereas the right atrial and pulmonary artery pressures normalize by 3 to 6 months. The more severe the pre-operative pulmonary hypertension, the longer it will take to normalize following transplant surgery. Hemodynamic abnormalities, however, return to normal by the end of the first posttransplant year. The most prevalent hemodynamic abnormality is an elevated left ventricular end-diastolic pressure. It may be related to the development of systemic hypertension and left ventricular hypertrophy.[29] Hemodynamic deterioration may occur without symptoms of acute cardiac rejection. The incidence of rejection is highest during the first 6 months following transplantation. Rejection is generally detected by routine surveillance endomyocardial biopsy, often before the appearance of any symptoms. Occasionally, rejection presents itself as malaise, fatigue, low-grade fever, loss of appetite, reduction in BP, or a reduced exercise capacity. Clinical evidence for ventricular dysfunction is sometimes seen, and hemodynamic disturbances such as elevated filling pressures and a reduced cardiac output can occur. Successful treatment of rejection often reverses the hemodynamic abnormalities. Because the risk of rejection is greatest during the first few months after cardiac transplantation, surveillance endomyocardial biopsies are performed more frequently during this period. Generally, weekly biopsies are done during the first 4 to 8 weeks, followed by monthly biopsies during the first 6 months. Approximately four biopsies are done during the second posttransplant year, and two biopsies are done every year thereafter. Right heart catheterization with measurement of hemodynamics and cardiac output is usually performed during endomyocardial biopsy, although most, but not all, cases of moderate rejection do not show hemodynamic abnormalities. Three to five samples are obtained from the apex and apical septum of the right ventricle for histologic grading. A standardized rejection grading system has been established by the International Society for Heart and Lung Transplantation.[30]

Restrictive hemodynamics characterized by diastolic equalization of filling pressures with a normal or slightly reduced cardiac output are sometimes seen after transplantation. This has generally been attributed to recurrent cardiac rejection or myocardial fibrosis. Cardiac tamponade may occur early following cardiac transplantation, particularly if the surgery is complicated by mediastinal bleeding. Large pericardial effusions with or without tamponade physiology can also occur (rarely) late after transplantation in association with cardiac rejection.[18] Serial hemodynamic assessment is therefore necessary to ensure adequate function of the cardiac allograft. The hemodynamic assessment can complement other findings obtained by noninvasive studies such as radionuclide ventriculography and echocardiography.

Cardiac Allograft Vasculopathy

Cardiac allograft vasculopathy is a unique form of coronary artery disease that develops in the cardiac allograft. Its development is the major limiting factor for the long-term survival of cardiac transplant recipients.[31] The prevalence of cardiac allograft vasculopathy increases progressively over time. It is present in approximately 10% to 15% of patients by the first posttransplant year, 20% to 25% by the second year, and 35% to 50% by the fifth year.[32] It accounts for almost all of the cardiac deaths after the fifth year posttransplant. The pathogenesis of cardiac allograft vasculopathy is unknown, but there is strong evidence that suggests that it results from immune-mediated injury to the coronary vascular endothelium.[33] Conventional risk factors for atherosclerotic coronary disease, such as diabetes, hyperlipidemia, or older donor age, do not appear to predispose to the development of this unique condition. The presence or absence of cardiac allograft vasculopathy also is not related to any particular use or avoidance of immunosuppressive agent. A direct association between frequency of cardiac rejection and prevalence of cardiac allograft vasculopathy has been reported (although not in all studies), strengthening the hypothesis that it is an immune-mediated phenomenon.[31] In animal studies, increased expression of vascular cell adhesion molecules (ICAM-1 and VCAM-1), both in the myocardium and coronary arteries of the allograft, has been observed.[34] These molecules promote adhesion and transendothelial migration of inflammatory cells. Morphologically, there are several differences between cardiac allograft vasculopathy and atherosclerosis of the coronary arteries in the nontransplanted heart. Generally, cardiac allograft vasculopathy is diffuse and involves the entire length of the coronary vessel. Both conductance and resistance vessels are involved.[35] Histologically, intimal proliferation, mononuclear cell infiltration, medial hypertrophy, and lipid-laden macrophages are present throughout the vessel wall.

Cardiac allograft vasculopathy usually is not suspected clinically because following cardiac transplantation, most patients remain denervated and do not have angina. Often the initial presentation is congestive heart failure or sudden cardiac death due to infarction or ischemia.[32] Noninvasive screening studies, such as stress thallium scintigraphy and stress echocardiography, are generally not sensitive or specific in making the diagnosis.[36] Coronary angiography is needed to establish the diagnosis and to assess its severity. Coronary angiography is typically performed annually following cardiac transplantation. Interim procedures may be indicated when new cardiac symptoms occur in the absence of histologic evidence for cardiac rejection. Findings on angiography may vary from discrete proximal concentric or eccentric lesions to diffuse involvement of the vessels throughout their course. Loss of branches and pruning of the vessels also may be noted. Another striking feature is the near total absence of collateralization.[35] Conventional coronary angiography (even with sophisticated quantitative angiographic techniques) may vastly underestimate the severity of cardiac allograft vasculopathy, because the disease is often diffuse and can cause concentric luminal narrowing of the entire vessel.[37] Autopsy studies have shown severe cardiac allograft vasculopathy in patients who had a normal-appearing angiogram shortly before their deaths.[32]

Intracoronary ultrasound imaging is utilized in many transplant centers as an adjunct to conventional angiography to define the severity and progression of vasculopathy (see Chapter 19). Abnormalities of coronary endothelial function may precede the development of anatomic cardiac allograft vasculopathy.

This abnormality is evidenced by paradoxical vasoconstriction to intracoronary administration of an endothelium-dependent vasodilator such as acetylcholine. Abnormalities in coronary vascular flow reserve also are observed in patients with advanced cardiac allograft vasculopathy. Measurement of flow reserve can be accomplished with intracoronary Doppler techniques (see Chapter 20). The precise utility of intracoronary ultrasound, assessment of coronary endothelial function, and measurement of coronary vascular flow reserve in cardiac transplant recipients needs to be more fully defined.

Medical therapy for cardiac allograft vasculopathy is empiric and unproven. There is some evidence that treatment with calcium channel blocking agents, antiplatelet agents, and HMGCoA reductase inhibitors may be beneficial.[38] Discrete proximal coronary stenoses can be successfully dilated by percutaneous transluminal coronary angioplasty, atherectomy, or intracoronary stenting.[39] Coronary artery bypass grafting has been used but is generally avoided because of the diffuse nature of the disease. Experimental procedures such as transmyocardial coronary laser revascularization are under investigation. Cardiac retransplantation offers the only definitive therapy for patients with advanced cardiac allograft vasculopathy. This strategy, of course, is markedly limited by the lack of availability of adequate donor organs.

The Cardiomyopathies

The cardiomyopathies are a group of disorders of known or unknown etiology that are characterized by primary involvement of the heart muscle. In general, these disorders are not due to ischemic, hypertensive, valvular, or congenital heart disease. Most cardiologists, however, use the term *cardiomyopathy* to describe the end stage of many cardiac disorders. For example, *ischemic cardiomyopathy* refers to a condition in which long-standing ischemic disease with multiple myocardial infarctions results in diffuse fibrosis, ventricular dilatation, and heart failure. A descriptive classification of cardiomyopathies is listed in Table 17-4. Availability of improved diagnostic techniques during the past decade, such as echocardiography and radionuclide ventriculography, has permitted early diagnosis of cardiomyopathies, sometimes even prior to the onset of clinical symptoms. The hemodynamic profile in the different types of cardiomyopathies is also distinctly different, thus aiding in appropriate diagnosis.

Dilated Cardiomyopathy

Dilated cardiomyopathy is characterized by dilatation of ventricular chambers, with increased end-diastolic and end-systolic volumes and decreased cardiac contractility. It is often accompanied by symptoms of systemic and pulmonary

Table 17-4 Classification of Cardiomyopathies

1. Dilated cardiomyopathy
   a. Idiopathic
   b. Postmyocarditis
   c. Peripartum
   d. Toxic; e.g., ethanol or anthracycline
   e. Metabolic; e.g., uremia, diabetes, pheochromocytoma
   f. Miscellaneous; e.g., sarcoidosis, autoimmune disorders, obesity, hemachromatosis
2. Hypertrophic cardiomyopathy
   a. Asymmetric septal hypertrophy
   b. Diffuse symmetric hypertrophy
   c. Apical hypertrophy
3. Restrictive cardiomyopathy
   a. Idiopathic
   b. Infiltrative; e.g., amyloidosis, hemochromatosis, sarcoidosis
   c. Endomyocardial fibrosis

congestion and the syndrome of congestive heart failure. Hence, it is sometimes used synonymously with the term *congestive cardiomyopathy*. Patients with dilated cardiomyopathy, however, do not always exhibit congestive symptoms early in the course of the disease or when they are receiving effective diuretic and vasodilator therapies.

Primary or idiopathic dilated cardiomyopathy refers to dilated cardiomyopathy of unknown cause. Known causes of dilated cardiomyopathy include myocarditis, toxic agents, metabolic and endocrine disorders, pregnancy, and other miscellaneous conditions. Dilated cardiomyopathy may be familial. Although the precise mode of transmission is unknown, autosomal dominant and x-linked inheritance have been reported.[40] The clinical course of dilated cardiomyopathy is generally characterized by gradual progressive deterioration of ventricular function, with a 60% mortality by 5 years from the onset of symptoms and 80% mortality by 10 years.[41] Improvements in cardiac function do occur in a minority of patients and are accompanied by a decrease in ventricular size and a longer survival.[42] Dilated cardiomyopathy often can be diagnosed noninvasively. Two-dimensional echocardiography can demonstrate the enlarged cardiac chambers and diminished ventricular systolic function. Ventricular and annular dilatation often results in mitral and tricuspid valvular regurgitation, which can be detected and quantified by Doppler studies. Radionuclide ventriculography, much like echocardiography, can also demonstrate increased end-diastolic and end-systolic left ventricular volumes and reduced ejection fraction. However, to maximize the probability of diagnosing the cause, cardiac catheterization with hemodynamic assessment, angiography, and often endomyocardial biopsy is usually necessary.

Hemodynamic Profile in Dilated Cardiomyopathy

Symptomatic patients with dilated cardiomyopathy often exhibit elevated right and left ventricular filling pressures and a reduced cardiac output. However, an asymptomatic patient or a patient who is on optimal medical therapy may demonstrate normal hemodynamics. In such patients, hemodynamic assessment during supine bicycle exercise can help unmask the lack of contractile reserve. With minimal exercise, profound increases in filling pressures and an inappropriate augmentation or, in some cases, a drop in cardiac output may be noted. Typically, in the early stage of dilated cardiomyopathy, elevation in left ventricular end-diastolic pressure is noted. Mild-to-moderate pulmonary artery hypertension may be present, and the severity of pulmonary hypertension generally increases as the disease progresses. In advanced cases, elevation in right atrial (right ventricular end-diastolic pressure) becomes evident. The cardiac output may be maintained within the normal range until the later stages of the disease.

The hemodynamic profile in an advanced case of dilated cardiomyopathy is shown in Figure 17-3. The left ventricular pressure tracing is quite abnormal in these patients and demonstrates a slow rate of rise and a slow rate of fall. The left ventricular end-diastolic pressure is increased, sometimes markedly. Normally, following closure of the aortic valve, the left ventricular pressure declines briskly. In dilated cardiomyopathy, left ventricular relaxation is slow and probably incomplete in some cases. The increased end-systolic volume as well as the increased stiffness of the left ventricle in many cases will elevate end-diastolic volume and end-diastolic pressure. In advanced cases of dilated cardiomyopathy, in which the loss of cardiac contractility is profound, the left ventricular systolic pressure may be reduced. Administration of inotropic agents such as beta-adrenergic agonists (e.g., dobutamine) and phosphodiesterase inhibitors (e.g., milrinone) may correct the abnormalities in the left ventricular pressure tracing by reducing end-diastolic volume and augmenting systolic pressure.[43] Accurate approximation of the left atrial pressure can be obtained from the pulmonary artery wedge pressure. In advanced cases of dilated cardiomyopathy, it is sometimes difficult to position the catheter far enough in the pulmonary circulation to obtain a true pulmonary artery wedge pressure tracing. Aspiration of a fully saturated arterialized blood sample from the pulmonary wedge position confirms the accuracy of the measurement obtained. Pulmonary hypertension of varying severity may be present in dilated cardiomyopathy, with advanced cases often demonstrating severe pulmonary hypertension. The PVR is elevated, but the transpulmonary pressure gradient is usually normal early in the disease and increased in the later stages. Right ventricular systolic and end-diastolic pressures are also elevated, particularly in the advanced cases. As with the left ventricular pressure tracing, the rate of rise and the rate of fall of the right ventricular pressure tracing is slowed. The right atrial pressure also may

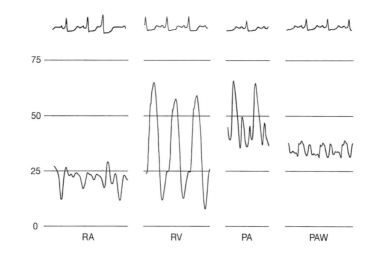

A   RA   RV   PA   PAW

Figure 17-3 Ilustrative hemodynamic profile in patients with advanced dilated cardiomyopathy. **(A)** Pressures in pulmonary
artery wedge position (PAW), pulmonary artery (PA), right ventricle (RV), and
right atrium (RA). **(B)** A second patient
shows characteristic left ventricular (LV)
pressure.

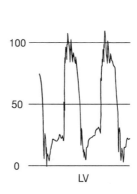

B   LV

be increased. The more advanced the disease is, the greater the reduction in
cardiac output. The resting heart rate is often increased but not to the extent
that an adequate cardiac output is maintained. The systemic vascular resistance,
like the PVR, is increased. The stroke volume is markedly reduced. Despite the
increase in systemic vascular resistance, the systemic arterial pressure either is
within the normal range or is decreased. Typically, pulse pressure is reduced
(<40 mm Hg); pulsus alternans may be seen.

Left ventriculography usually reveals a dilated left ventricle with generalized hypokinesis. The end-diastolic and end-systolic volumes are increased, with
consequent reduction in ejection fraction. Although the wall motion abnormality is usually diffuse in nature, sometimes regional systolic dysfunction is
present. This asymmetry in regional wall motion function is probably related to

the involvement of various parts of the left ventricle by the disease process, causing the dilated cardiomyopathy. Typically, the basal segments show the most vigorous contraction, and apical areas show the least. Intracavity filling defects indicative of left ventricular mural thrombi may be present. Mitral regurgitation of varying severity (ranging from mild to severe) is often present. Coronary arteriography generally reveals normal epicardial coronary arteries. Sometimes mild-to-moderate coronary disease is noted, but the extent of this disease is not severe enough to explain the degree of left ventricular systolic dysfunction or all of the wall motion abnormalities. The maximal coronary vasodilatory capacity measured by intracoronary angiometry may be reduced in spite of normal-appearing epicardial vessels on angiography.[44] The reduced coronary flow reserve might explain the presence of chest pain and Q waves on the surface ECG in some patients with dilated cardiomyopathy.

An endomyocardial biopsy (see Chapter 11) may aid in ascertaining the cause of dilated cardiomyopathy. Histologic findings can confirm the following diagnoses: myocarditis, sarcoidosis, hemachromatosis, amyloidosis, scleroderma, vasculitis, and anthracycline cardiomyopathy. Acute myocarditis is characterized histologically by dense interstitial and perivascular cellular infiltrates, myocyte necrosis, and interstitial fibrosis. In hemachromatosis, iron can be demonstrated in the myocardium by using special stains. Myocardial sarcoidosis is characterized by the presence of noncaseating granulomas. Myocardial deposition of amyloid protein can be detected using the Congo red stain, a positive birefringence appearance being pathognomonic of cardiac amyloidosis. In idiopathic dilated cardiomyopathy, the endomyocardial biopsy findings are nonspecific and include interstitial and perivascular fibrosis, myocyte hypertrophy, myocyte degeneration, and very scant or no cellular infiltrate. In addition to its diagnostic utility, histologic and histomorphometric assessment of biopsy samples may provide useful prognostic information about patients with dilated cardiomyopathy, although not all studies have confirmed these data.[45]

Hypertrophic Cardiomyopathy

Hypertrophic cardiomyopathy is characterized by inappropriate cardiac hypertrophy in the absence of an obvious stimulus. The typical features of this disorder include myocardial hypertrophy, which may be asymmetric, symmetric, or apical; a nondilated left ventricle; and hyperdynamic left ventricular function. The disorder may be transmitted genetically as an autosomal dominant trait with variable expression and penetrance, although sporadic cases do occur. In familial hypertrophic cardiomyopathy, there is a point mutation in the gene encoding for beta-myosin heavy chain that is located in the long arm of the fourteenth chromosome.[46] In asymmetric hypertrophic cardiomyopathy, the hypertrophy is restricted to the high interventricular septum such that the ratio of the thickness of the diastolic septal wall to that of the posterior wall is greater than 1.3. Symmetric hypertrophic cardiomyopathy is characterized by concentric left ventricular hypertrophy. Apical hypertrophic cardiomyopathy, described initially in Japan, shows massive apical hypertrophy accompanied by giant T-wave inversions in the precordial electrocardiographic leads.

The physiology of hypertrophic cardiomyopathy is distinctly different from that of dilated cardiomyopathy. The predominant abnormality is diastolic dysfunction due to an excessive stiffness of the ventricular chamber, resulting in impaired ventricular relaxation and filling. The ventricular chamber size is small and the myocardial mass is greatly increased. The hypertrophic process always involves the left ventricle, but in some cases, the right ventricle is also affected. The atria are often dilated and sometimes hypertrophic. Histologically, the cardinal features are myocyte hypertrophy and disarray. There is disorganization of the myocyte arrangement as well as the myofibrillar architecture within the myocyte. Interstitial fibrosis also is present. The intramural coronary arteries demonstrate thickening of the tunica media and adventitial fibrosis, resulting in a substantial reduction of the lumen size. Generally, foci of disarray are interspersed with foci of normally arranged myocytes.

The clinical spectrum of hypertrophic cardiomyopathy can range from an asymptomatic patient to one with incapacitating symptoms. Dyspnea is the most common symptom, followed by angina, palpitations, paroxysmal nocturnal dyspnea, and dizziness. Congestive heart failure may be present, and transmural myocardial infarctions can occur in the absence of significant coronary artery disease. Syncope may occur, particularly during exertion, and is usually a result of inadequate augmentation of cardiac output or of cardiac arrhythmias. Diagnosis of hypertrophic cardiomyopathy usually can be made noninvasively with two-dimensional echocardiography and Doppler examinations. The cardinal echocardiographic feature is left ventricular hypertrophy, which may be diffuse symmetric, apical, or asymmetric, that is often restricted to the high or mid-interventricular septum. Often, the septum is greater than 15 mm in thickness (normal thickness less than or equal to 11 mm), and the hypertrophic myocardium demonstrates a ground-glass appearance. If asymmetric septal hypertrophy is present, the left ventricular outflow tract may be narrowed. A pressure gradient across the left ventricular outflow tract associated with an abnormal systolic anterior motion (SAM) of the anterior leaflet of the mitral valve may be present. The greater the degree of SAM, the higher the outflow tract gradient. Other echocardiographic findings include a small left ventricular chamber size, normal systolic wall motion with the exception of septal hypokinesis, reduced rate of closure of the mitral valve during diastole, and coarse systolic fluttering of the aortic valve. Cardiac catheterization with hemodynamic assessment and angiography is often necessary for accurate assessment of the left ventricular outflow tract gradient and for delineation of the coronary anatomy.

Hemodynamic Profile in Hypertrophic Cardiomyopathy

The main hemodynamic feature is an elevated left ventricular end-diastolic pressure due to a reduced diastolic compliance. The reduced compliance results from increased stiffness of the hypertrophic left ventricular wall and a reduced rate and extent of myocardial relaxation. The pulmonary artery wedge pressure is also elevated, particularly when mitral regurgitation is present. The a and v waves on the pulmonary artery wedge pressure tracing may be prominent. Cardiac output is usually normal, but in the later stages of the disease, it may be reduced because of reduced left ventricular contractility or decreased end-diastolic volume from cavity obliteration. Patients who have advanced hypertrophic cardiomyopathy also may demonstrate pulmonary hypertension, which may range from mild to severe with elevations in right ventricular end-diastolic and right atrial pressures.

When asymmetric septal hypertrophy is present, the classic hemodynamic feature is the systolic intraventricular (outflow tract) pressure gradient. This gradient is often dynamic and labile, that is, present on one occasion but absent at another time in the same patient. If the gradient is absent at rest, provocative maneuvers are necessary to demonstrate its presence. The symmetric and apical forms of hypertrophic cardiomyopathy do not demonstrate this gradient. Sometimes a gradient also may be observed across the right ventricular outflow tract in patients who demonstrate a left ventricular outflow tract gradient.[47] The precise mechanism for this gradient is the marked narrowing of the outflow tract as a result of hypertrophy of the septum and the apposition of the anterior mitral leaflet against the septum during systole. Increased contractility and decreased preload and afterload that reduce left ventricular volume and exaggerate the apposition of the anterior mitral leaflet against the septum markedly increase the gradient. For accurate measurement of this gradient, the left ventricular catheter with a single end hole or several holes 1 to 2 mm from the tip (e.g., multipurpose A_1 or A_2) is advanced close to the left ventricular apex and a gradual pullback maneuver is performed under continuous hemodynamic pressure recording. As the catheter is withdrawn from the left ventricular cavity into the outflow tract, the presence of this systolic gradient is demonstrated (Fig 17-4). Another hemodynamic feature of asymmetric hypertrophic cardiomyopathy is the presence of a spike-and-dome configuration in the arterial pressure tracing. This pattern is seen in the central aortic as well as the peripheral arterial pressure tracings. It is the result of an initial rapid rise in aortic pressure due to the hyperdynamic systolic ejection, followed by a sudden drop in pressure and a dome-shaped tidal wave prior to the dicrotic notch. The dome-shaped wave is the result of the pulling of the anterior mitral leaflet into the outflow tract, resulting in the obstruction to the mid- and late-systolic ejection. This spike-and-dome configuration is seen only in association with a left ventricular outflow tract gradient. Provocative maneuvers that are typically used to demonstrate the left ventricular outflow tract gradient (if it is absent at rest) include the Valsalva maneuver, leg exercise, isoproterenol infusion, amyl nitrate inhalation, and induction of ventricular extrasystoles. In addition to the increase in gradient, the Valsalva maneuver also results in a change in the femoral arterial pressure configuration to the spike-and-dome pattern. Similar augmentation of the left ventricular outflow tract gradient can be seen with leg exercise (due to increased contractility and reduced afterload), isoproterenol infusion (due to decreased preload), and amyl nitrate inhalation (due to reduced preload and afterload).

An additional feature of the arterial pressure tracing in asymmetric hypertrophic cardiomyopathy is the failure of the pulse pressure to augment in a postextrasystolic beat. Typically, the beat following a premature ventricular contraction demonstrates a higher pulse pressure. In hypertrophic cardiomyopathy, the beat following an extrasystole demonstrates either the same or, occasionally, a reduced pulse pressure. This finding was first described by Brockenbrough and is referred to as the Brockenbrough sign (see Fig 17-4). It is thought to be due to worsening of the outflow tract obstruction during the potentiated beat, resulting in a reduced stroke volume and a diminished pulse pressure. The precise mechanism for the increased outflow tract obstruction is debated but is felt to be from a reduced afterload during the potentiated extrasystolic beat.

Abnormalities in diastolic function seen in hypertrophic cardiomyopathy are thought to be related to abnormal calcium fluxes with a consequent increase in intracellular calcium concentration. Calcium channel blocker therapy appears to be effective, in some cases, in reversing these diastolic abnormalities. The acute response to calcium channel blockade can be assessed during cardiac catheterization. Administration of sublingual nifedipine or IV verapamil often results in a reduction in left ventricular end-diastolic pressure and a restoration of normal left ventricular relaxation. Normally, the left ventricular pressure rapidly declines to a nadir near 0 mm Hg, followed by a gradual increase during diastole to an end-diastolic pressure of 3 to 12 mm Hg. In hypertrophic cardiomyopathy, the left ventricular pressure often declines to approximately 3 to 5 mm Hg during early diastole, with a slowed relaxation followed by the continued gradual decrease during mid-diastole.[48] During late-diastole, when atrial systole occurs, the diastolic pressure rises coincident with the a wave. Calcium channel blockers have been reported to decrease early and late diastolic pressures and improve the speed of ventricular relaxation.[49]

Left ventriculography in hypertrophic cardiomyopathy demonstrates a small left ventricular cavity. If asymmetric septal hypertrophy is present, the

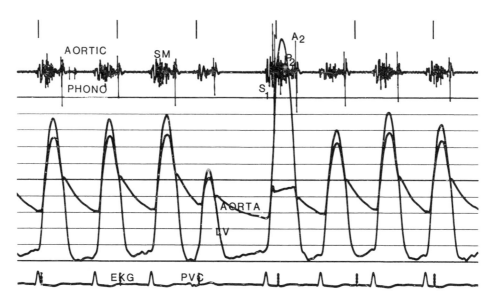

Figure 17-4 Simultaneous left ventricular (LV) and aortic pressure, EKG, and phonocardiogram in a patient with hypertrophic cardiomyopathy. There is a small (<20 mm Hg) LV-aortic gradient (scale 0–200 mm Hg). With postpremature ventricular contraction (PVC), there is a large provoked gradient (>140 mm Hg), a spike and dome appearance in the aortic tracing, and a decrease in aortic pulse pressure (Brockenbrough sign). (Illustration courtesy of Dr. James A. Shaver.)

thickened interventricular septum may be seen bulging into the left ventricular outflow tract during systole. Systolic anterior motion of the anterior leaflet of the mitral valve also may be seen. In apical hypertrophic cardiomyopathy, the marked thickening of the anteroapical wall gives the left ventricle a characteristic spade-like appearance. Mitral regurgitation of varying severity may be observed during left ventriculography. The end-systolic and end-diastolic volumes are lower than normal, and the ejection fraction is often higher. In advanced cases, the end-systolic volume actually may be increased, resulting in a reduced systolic function. Coronary angiography usually reveals normal coronary arteries. When asymmetric septal hypertrophy is present, systolic narrowing of the left anterior descending coronary artery or phasic narrowing of the septal perforator branches of the left anterior descending coronary artery (myocardial bridging) may be evident.

Dual-chamber sequential pacing with optimal atrioventricular conduction interval has been shown to reduce resting left ventricular outflow tract gradient and prevent the augmentation of this gradient during exercise in patients with asymmetric hypertrophic cardiomyopathy.[50] Determination of atrial and ventricular pacing rates as well as the optimal atrioventricular conduction time may be performed during cardiac catheterization. Temporary pacing catheters are inserted into the right atrium and the right ventricle. The atrial pacemaker catheter is positioned on the right atrial free wall and the ventricular catheter at the right ventricular apex. The position of these two catheters is confirmed by the electrogram and/or fluoroscopy. The resting left ventricular outflow tract gradient is measured and the increase in the gradient following provocations such as leg exercise is documented. The left ventricular outflow tract gradient is then remeasured at different atrial and ventricular pacing rates and atrioventricular conduction times to determine which pacing rate and atrioventricular conduction interval provides the lowest resting and exercise gradients. This information is utilized to establish the appropriate criteria for chronic pacing.

Restrictive Cardiomyopathy

Restrictive cardiomyopathy refers to a group of disorders in which the predominant cardiac impairment is ventricular diastolic dysfunction. The ventricular walls are stiff and noncompliant and restrict ventricular filling. The systolic function is usually normal or only modestly impaired. This form of cardiomyopathy is often confused with constrictive pericarditis, in which the thickened pericardium restricts ventricular filling. It is, however, important to differentiate between these two conditions, because constrictive pericarditis often can be cured with pericardial stripping.

Restrictive cardiomyopathies can be classified as idiopathic noninfiltrative, infiltrative, and endomyocardial fibrosis. The cause of idiopathic noninfiltrative restrictive cardiomyopathy is unknown. Familial cases have been reported, but the mode of genetic transmission is not clear. It is often associated with atrioventricular conduction abnormalities and sudden cardiac death due to recurrent ventricular arrhythmias. The most common causes of infiltrative restrictive cardiomyopathy are amyloidosis and hemachromatosis. Amyloidosis may be (1) primary, in which the amyloid protein infiltrating the myocardium is composed of immunoglobulin light chain (termed *AL*) produced by plasma cells in the reticulo-endothelial system; (2) secondary, in which the amyloid protein is a nonimmunoglobulin (termed *AA*); (3) familial, in which transthyretin produced predominantly in the liver is the amyloid protein; or (4) senile, in which the amyloid protein is a pre-albumin that is produced in excess, generally in patients over 80 years old.[51] Hemachromatosis may be (1) primary or idiopathic, (2) familial, or (3) secondary.[52] It is characterized by excessive deposition of iron in the myocardium along with a number of other organs. Secondary causes of hemachromatosis include beta-thalassemia and similar conditions associated with ineffective erythropoiesis and chronic liver disease. Endomyocardial fibrosis is a disorder of unknown cause in which extensive fibrosis of the endocardium and myocardium predominantly involves the inflow portions of the right and left ventricles.[53]

The predominant symptom of restrictive cardiomyopathy is progressive exercise intolerance. The impaired ventricular filling at rest is further compromised during exercise when the heart rate rises. In advanced cases, jugular venous distention, peripheral edema, ascites, and hepatomegaly are often present. Regurgitation of the mitral and tricuspid valves is common. Radionuclide ventriculography and Doppler echocardiography can demonstrate the presence of impaired ventricular filling and thus help to confirm the diagnosis. Reduced peak ventricular filling rate, prolonged time to peak filling, increased atrial filling period, and augmented atrial contribution to filling can be shown with these noninvasive methods.[54] Thickened ventricular walls with a characteristic granular sparkling texture may be seen on echocardiography in cardiac amyloidosis.[55] Computed tomography scanning and magnetic resonance imaging can sometimes help distinguish constrictive pericarditis from restrictive cardiomyopathy by demonstrating the presence of pericardial thickening, fibrosis, and calcification. The pattern of left ventricular filling on Doppler echocardiography or radionuclide ventriculography also may help to differentiate between restrictive cardiomyopathy and constrictive pericarditis.[56] In restrictive cardiomyopathy, the time to peak filling as well as the atrial filling period are prolonged, whereas in constrictive pericarditis, the time to peak filling is normal, while the atrial filling period is markedly increased.[57] Despite this utility of the noninvasive techniques, cardiac catheterization with hemodynamic assessment, ventriculography, and endomyocardial biopsy is often necessary for the demonstration of left ventricular diastolic dysfunction, normal systolic function, and presence of myocardial infiltration and fibrosis.

Hemodynamic Profile in Restrictive Cardiomyopathy

The classic hemodynamic feature of restrictive cardiomyopathy is the dip and plateau of the left ventricular pressure tracing, referred to as the square root sign (Fig 17-5). The left ventricular pressure declines rapidly at the onset of ventricular diastole. This is followed by a rapid rise to a plateau during the early part of diastole. The left ventricular diastolic pressure is markedly increased because of the stiff, noncompliant left ventricle, which requires a higher pressure to fill. Because of the profound ventricular stiffness, little filling occurs after early diastole, reflected in minimal change of ventricular pressure with atrial systole. The pulmonary artery wedge pressure is also increased and corresponds to the left ventricular end-diastolic pressure. Moderate-to-severe pulmonary hypertension is usually present. The dip-and-plateau configuration also may be seen in the right ventricular pressure tracing, when the right ventricle is involved in the restrictive entity. The right atrial pressure is elevated, and the atrial pressure tracing may demonstrate a prominent y descent. The x descent also may be prominent. The a wave is usually prominent, and its height is either the same or greater than the v wave. The cardiac output is usually normal in

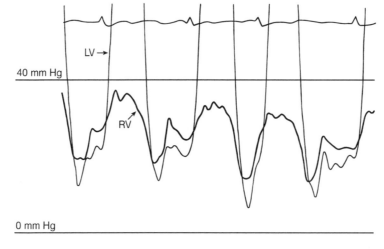

Figure 17-5 Hemodynamic profile in a 60-year-old man with restrictive cardiomyopathy due to hemochromatosis. The simultaneous pressure recordings from the left (LV) and right ventricles (RV) are shown. The diastolic pressures are increased in both ventricles and a dip and plateau configuration is seen particularly in the right ventricular tracing. This case is particularly unusual in that the RV diastolic pressure is higher than the LV pressure suggesting more severe involvement of the RV than the LV. Note that in Figure 17-3A the right ventricular tracing has somewhat of a square root sign, illustrating that this finding cannot be considered pathognomonic for restrictive physiology.

restrictive cardiomyopathy, but an increased heart rate is typical because of reduction in the stroke volume. In the later stages of the disease, cardiac output is usually reduced.

Distinction between restrictive cardiomyopathy and constrictive pericarditis often can be suggested during cardiac catheterization. It is imperative to obtain simultaneous recordings of both the right and the left ventricular diastolic pressures to demonstrate a true difference. The hemodynamic differences between restrictive cardiomyopathy and constrictive pericarditis are listed in Table 17-5. Typically, in restrictive cardiomyopathy, the left ventricular end-diastolic pressure exceeds the right ventricular end-diastolic pressure by more than 5 mm, and the right ventricular end-diastolic pressure is less than one third of the peak right ventricular systolic pressure. Pulmonary hypertension is often mild in constrictive pericarditis, and the pulmonary artery systolic pressure often does not exceed 50 mm Hg. Both the x and the y descents in the right atrial pressure tracing are prominent in constrictive pericarditis, giving a characteristic m or w waveform of the right atrial pressure tracing. In restrictive cardiomyopathy, the y descent is usually more prominent. In some cases, however, these hemodynamic differences may not be obvious. Exercise testing or volume challenge may be necessary to bring out the difference. There is no

Table 17-5 Hemodynamic Differences Between Restrictive
Cardiomyopathy and Constrictive Pericarditis

Restrictive cardiomyopathy	*Constrictive pericarditis*
1. LVEDP − RVEDP > 5-mm Hg difference	LVEDP − RVEDP 0–5 mm Hg
2. RVEDP < 1/3 RVSP	RVEDP > 1/3 RVSP
3. PA systolic > 50 mm Hg	PA systolic < 50 mm Hg
4. Prominent y descent in RA pressure	Prominent x and y descent in RA pressure tracing

Abbreviations: LVEDP, left ventricular end-diastolic pressure; RVEDP, right ventricular end-diastolic pressure; RVSP, right ventricular systolic pressure; PA, pulmonary artery; RA, right atrial.

pathognomonic sign to differentiate these two entities. Diagnosis requires synthesis of clinical, noninvasive, and invasive data. Even then, thoracotomy may be necessary and is considered the approach when the suspicion of constriction is high.

Left ventriculography in restrictive cardiomyopathy demonstrates normal contractile function, except in the later stages of the disease when the systolic function may be reduced diffusely. Mitral regurgitation of varying severity is often present. Filling defects due to intracavitary thrombus are sometimes present. Coronary arteriography usually demonstrates normal coronary arteries.

Endomyocardial biopsy may help to identify the etiology of restrictive cardiomyopathy and help to differentiate this disorder from constrictive pericarditis.[58] Idiopathic noninfiltrative restrictive cardiomyopathy is characterized by extensive interstitial fibrosis in the myocardium. There is no cellular infiltrate. In amyloidosis, the deposition of amyloid protein in the interstitium can be demonstrated using the Congo red stain (see earlier discussion). The deposition may sometimes be focal, and the diagnosis may be missed unless multiple biopsy samples are obtained. Occasionally, amyloid deposits are seen in the tunica media and adventitia of intramural coronary arteries with narrowing of the lumen size. In hemachromatosis, myocardial iron deposits can be demonstrated by using special stains for iron. The iron deposits are usually either subepicardial or located within the sarcoplasmic reticulum. The subepicardial myocardium tends to be involved later in the disease. Myocyte degeneration and interstitial fibrosis may occasionally coexist. In endomyocardial fibrosis, there is extensive endocardial fibrosis extending into the myocardium accompanied by interstitial edema. No cellular infiltration is present. Occasionally, endomyocardial fibrosis may involve only the left ventricle, and a right ventricular biopsy may miss the diagnosis. Because intramural ventricular thrombi are sometimes present in restrictive cardiomyopathy (particularly endomyocardial fibrosis), endomyocardial biopsy must be performed with utmost caution. The absence of an intramural thrombus must be demonstrated on either echocardiography or contrast ventriculography before the biopsy procedure is attempted.

Because there is no specific therapy for restrictive cardiomyopathy, treatment is often aimed at relieving symptoms. Occasional benefit from chemotherapy has been noted in patients with cardiac amyloidosis.[59] Familial cardiac amyloidosis, in which the amyloid protein transthyretin is produced predominantly in the liver, may be cured by hepatic transplantation.[60] Hemochromatosis may respond to phlebotomy or chelation therapy with desferrioxamine.[61] Surgical excision of the fibrotic endocardium along with replacement of the mitral valve may be effective in patients with endomyocardial fibrosis. Calcium channel blocker therapy can improve the impaired left ventricular diastolic function, but data are mixed on this point.[62] Symptoms of congestive heart failure, however, may be exacerbated due to the negative inotropic effects of these agents. Acute responses to calcium channel blocker therapy can be determined by cardiac catheterization, during which the hemodynamic response to either IV verapamil or sublingual nitroglycerin on left ventricular and right ventricular end-diastolic pressures can be evaluated.

Hemodynamic Assessment During Isotonic and/or Isometric Exercise

In patients studied in the catheterization laboratory who demonstrate normal resting hemodynamics, an exercise study may add diagnostic information. Hemodynamic assessment during exercise may identify abnormalities of cardiac performance that explain symptoms and direct appropriate therapy. Exercise hemodynamic testing also may be helpful in clarifying prognosis. Isotonic leg exercise has utilized a supine bicycle and for upper extremity exercise an arm ergometer.[63] Straight leg raising also has been utilized. Isometric exercise using a hand dynamometer may be helpful but has been less frequently employed, so data are limited.

Indications for Obtaining Exercise Hemodynamics

The indications for exercise hemodynamic measurement are listed in Table 17-6. In patients with exercise intolerance and normal resting cardiac function, exercise hemodynamic testing may provide the diagnosis and assist in understanding the mechanism for reduced exercise capacity.[63] When cardiac and pulmonary diseases coexist, exercise hemodynamic assessment may help to differentiate the mechanism so that appropriate therapy can be prescribed. Exercise hemodynamic testing has been used in an attempt to differentiate restrictive cardiomyopathy from constrictive pericarditis. Hemodynamic assessment during exercise also may help to define prognosis and therapy in patients with asymptomatic left ventricular dysfunction, mild valvular stenosis with a low resting transvalvular pressure gradient, valvular insufficiency that is mild at rest, in-

Table 17-6   Indications for Exercise Hemodynamic Testing

A. For diagnosis
    Evaluation of
    - Exertional dyspnea or fatigue of unknown cause in the presence of normal resting cardiac function
    - Etiology of dyspnea in the presence of both cardiac and pulmonary disease
    - Restrictive cardiomyopathy and constrictive pericarditis
B. For prognosis and therapy
    Evaluation of
    - Left ventricular dysfunction
    - Valvular stenosis and insufficiency
    - Intracardiac shunt
    - Pulmonary hypertension

tracardiac shunt that is small or insignificant at rest, and pulmonary hypertension that is mild at rest.[64]

Exercise Protocol

After baseline hemodynamic assessment, the appropriate exercise protocol should be initiated. It is important to perform exercise hemodynamic testing prior to angiography, because contrast agents modify hemodynamics. If bicycle ergometer exercise is utilized, baseline resting hemodynamics should be measured with the patient's feet strapped to the bicycle pedals. During exercise, the heart rate and BP are recorded continuously. At peak exercise, all of the hemodynamic measurements, including cardiac output, are repeated. Serial oximetry and simultaneous pressure recordings at various exercise stages are performed as indicated.

Normal Hemodynamic Response to Exercise

During isotonic exercise, oxygen consumption increases to match the augmented oxygen demand of the exercising skeletal muscles. Oxygen consumption is expressed as metabolic equivalents (METs), such that the oxygen consumption at rest ($\sim$ 4.5 ml O_2/kg/min) is defined as 1 MET. During maximal exercise, the oxygen consumption can increase up to 12-fold; that is, the maximal exercise oxygen consumption may rise to 12 METs. Maximal oxygen consumption is influenced by age, gender, fitness level, metabolic state, body temperature, and hemoglobin concentration, and it is lower in women, older and sedentary persons, or patients with anemia. Exercise training and improved fitness can increase maximal exercise oxygen consumption. The increase in oxygen consumption during exercise is brought about by an increase in cardiac output (oxygen delivery) and by augmented oxygen extraction at the tissue level. The difference between the arterial and venous oxygen content is therefore widened. The 12-fold increase in oxygen consumption is brought about by a fourfold rise in cardiac output and a threefold increase in the arteriovenous oxygen difference. The increase in cardiac output results from an increase in heart rate and an increase in stroke volume. There is a strong linear relationship between cardiac output and oxygen consumption during exercise. Systemic arterial pressure increases during exercise mainly because of the augmented cardiac output. The systemic vascular resistance, on the other hand, decreases due to vasodilation in the vascular bed of the exercising skeletal muscles. The left ventricular systolic performance improves with augmented left ventricular contractility and ejection fraction. The left ventricular end-diastolic volume does not change, but the end-systolic volume decreases, resulting in an increase in stroke volume. During upright isotonic exercise, the left ventricular end-diastolic volume may increase. The left ventricular end-diastolic pressure may remain unchanged or decrease during exercise. Thus, a normal heart is capable of augmenting left ventricular systolic performance despite a decrease in filling pressure. There is little or no change in pulmonary artery pressures during exercise in normal subjects, although a transient pressure increase has been noted, but it decreases over time. This transient increase probably is related to an increased pulmonary blood flow and unchanged pulmonary resistance, which then decreases over time, either by decreasing arteriolar tone or recruiting more pulmonary arterioles.

Isometric exercise in normal subjects also increases both the heart rate and the BP. The cardiac output augmentation is predominantly from an increase in heart rate, because the stroke volume changes very little. The systemic vascular resistance increases, and there is little change in the end-diastolic and end-systolic left ventricular volumes. The left ventricular end-diastolic pressure and the pulmonary artery pressure usually remain unchanged. The maximal oxygen consumption achieved during isometric exercise is smaller when compared with isotonic exercise.

The increasing metabolic needs of the skeletal muscles during exercise augment gluconeogenesis, and the hepatic and skeletal muscle glycogen stores are broken down in an accelerated manner. The resultant excessive production of carbon dioxide increases the rate and depth of ventilation. When the oxygen supply is no longer able to keep up with demand during exercise, anaerobic metabolism of glycogen ensues, resulting in metabolic acidosis from lactic acid production. This causes a feeling of exhaustion and breathlessness, resulting in the cessation of exercise.

Exercise Hemodynamic Response in Left Ventricular Dysfunction

Unlike normal subjects, patients with left ventricular dysfunction increase left ventricular end-diastolic, pulmonary artery wedge, and pulmonary artery pres-

Table 17-7   Hemodynamic Data at Rest and After
Seven Minutes of Supine Bicycle Exercise in a Patient
with Severe Left Ventricular Systolic Dysfunction

	Rest	Exercise
HR	90	140
MAP	90	102
RAP	6	10
PAP	32	45
PAW	16	30
LVEDP	18	32
CO	4.3	7.0
AVO_2	5.9	12.2
SV	48	50

Abbreviations: AVO_2, arteriovenous oxygen difference (vols O_2%); CO, cardiac output (l/min); HR, heart rate (beats per minute); LVEDP, left ventricular end-diastolic pressure (mm Hg); MAP, mean arterial pressure (mm Hg); PAP, mean pulmonary artery pressure (mm Hg); PAW, mean pulmonary artery wedge pressure (mm Hg); RAP, mean right atrial pressure (mm Hg); SV, stroke volume (ml/beat).

sures during supine bicycle exercise (Table 17-7). The heart rate increases with little change in stroke volume, such that the maximal exercise cardiac output is lower than predicted. The left ventricular end-diastolic volume increases, and in severe cases, the left ventricular end-systolic volume increases as well. The ejection fraction either does not change or actually may decrease. The systemic arterial pressure increases and is often accompanied by an increase in the systemic vascular resistance.

Isometric exercise in left ventricular dysfunction can result in marked augmentation of heart rate, left ventricular end-diastolic pressure, and pulmonary artery pressure. The systemic arterial pressure increases along with a marked increase in systemic vascular resistance. The left ventricular end-diastolic volume is unchanged, but the end-systolic volume increases, thereby reducing stroke volume and ejection fraction.

Exercise Hemodynamic Response in Coronary Artery Disease

Patients with coronary artery disease may demonstrate myocardial ischemia during exercise hemodynamic testing. Ischemia will result in a marked augmentation of left ventricular end-diastolic pressure and often a reduction in cardiac output. Both the heart rate and BP may increase, along with an increase in left ventricular end-diastolic and end-systolic volumes. The stroke volume and ejection fraction may therefore fall during exercise. These hemodynamic abnormalities may be accompanied by electrocardiographic changes of myocardial ischemia and angina.

Exercise Hemodynamic Response in Valvular Heart Disease, Congenital Heart Disease, and Pulmonary Hypertension

In patients with mitral stenosis, the augmented heart rate during exercise reduces the diastolic filling period in the face of increased transmitral blood flow.[63] The pressure gradient across the mitral valve therefore increases markedly, resulting in augmented left atrial and pulmonary artery wedge pressures along with significant pulmonary hypertension (Table 17-8). In aortic stenosis, the systolic gradient across the aortic valve also increases with exercise as the transvalvular flow is augmented. The left ventricular end-diastolic pressure and pulmonary artery wedge pressure may increase and, as in mitral stenosis, significant pulmonary hypertension may result.[64] The calculated valve area during exercise may be slightly larger than the resting values due to augmented transvalvular flows and pressure gradients (see Chapter 9). This variance is, however, relatively small.[65] In valvular regurgitation, exercise increases regurgitant fraction. In advanced cases, the left ventricular end-diastolic and end-systolic volumes increase, with a fall in ejection fraction.

In congenital heart disease, exercise causes augmented flow across the intracardiac shunt, which may result in a substantial oxygen step-up in the chamber distal to the shunt and a significant increase in pulmonary pressure (with left-to-right shunts). An increase in right-to-left shunting may cause hypoxemia. In patients with pulmonary hypertension, exercise results in marked augmentation of pulmonary artery, right ventricular end-diastolic, and right atrial pressures. The cardiac output declines in the face of increasing heart rate, with a marked reduction in stroke volume. Arterial hypoxemia also may occur. Thus, exercise in patients with congenital heart disease and pulmonary hypertension should be performed carefully for clear indications.

Table 17-8   Hemodynamic Data at Rest and After Five Minutes of Supine Bicycle Exercise in a Patient with Moderate Mitral Stenosis

	Rest	Exercise
HR	76	110
MAP	86	95
RAP	7	10
PAP	36	50
PAW	13	27
LVEDP	5	5
CO	5.2	8.4
AVO$_2$	5.4	10.1
MVG	8	21
MVA	1.6	1.7

Abbreviations: MVA, mitral valve area (cm^2); MVG, mitral valve gradient (mm Hg); other abbreviations as in Table 17-7.

SELECTED READINGS

1. Salerni R, Rodnan GP, Leon DS, Shaver, JA. Pulmonary hypertension in the CREST variant of progressive systemic sclerosis (scleroderma). Ann Intern Med 1977;86: 394–399.
2. Asherson RA, Macworth-Young CG, Boey ML. Pulmonary hypertension in systemic lupus erythematosus. Br Med J 1983;287:1024–1025.
3. Staub NC. Pulmonary edema-hypoxia and overperfusion. N Engl J Med 1980;302: 1085–1090.
4. Segel N, Kay JR, Bayley JJ, Paton A. Pulmonary hypertension in hepatic cirrhosis. Br Heart J 1968;30:575–578.
5. D'Alonzo GG, Barst RJ, Ayres SM. Survival in patients with primary pulmonary hypertension: results from a national prospective registry. Ann Intern Med 1991; 115:343–349.
6. Rich S, Kaufman E, Levy PS. The effect of high doses of calcium channel blockers on survival in primary pulmonary hypertension. N Engl J Med 1992;327:76–81.
7. Rich S, D'Alonzo GG, Dantzker DR. Magnitude and implications of spontaneous hemodynamic variability in primary pulmonary hypertension. Am J Cardiol 1985; 55:159–163.
8. Rich S, Brundage BH. High-dose calcium channel blocking therapy for primary pulmonary hypertension: evidence for long-term reduction in pulmonary arterial pressure and regression of right ventricular hypertrophy. Circulation 1987;76:135–141.
9. Rubin LJ, Mendoza J, Hood M, et al. Treatment of primary pulmonary hypertension with continuous intravenous prostacyclin (epoprostenol). Result of a randomized trial. Ann Intern Med 1990;112:485–491.
10. Barst RJ, Rubin LJ, McGoon MD, et al. Survival in primary pulmonary hypertension with long-term continuous intravenous prostacyclin. Ann Intern Med 1994;121: 409–415.
11. Morgan JM, McCormack DG, Griffiths MJ, et al. Adenosine as a vasodilator in primary pulmonary hypertension. Circulation 1991;84:1145–1149.
12. Furchgott RF, Zawadzki JV. The obligatory role of endothelial cells in the relaxation of arterial smooth muscle by acetylcholine. Nature 1980;288:373–375.
13. Giaid A, Saleh D. Reduced expression of endothelial nitric oxide synthase in the lungs of patients with pulmonary hypertension. N Engl J Med 1995;333:214–221.
14. Yanagisawa M, Kujihara H, Kimura S, et al. A novel potent vasoconstrictor peptide produced by vascular endothelial cells. Nature 1988;332:411–415.
15. Stewart DJ, Levy RD, Cejnacek P, Langleben D. Increased plasma endothelin-1 in pulmonary hypertension: marker or mediator of disease? Ann Intern Med 1991; 114:464–469.
16. Giaid A, Yanagisawa M, Langleben D, et al. Expression of endothelin-1 in the lungs of patients with pulmonary hypertension. N Engl J Med 1993;328:1732–1739.
17. Hosenpud JD, Novick RJ, Keck B, Darby P. The Registry of the International Society for Heart and Lung Transplantation: twelfth official report—1995. J Heart Lung Transplant 1995;14:805–815.
18. O'Connell JB, Bourge RC, Costanzo-Nordin MR, et al. Cardiac transplanation: recipient selection, donor procurement, and medical follow-up. Circulation 1992; 86:1061–1079.
19. Murali S, Kormos RL, Uretsky BF, et al. Preoperative pulmonary hemodynamics and early mortality after orthotopic heart transplantation: the Pittsburgh experience. Am Heart J 1993;126:896–904.
20. Kirklin JK, Naftel DC, Kirklin JW, et al. Pulmonary vascular resistance and the risk of heart transplantation. J Heart Transplant 1988;7:331–336.
21. Erickson KW, Costanzo-Nordin MR, O'Sullivan EJ, et al. Influence of preoperative transpulmonary gradient on late mortality after orthotopic heart transplantation. J Heart Transplant 1990;9:526–537.

22. Costard-Jackle A, Fowler MB. Influence of preoperative pulmonary artery pressure on mortality after heart transplantation: testing of potential reversibility of pulmonary hypertension with nitroprusside is useful in defining a high risk group. J Am Coll Cardiol 1992;19:48–54.
23. Murali S, Uretsky BF, Reddy PS, et al. Reversibility of pulmonary hypertension in congestive heart failure patients evaluated for cardiac transplantation: comparative effects of various pharmacologic agents. Am Heart J 1991;122:1375–1381.
24. Murali S, Uretsky BF, Armitage JM, et al. Utility of prostaglandin E-1 in the pretransplantation evaluation of heart failure patients with significant pulmonary hypertension. J Heart Lung Transplant 1992;11:716–723.
25. Haywood GA, Jennison SM. Adenosine infusion for the reversal of pulmonary vasoconstriction in biventricular failure. Circulation 1992;86:896–902.
26. Kieler-Jensen N, Ricksten S, Stenqvist O, et al. Inhaled nitric oxide in the evaluation of heart transplant candidates with elevated pulmonary vascular resistance. J Heart Lung Transplant 1994;13:366–375.
27. Stevenson LW, Warner SL, Steimle AE. The impending crisis awaiting cardiac transplantation. Modeling a solution based on selection. Circulation 1994;89:450–457.
28. Stevenson LW. Tailored therapy before transplantation for treatment of advanced heart failure: effective use of vasodilators and diuretics. J Heart Lung Transplant 1991;10:468–476.
29. Murali S, Uretsky BF, Reddy PS, et al. Hemodynamic abnormalities following cardiac transplantation: relationship to hypertension and survival. Am Heart J 1989; 118:334–341.
30. Billingham ME, Cary NR, Hammond ME, et al. A working formulation for the standardization of nomenclature in the diagnosis of heart and lung rejection: heart rejection study group. J Heart Transplant 1990;9:587–593.
31. Uretsky BF, Murali S, Reddy PS, et al. Development of coronary artery disease in cardiac transplant patients receiving immunosuppressive therapy with cyclosporine and prednisone. Circulation 1987;76:827–834.
32. Uretsky BF, Kormos RL, Zerbe TR, et al. Cardiac events after heart transplantation: incidence and predictive value of coronary arteriography. J Heart Lung Transplant 1992;11:S545–S551.
33. Billingham ME. Cardiac transplant atherosclerosis. Transplant Proc 1987;19:19.
34. Molossi S, Clausell N, Sett S, et al. ICAM-1 and VCAM-1 expression in accelerated cardiac allograft arteriopathy and myocardial rejection are influenced differently by Cyclosporin A and tumor necrosis factor-alpha blockade. J Pathology 1995; 176:175–182.
35. Schroeder JS, Gao SZ, Hunt SA, Stinson EB. Accelerated graft coronary artery disease: diagnosis and prevention. J Heart Lung Transplant 1992;11:S258.
36. Smart FW, Ballantyne CM, Cocanougher B, et al. Insensitivity of non-invasive tests to detect coronary artery vasculopathy after heart transplant. Am J Cardiol 1991; 67:243–247.
37. O'Neill BJ, Pflugfelder PW, Singh NR, et al. Frequency of angiographic detection and quantitative assessment of coronary arterial disease one and three years after cardiac transplantation. Am J Cardiol 1989;63:1221–1226.
38. Schroeder JS. A preliminary study of diltiazem in the prevention of coronary artery disease in heart-transplant recipients. N Engl J Med 1993;326:164–170.
39. Halle AA, Wilson RF, Marsin EK, et al. Coronary angioplasty in cardiac transplant patients: results of a multicenter study. Circulation 1992;86:458–462.
40. Berko BA, Swift M. X-linked dilated cardiomyopathy. N Engl J Med 1987;316: 1186–1191.
41. Diaz RA, Obasohan A, Oakley CM, et al. Prediction of outcome in dilated cardiomyopathy. Br Heart J 1987;58:393–399.
42. Stevenson LW, Fowler MB, Schroeder JS, et al. Poor survival of patients with idiopathic cardiomyopathy considered too well for transplantation. Am J Med 1987; 83:871–876.

43. Baim DS, McDowell AV, Chernilles J, et al. Evaluation of a new bipyridine inotropic agent—milrinone in patients with severe congestive heart failure. N Engl J Med 1983;309:748–756.
44. Treasure CB, Vita A, Cox DA, et al. Endothelium-dependent dilation of coronary micro vasculature is impaired in dilated cardiomyopathy. Circulation 1990;81:772.
45. Figulla HR, Rahlf A, Nieger M, et al. Spontaneous hemodynamic improvement or stabilization and associated biopsy findings in patients with congestive cardiomyopathy. Circulation 1985;71:1095–1104.
46. Jarcho JA, McKenna W, Pare JAP, et al. Mapping a gene for familial hypertrophic cardiomyopathy to chromosome 14 q 1. N Engl J Med 1989;321:1372–1378.
47. Braunwald E, et al. Idiopathic hypertrophic subaortic stenosis. Clinical analysis of 126 patients with emphasis on natural history. Circulation 1968;759–788.
48. Murgo JP, Alter BR, Dorethy JF, et al. Dynamics of left ventricular ejection in obstructive and non-obstructive hypertrophic cardiomyopathy. J Clin Invest 1980; 66:1369–1382.
49. Lorell BH, et al. Improved diastolic function and systolic performance in hypertrophic cardiomyopathy after nifedipine. N Engl J Med 1980;303:801–803.
50. Spirito P, McKenna WJ, Schultheiss HP. DDD pacing in obstructive hypertrophic cardiomyopathy. Circulation 1995;92:1670–1673.
51. Falk RH. Cardiac amyloidosis. In: Zipes DP, Rowlands DJ, eds. Progress in Cardiology. Philadelphia: Lea & Febiger, 1989:143–177.
52. Cutler DJ, Isner JM, Bracey AW, et al. Hemachromatosis heart disease. An unemphasized cause of potentially reversible restrictive cardiomyopathy. Am J Med 1980;69:923–928.
53. Valiathan MS, Kastha CC, Eapen JT, et al. A geochemical basis for endomyocardial fibrosis. Cardiovasc Res 1989;23:647–648.
54. Aroney CN, Ruddy TD, Dighjo H, et al. Differentiation of restrictive cardiomyopathy from pericardial constriction: assessment of diastolic function by radionuclide angiography. J Am Coll Cardiol 1989;13:1007–1014.
55. Falk RH, Plehn JF, Deesing T, et al. Sensitivity and specificity of the echocardiographic features of cardiac amyloidosis. Am J Cardiol 1987;59:418–422.
56. Hatle LK, Appleton CP, Popp RL. Differentiation of constrictive pericarditis and restrictive cardiomyopathy by Doppler echocardiography. Circulation 1989;79: 357–370.
57. Gerson MC, Colthar MS, Fowler NO. Differentiation of constrictive pericarditis and restrictive cardiomyopathy by radionuclide ventriculography. Am Heart J 1989; 118:114–120.
58. Schoenfeld MH, Supple EW, Dec GW, et al. Restrictive cardiomyopathy versus constrictive pericarditis: role of endomyocardial biopsy in avoiding unnecessary thoracotomy. Circulation 1987;75:1012–1017.
59. Olson LJ, Gertz MA, Edwards WD, et al. Senile cardiac amyloidosis with myocardial dysfunction: diagnosis by endomyocardial biopsy and immunohistochemistry. N Engl J Med 1987;317:738–742.
60. Holmgren A, Ericzon GA, Groth CA, et al. Clinical improvement and amyloid regression after liver transplantation in hereditary transthyretin amyloidosis. Lancet 1993;341:1113–1116.
61. Rakho PS, Salerni R, Uretsky BF. Successful reversal by chelation therapy of congestive cardiomyopathy due to iron overload. J Am Coll Cardiol 1986;8:436–440.
62. Benotti JS, Grossman W, Cohn PF. The clinical profile of restrictive cardiomyopathy. Circulation 1980;61:1206–1212.
63. Epstein SE, et al. Characterization of the circulatory response to maximal upright exercise in normal subjects and patients with heart disease. Circulation 1967;35: 1049–1062.
64. Bache RJ, Wang Y, Jorgenson CR. Hemodynamic effects of exercise in isolated valvular aortic stenosis. Circulation 1971;44:1003–1013.
65. Richardson JW, Anderson FL, Tsargaris TJ. Rest and exercise hemodynamic studies in patients with isolated aortic stenosis. Cardiology 1979;64:1–11.

18

CONGENITAL HEART DISEASE IN THE ADULT

Lee Beerman

O
VER THE PAST decade it has become increasingly important for adult cardiologists to have a familiarity with various aspects of congenital heart disease. Not only are adults with the common forms of congenital heart disease occasionally encountered, but there is a growing population of young adults who have survived palliative or curative surgery for more complex anomalies. An extensive discussion of this topic is beyond the scope of this text. However, some of the important considerations in dealing with this group of patients are discussed.

Common Unoperated Lesions

Atrial Septal Defect

Atrial septal defects are a common form of congenital heart disease comprising approximately 15% of all congenital anomalies of the heart. The physical signs are subtle, and symptoms are rare prior to adulthood. These two aspects result in this lesion being the most common one to receive initial cardiovascular evaluation by an adult cardiologist.

Anatomy

There are generally three types of atrial communications. The most prevalent, occurring 65% of the time, is a defect in the central portion of the atrial septum in the fossa ovalis region, known as a secundum defect. The next most common type, occurring with a frequency of 30%, is a defect between the inferior free edge of the atrial septum and the plane of the atrioventricular (AV) valves, namely an ostium primum defect. This anomaly is more properly thought of as being part of the spectrum of AV septal (also known as endocardial cushion) defects that involve both atrial and ventricular defects and a common AV valve with or without partitioning. When only an ostium primum atrial defect is present, this entity is usually referred to as a partial AV septal defect and is always accompanied by a cleft in the mitral valve. The least common type of defect, which occurs 5% of the time, is the sinus venosus defect. It is located in the most posterior and superior aspect of the septum. In this entity, the superior vena cava (SVC) overrides the atrial septum, and there is partial anomalous return of the right upper lobe pulmonary vein to the distal SVC near its junction with the right atrium. The right middle lobe vein may also occasionally drain into the same region. There are other exceedingly rare types of atrial defects that include an inferior form of a sinus venosus defect (the inferior vena cava [IVC] overrides a posterior inferior defect) or a coronary sinus defect ("unroofing" of the coronary sinus, allowing direct left atrial shunting into this structure).

Associated Defects

Associated defects are valvular pulmonic stenosis, ventricular septal defect, partial anomalous pulmonary venous return, and mitral valve prolapse.

Physiology

Atrial defects are associated with a left-to-right shunt at the atrial level, the magnitude of which depends on the size of the defect and the relative compliance of the right and left ventricles. Thus, for any given defect size, shunt flow tends to increase during the first year of life as right ventricular compliance physiologically increases due to regression of neonatal right ventricular hypertrophy. Similarly, during mid to late adulthood, the atrial shunt increases as left ventricular compliance falls secondary to acquired processes such as coronary artery disease, systemic hypertension, or aging. The main complications of an uncorrected atrial septal defect are congestive heart failure secondary to chronic volume overload, pulmonary hypertension, and atrial arrhythmias.

Indications for Catheterization

Although the diagnosis is almost always definitively made by echo/Doppler studies, catheterization may be helpful in quantitating shunts of borderline significance. Furthermore, measurement of pulmonary artery pressure becomes important after the second or third decade of life, because the prevalence of pulmonary hypertension steadily increases after that age.

Catheterization and Technical Approach

This procedure is most easily performed by a femoral venous approach. Arterial access is not necessary unless coronary arteriography is indicated. After a catheter is advanced through the right side of the circulation in the usual manner, a rapid oximetric shunt run is performed. Entering both branch pulmonary arteries is not necessary unless the main pulmonary artery pressure is elevated and branch pulmonary artery stenosis is suspected. The catheter is then passed across the atrial defect by advancing it leftward and superiorly from the IVC at the right atrial junction, with the tip rotated slightly posterior. In the case of a secundum defect, the natural course of the catheter takes it directly into the left atrium. In fact, it is often difficult to keep it out of this chamber. With an ostium primum defect, however, the catheter must be manipulated into a lower and somewhat more posterior position to traverse the defect. The most difficult defect to traverse is the sinus venosus defect. This lesion is best approached by advancing the catheter to the SVC and withdrawing it to the right atrial border, using the tip of the catheter to explore the posterior and superior aspect of the atrial septum. In rare cases, this defect can be traversed only from above by an approach from the internal jugular or subclavian veins. Once the catheter is in the left atrium, right- and left-sided pulmonary veins should be entered to confirm their normal drainage. With a sinus venosus defect, the right upper pulmonary vein is usually easily entered from the right heart border at the right atrial superior vena caval junction, although occasionally this vein may drain higher directly into the SVC. The left ventricle also may be entered from the left atrium to record left ventricular diastolic pressure and perform angiography if indicated.

Hemodynamic Findings

Oximetry generally reveals a step-up of 5% or more going from the SVC to the right atrium. There often will be a further increase in saturation in the right ventricle as mixing becomes more complete. An important caveat is that an elevated saturation in the SVC of 85% or more is probably indicative of partial anomalous pulmonary venous return to this vessel and requires accurate definition of pulmonary venous drainage. This finding also complicates the Qp/Qs ratio calculation (see Chapter 10), because the SVC cannot be used for the mixed venous saturation. Sampling more proximally in the innominate vein, right internal jugular vein, and subclavian veins may allow a reasonable estimate of mixed venous saturation. The left side of the circulation should be fully saturated unless there is a right-to-left atrial shunt due to abnormal right ventricular compliance or severe pulmonary hypertension. A Qp/Qs ratio of greater than 1.5 : 1.0 is considered a physiologically important shunt.

Pressure data reveal equalization of the mean right and left atrial pressures with loss of the usual right atrial a wave dominance. In some cases, with very large left-to-right shunts, there may be a mean gradient up to 3 mm Hg between the atria. However, a significant left atrial to right atrial pressure differential implies that the atrial communication is not large and may be only a patent foramen ovale rather than a true defect. Left ventricular, right ventricular, and pulmonary artery pressures are uniformly normal in the first two decades, but various degrees of pulmonary hypertension occur later in life. The incidence of pulmonary hypertension is as follows: less than 20 years, 5%; 20 to 40 years, 20%; and greater than 40 years, 50%. Pulmonary vascular resistance also may become elevated in adults.

There is usually no gradient between the right ventricle and the pulmonary artery. However, with a large left-to-right shunt, there may be a systolic pressure difference across the right ventricular outflow tract up to 25 mm Hg due to "relative pulmonic stenosis" in the presence of a structurally normal pulmonary valve. See Chapter 10, Example 2 for typical hemodynamic data in a patient with an atrial septal defect.

Angiography

If the defect is well visualized by echocardiography, angiography is not necessary. Occasionally, a pulmonary artery injection is of value to define pulmonary venous return and give an estimate of the magnitude of the left-to-right shunt. The defect itself is best visualized with an injection in the right upper lobe pulmonary vein in the left anterior oblique (LAO) projection at 20 to 45 degrees, with craniocaudal angulation (the position of the image intensifier and x-ray tube, respectively) of 25 degrees. A retrograde left ventriculogram may be useful if there is concern about contractility or mitral regurgitation. It is generally advisable to perform a left ventricular injection for a partial AV septal defect to visualize the outflow tract with its elongated appearance (so-called goose neck deformity) and mitral valve function, and to rule out associated ventricular defects. The most useful views are anteroposterior (AP) and LAO 60 to 70 degrees, with craniocaudal angulation of approximately 25 degrees.

Ventricular Septal Defect

Ventricular septal defects make up 20% of congenital defects and are the most common of the clinically recognized anomalies. The presentation varies with the size of the defect, but if symptoms of congestive heart failure occur, it is almost always in early infancy. Otherwise, this lesion will be discovered because of a loud systolic murmur.

Anatomy

Many classifications of ventricular defects have been proposed, but it is useful to think of defects as being perimembranous, muscular, or subarterial. Perimembranous defects are most common, include the membranous septal region, and are located adjacent to the septal leaflet of the tricuspid valve. These may extend inferiorly, anteriorly, or posteriorly into the inlet septum (i.e., location of a defect seen in an AV septal defect). These defects often are associated with a pouch of tricuspid valve tissue around their margins (also known as aneurysm of the membranous septum), which may contribute to partial or complete closure of the defect. Muscular defects may occur anywhere in the septum and are completely surrounded by a rim of muscle. A frequent site of these defects is the apical trabecular septum. The subarterial classification refers to a defect whose superior border comprises both the pulmonary and aortic valves (also known as supracristal defect). The importance of this defect resides in its association with aortic leaflet prolapse and aortic regurgitation.

Associated Lesions

Associated lesions are subpulmonic stenosis, valvular pulmonic stenosis, tricuspid regurgitation, direct left ventricular to right atrial shunt, and discrete membranous subaortic stenosis.

Physiology

The magnitude of the shunt in a ventricular septal defect is determined by the size of the defect and resistance to flow across the right ventricular outflow tract or pulmonary vascular bed. Pulmonary vascular disease and Eisenmenger's reaction (elevation in pulmonary vascular resistence leading to a reversal of initial left-to-right to predominant right-to-left shunt) may occur if a large defect is not corrected early in life.

Indications for Catheterization

Whenever a ventricular defect is associated with findings of significant left ventricular volume overload (cardiomegaly, diastolic murmur at the apex, congestive heart failure) or pulmonary hypertension, it is important to document the degree of shunting, pulmonary artery pressure, and pulmonary vascular resistance. Important associated anomalies such as aortic regurgitation, right ventricular outflow tract obstruction, or subaortic stenosis also may provide indications for invasive studies.

Catheterization and Technical Approach

Right heart catheterization is performed in the usual manner. Because a left ventriculogram should be performed in most cases, the left heart will need to be entered via an atrial communication, by directly crossing the ventricular defect, or by the retrograde arterial approach. When the defect is perimembranous, it may be possible to advance a venous catheter across it by rotating the tip upward and posterior immediately after traversing the tricuspid valve. Frequently, the catheter will pass into the aorta, and the left ventricle can then be entered by withdrawing it across the valve and advancing the catheter while rotating the tip posteriorly.

Hemodynamics

Oximetry will show an initial step-up in the right ventricle unless there is tricuspid regurgitation, an associated atrial septal defect, or a left ventricular to right atrial shunt. Complete mixing will not be present until the pulmonary artery level, and in fact, with a supracristal defect, the increase in saturation may not be encountered until the pulmonary artery. Pulmonary artery pressures will vary, depending on the size of the defect and pulmonary vascular resistance. If pulmonary vascular resistance is elevated, reactivity should be assessed by administering oxygen (or a pulmonary vasodilator) and the oximetric run and pressure recordings repeated.

Angiography

A left ventriculogram should be performed to define the position and size of the defect and rule out unsuspected multiple defects. The most useful projection is the LAO view at 45 to 70 degrees, with 25-degree craniocaudal angulation. The degree of obliquity should be varied based on the presumed position of the defect. Perimembranous defects are shown well with LAO 60- to 70-degree angulation. More posterior or inlet defects are best visualized at LAO 45 degrees, and anterior defects, such as a supracristal one, may be seen best in the direct lateral or even right anterior oblique (RAO) view. Aortic root angiography should also be performed if there is a supracristal defect or aortic regurgitation. A right ventriculogram may be necessary if there is associated right ventricular outflow tract obstruction or to help discriminate between a direct left ventricular–right atrial shunt and a ventricular septal defect associated with tricuspid regurgitation.

Patent Ductus Arteriosus

In most patients with a patent ductus arteriosus, the shunt is relatively small and no symptoms occur. Detection of this defect is usually accomplished by recognizing a continuous murmur, or rarely, during the course of working up bacterial endocarditis.

Anatomy

The ductus normally arises from the aortic arch just distal to the left sub-clavian artery and inserts into the main pulmonary artery at its junction with the left pulmonary artery. The ductus is of variable length and may be associated with dilatation of the aortic diverticulum. When a right aortic arch is present, the ductus may arise anteriorly from the mirror-image left innominate artery, posteriorly from an anomalous left subclavian artery, or rarely, from the right-sided descending aorta.

Physiology

The left-to-right shunt is usually small, but occasionally, a large patent ductus arteriosus may lead to congestive heart failure or pulmonary hypertension and Eisenmenger's reaction.

Associated Lesions

Associated lesions are coarctation of the aorta and pulmonary artery stenosis (particularly in the rubella syndrome).

Indications for Catheterization

One indication for catheterization is failure of the echo/Doppler studies to define the source of a continuous murmur or the cause of pulmonary hypertension. Another indication is if transcatheter closure is being considered.

Catheterization and Technical Approach

A non–balloon-tipped catheter passing from the right ventricle to the pulmonary artery will usually advance easily across the ductus into the descending aorta, because this course mimics the normal fetal flow pattern. In fact, it is sometimes necessary to use a guidewire to manipulate the catheter into the branch pulmonary arteries. It is important to enter the distal right and left pulmonary artery, because the ductal shunt is usually eccentric, making the main pulmonary artery and proximal branch pulmonary artery saturations unreliable indicators of mixed pulmonary artery saturation. If pulmonary hypertension is present, "test" occlusion of the ductus, using a balloon-tipped catheter, may yield useful data.

Hemodynamics

Step-up in oxygen saturation occurs in the pulmonary artery. Distal pulmonary artery saturations should be averaged and used for the Q_p/Q_s calculation because the ductal jet is eccentric and usually directed preferentially into the left pulmonary artery. Although most ducts are relatively small and associated with normal pulmonary artery pressures, pulmonary hypertension may be present in patients with large ducts. If there is a significant elevation of pulmonary artery pressure, potential reversibility should be assessed by test occlusion with a balloon-tipped catheter with side holes. This maneuver allows sampling of the oxygen saturation and pressure in the main pulmonary artery when ductal flow is temporarily eliminated by balloon inflation. If Eisenmenger's reaction is present, there will be a right-to-left shunt across the ductus, with the descending aortic saturation being lower than the ascending aorta.

Angiography

An injection in the proximal descending aorta in the direct lateral view is best for imaging the ductus arteriosus, and this projection will effectively rule out an associated coarctation of the aorta.

Pulmonic Stenosis

Pulmonic stenosis usually presents with a systolic murmur, but right heart failure or cyanosis from right-to-left atrial shunting may occur in infancy if the stenosis is critical. Most cases of valvular pulmonic stenosis are amenable to balloon valvuloplasty.

Anatomy

Pulmonic stenosis occurs at the valvular level more than 80% of the time and is usually associated with a normal-sized annulus, mild to moderate thickening of the leaflets, and commissural fusion. Occasionally, the valve may be dysplastic, with a small annulus, marked thickening and dysplasia of the leaflets, and minimal or no commissural fusion. Less commonly, the obstruction may be subvalvular due to an anomalous muscle bundle.

Physiology

Outlet obstruction leads to right ventricular hypertrophy, which may be progressive. Right-to-left atrial shunting may occur across a patent foramen ovale or atrial septal defect as right ventricular compliance decreases and end-diastolic pressure increases.

Associated Defects

Associated defects are atrial septal defect and ventricular septal defect.

Indications for Catheterization

The major indications are as follows: suspected gradient as estimated by Doppler studies across the right ventricular outflow tract of greater than 50 mm Hg or a right ventricular to left ventricular systolic pressure ratio greater than

0.75, evidence of severe right ventricular hypertrophy, or right-to-left atrial shunting secondary to abnormal right ventricular compliance. All of these findings would suggest that either balloon valvuloplasty or a surgery should be undertaken.

Catheterization and Technical Approach

The femoral venous approach is preferred. A right heart catheterization is performed with determination of cardiac output by the Fick technique. Entering the pulmonary artery from the right ventricle may be more difficult than usual when severe pulmonic stenosis is present. However, it can usually be accomplished by gentle manipulation of the catheter in the right ventricular outflow tract. An end-hole catheter (with or without a balloon tip) should be advanced to a point just proximal to the pulmonic valve. If the catheter does not easily advance across the valve with gentle buckling in the outflow tract, a guidewire with a soft tip should be passed through the end-hole and across the valve into a branch pulmonary artery. The catheter can then be easily advanced over the wire into position. Pressures and oximetry data are obtained from the right side of the circulation. If there is a patent foramen ovale or atrial septal defect, the left atrium and left ventricle should be entered to complete the hemodynamic assessment. A right ventriculogram is done, and if indicated, balloon valvuloplasty of the pulmonic valve should be performed.

Hemodynamics

Oximetry will be normal unless there is an associated atrial septal defect. If an atrial communication is present, a right-to-left shunt may occur if right ventricular compliance is significantly decreased, or a left-to-right shunt may be present if right ventricular compliance is normal. Pressure data will show an increased right ventricular systolic pressure with a normal to low pulmonary artery pressure, normal to increased right atrial pressure with an exaggerated a wave, and normal left heart pressures.

Angiography

If valvular pulmonic stenosis is suspected, a right ventriculogram should be performed in the AP projection, with 20- to 25-degree craniocaudal angulation, and in the lateral view. These will show right ventricular size, function, presence of tricuspid regurgitation, the anatomy of the valve, and size of the annulus. A relatively thin doming valve is generally much more amenable to balloon dilatation than a thick dysplastic valve. If subvalvular obstruction is seen, the RAO craniocaudal projection should be substituted for the AP view because this will best demonstrate anomalous muscle bundles and the site of subvalvular obstruction. Levophase should be observed for pulmonary venous return, evidence of left-to-right intracardiac shunting, and assessment of left ventricular size and function.

Aortic Stenosis

This common congenital defect tends to be progressive through childhood. Symptoms are uncommon unless the obstruction is very severe. Valvular stenosis in the child and young adult may be treatable by balloon valvuloplasty.

Anatomy

Nearly all congenitally stenotic aortic valves are bicuspid or, occasionally, unicommissural. The leaflets are usually very mobile despite commissural fusion, and calcification is rare in the first two to three decades of life. Therefore, unlike the adult with acquired aortic valve stenosis, congenital aortic valvular stenosis in the young is generally amenable to balloon dilatation. Left ventricular outflow tract obstruction may also occur in the subvalvular region with a discrete membrane or a fibromuscular ridge. Discrete or diffuse supravalvular aortic stenosis is infrequently the site of the aortic obstruction.

Associated Defects

Associated defects are coarctation of the aorta; multiple left heart obstructions such as discrete subaortic stenosis, mitral stenosis, or supravalvar mitral ring; and aortic and mitral regurgitation.

Physiology

Left ventricular outflow tract obstruction leads to left ventricular hypertrophy, hypercontractility of the left ventricle, diastolic dysfunction, and eventual left ventricular failure. Pulmonary venous hypertension with secondary pulmonary artery hypertension progresses along with the diastolic and systolic dysfunction of the left ventricle.

Indications for Catheterization

A Doppler-predicted gradient greater than 50 to 70 mm Hg, severe left ventricular hypertrophy, or left ventricular dysfunction is an indication for catheterization. Although symptoms are rare in the first two decades, unless aortic stenosis is extremely severe, syncope, angina, and dyspnea on exertion are also clear indications for intervention.

Catheterization and Technical Approach

A right heart catheterization should be done to determine pulmonary artery and wedge pressures and measure cardiac output. The most critical aspect of the catheterization is the measurement of the left ventricular to aortic gradient. The femoral or brachial artery pressure should not be substituted for the central aortic pressure, because there may be a significant distal augmentation of the systolic pressure. The left ventricle may be entered via a transseptal approach to the left atrium and mitral valve, or retrograde from the aortic root.

If the transseptal approach is used, simultaneous left ventricular and aortic pressures can be recorded. Crossing the aortic valve from the root may be difficult, but can usually be accomplished with the aid of a soft-tipped guidewire. A left ventricular to aortic pullback can then be performed. When subaortic stenosis is suspected, an end-hole catheter should be used to define a subvalvular lower pressure chamber on pullback. Balloon dilatation should be considered if the stenotic aortic valve appears mobile and there is either minimal or no aortic regurgitation.

Hemodynamics

Oximetry is generally normal. Elevation of left ventricular systolic and end-diastolic pressures is usually present. If the end-diastolic pressure is increased, the wedge and pulmonary artery pressures also will be elevated. A gradient of greater than 70 mm Hg is an indication for intervention, either with balloon dilatation or an open surgical approach. A 50- to 70-mm Hg gradient is borderline, and other factors need to be considered before proceeding with intervention.

Angiography

A left ventriculogram in the RAO and LAO views elucidates left ventricular function, left ventricular outflow tract morphology, and the size, mobility, and thickness of the aortic valve. If a discrete subaortic membrane is suspected, the AP and the RAO and LAO 70-degree views, with the craniocaudal 25-degree angulation, are also useful. An aortic root injection should be done to assess the presence and degree of aortic regurgitation.

Coarctation of the Aorta

A patient with coarctation of the aorta may present as a critically ill infant in the first 2 to 3 weeks of life, particularly when there is an associated left-to-right shunt. Isolated coarctations are more likely to be detected on routine examination during childhood or later with findings of upper extremity hypertension and decreased or absent femoral pulses.

Anatomy

The vast majority of coarctations occur in the juxtaductal position, that is, adjacent to the ductal insertion in the descending aorta. There is usually a discrete curtain or shelf of tissue on the posterior aortic wall in addition to constriction of the aorta at this site. Variable degrees of hypoplasia of the isthmus may occur, but this is more common when coarctation presents with congestive heart failure in infancy. The left subclavian artery often has a more distal takeoff, and its origin may be narrowed by the coarctation. In rare cases, the site of obstruction may be in the mid-thoracic or abdominal aorta.

Associated Defects

Associated defects are bicuspid aortic valve (approximately 50%), subaortic stenosis, mitral valve morphologic abnormalities, ventricular septal defect, and anomalous origin of the right subclavian artery.

Physiology

The sequelae of coarctation include upper extremity hypertension with a differential in the upper extremity and lower extremity systolic BPs. Left ventricular hypertrophy develops as an adaptive response to increased afterload on the left ventricle. Furthermore, extensive chest wall collateral vessels to the descending thoracic aorta develop to compensate for impaired flow through the coarctation.

Indications for Catheterization

Intervention is indicated for all but the mildest of clinically detectable coarctations. Although some centers advocate balloon angioplasty for native coarctations, the majority opinion currently favors the surgical approach initially and utilization of balloon angioplasty for recurrent or residual coarctations. Prior to any procedure, the region of the coarctation must be visualized in some fashion. Echo/Doppler studies are excellent and usually sufficient in infants. Magnetic resonance imaging provides excellent images in older individuals. However, cardiac catheterization and aortography are recommended when there are important associated defects, noninvasive studies are inadequate, or there is local surgical preference for the detailed vascular imaging that only angiography can provide, including definition of collateral vessels.

Catheterization and Technical Approach

A right heart catheterization is done if there are suspected associated intracardiac abnormalities. A retrograde arterial approach is used to obtain a pressure differential across the coarctation and to perform angiography.

Hemodynamics

The unique finding with a coarctation is a BP difference of greater than 10 mm Hg between the ascending and descending aortas. The magnitude of the gradient is not directly related to the severity of the aortic narrowing, because extensive collateral vessels may develop and ameliorate the gradient.

Angiography

An injection with the catheter tip placed just proximal to the coarctation in the RAO and LAO projections will demonstrate the coarctation. Collateral vessels are best visualized with an aortic root injection. Other angiograms should be performed as indicated by the presence of associated anomalies.

Defects Undergoing Operation in Childhood

Tetralogy of Fallot

Tetralogy of Fallot is the most common form of cyanotic congenital heart disease and usually presents in the first 6 months of life. Occasionally, the diagnosis is delayed because of the relatively mild degree of aortic desaturation. Today, it is rare that an adult cardiologist will encounter an untreated patient with tetralogy of Fallot.

Anatomy

The basic defect is anterior deviation of the outlet septum, which divides the aortic and pulmonary outflow tracts. This structural abnormality results in right ventricular outflow tract obstruction at multiple levels, including subvalvular muscular obstruction and valvular stenosis. Supravalvular and branch pulmonary artery stenosis also are commonly present. In addition to this abnormality, there is a large aortic root that overrides a ventricular septal defect. The ventricular defect is virtually always large and unrestrictive and is perimembranous in location in 80% of the patients, with the remainder having a thin muscular rim around its margins. The fourth component of tetralogy of Fallot, in addition to the pulmonic stenosis, ventricular defect, and overriding aorta, is the obligatory right ventricular hypertrophy.

Associated Defects

Associated defects are right aortic arch (25%), pulmonary artery stenosis (10%–20%), pulmonary atresia with systemic to pulmonary collateral vessels (5%–10%), additional muscular ventricular septal defects (5%–10%), systemic to pulmonary artery collateral vessels (5%–10%), and coronary artery anomalies (1%–2%). Variation in coronary anatomy deserves special mention. One of the more common abnormalities is the origin of the anterior descending coronary from the right coronary artery. This vessel courses across the right ventricular outflow tract and may complicate the surgical approach.

Physiology

The right ventricle has pressure overload because of the pulmonic stenosis. This feature is well tolerated, however, because the large ventricular septal defect prevents the right ventricular systolic pressure from becoming suprasystemic. Furthermore, there is no volume overload of this chamber because the pulmonic stenosis limits pulmonary blood flow. The direction and magnitude of the shunt across the ventricular defect depends on the relative degree of pulmonic stenosis and systemic vascular resistance. As right ventricular outflow tract obstruction increases (the natural history of muscular obstruction) and/or systemic vascular resistance falls (e.g., during exercise), the amount of right-to-left shunting and systemic desaturation will increase. Volume overload and eventual congestive heart failure may occur after palliation with a systemic to pulmonary artery shunt that leads to increased pulmonary blood flow.

Indications for Catheterization

Precise angiographic definition of the right ventricular outflow tract and of proximal and distal pulmonary arteries and assessment of any coronary artery anomalies are essential before surgical intervention.

Catheterization and Technique Approach

Using a femoral venous approach, the catheter may pass from the right ventricle across the outflow tract to the pulmonary artery in the usual manner. A non–balloon-tipped catheter is preferred because flow-directed catheters are not an advantage when a bidirectional or right-to-left shunt is present. This pass may prove difficult because of induced ventricular arrhythmias or increased infundibular hypercontractility. Persistent efforts to enter the pulmonary artery may be unwise and precipitate a hypercyanotic spell. Obtaining a pulmonary artery pressure is generally not necessary if Doppler studies have shown a large right ventricular to pulmonary artery gradient and if the patient has not had a previous systemic artery to pulmonary artery shunt. In the latter case, it is important to obtain a pulmonary artery pressure to rule out pulmonary hypertension from the increased flow resulting from the shunt. A patent foramen ovale is present, with a higher prevalence in tetralogy of Fallot than in normals, which allows access to the left atrium and left ventricle from this approach. It also may be possible to enter the aorta and left ventricle by anterogradely traversing the ventricular defect. To accomplish this maneuver, the catheter is rotated clockwise and superiorly in a manner similar to the usual pass toward the pulmonary outflow tract. In this case, however, the catheter tip should be maneuvered superiorly from a more medial position just after passing across the tricuspid valve.

Hemodynamics

Oximetry will show bidirectional shunting across the ventricular septal defect with a step-up in oxygenation in the right ventricular outflow tract and a step-down in the left ventricle and/or the aorta. Right ventricular, left ventricular, and aortic systolic pressures are always identical because the large ventricular septal defect ensures equalization of ventricular pressures. The pulmonic stenosis is usually at least moderately severe and results in normal to low pulmonary artery pressures. See Chapter 10, Example 4 for an illustration of typical oximetry data.

Angiography

A right ventriculogram in the RAO 30-degree and craniocaudal 25-degree views and the LAO 60- to 70-degree view, with a craniocaudal 25-degree angle, will show the right ventricular outflow tract and pulmonary artery (RAO view) and the ventricular septal defect (LAO view). If necessary, a right ventricular outflow tract injection in a very shallow (30-degree) LAO with a 25-degree craniocaudal tilt will show the pulmonary arteries and bifurcation. A left ventriculogram (RAO and LAO 60- to 75-degree view with craniocaudal 25-degree angle) is indicated if there is suspicion of left ventricular dysfunction or multiple ventricular septal defects. An aortic root injection in the RAO and LAO views or selective coronary arteriography is very important and should be performed in all cases to rule out the presence of anomalous origin of the coronary arteries. In particular, the origin of the anterior descending artery should be clearly defined. If a previous aortic to pulmonary artery shunt has been performed, an angiogram should be performed to visualize this structure.

Postoperative

Adult cardiologists will more frequently see patients who have already had a repair of tetralogy of Fallot. The important residual hemodynamic abnormalities that should be sought include residual pulmonic stenosis, a residual ventricular septal defect, hemodynamically important pulmonic regurgitation, marked right ventricular enlargement, right ventricular dysfunction, and tricuspid regurgitation. A catheterization may be indicated if the residual defects are severe enough to require re-operation. Ventricular arrhythmias are also important long-term sequelae and may provide an indication for electrophysiologic studies.

Transposition of the Great Arteries

The most common type of cyanotic congenital heart disease presenting in the newborn period is transposition of the great arteries. Because the natural history is so devastating, some form of surgical intervention is required for survival of the patient into adulthood.

Anatomy

The basic defect in transposition is that the right ventricle gives rise to an anterior aorta, whereas the left ventricle connects to the more posterior pulmonary artery. This results in parallel circulations, with survival depending on mixing at the atrial, ventricular, or great vessel level. Early surgical intervention is required. Until the past 10 years, this group of patients was treated with an atrial redirection procedure—the Mustard or Senning operation. These procedures involve removal or redirection of the atrial septum and placement of an intra-atrial baffle so that the superior and inferior venae cavae drain posterior and to the left of the baffle so as to enter the left ventricle, and the pulmonary venous return is directed anterior and to the right of the baffle, eventually reaching the right ventricle (Fig 18-1). Over the past 10 years, a more direct approach to repair has been the arterial switch procedure with the establishment

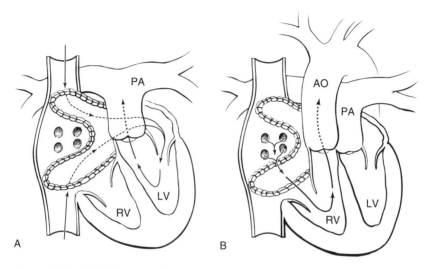

Figure 18-1 **(A)** The systemic venous return as it is directed posterior to the intra-atrial baffle, eventually entering the left ventricle (LV) and pulmonary circuit. **(B)** Pulmonary venous return rightward and anterior to the baffle, which results in oxygenated blood entering the right ventricle (RV) and systemic arterial circuit. PA, pulmonary artery; AO, aorta.

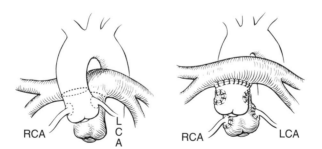

Figure 18-2 (Left) The AP view of the typical great vessel relationships of transposition of the great vessels. (Right) The AP view of surgically reconstructed great vessels, including translocation of the coronary arteries to the neo-aortic root. LAT, lateral; RCA, right coronary artery; LCA, left coronary artery.

of right ventricular to pulmonary artery and left ventricular to aortic continuity. The most demanding aspect of this latter operation is the translocation of the coronary ostia from the anterior great vessel to the new aortic root (native pulmonary artery stump), which arises from the left ventricle (Fig 18-2).

Associated Defects

Ventricular septal defect and pulmonary stenosis (usually subvalvular) occur in 40% and 30% of patients, respectively. Many postoperative abnormalities can occur and are directly related to the type of operation. After an atrial redirection procedure, systemic or pulmonary venous obstruction, baffle shunting, and right ventricular dysfunction with or without tricuspid regurgitation are commonly found. Following an arterial switch procedure, supravalvular pulmonic stenosis is the most common structural defect, with distortion of the proximal coronary arteries less frequently noted.

Indications for Catheterization

Preoperative catheterization may need to be performed in the newborn period to enlarge the atrial communication with a balloon septostomy, assess associated anomalies, and define the coronary arterial pattern. In the adult who has had a Mustard or Senning repair, catheterization may be indicated to assess factors causing progressive failure of the systemic ventricle, associated defects such as pulmonic stenosis, baffle leaking, or obstruction of the systemic or pulmonary venous return. Late-onset arrhythmias are extremely common and include sinus node dysfunction, bradycardia/tachycardia syndrome, and ventricular ectopy. These arrhythmias may make electrophysiologic investigations advisable. After an arterial switch procedure, catheterization may be necessary for significant pulmonary artery stenosis, aortic insufficiency, or evidence of compromised coronary circulation or left ventricular dysfunction.

Catheterization and Technique Approach

The approach to the patient who has had a Mustard or Senning repair is somewhat complex because of the circuitous course the catheter must take through the right side of the circulation. A balloon-tipped catheter is most helpful. It is advanced to the IVC, to the systemic venous atrium behind the baffle, and across the mitral valve into the left ventricle. The balloon is then inflated and the catheter tip must be encouraged to take a 180-degree turn medially and superiorly to enter the pulmonary outflow tract and pulmonary artery. The use of a tip-deflecting wire is very helpful in this situation. The systemic circulation is assessed by passing an arterial catheter retrograde around the arch and across the aortic valve into the right (systemic) ventricle. It is important to compare the wedge pressure with the right ventricular end-diastolic pressure to rule out pulmonary venous obstruction. If this is present, it may be important to pass the tip of the catheter from the right ventricle retrogradely across the tricuspid valve into the distal and proximal pulmonary venous atria to determine the site of obstruction.

Hemodynamics

The characteristic and virtually unique finding in transposition of the great vessels is that the pulmonary artery saturation is higher than the aortic saturation. A step-up in saturation from the SVC going into the right atrium (due to a left-to-right atrial shunt) is essential to achieve a satisfactory aortic saturation. Pulmonary artery pressure varies, depending on the presence of associated defects such as a ventricular septal defect or pulmonic stenosis. After a Senning or Mustard procedure, oximetry should be normal unless there is a residual shunt. Depending on the site of baffle defect, the shunt could be left to right, right to left, or bidirectional. Pulmonary artery pressure is expected to be normal, and left ventricular pressure should be considerably lower than right ventricular systolic pressure, which will equal aortic systolic pressure. It is important to obtain the following pressure gradients: SVC and IVC to the systemic venous atrium, left ventricle to pulmonary artery, and pulmonary artery wedge to right ventricular end-diastolic pressure. The most common abnormalities seen in patients after the arterial switch procedure are a pressure gradient going from the main pulmonary artery to the branch pulmonary arteries and an elevated end-diastolic pressure in the left ventricle. This latter abnormality may result from left ventricular systolic or diastolic dysfunction as a function of coronary artery obstruction related to their surgical translocation.

Angiography

The diagnostic injection pre-operatively is the left ventriculogram, which demonstrates connection of this chamber to the pulmonary artery. An aortic injection should be done to visualize the coronary arteries. Following atrial redirection surgery, a left ventriculogram with follow-through on levophase will show the left ventricular outflow tract and visualize the pulmonary venous return. The best views for this injection are the AP and LAO 75-degree views, with a craniocaudal 25-degree tilt. A right ventriculogram in the AP and lateral views is important to show right ventricular function and assess for tricuspid regurgitation. The systemic venous return chambers are well visualized by injections in the SVC and IVC near their junction with the right atrium. After an arterial switch procedure, an injection in the right ventricle or main pulmonary artery should be done in the LAO 20- to 30-degree view, with craniocaudal 25-degree tilt, to show the main pulmonary artery and bifurcation. An aortic root injection, usually in the AP and shallow LAO views, with craniocaudal angulation or selective coronary arteriography, should be performed to evaluate the origin and course of the proximal coronary arteries.

Anomalous Pulmonary Venous Return

Total anomalous pulmonary venous return presents early in life either with congestive heart failure secondary to volume overload or with severe cyanosis in the newborn period when there is associated obstruction to pulmonary venous return.

Anatomy

The three most common sites of return are to a left vertical vein leading to the innominate vein, an infradiaphragmatic vein that connects to the portal circulation, and direct connection to the coronary sinus. Partial anomalous pulmonary venous return may be isolated, usually one or two veins draining to the SVC or innominate vein, or associated with a sinus venosus atrial septal defect. With a sinus venosus defect, the right upper lobe and sometimes the right middle lobe will drain to the superior vena caval–right atrial junction or sometimes more proximally directly into the SVC. A right lower lobe pulmonary vein and/or right middle vein may drain to the right atrium in the presence of an inferior type of sinus venosus defect. Occasionally, an isolated left upper lobe pulmonary vein will drain directly to the innominate vein.

Associated Defects

Associated defects are atrial septal defect and scimitar syndrome, which includes hypoplastic right lung, anomalous drainage of the right lung to the IVC, and a sequestered pulmonary lobe with an anomalous arterial supply.

Physiology

Total anomalous pulmonary venous connection results in the complete admixture of systemic and pulmonary venous return in the right atrium. All systemic blood flow results from a right-to-left shunt across an atrial defect, because there is no other way for blood to enter the left heart. Partial anomalous pulmonary venous return is a very different situation and results in an obligatory left-to-right shunt, the size of which depends on the number and territory drained by the anomalous veins. If only a single vein is involved and there is no associated atrial defect, the left-to-right shunt is modest and usually not hemodynamically important.

Indications for Cardiac Catheterization

For total anomalous pulmonary venous return, the indication for study is to measure the pulmonary artery pressure and accurately define the anatomy of the pulmonary venous connection, particularly when mixed venous return to various sites is suspected. The major indications for catheterization with partial anomalous pulmonary venous return are to evaluate an unexplained left-to-right shunt and to assess the magnitude of the shunt when an anomalous vein is identified by noninvasive techniques.

Catheterization and Technique Approach

A right heart catheterization and pulmonary arteriogram are done in the usual manner. Selective right or left pulmonary arteriograms also may be helpful. In the setting of partial anomalous pulmonary venous return, it is valuable to directly enter and inject the anomalously draining veins. These veins are usually easily entered with exploration by the catheter tip in the right atrium, SVC, or innominate vein.

Hemodynamics

A saturation of 85% or greater in the SVC or innominate vein should strongly suggest anomalous drainage of pulmonary veins. When the vein is directly entered, a saturation of 95% should be obtained. An accurate Qp/Qs ratio is often impossible to determine because of uncertainty about the true value of the mixed venous saturation. Pulmonary artery pressure is usually elevated with total anomalous pulmonary venous return. With partial anomalous return, however, the pressure is generally normal.

Angiography

A pulmonary arteriogram in the AP and lateral views will visualize the pulmonary venous return. Selective branch pulmonary artery injections are preferred in the setting of partial anomalous return. A direct injection into the anomalous veins gives the most definitive picture of the anatomy.

Ebstein's Anomaly

Ebstein's anomaly is a relatively rare defect with an incredibly wide spectrum of clinical presentations, ranging from a cyanotic newborn to unexpected cardiomegaly or dyspnea on exertion in childhood, or new-onset supraventricular arrhythmia in an adult.

Anatomy

The hallmark of this abnormality is apical displacement of the septal and/or inferior leaflets of the tricuspid valve; that is, these leaflets arise distal to the normal site of the annulus. This results in a portion of the right ventricle proximal to the effective valve orifice becoming "atrialized." The anterior leaflet always arises normally from the annulus, but generally has an abnormal distal attachment such as a direct linear attachment into the body of the right ventricle. Associated dysplasia of the leaflets is a common finding. The result is that right ventricular function is variably compromised based on the size of the chamber distal to the effective orifice and tricuspid valve function. In addition to these structural abnormalities, there is a high prevalence of accessory AV bypass tracts and a high incidence of recurrent supraventricular tachycardia.

Associated Defects

Associated defects are atrial septal defect or incompetent foramen ovale, pulmonic stenosis, and left ventricular dysfunction.

Physiology

The abnormal physiology correlates with the degree of anatomic abnormalities. Severe tricuspid insufficiency, tricuspid stenosis, or marked displacement of the tricuspid orifice results in inadequate right ventricular pump function, with secondary elevation of the right atrial pressure. This leads to systemic desaturation with a right-to-left atrial shunt if an atrial communication is present. If the atrial septum is intact, cardiac output may be decreased. The combination of right atrial hypertension and increased incidence of AV bypass tracts leads to a high likelihood of supraventricular arrhythmias, which include re-entrant supraventricular tachycardia, atrial ectopic tachycardia, atrial flutter, and atrial fibrillation.

Indications for Catheterization

Invasive studies should be considered to provide supplementary information to the echo/Doppler studies in patients who are to undergo surgical intervention. Electrophysiologic studies are indicated in patients with severe arrhythmias.

Catheterization and Technique Approach

A right heart catheterization is usually more easily done with a non–balloon-tipped catheter. An end-hole catheter allows determination of the point of entry into the ventricular pressure zone in the right ventricle, and tip entrapment is more readily detected. This type of catheter can often be advanced from the right ventricle into the pulmonary artery easier than a flow-directed catheter because of the tricuspid regurgitation or stenosis. There is a high incidence of either an atrial septal defect or a patent foramen ovale, which allows easy access to the left atrium and left ventricle.

Hemodynamics

Oximetry may show evidence of right-to-left or occasionally left-to-right shunting across an atrial defect. Pressure data usually show low or normal right ventricular systolic pressure and elevated right ventricular end-diastolic and right atrial pressures. There is usually only a minimal right atrial to right ventricular diastolic gradient, even with significant tricuspid stenosis. The a and v waves in the right atrium are often blunted and lose their diagnostic value because of the large compliant right atrium that is usually present. Right atrial pressure will commonly exceed left atrial pressure. However, they tend to equalize in the presence of an atrial defect.

Angiography

A right ventriculogram in the AP or RAO view will define the size and function of the right ventricle distal to the tricuspid orifice, as well as help to evaluate the amount of tricuspid regurgitation. A right atrial injection is useful to show the size of the right atrium and atrialized ventricle if there is no tricuspid regurgitant jet to fill these chambers on the right ventriculogram. A left ventriculogram may help clarify the function of this chamber, because there is frequently a dyskinetic pattern of contraction that may give misleading information by echocardiography alone.

Single Ventricle

Among the more complex forms of congenital heart disease is a spectrum of anomalies that is unified by having a single functioning ventricle. In years past, an adult cardiologist would be unlikely to encounter patients with these abnormalities. Innovative palliative surgical procedures, however, have been performed over the past 15 years, resulting in increasing survival into adulthood.

Anatomy

Three prototypes representative of the spectrum of these anomalies include the hypoplastic left heart syndrome, tricuspid atresia, and double-inlet left ventricle. The hypoplastic left heart syndrome is usually secondary to aortic atresia and results in a diminutive left ventricle incapable of supporting the systemic circulation. The right ventricle, by default, becomes the only functioning ventricle and is required to support both the systemic and pulmonary artery circulations. The converse situation occurs with tricuspid atresia, in which the right ventricle is hypoplastic and the left ventricle is the only ventricle capable of supporting the circulation. In patients with double-inlet left ventricle, the right and left atria empty into a large morphologic left ventricle, which then gives rise to a rudimentary outflow chamber and both great vessels. Early palliation is designed to establish a balance of systemic and pulmonary blood flow. If no natural pulmonic stenosis is present, pulmonary artery banding or complex aortopulmonary reconstruction is performed. If severe pulmonic stenosis is present, pulmonary blood flow becomes inadequate and a systemic to pulmonary artery shunt must be performed. Secondary palliation then consists of a modified Fontan operation. This operation, which is now the most common open-heart surgical procedure done in children over 2 years of age, consists of

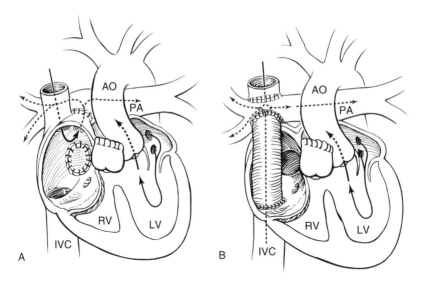

Figure 18-3 Two of the more common techniques to baffle the systemic venous return directly to the pulmonary arteries in the Fontan procedure. **(A)** An atriopulmonary connection with closure of the atrial septal defect in a patient with tricuspid atresia. **(B)** A total cavopulmonary connection with a lateral tunnel in the same lesion. AO, aorta; PA, pulmonary artery; RV, right ventricle; LV, left ventricle; IVC, inferior vena cava.

separating the circulations by diverting the systemic venous return to the pulmonary arteries without an intervening ventricular pump (Fig 18-3).

Associated Defects

Associated defects are valvular atresias, AV valve insufficiency, pulmonic stenosis, and coarctation of the aorta.

Physiology

Pre-operative physiology varies widely based on the underlying anatomy and relative distribution of pulmonary and systemic blood flow. Post-Fontan physiology is dominated by elevated pressure in the right atrium and venae cavae, which is required to drive flow through the pulmonary vascular bed. Cardiac output is normal to low at rest, and the increase during exercise is markedly limited.

Indications for Catheterization

Catheterization is indicated for pre-operative evaluation and for evaluation of postoperative patients who develop evidence of right heart failure or inadequate cardiac output.

Catheterization and Technical Approach

The most important aspect of catheterization in this group of patients is to have a detailed knowledge and understanding of the anatomy of the particular lesion and, where applicable, the type of repair that has been done. (The reader is referred to other sources for discussion of this subject in detail.) In the preoperative situation, there are critical data that must be obtained to determine whether a patient is a candidate for a Fontan procedure. These include measurement of pulmonary artery pressure, cardiac output, and pulmonary vascular resistance and angiographically defining pulmonary artery anatomy, size, and any distortion of the pulmonary arterial bed. It is frequently necessary to enter shunts to directly catheterize the pulmonary artery to obtain pressure in this vessel. Assessment of the systemic ventricular and AV valve function also is critical. With regard to the postoperative patient, there are numerous modifications of the technique of the Fontan operation that have been utilized over the past several years, and these modifications will greatly affect catheter courses through the right side of the circulation. The postoperative study should carefully evaluate the presence of any gradients between the systemic veins and the pulmonary artery, as well as assessing left ventricular systolic and diastolic function.

Hemodynamics

Preoperative hemodynamics vary with the physiology. An aortic saturation of greater than 85% indicates the presence of increased pulmonary blood flow, whereas an aortic saturation less than 75% indicates decreased pulmonary artery flow. As already mentioned, pulmonary pressure and pulmonary vascular resistance are variables that are extremely important to define. Post-Fontan hemodynamics are characterized by variably elevated right atrial pressure. Pulmonary artery pressure resembles right atrial pressure, and there should be no gradient between the atrium and pulmonary arteries. The a wave is dominant throughout the right side of the circulation if sinus rhythm is present. Mean right atrial pressure is generally in the range of 12 to 18 mm Hg. Wedge pressure should correlate with left ventricular end-diastolic pressure and will be normal to low in a well-functioning Fontan procedure. However, elevation of these pressures may occur and be partly responsible for inadequate cardiac output and marked elevation of the right heart pressures.

Angiography

Pre-operatively, it is very important to obtain a pulmonary arteriogram so that the size and anatomy of these arteries are well demonstrated. Ventricular contractility and AV valve function also should be assessed angiographically. In patients who have had a Fontan operation, injections in the SVC, IVC, or right atrium (depending on the type of connection) are performed to visualize surgical anastomoses and flow patterns through the right side of the circulation. A left ventriculogram is performed as indicated to assess left ventricular systolic and AV valve function.

Systemic Venous Anomalies

The most common systemic venous anomaly is a persistent left SVC that drains into the coronary sinus (occurring in 0.3% of procedures performed in adults). It may often be suspected when the echocardiogram demonstrates a large coronary sinus. During catheterization of patients with congenital heart disease, it is advisable to document the presence of a normal innominate vein. A persistent left SVC does not perturb the physiology, but it is important to identify if the left subclavian approach to the heart is contemplated. This issue is particularly relevant in the case of pacemaker implantation. During a right heart catheterization from the femoral venous approach, the catheter may preferentially enter the coronary sinus when it is dilated due to drainage of a persistent left SVC. A low leftward pass of the catheter without encountering a ventricular pressure zone should raise suspicion regarding the possible existence of this entity. By gently advancing the catheter and directing the tip superiorly with clockwise rotation, it should pass easily into a left SVC. If surgical intervention or pacemaker insertion is a consideration, an injection in the high left SVC (AP view) may be important to document its drainage and determine if there is a bridging innominate vein.

Other rare systemic venous anomalies include a left SVC that directly enters the left atrium (this leads to aortic desaturation), congenital absence of the right SVC, and absence of the intrahepatic portion of the IVC. This latter anomaly often may occur in association with complex congenital heart defects. The catheter course from the femoral vein includes posterior diversion into the azygous system, with subsequent passage of the catheter above the diaphragm into the thoracic cavity using the azygous vein, which then enters into the SVC. A right heart catheterization may still be done from this approach if a balloon-tipped flow-directed catheter is utilized.

SELECTED READINGS

Beerman LB, Zuberbuhler JR. Atrial septal defect. In: Anderson RH, Shinebourne EA, Macartney FJ, Tynan M, eds. Pediatric cardiology. Edinburgh: Churchill Livingstone, 1987:541–562.

Epstein M. The adult patient with known or suspected congenital heart disease. In: Pepine CJ, Hill JA, Lambert CR, eds. 2nd ed. Diagnostic and therapeutic cardiac catheterization. Baltimore: Williams & Wilkins, 1994:765–782.

Lock JE, Perry SB, Keane JF. Profiles in congenital heart disease. In: Grossman W, Baum DS, eds. 4th ed. Cardiac catheterization, angiography and intervention. Philadelphia: Lea & Febiger, 1991:655–675.

Neches WH, Park SC, Zuberbuhler JR, eds. Perspectives in pediatric cardiology. Pediatric cardiac catheterization. vol. 3. Mount Kisco, NY: Futura Publishers; 1991.

III

NEWER CATHETER DIAGNOSTIC MODALITIES

19

INTRAVASCULAR ULTRASOUND IMAGING

E. Murat Tuzcu
Anthony C. De Franco
Steven E. Nissen

T HE DEVELOPMENT OF coronary angiography, by Mason Sones
in 1958 heralded a new era in the diagnosis and treatment of coronary artery disease.[1] Coronary angiography remains the major technique for the diagnosis of coronary artery disease. Effective treatment strategies have been developed based on angiographic findings. As
experience with coronary angiography increased, however, so did appreciation
of its shortcomings. The development of quantitative coronary angiography has
overcome some of these limitations.[2] The accuracy and reproducibility of quantitative coronary angiographic systems and their on-line applications have been
established.[3] Nevertheless, a carefully performed coronary angiography may
still be inadequate for a definitive diagnosis. A newer imaging modality, intravascular ultrasound, which has grown rapidly in the 1990s, provides cross-
sectional images of the coronary arteries, adding valuable information to standard angiographic studies.

Angiography displays a planar image of the coronary artery as the silhouette
of the contrast-filled lumen, whereas intravascular ultrasound displays the artery as a cross-sectional tomographic image. Ultrasound directly visualizes the
atherosclerotic plaque and the structures of the vascular wall, whereas arteriog-

raphy images the plaque inferentially when the lumen is encroached upon by atheroma. Intravascular ultrasound is not an alternative to angiography, but complements its "road-mapping" characteristics by providing tomographic visualization of the lumen and vessel wall. This new technique provides insights into the pathophysiology of coronary atherosclerosis, as well as into the mechanism and outcome of various coronary interventions.

Limitations of Angiography

The accuracy of coronary angiography in the assessment of stenosis has been questioned for many years. Angiographic and necropsy studies have demonstrated significant differences between lesion severity by angiography and by histology.[4-8] Visual assessment of coronary stenosis is limited by interobserver and intra-observer variability.[9] Although quantitative coronary angiography overcomes some of these inconsistencies, calibration requirements remain as potential sources of error in achieving accurate measurements.[10] The difference between angiographic and histologic severity of coronary stenosis is multifactorial. Angiographic percent diameter stenosis and absolute diameter (in millimeters) are based on a comparative assessment of the narrowest site and a reference segment. However, normal-appearing reference segments frequently are involved by atherosclerosis. Postmortem studies have demonstrated that atherosclerosis often is a diffuse process rather than a discrete phenomenon.[7] Unless the reference segment truly is normal, the calculated percent diameter stenosis will be an underestimation of true stenosis. Thus, as the plaque burden in the reference segment increases, so does the underestimation of the lesion severity. Atherosclerotic involvement of the angiographically normal segments may have implications for the interventional cardiologist.[11,12]

Remodeling of coronary arteries is another cause of negative results of coronary arteriography. During the early and mid stages of atheroma growth, the vessel wall may enlarge to accommodate the growing atheroma.[13] The local change in arterial size and shape hides the growing atheroma from angiographic detection by preserving the lumen area.

The limitations of angiography are particularly important for the interventional cardiologist. The complex luminal geometry that is created by various interventional techniques is displayed as a planar silhouette of the contrast-filled vessel. The fractured atheroma and displaced structures allow extravasation of contrast material into the atheroma and to the deeper layers of the vessel wall. The contrast material occupying these cracks and crevices creates an appearance of enlarged lumen. Thus, quantitative measurements of the enlarged angiographic silhouette after balloon angioplasty frequently overestimates the true vessel cross-sectional area.[14]

Intravascular Ultrasound

Equipment

Intracoronary ultrasound systems employ a catheter that is attached to a dedicated scanner. The miniaturized transducers permit the use of ultrasound catheters in the range of 2.9 to 3.5 Fr (0.96–1.17 mm in diameter). These flexible catheters can be placed safely in most arteries and consistently generate high-quality images. There are two different systems employed in the intravascular ultrasound devices: the single-element mechanical system and the multi-element electronic system (Fig 19-1). In the single-element mechanical system, one ultrasound transducer is mounted on the tip of the catheter and connected via a flexible shaft to an external motor. In some systems, the transducer is rotated by the external motor, creating a rotating sound beam to build a cross-sectional real-time image. Other mechanical systems use a fixed element with a rotating mirror.

Multi-element electronic systems consist of multiple small transducer elements with circumferential configuration at the catheter tip. The ultrasound signals that are generated from sequentially working individual transducer elements create the 360-degree real-time ultrasound image. The ultrasound signal is processed at the site via integrated circuits. Although the earlier models had suboptimal resolution, recent developments in transducer design have led to considerable improvement in image quality. The advantage of multi-element electronic systems is the absence of a rotating part (the drive shaft) and, thus, a lack of rotational artifacts. On the other hand, rotating mechanical devices

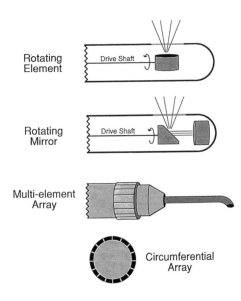

Figure 19-1   Different intravascular catheter designs. The upper two illustrations show the mechanical system with single element. The lower two illustrations show the multi-element electronic systems.

have a higher acoustic power, greater dynamic range, and better tissue penetration. However, they are sometimes limited by a nonuniform rotation in tortuous arterial segments and continuous circular movement of the transducer and the shaft.

Technique

The laboratory techniques required for intravascular ultrasound imaging are similar to those required for percutaneous coronary interventions. The ultrasound catheters with larger shafts require 8-Fr guiding catheters, whereas smaller catheters can be introduced through a 7- or 6-Fr catheter. All the catheters can be advanced over a standard 0.014″ steerable angioplasty guidewire. Most of the ultrasound catheters have a monorail design, although coaxial over-the-wire catheters with multi-element electronic systems also are available.[15] Despite improved handling characteristics, the trackability of ultrasound catheters is not as good as the state-of-the-art balloon angioplasty catheters. As a result, distal segments of heavily calcified tortuous arteries or severely obstructed segments may occasionally be inaccessible to ultrasound imaging. Nevertheless, currently available catheters can safely cross most diseased segments. In addition to the over-the-wire and monorail designs, a new ultrasound catheter design employs a sheath system; the distal portion of these catheters are ultrasound-transparent sheaths. After the catheter is placed into the coronary artery, with the tip beyond the obstruction site, the guidewire is withdrawn to a proximal site, and the ultrasound transducer, which is on a moving wire within the catheter, is advanced into the sheath. The ultrasound transducer remains in the sheath, but allows high-resolution images along the length of the sheath.

Safety

Intravascular ultrasound imaging has the potential for complications. Coronary spasm is the most frequent complication of intravascular imaging and usually responds promptly to intracoronary nitroglycerin. The imaging catheter may obstruct a stenosed coronary artery segment and lead to myocardial ischemia. Rarely, severe ischemia may prohibit imaging or limit the imaging time. The separation of the guidewire and the ultrasound catheter in the coronary artery can occur in systems that have a short monorail design. This separation occasionally may lead to plaque disruption. Movement of the guidewire or the transducer through the sheath may be difficult in tortuous arteries when intravascular ultrasound catheters with distal sheaths are used. Despite these limitations, the number of serious complications associated with intravascular ultrasound, such as coronary dissections, abrupt closure, acute myocardial infarction, emergency bypass surgery, or death, is very low when it is performed by physicians with expertise in intracoronary procedures.[16,17]

Normal Morphology

The circular catheter is surrounded by a narrow circle of near-field artifact or ring-down artifact, which varies in size among ultrasound systems. The surrounding lumen is echolucent, with speckles originating from blood elements. The vessel wall may appear as a monolayered or a trilayered structure (Fig 19-2).[18] Imaging performed with a 30-MHz catheter more often reveals a triluminal structure than that performed with a 20-MHz catheter. The differentiation of the layers in the vessel wall depends on the thickness and refractile characteristics of the layers, the frequency of the ultrasound system, and the proximity of the transducer to the vessel wall.[19–21] The intima is represented by the innermost layer, which appears as an echogenic circular structure. The thin echolucent circular layer beyond the intima is thought to represent the media. The bright echos beyond the media originate from the adventitia. A number of histologic and ultrasound studies have made quantitative measurements of these structures.[22,23] The intima is very thin in early life and becomes thicker with age.[24] Ultrasound images from a child or a young person generally show a monolayer vessel wall because the thin intima is not differentiated, even with 30-MHz transducers. Higher-frequency ultrasound transducers may be able to

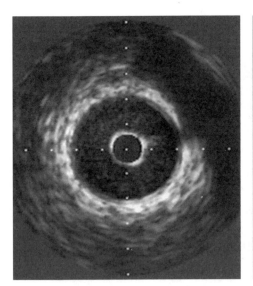
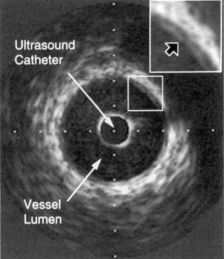

Figure 19-2 Intravascular ultrasound appearance of a normal coronary artery. The ultrasound catheter is at the center. There is a thin bright halo of ring-down artifact. The echolucent zone around the catheter is the vessel lumen. The layers of the vessel wall are shown in a magnified view in the upper-right hand corner. The echodense innermost layer represents intima. The echolucent layer in the middle corresponds to the media, and the bright echos beyond the intima originate from the adventitia.

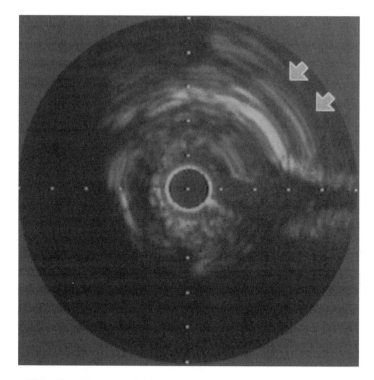

Figure 19-3 An ultrasound image of an atherosclerotic coronary artery, which is distorted by nonuniform rotation. The information from tissues from 12 o'clock to 3 o'clock (indicated by the arrows) is uninterpretable due to artifact.

detect very thin intimal layers. In a middle-aged adult, normal intimal thickness is less than 300 μg.[24] The media is thin and may extend beyond the central echolucent layer, making accurate measurement difficult.[25]

Imaging artifacts that distort the normal vessel morphology are seen commonly with the currently available intravascular ultrasound devices. Single-element mechanical systems are prone to cyclical oscillations due to inequalities in rotational speed along the flexible driveshaft. This irregular motion leads to nonuniform rotational distortion, which is common when the catheter is positioned in a tortuous vessel. The arterial wall appears stretched on one side and "compressed" on the other, and shape of the artery and the image of the tissues appear distorted (Fig 19-3). This artifact can sometimes be corrected by minor manipulations of the catheter and relieving the torque. Another artifact that is seen during the interpretation of ultrasound images is the transducer ring-down artifact. This artifact, which appears as a halo around the transducer that obscures all the ultrasound signals, originates from the affected field near the transducer. High-amplitude signals created by the acoustic oscillations of the transducer obscure the near-field imaging. In small arterial segments, a ring-down artifact may cover the echos from the vessel wall structures adjacent to the catheter and make accurate assessment impossible.

Quantitative assessment of the maximum and minimum diameters and area of the lumen, intimal thickness, plaque thickness and plaque area, and vessel diameter and area can be measured on-line or off-line. These measurements are based on the assumption that the ultrasound catheter is located co-axially in the coronary artery. If the catheter is not co-axial, the beams emitted from the transducer are directed to the vessel wall obliquely. This oblique angle will distort the true shape of the vessel and lead to errors in measurements.

Abnormal Morphology

Intravascular ultrasound allows direct assessment of the severity, location, and distribution of atherosclerosis and the composition of atheroma.[26,27] Early atherosclerotic plaques appear as intimal thickening, whereas advanced lesions appear as large echogenic masses (Fig 19-4). Dimensions of the lumen and atheroma can be quantified accurately from the tomographic images provided by intravascular ultrasound. The ultrasound measurements correlate closely with angiographic measurements in normal coronary arteries. In patients with advanced atherosclerosis, angiographic assessment of lesion severity does not correlate with ultrasound measurements because disease-free segments with circular lumens are uncommon in atherosclerotic arteries. The complex geometry

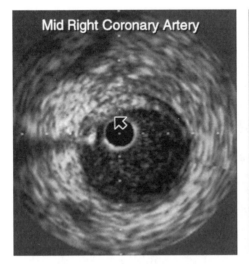
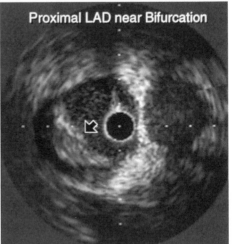

Figure 19-4   Two ultrasound images from the same patient, illustrating (left) early atherosclerosis manifested by a small eccentric plaque (at 11 o'clock). More advanced atherosclerosis is manifested by a large eccentric plaque at the ostium of the left anterior descending (LAD) coronary artery, typically located opposite the flow-dividing wall.

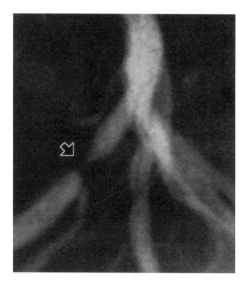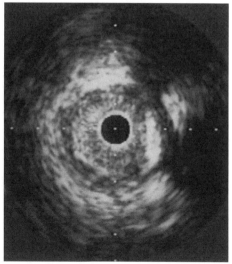

Figure 19-5   (Left) The left coronary angiogram in the left anterior oblique projection, showing an eccentric lesion in the left anterior descending coronary artery (arrow). (Right) Intravascular ultrasound image of the lesion shows a concentric atheroma involving the entire circumference of the vessel.

of the lumen is readily appreciated by intravascular ultrasound, whereas angiography reduces the irregular lumen to a two-dimensional planar silhouette. The shape of the lumen becomes more complex following percutaneous interventions, making accurate assessment by angiography more difficult. The minimal luminal diameter and the percent diameter stenosis, which are standard measurements in quantitative angiography, are based on this planar silhouette; these measurements do not take into account noncircular characteristics of the narrowed coronary lumen. The relative location of the atheroma in the circumference of the vessel wall, which is important in the planning of percutaneous coronary interventions, is traditionally judged by angiography as eccentric or concentric. Ultrasound imaging, however, has shown that angiography is an insensitive tool in the determination of circumferential location of the atheroma.[28,29] Many angiographically eccentric lesions are found to be large atheroma occupying the entire circumference of the artery (Fig 19-5).

Comparative ultrasound histologic studies have demonstrated that plaque textures observed with ultrasound imaging correlate well with atheroma content.[19,20,30] Generally, plaques are defined as "soft" if they are less echogenic (sonolucent) than the surrounding adventitia (Fig 19-6). These plaques are likely to have a higher lipid content. Plaques that are defined as "fibrous" appear as dense as the adventitia. Increasing fibrous elements create this echodense texture. These are very broad and overlapping classifications. With currently available technology, the composition of the plaque cannot be assessed

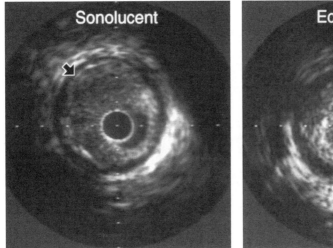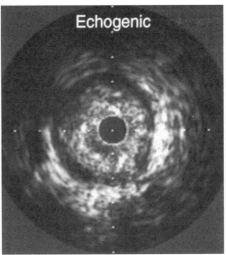

Figure 19-6   (Left) Intravascular ultrasound picture of a "soft" plaque due to the sonolucent appearance indicated by the arrow. (Right) Intravascular ultrasound of a "fibrous" plaque that appears as echogenic as the adventitia.

more accurately. In most instances, a layered thrombus cannot be differentiated from a soft plaque. The ongoing work with tissue characterization may provide more accurate analysis of atheroma content. Nevertheless, ultrasound imaging provides the interventional cardiologist a better understanding of the target lesion, especially by identifying calcium. Calcium deposits appear typically as bright echoes, more echogenic than the surrounding adventitia, and produce acoustic shadowing of deeper tissues (Fig 19-7). The shadowing, which is accepted as the hallmark of calcified plaques, occurs because of attenuated transmission of the ultrasound segment. Calcified plaque detected by angiography is associated with an increased risk of dissection following balloon angioplasty, typically occurring adjacent to the calcified area.[31,32] Cutting and retrieval of calcified plaques with currently available directional coronary atherectomy catheters are very difficult.[33] Stent deployment in heavily calcified arteries also is difficult because of the resistance to the full expansion of stents, even with high pressure. Rotational ablation is recommended as the treatment of choice for arteries with extensive superficial calcification.[34] The conventional way of identifying coronary calcium utilizes fluoroscopy to visualize opacities in close proximity to the vessel, but even careful inspection of angiograms combined with clinical and demographic information prior to intervention cannot identify patients with significant calcification of target lesions. In a series of 185 consecutive patients, we found that angiography identifies less than half of the patients with calcified plaques detected by ultrasound. The sensitivity of angiography and fluoroscopy increases to 52% at sites where calcification involved

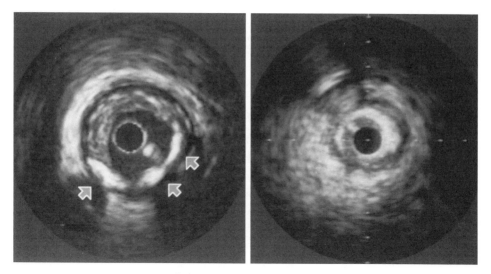

Figure 19-7 (Left) Two large areas of calcification (arrows) obscure the underlying structures of the vessel wall by accoustic shadowing. (Right) A fibrotic plaque that exhibits greater echogenicity than adventitia, but without acoustic shadowing.

more than one quadrant and to 63% where calcification involved two or more quadrants of the circumference.[35] Angiography also is not an effective method for localizing the depth of calcium deposits. In our study, only one third of the patients with superficial and 25% with deep calcium were identified correctly by angiography. Despite a low sensitivity, angiography has a high specificity. When angiography is positive for coronary artery calcium, the target lesion usually contains a relatively large arc of calcium and is likely to be superficial in location. Even if calcium is not detected at the target lesion site, the presence of calcium at a remote site in the coronary tree increases the likelihood of calcium at the site of interest. Mintz et al. reported similar findings in a very large series.[36]

Clinical Applications

Ambiguous Lesions

Angiographic examination cannot assess precisely all of the stenoses in the coronary tree. Stenoses at the ostia of the coronary arteries, those near bifurcations, or those at sites where multiple branches overlap are typical examples of angiographically ambiguous lesions. Suboptimal angiographic pictures due to poor injections, obscuring of the lesion by sinus of Valsalva opacification, wedging of the catheter, or patient characteristics such as obesity, emphysema, and thoracic deformities are not infrequent occurrences in a busy catheterization laboratory. Some stenoses appear to be severe on only one view and seem to be mild in other views. Angiography may demonstrate abnormal areas that are impossible to quantitate, such as "napkin ring" lesions, dynamic obstructions (kinks and bridges), or hazy arterial sites. Intravascular ultrasound is an excellent tool for identifying cross-sectional vessel wall morphology in these difficult cases.[37–39]

The Left Main Coronary Artery

The left main coronary artery can be the most difficult arterial segment to visualize adequately by angiography. This may be due to diffuse atherosclerotic involvement, angulation leading to inadequate angiographic projections, or inability to selectively cannulate the vessel. Autopsy studies have shown the relative insensitivity of angiography in the detection of left main atherosclerosis.[6] Because of the serious clinical consequences of left main coronary artery stenosis, complementary information provided by intravascular ultrasound imaging can be very valuable.

The functional significance of a lesion cannot be determined in the conventional sense by intravascular ultrasound. In the setting of ambiguous lesions in the left main trunk or coronary ostia, however, ultrasound offers incremental diagnostic value. A narrowed lumen with a large atheroma demonstrated by ultrasound in the angiographically suspicious but poorly defined arterial segment facilitates decision making.

In two ultrasound studies, high prevalence of atherosclerosis was reported in the angiographically normal-looking left main coronary arteries.[37,38] We routinely use ultrasound imaging in the evaluation of left main coronary lesions if angiographic findings are uncertain. On such occasions, we make major management decisions regarding revascularization versus medical therapy with the help of ultrasound findings.[40] In this circumstance, findings of the ultrasound imaging are not used independently, but as adjunctive information to the available data from clinical evaluation, coronary angiography, and noninvasive tests.

The only unusual aspect of a left coronary angiogram may be the relatively small vessel caliber. Due to lack of a discrete abnormality, there would be no measurable obstruction. In these cases, although the left main appears "not normal," it eludes further characterization by angiography. In an ultrasound study, a ratio of diameters of the left main coronary artery to its daughter branches (left anterior descending and left circumflex coronary arteries) was proposed to identify such patients who might have a high likelihood of angiographically unrecognized left main coronary atherosclerosis.[41] An abnormal left main ratio was defined as less than 0.58. This index was prospectively evaluated in 64 consecutive patients with coronary disease and found to have a specificity of 93% and a sensitivity of 44%. Thus patients with a left main ratio of less than 0.58 may warrant further investigation for possible unrecognized left main atherosclerosis.

Ultrasound in Interventional Cardiology

Balloon Angioplasty

The role of intravascular ultrasound imaging in balloon angioplasty is still evolving. Ultrasound examination aids in the patient selection process. The length of the lesion, circumferential distribution, composition of plaque, and true vessel size all play important roles in choosing the right device for percutaneous intervention. Longer lesion lengths may require 30- to 40-mm balloons. The presence of extensive calcification indicates a potential high risk of complications or suboptimal result. Although previous angiographic studies have shown that oversized balloons lead to dissection more frequently, a group of in-

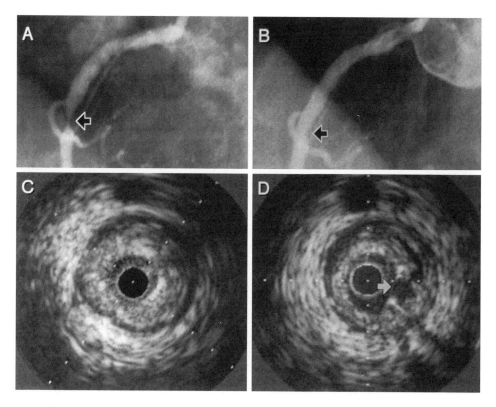

Figure 19-8 Angiographic and ultrasound appearance of right coronary artery before and after balloon angiography: (**A**) Severe stenosis of the mid right coronary artery; (**B**) enlarged coronary lumen following a successful balloon angioplasty; (**C**) concentric fibrous plaque occupying most of the lumen; and (**D**) the enlarged coronary lumen following balloon angioplasty, which is due mainly to a deep dissection. Contrast filling this dissection appears as an enlarged, smooth lumen on the angiogram shown in panel b.

vestigators have recommended using ultrasound measurements for choosing the appropriate balloon size.[42,43] This study suggests that larger balloon sizes may be used safely with ultrasound guidance and lead to better outcomes.[43]

Ultrasound provides valuable follow-up information after balloon angioplasty, and it provides insights into the mechanism of lumen dilatation.[22,44–47] Stretching of the vessel wall, compression and redistribution of the plaque mass, plaque fractures, and dissections all contribute to lumen enlargement. The extent of coronary dissections is best evaluated by intravascular ultrasound[43,44,47,48] (Fig 19-8). Ultrasound assessment of the target lesion site after balloon angioplasty may provide information about the need for further treatment (e.g., stenting) before the patient leaves the catheterization laboratory. Postangioplasty ultrasound assessment provides clues about the long-term outcome of the procedure. Several preliminary studies have suggested that vessel stretching and plaque compression, in contrast to plaque fracture and large dissections, increase the risk of restenosis. Mintz et al. evaluated 284 lesions by intravascular ultrasound following various coronary interventions and found that residual cross-sectional area was an independent predictor of restenosis.[49] Similar results have been reported in the interim analysis of the GUIDE II trial.[50] Clinical restenosis was more frequent in patients who had larger plaque burdens and smaller lumen areas following percutaneous interventions. In contrast, the PICTURE study, which analyzed 200 patients prospectively, revealed no ultrasound characteristic as a predictor of restenosis.[51] Clearly, further study is needed in this area. If intravascular ultrasound provides definite predictors of restenosis in the immediate postinterventional period, the interventionist may use other techniques to improve long-term outcome. To reach this goal, predictors of restenosis should be easily detectable by on-line approaches with consistency, as well as high sensitivity and specificity.

Directional Atherectomy

The tomographic images of intravascular ultrasound, which clearly show the extent and distribution of atheroma, may help improve the efficacy of debulking procedures (Fig 19-9). Ultrasound imaging following directional atherectomy has shown that excellent angiographic results can be achieved either by extensive debulking or by vessel stretching and plaque compression while a minimal amount of plaque is removed.[52–54] Pre-intervention imaging of the target lesions will help in planning the procedure according to the location, composition, and distribution of the atheroma.[55] Lesions that have extensive calcifications, particularly at or near the intimal surface, are unsuitable for directional atherectomy with currently available catheters. Lesions that appear eccentric on angiogram may be more concentric by ultrasound, and will require cutting in all four quadrants. On the other hand, with eccentric plaques, cuts should be made at the site of the atheroma but not in the direction of disease-free quadrants.

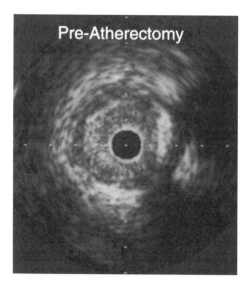
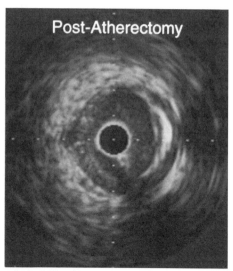

Figure 19-9   Intravascular ultrasound shows a concentric atheroma with a small fibrocalcific element between 1 o'clock and 4 o'clock occupying most of the lumen. Postatherectomy imaging reveals a markedly enlarged lumen due to plaque debulking. The fibrocalcific element of the plaque remained despite aggressive atherectomy.

After planning the intervention, imaging can be repeated during the procedure for further guidance. Nevertheless, ultrasound guidance of directional atherectomy can be a challenge. It requires experience, patience, and repeated catheter exchanges. Target lesion sites and the neighboring segments are examined carefully by intravascular ultrasound for landmarks such as side branches. The location of the plaque and changes in the plaque thickness are defined according to these landmarks. Atherectomy is then directed toward the atheroma based on these landmarks. In our experience, this technique is helpful in achieving better plaque removal in a safe manner. However, the limited accuracy of rotation, imprecise determination of the side branch ostia by angiography, and the lack of landmarks in some atherectomy cases limit this method. More elaborate methods for ultrasound guidance have been proposed, but these have not gained widespread use.[56] The final ultrasound assessment after atherectomy is useful in determining the amount of plaque removed, the lumen shape, and the surface characteristics. We have found that directional atherectomy leaves the most irregular surfaces among all interventional devices.[57] Postatherectomy ultrasound evaluation, in addition to angiographic assessment, helps to determine the need for adjunctive balloon angioplasty. Ongoing trials of ultrasound-guided atherectomy will establish the value of intravascular ultrasound as a guide to directional coronary atherectomy.

Rotational Ablation

Rotational atherectomy consists of a catheter with a high-speed diamond-coated burr at the tip and an external motor that drives the burr at 200,000 rpm. The major indication for "rotablation" is a calcified coronary artery lesion (Fig 19-10). Balloon angioplasty and directional atherectomy are often ineffective and are associated with higher complication rates in the setting of heavy calcification. On the other hand, rotablation is effective in removing calcification (see Fig 19-10). The detection of coronary calcification and its relative location in the vessel wall cannot be determined accurately by angiography alone.[35,36] The major role of intravascular ultrasound in rotational ablation is the selection of lesions that will benefit most from this technique compared

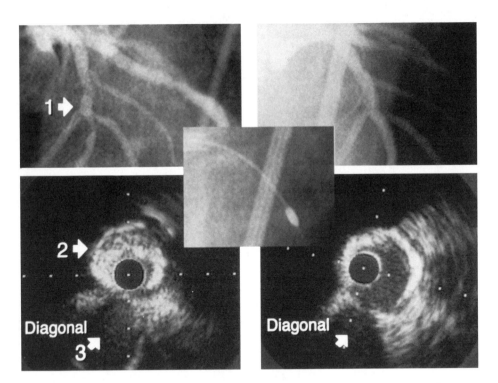

Figure 19-10 Coronary angiography. Coronary angiogram and intravascular ultrasound imaging of the left anterior descending coronary artery before and after rotablation. In the upper left panel, the white arrow (site 1) indicates the target lesion. The upper right-hand panel shows the same site following rotablation. In the lower left frame, the dense calcified plaque occupying the lumen is illustrated (site 2). The diagonal branch is seen between 6 o'clock and 8 o'clock (site 3). In the bottom right panel, the ultrasound image that is obtained after rotablation demonstrates the smooth, circular lumen achieved by the ablation of calcified atheroma.

with other interventional devices. Ultrasound studies have shown that rotational ablation leaves a smooth, round, ellipsoid lumen.[57,58] The concept of preferential ablation of the atheroma, but not the normal vessel wall, has been demonstrated by intravascular ultrasound imaging. Although rotational atherectomy preferentially removes a hard layer of calcium, it also achieves comparable debulking in noncalcified atherosclerotic sites as well.[59] Postrotablation assessment by ultrasound may lead to another intervention with a different device to further enlarge the lumen, or to obviate the need for an adjunctive device if the lumen size is adequately enlarged and if there is no significant residual atheroma.

Stents

Stents have had a major impact on interventional cardiology.[60,61] Intravascular ultrasound has played an important role in the development of this technology by improving the technique used for stent implantation. Until recently, patients were aggressively anticoagulated with warfarin as well as antiplatelet agents. These regimens led to a high rate of bleeding complications.[60,61] Despite these aggressive efforts, subacute thrombosis, with serious clinical consequences within the first 2 weeks of the procedure, has been reported to be as high as 15%. The requirement for vigorous anticoagulation initially limited the widespread application of stents. Intravascular ultrasound imaging shed new light on the technique of stent deployment. These examinations demonstrated that stent implantation was often suboptimal, despite a satisfactory angiographic appearance.[62] Observations from ultrasound studies have shown that reasons for suboptimal stent deployment include incomplete strut apposition, small residual lumen, irregular surface characteristics, and diffuse atherosclerotic involvement in adjacent arterial sites. At least one of these findings was observed in 80% to 90% of the patients, even though angiographic assessment was described as optimal by the interventionist.

These unfavorable findings can be detected easily by ultrasound examination. Metallic struts of the coronary stents produce a distinct appearance with bright reflections. The site and extent of strut apposition can be remedied either by high-pressure inflations or larger balloons (Fig 19-11). Similarly, small lumen size or irregular surface characteristics can be improved by additional balloon inflations. Caution is necessary while enlarging the lumen, however, because oversized balloons increase the risk of arterial rupture.[63,64] Thus, a balance must be struck between optimal lumen appearance versus the risk of serious complications. The total vessel size measured by ultrasound before the intervention can help in the selection of appropriate stent size. After stent deployment, measurement of the total vessel dimension at the stented site is difficult because of reverberations of the metal struts. Adjacent arterial sites

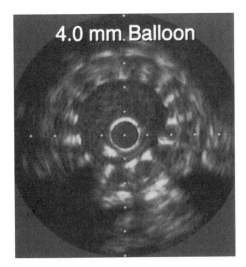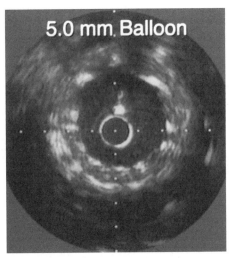

Figure 19-11   (Left) Ultrasound appearance of the an inadequately deployed Palmaz-Schatz stent in a coronary artery. The struts that are seen as bright echos are well apposed to the vessel wall between 7 o'clock and 3 o'clock, but not well expanded between 3 o'clock and 7 o'clock. (Right) Dilation with a larger balloon led to uniform opposition of the stent struts and a large circular lumen.

proximal and distal to the stented segment are used as references for the optimal lumen size. Empirically defined ratios are used to achieve the optimal intrastent area. In the setting of a hard calcific plaque, it may be impossible to expand the stent to achieve a lumen area comparable to the reference site. Ablation before stent placement may be needed in such cases.

Intravascular ultrasound is useful in determining the extent of coronary dissections that are created by balloon inflations. Residual dissections that are left uncovered by the stent are thought to increase the risk of thrombus development. Multiple stents may be necessary if dissection is not fully covered by a single stent. Multiple stenting is also used when segments neighboring to the stented site show large atheroma burdens. In the experience of one center, multiple stents were implanted in 40% of the cases to relieve the inflow or outflow obstructions, or to remedy the complications of stent deployment.[65] Subacute thrombosis rate has decreased dramatically with new ultrasound-guided strategies, including high-pressure balloon inflations, complete strut apposition, and large intrastent lumens. Currently, many centers utilize only antiplatelet agents following stent deployment and have less than a 2% subacute thrombosis rate. Intravascular ultrasound will continue to play an important role in the evaluation of new stent designs, stenting in smaller vessels, or evaluation of arteries with diffuse disease.

Intravascular Ultrasound in the Evaluation of Cardiac Transplant Recipients

Cardiac transplantation has been a major step forward in the treatment of patients with end-stage heart failure, and has led to improved survival rates and quality of life.[66,67] Transplant coronary artery disease is a leading cause of mortality and morbidity beyond the first year posttransplantation.[68] Conventional methods of diagnosis have low sensitivity in the early detection of this disease.[69] Although annual screening coronary angiograms are performed to overcome this diagnostic difficulty, these surveillance studies often fail to detect atherosclerosis prior to a clinical event. Necropsy studies have demonstrated that angiography underestimates atherosclerosis after cardiac transplantation.[70]

Intravascular ultrasound imaging is uniquely capable of detecting early phases of atherosclerosis as well as rapidly progressive arterial changes in these patients. Using this technology, we and others have demonstrated a high prevalence of donor-transmitted atherosclerosis in patients who were imaged within weeks of cardiac transplantation.[71–73] In a series of patients examined 1 to 9 years after transplantation, we have also shown the heterogeneous nature of coronary artery disease seen in transplant patients.[74] These studies revealed proximal focal, eccentric plaques similar to native atherosclerosis as well as diffuse, concentric lesions characteristic of classic transplant vasculopathy. In many of these patients, angiography appeared completely normal. In a preliminary study, abnormal ultrasound findings were predictors of angiographically detectable coronary artery disease. Currently, in many centers, intravascular ultrasound imaging is used routinely in conjunction with annual cardiac catheterization after cardiac transplantation.

Future Directions

A single intravascular ultrasound cross-section provides information from a highly selected site. To gather information from the entire arterial segment, three-dimensional reconstruction of a sequence of two-dimensional images is performed. The quality of qualitative and quantitative assessment of atherosclerotic arterial segments by three-dimensional reconstruction will be possible as better edge detection algorithms are developed and problems originating from tortuosity of the coronary arteries are resolved. Currently available ultrasound catheters have a distal shaft size of 2.9 to 3.5 Fr. Ongoing studies are exploring the possibility of even smaller ultrasound systems mounted on a core wire. This will allow the imaging of small, distal vessels as well as severely obstructed arterial segments. Another development that is being tested is the ultrasound catheter with a micromotor at the tip. This design aims to avoid the problems associated with a drive motor and flexible shaft connecting the motor to the transducer. While better image quality is sought by improved transducer design, higher-frequency transducers also are being investigated. The 50-MHz transducers produce higher-resolution images, but limited penetration and echoes from blood particles are important obstacles for their clinical application. Some investigators are exploring the possibility of better tissue characterization through image processing methods. Most of these are based on radio-frequency signal processing. Some of the advances are close to widespread clinical applications; others are in the early developmental phase.

Acknowledgment

The authors wish to thank Robert E. Hobbs, M.D., for his review of the manuscript and Karen L. Howell for her valuable assistance in the preparation of this chapter.

SELECTED READINGS

1. Sones FM, Shirey EK. Cine coronary arteriography. Mod Concepts Cardiovasc Dis 1962;31:735.
2. Foley DP, Escaned J, Strauss BH, et al. Quantitative coronary angiography in interventional cardiology. Application to scientific research and clinical practice. Prog Cardiovasc Dis 1994;36:363–384.
3. Keane D, Haase J, Slager C, et al. Comparative validation of quantitative coronary angiographic systems: results and implications from a multicenter study using standardized approach. Circulation 1995;91:2174–2183.
4. Arnett EN, Isner JM, Redwood DR, et al. Coronary artery narrowing in coronary heart disease: comparison of cineangiographic and necropsy findings. Ann Intern Med 1979;91:350–356.
5. Grodin C, Dydra I, Pasternac A, et al. Discrepancies between cineangiographic and post-mortem findings in patients with coronary artery disease and recent myocardial revascularization. Circulation 1974, 49:703–709.
6. Isner J, Kishel J, Kent K. Accuracy of angiographic determination of left main coronary arterial narrowing. Circulation 1981;63:1056–1061.
7. Roberts W, Jones A. Quantitation of coronary arterial narrowing at necropsy in sudden coronary death. Am J Cardiol 1979;44:39–44.
8. Vlodaver Z, French R, van Tassel RA, Edwards JE. Correlation of the antemortem coronary angiogram and the postmortem specimen. Circulation 1973;47:162–168.
9. Goldberg RK, Kleiman NS, Minor ST, et al. Comparison of quantitative coronary angiography to visual estimates of lesion severity pre and post percutaneous transluminal coronary angioplasty. Am Heart J 1990;1:178–184.
10. Fortin DF, Spero LA, Cusma JT, et al. Pitfalls in the determination of absolute dimensions using angiographic catheters as calibration devices in quantitative coronary angiography. Am J Cardiol 1991;68:1176–1182.
11. Nissen SE, De Franco AC, Raymond RE, et al. Angiographically unrecognized disease at normal reference sites: a risk factor for suboptimal results after coronary interventions. Circulation 1993;88:I-412A.
12. Mintz GS, Painter JA, Pichard AD, et al. Atherosclerosis in angiographically "normal" coronary artery reference segments: an intravascular ultrasound study with clinical correlations. J Am Coll Cardiol 1995;25:1479–1485.
13. Glagov S, Weisenberg E, Zarins C, et al. Compensatory enlargements of human coronary arteries. N Engl J Med 1987;316:1371–1375.
14. De Franco AC, Tuzcu EM, Abdelmeguid A, et al. Intravascular ultrasound assessment of percutaneous transluminal coronary angioplasty results: insights into the mechanisms of balloon angioplasty. J Am Coll Cardiol 1993;21:485A.
15. Hodgson J, Graham SP, Savakus AD, et al. Clinical percutaneous imaging of coronary anatomy using an over-the-wire ultrasound catheter system. Int J Cardiac Imaging 1989;4:187–193.
16. Hausmann D, Erbel R, Alibelli-Chemarin M-J, et al. The safety of intracoronary ultrasound. A multicenter survey of 2207 examinations. Circulation 1995;91:623–630.
17. Nissen SE, Tuzcu EM, De Franco AC. Coronary intravascular ultrasound: diagnostic and interventional applications. In: Topol EJ, ed. Textbook of interventional cardiology. St. Louis: Mallinckrodt Medical, 1994:207.
18. Fitzgerald PJ, St. Goar FG, Connolly AJ, et al. Intravascular ultrasound imaging of coronary arteries. Is three layers the norm? Circulation 1992;86:154–158.
19. Di Mario C, The SH, Madretsma S, et al. Detection and characterization of vascular lesions by intravascular ultrasound: an in vitro study correlated with histology. J Am Soc Echocardiogr 1992;5:135–146.

20. Gussenhoven EJ, Essed CE, Lancee CT, et al. Arterial wall characteristics determined by intravascular ultrasound imaging: an in vitro study. J Am Coll Cardiol 1989;14:947–952.
21. Potkin BN, Bartorelli AL, Gessert JM, et al. Coronary artery imaging with intravascular high-frequency ultrasound. Circulation 1990;81:1575–1585.
22. Nissen SE, Gurley JC, Grines CL, et al. Intravascular ultrasound assessment of lumen size and wall morphology in normal subjects and coronary artery disease patients. Circulation 1991;84:1087–1099.
23. Mallery JA, Tobis JM, Griffith J, et al. Assessment of normal and atherosclerotic arterial wall thickness with an intravascular imaging catheter. Am Heart J 1990; 119:1392–1400.
24. Velican D, Velican C. Comparative study on age related changes and arteriosclerosis involvement of the coronary arteries of male and female subjects up to 40 years of age. Arteriosclerosis 1981;38:39–50.
25. Porter TR, Radio SJ, Anderson JA, Michels A. Composition of coronary atherosclerotic plaque in the intima and media affects intravascular ultrasound measurements of intimal thickness. J Am Coll Cardiol 1994;23:1079–1084.
26. Sheikh KH, Harrison JK, Harding MB, et al. Detection of angiographically silent coronary artery disease by intravascular ultrasonography. Am Heart J 1991;121: 1803–1807.
27. Porter TR, Sears T, Xie F, et al. Intravascular ultrasound study of angiographically mildly diseased coronary arteries. J Am Coll Cardiol 1993;22:1858–1865.
28. Hausmann D, Lundkvist JS, Friedrich G, et al. Lumen and plaque shape in atherosclerotic coronary arteries assessed by in vivo intravascular ultrasound. Am J Cardiol 1994;74:857–863.
29. De Franco AC, Tuzcu EM, Moliterno DJ, et al. "Directional" coronary atherectomy removes atheroma more effectively from concentric than eccentric lesions: intravascular ultrasound predictors of lesional success. J Am Coll Cardiol 1995; Special Issue:137A.
30. Tobis JM, Mallery J, Mahon D, et al. Intravascular ultrasound imaging of human coronary arteries in vivo. Analysis of tissue characterization with comparison to in-vitro histological specimens. Circulation 1991;83:913–926.
31. Fitzgerald PJ, Ports TA, Yock PG. Contribution of localized calcium deposits to dissection after angioplasty in vivo assessed by intravascular ultrasound imaging. Circulation 1992;86:64–70.
32. De Franco AC, Nissen S, Tuzcu E, et al. Ultrasound plaque morphology predicts major dissections following stand-alone and adjunctive balloon angioplasty. Circulation 1994;90:I–50. Abstract.
33. Hinohara T, Robertson GC, Simpson JB. Directional coronary atherectomy. In: Topol EJ, ed. Textbook of interventional cardiology. 2nd ed. Philadelphia: WB Saunders, 1994:641–658.
34. Betrand ME, Bauters C, Lablanche JM. Percutaneous coronary rotational angioplasty with rotablator. In: Topol EJ, ed. Textbook of interventional cardiology. 2nd ed. Philadelphia: WB Saunders, 1994:659–667.
35. Tuzcu EM, Berkalp B, De Franco AC, et al. The dilemma of diagnosing coronary calcification: angiography vs. intravascular ultrasound. J Am Coll Cardiol 1996;27: 832–838.
36. Mintz GS, Douek P, Pichard AD, et al. Target lesion calcification in coronary artery disease: an intravascular ultrasound study. J Am Coll Cardiol 1992;20:1149–1155.
37. De Franco AC, Tuzcu EM, Eaton G, et al. Detection of unrecognized LMCA disease by intravascular ultrasound in patients undergoing interventions: prevalence and severity. Circulation 1993;88:I-411A.
38. Gerber TE, Erbel R, Gorge G, et al. Extent of atherosclerosis and remodeling of the left main coronary artery determined by intravascular ultrasound. Am J Cardiol 1994;73:666–671.

39. Ge J, Erbel R, Rupprecht HJ, et al. Comparison of intravascular ultrasound and angiography in the assessment of myocardial bridging. Circulation 1994;89: 1725–1732.

40. Goodhart DM, Nissen SE, DeFranco AC, et al. Diagnosis of angiographically elusive left main and ostial left anterior descending lesions by intravascular ultrasound. Circulation 1994;90:I-450A.

41. Elliott JM, Tuzcu EM, De Franco AC, et al. The left main diameter ratio: a specific index of left main coronary artery disease as validated by intravascular ultrasound. In press.

42. Roubin GS, Douglas JS Jr, King SB III, et al. Influence of balloon size on initial success, acute complications, and restenosis after percutaneous transluminal coronary angioplasty. A prospective randomized study. Circulation 1988;78:557–565.

43. Hodgson J McB, Stone GW, St. Goar FG, et al. Can intravascular ultrasound improve percutaneous transluminal coronary angioplasty results? Preliminary Core Lab Ultrasound analysis from the CLOUT pilot study. J Am Coll Cardiol 1995; 25:143A.

44. Tobis JM, Mahon DJ, Moriuchi M, et al. Intravascular ultrasound imaging following balloon angioplasty. Int J Cardiol Imaging 1991;6:191–205.

45. Yock PG, Fitzgerald PJ, Linker DT, Angelsen BAJ. Intravascular ultrasound guidance for catheter-based coronary interventions. J Am Coll Cardiol 1991;17:39B–45B.

46. Honye J, Mahon DJ, White CJ, et al. Morphological effects of coronary balloon angioplasty in vivo assessed by intravascular ultrasound imaging. Circulation 1992; 85:1012–1025.

47. Hodgson JMcB, Reddy KG, Suneja R, et al. Intravascular ultrasound imaging: correlation of plaque morphology with angiography, clinical syndrome and procedural results in patients undergoing coronary angioplasty. J Am Coll Cardiol 1993;21: 35–44.

48. Pasterkamp G, Borst C, Gussenhoven EJ, et al. Remodeling of de novo atherosclerotic lesions in femoral arteries: impact of mechanism of balloon angioplasty. J Am Coll Cardiol 1995;26:422–428.

49. Mintz GS, Pichard AD, Satler LF, et al. Intravascular ultrasound predictors of angiographic restenosis. Circulation 1994;90:I-163A.

50. The GUIDE Trial Investigators. Intravascular ultrasound-determined predictors of restenosis in percutaneous transluminal coronary angioplasty and directional coronary atherectomy: an interim report from the GUIDE Trial, Phase II. Circulation 1994;90:4:I-23A.

51. Peters RJG, for the PICTURE study group. Prediction of risk of angiographic restenosis by intravascular ultrasound imaging after coronary balloon angioplasty. J Am Coll Cardiol 1995;25:35A.

52. Tenaglia AN, Buller CE, Kisslo BK, et al. Mechanisms of balloon angioplasty and directional coronary atherectomy as assessed by intracoronary ultrasound. J Am Coll Cardiol 1992;20:685–691.

53. Suarez de Lezo J, Romero M, Medina A, et al. Intracoronary ultrasound assessment of directional coronary atherectomy immediate and follow-up findings. J Am Coll Cardiol 1993;21:298–307.

54. Popma JJ, Mintz GS, Satler LF, et al. Clinical and angiographic outcome after directional coronary atherectomy: a qualitative and quantitative analysis using coronary arteriography and intravascular ultrasound. Am J Cardiol 1993;72:55E–64E.

55. Mintz GS, Pichard AD, Kovach JA, et al. Impact of preintervention intravascular ultrasound imaging on transcatheter treatment strategies in coronary artery disease. Am J Cardiol 1994;73:423–430.

56. Bauman RP, Morris KG, Krucoff MW, et al. Maximizing plaque removal with directional coronary atherectomy: a new method using ultrasound guidance. J Am Coll Cardiol 1994;23:386A.

57. Berkalp B, Nissen SE, DeFranco AC, et al. Intravascular ultrasound demonstrates

marked differences in surface and lumen shape following interventional devices. Circulation 1994;90:I-58A.

58. Kovach JA, Mintz GS, Pichard AD, et al. Sequential intravascular ultrasound characterization of the mechanisms of rotational atherectomy and adjunct balloon angioplasty. J Am Cardiol 1993;22:1024–1032.

59. Tuzcu EM, De Franco AC, Moliterno DJ, et al. Rotational ablation produces comparable luminal gain and plaque removal in both calcified and non-calcified coronary lesions: evidence from intravascular ultrasound. Eur Heart J 1995;16:429A.

60. Fischman DL, Leon MB, Baim DS, et al, for the Stent Restenosis Study Investigators. A randomized comparison of coronary-stent placement and balloon angioplasty in the treatment of coronary artery disease. N Engl J Med 1994;331:496–501.

61. Serruys PW, de Jaegere P, Kiemaneij F, et al. A comparison of balloon-expandable stent implantation with balloon angioplasty in patients with coronary artery disease. N Engl J Med 1994;331:489–495.

62. Serruys PW, Di Mario C. Who was thrombogenic: the stent or the doctor? Circulation 1995;91:1891–1893.

63. Nakamura S, Colombo A, Gaglione A, et al. Intracoronary ultrasound observations during stent implantation. Circulation 1994;89:2026–2034.

64. Goldberg SL, Colombo A, Nakamura S, et al. Benefit of intracoronary ultrasound in the deployment of Palmaz-Schatz stents. J Am Coll Cardiol 1994;24:996–1003.

65. Colombo A, Hall P, Nakamura S, et al. Intracoronary stenting without anticoagulation accomplished with intravascular ultrasound guidance. Circulation 1995;91:1676–1688.

66. Kaye MP. The registry of the International Society for Heart and Lung Transplantation: tenth official report: 1993. J Heart Lung Transplant 1993;12:541–548.

67. Bourge RC, Naftel DC, Constanzo-Nordin MR, et al, for the Transplant Cardiologists Research Database Group. Pretransplantation risk factors for death after heart transplantation: a multi-institutional study. J Heart Lung Transplant 1993;12:549–562.

68. Olivari MT, Homans DC, Wilson RF, et al. Coronary artery disease in cardiac transplant patients receiving triple drug immunosuppressive therapy. Circulation 1989;80:III-111–III-115.

69. Uretsky BF, Kormos RL, Zerbe TR, et al. Cardiac events after heart transplantation: incidence and predictive value of coronary arteriography. J Heart Lung Transplant 1992;11:S45–S51.

70. Dressler FA, Miller LW. Necropsy versus angiography: how accurate is angiography? J Heart Lung Transplant 1992;11(part 2):S56–S59.

71. St. Goar FG, Pinto FJ, Alderman EL, et al. Detection of coronary arteriosclerosis in young adult hearts using intravascular ultrasound. Circulation 1992;86:756–763.

72. St. Goar FG, Pinto FJ, Alderman EL, et al. Intracoronary ultrasound in cardiac transplant recipients. In vivo evidence of "angiographically silent" intimal thickening. Circulation 1992;85:979–987.

73. Tuzcu EM, Hobbs RE, Rincon G, et al. Occult and frequent transmission of atherosclerotic coronary disease with cardiac transplantation: insights from intravascular ultrasound. Circulation 1995;91:1706–1713.

74. Tuzcu EM, De Franco AC, Goormastic M, et al. Dichotomous pattern of coronary atherosclerosis 1 to 9 years after transplantation: insights from systematic intravascular ultrasound imaging. J Am Coll Cardiol 1996;27:839–846.

20

FUNCTIONAL ANGIOMETRY

Richard G. Bach

I SCHEMIC CARDIAC SYNDROMES are the result of varying degrees of impairment of coronary blood flow by fixed or dynamic coronary artery obstructions. Coronary angiography is currently the standard by which physicians routinely determine the severity of obstructive coronary disease. Despite the introduction of computer-assisted digital analysis, however, the functional significance of coronary artery disease is often inadequately diagnosed by solely the anatomic information provided by coronary angiography, especially with respect to stenoses of intermediate severity and the complex lesions that result from percutaneous coronary intervention. *Functional angiometry* is a term coined to describe technology that has recently been developed for the translesional measurement of coronary blood flow, and that has been applied for the functional characterization of coronary pathophysiology. Specifically, these techniques, involving a practical means for assessment of coronary blood flow velocity by a Doppler-tipped angioplasty guidewire, have advanced our understanding of normal and abnormal coronary physiology, especially in patients with coronary artery disease. The clinical application of coronary flow velocity measurements using the Doppler flow wire during cardiac catheterization represents a promising means for providing immediate physiologic assessment of coronary artery lesion significance. Recent correlations with translesional hemodynamics and noninvasive stress perfusion imaging have confirmed the accuracy and reliability of Doppler translesional flow velocity assessment.

Use of intracoronary flow velocity for functional assessment can refine the selection of cases for revascularization. Translesional and distal coronary flow velocity dynamics during interventional procedures provide immediate data regarding the physiologic adequacy of intervention.

Appreciation of the advances provided by this technology, and of its potential applications, requires review of the physiology of coronary blood flow, the theory behind intravascular Doppler, and the limitations of currently utilized diagnostic modalities for coronary artery disease, especially coronary angiography.

Coronary Blood Flow: General Principles

In comparison to flow within arteries supplying blood to skeletal muscles and other organs, the flow of blood within the coronary arteries represents a relatively unique physiologic circumstance. Like other vessels, coronary flow depends on driving pressure and vascular resistance. Coronary resistance, however, is determined not only by vascular tone but also by cyclic compression of intramyocardial vessels by contracting cardiac muscle. As a result, coronary blood flow has a characteristic phasic pattern, and unlike peripheral vessels, the majority of blood delivery occurs during diastole.

Coronary blood flow is tightly regulated in response to myocardial oxygen demand. For normal function, the myocardium relies almost exclusively on oxidative metabolism and must extract near-maximal levels of available oxygen from blood, even under resting conditions. Changes in myocardial oxygen demand, therefore, can be met only by proportionate changes in myocardial blood flow. The epicardial coronary arteries contribute slightly to coronary vascular resistance but serve primarily as conductance vessels. The predominant resistance to coronary flow arises from smaller intramyocardial arterioles (10–140 μm in diameter) beyond the resolution of coronary arteriography. Alterations in coronary blood flow delivery are thus achieved chiefly by changes in coronary arteriolar resistance. Adjustment of coronary resistance in response to variation in myocardial demand and the resultant maintenance of steady-state blood flow over a wide range of driving pressure are known as *coronary autoregulation*. Basal coronary resistance in normal vessels can be reduced, and coronary blood flow therefore increased, two- to fivefold by potent arteriolar vasodilators, indicating a substantial reserve capacity within the coronary circulation to deliver increased blood flow to the myocardium. This ability to increase flow in response to a stimulus has been termed the *coronary flow reserve* or *coronary vasodilator reserve,* and is numerically expressed as the ratio of hyperemic to basal flow.

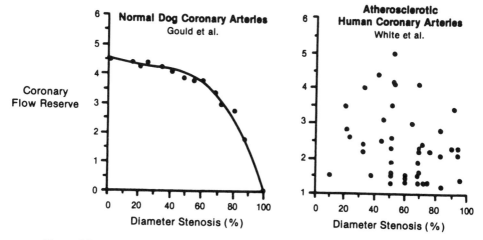

Figure 20-1   (Left panel) Illustration of the predictable relationship in experimental animals between increasing lesion severity expressed as percent diameter stenosis and reduction in coronary vasodilator reserve (original studies by Gould and colleagues). (Right panel) In patients assessed using proximally positioned 3-Fr Doppler catheters (original studies by White and colleagues), diameter stenosis shows poor correlation with impaired proximal coronary flow reserve. (Reproduced with permission of Marcus ML, Harrison DG, White CW, Hiratzka LF. Can J Cardiol 1986;2[suppl A]:195A.)

As a consequence of the autoregulatory capabilities of the coronary circulation, at least in patients without resting ischemia, coronary blood flow appears to remain at a fairly constant steady-state level over increasing degrees of epicardial coronary stenosis up to a critical level. Hyperemic coronary blood flow, however, becomes increasingly impaired in direct relation to stenosis severity above approximately 40% diameter narrowing. This has led to certain fundamental concepts: Levels of absolute resting blood flow are generally not sufficiently able to adequately discriminate the severity of coronary lesions, but coronary flow reserve, as a parameter normalizing maximal hyperemic flow to resting flow, can serve as a sensitive measure of the severity of coronary stenoses. In fact, in experimental animal models, impaired coronary flow reserve has been shown to correlate well with cross-sectional area reduction and physiologic severity of coronary stenoses (Fig 20-1, left panel). Notably, early studies of coronary flow reserve in patients with obstructive coronary artery disease showed a poor correlation with angiographic coronary stenosis, highlighting an inability to predict the degree of physiologic impairment due to a particular lesion from the geometric information provided by angiography (Fig 20-1, right panel).

Measurement of Coronary Blood Flow

Various methods have been developed to measure blood flow within the coronary arteries during cardiac catheterization, including coronary sinus thermodilution, contrast videodensitometry, and impedance catheter techniques. These techniques have substantial practical limitations. The application of Doppler theory to the measurement of blood flow velocity has represented a significant technical advance. Doppler technology was developed based on a theory originally derived in the mid-nineteenth-century. Christian Johann Doppler made the observation that sound frequency changes as a transmitter moves toward or away from a receiver, and that the change in frequency is related to the transmitter velocity. Applying this theory by constructing catheters with miniaturized transducers (piezoelectric crystals) that emit and receive high-frequency sound waves has allowed measurement of the velocity of RBC flowing within an instrumented artery. Velocity is calculated from the Doppler frequency shift by the equation

$$V = \frac{(f_1 - f_0)\ (C)}{(2\,f_0)\ (\cos\theta)}$$

where V = velocity of blood flow, f_0 = transmitting frequency, f_1 = returning frequency, C = speed of sound in blood (constant), and θ = angle of incidence. To yield velocity quantitation, Doppler signals are analyzed by one of two methods: zero-crossing frequency analysis and fast Fourier transform spectral analysis. Although the details of these methods are beyond the scope of this discussion, recent comparative studies have suggested an improvement in sensitivity and accuracy using spectral analysis, which produces a gray-scale display of all RBC velocities within the sample volume and which yields an output accurately representing the phasic components of blood flow velocity in real time.

Intracoronary Doppler has advantages over other techniques for assessing coronary blood flow. Doppler velocimeters directly measure the velocity of RBC, so that indicator-dilution markers or indirect contrast-based methods are not required. Changes in blood flow velocity will accordingly alter quantitatively the Doppler frequency shift, allowing quantitation of absolute velocities and instantaneous detection of changes in these velocities. Subselective catheter insertion in epicardial vessels permits individual lesion, vessel, or region assessment. Digitized spectral analysis allows accurate quantitative measurement not only of overall flow velocity, but also of the individual phasic components.

For comparative analyses within the coronary circulation, the measurement of blood flow velocity has advantages over the measurement of volumetric blood flow. The coronary tree represents a system of frequently branching conduit vessels (Fig 20-2). In branching arterial systems like the coronary arteries,

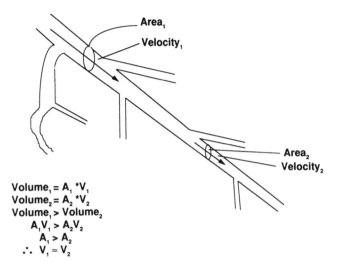

$$Volume_1 = A_1 \, {}^*V_1$$
$$Volume_2 = A_2 \, {}^*V_2$$
$$Volume_1 > Volume_2$$
$$A_1V_1 > A_2V_2$$
$$A_1 > A_2$$
$$\therefore \; V_1 \approx V_2$$

Figure 20-2 Diagram of coronary artery illustrating that coronary arteries normally branch frequently and taper, that volumetric flow is proportional to velocity and cross-sectional area, and that as vessels taper, both cross-sectional area and volumetric flow are reduced, whereas velocity is therefore relatively preserved. (Reproduced with permission from Kern MJ, Aguirre FV, Bach RG, et al. Translesional pressure-flow velocity assessment in patients: part I. Cathet Cardiovasc Diagn, 1994;31:49–60. Copyright © 1994 by Wiley-Liss, Inc.)

physiologic mechanisms produce, and tend to maintain, vessel size in proportion to the muscle mass subtended. Although volumetric flow and vessel cross-sectional area decrease from proximal to distal locations with branching, flow velocity remains relatively preserved, allowing better comparison of velocities than volume flows at different locations. Volumetric blood flow can nonetheless be calculated from vessel cross-sectional area and flow velocity with correction for the parabolic flow profile. If vessel cross-sectional area at the site of measurement remains constant, relative changes in flow velocity reliably represent relative changes in absolute coronary flow.

As originally developed, the application of Doppler ultrasound for intracoronary analysis of blood flow required the use of relatively large catheters (≥ 3 Fr) or nonselective angiographic catheters modified with tip-mounted transducers (Fig 20-3). Signals were typically processed by zero-crossing frequency analysis. Given their size and design, these catheters were limited to the very proximal coronary arteries, and they were somewhat difficult to incorporate into interventional procedures. Due to the significant diameter of the catheter in relation to coronary artery diameter, flow profile disturbance and potential flow obstruction in smaller arteries presented additional limitations. Likely due to their limitations, these catheter techniques were not widely adopted into clinical practice.

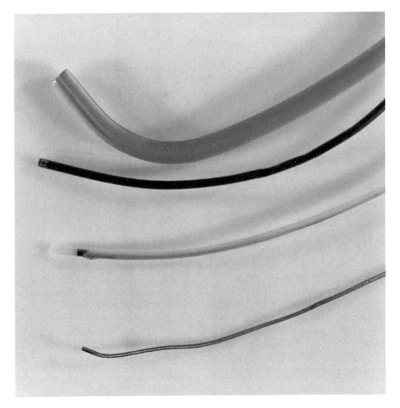

Figure 20-3   Comparison of Doppler catheters and guidewire. (From top to bottom): Judkins 8-Fr Doppler-tipped angiographic catheter (Cordis Corp., Miami, FL); Millar 3-Fr end-mounted Doppler catheter (Millar Instruments, Houston, TX); NuMed 3-Fr side-mounted Doppler catheter (NuMed, Hopkinton, NY); 0.018″ angioplasty-style Doppler guidewire (Cardiometrics, Inc., Mountain View, CA). (Reprinted by permission of the publisher from Ofili EO, Labovitz AJ, Kern MJ. Coronary flow velocity dynamics in normal and diseased arteries. Am J Cardiol 1993;71:3D–9D. Copyright © 1993 by Excerpta Medica Inc.)

The development of an angioplasty guidewire with a forward-directed Doppler crystal incorporated into the tip (FloWire, Cardiometrics, Inc., Mountain View, CA) has overcome many of the limitations of previous-generation devices. A comparison of available Doppler catheters and the Doppler guidewire is shown in Figure 20.3. Use of the Doppler wire has provided the first method by which *poststenotic* coronary blood flow can be practically and directly measured in the catheterization laboratory. In brief, the FloWire is a 175-cm-long, 0.018″- or 0.014″-diameter flexible, steerable guidewire with a piezoelectric ultrasound transducer integrated into the tip. Velocity signals are acquired from a sample volume diverging over a 27-degree arc 0.5 cm forward of the wire (Fig 20-4). Over the normal size range of coronary arteries, the Doppler signal interrogates the majority of the coronary flow profile. Velocity data are processed by on-line fast Fourier transformation and quantitative digitized analyses generated from a real-time scrolling spectral gray-scale display. The output allows quantitation of blood flow velocity and of the individual phasic components of flow velocity. An example of flow velocity signals acquired using the Doppler guidewire in a normal left anterior descending artery is shown in Figure 20-5. The most commonly employed velocity parameter is the time average of the digitized instantaneous spectral peak velocity, which is called the average peak velocity. The velocity integrals and diastolic-to-systolic velocity ratio, a measure of the normalcy of the phasic pattern of coronary blood flow, are also automatically quantitated. In conjunction with pharmacologic vasodilators, coronary hyperemic responses can also be quantified for determination of coronary flow reserve (Fig 20-6).

There are certain important advantages of functional angiometry employing the Doppler guidewire for practical assessment of coronary flow during cardiac catheterization. The Doppler wire can be used with any angioplasty balloon and can serve as a "workhorse" guidewire during percutaneous transluminal coronary angioplasty (PTCA), allowing easy incorporation of physiologic data into interventional procedures. During routine PTCA, we have found the Doppler guidewire effective as a primary wire in more than 85% of attempts. Like other angioplasty guidewires, the Doppler wire has a soft, flexible tip that is unlikely to cause arterial injury during use. The wire tip can be shaped and steered selectively into almost any branch of the epicardial coronary tree. A 0.018"-diameter guidewire has a cross-sectional area of 0.16 mm^2, which is less than 25% of the cross-sectional area of a 1-mm vessel. The wire thus provides access to flow measurements in the relevant poststenotic zone, and yet avoids the potential problem of catheter-induced flow disturbance in most large or small coronary arteries.

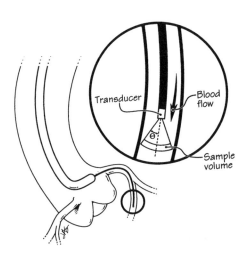

Figure 20-4 Illustration of a Doppler guidewire positioned in the proximal coronary artery with the transducer beam parallel with blood flow. The beam spread angle of incidence is approximately 27 degrees; the range gate, 0.5 cm; and the sample volume thickness, 1.2 mm. Reprinted with permission from the American College of Cardiology (Ofili EO, Kern MJ, Labovitz AJ, et al. J Am Coll Cardiol 1993, 21:308–316).

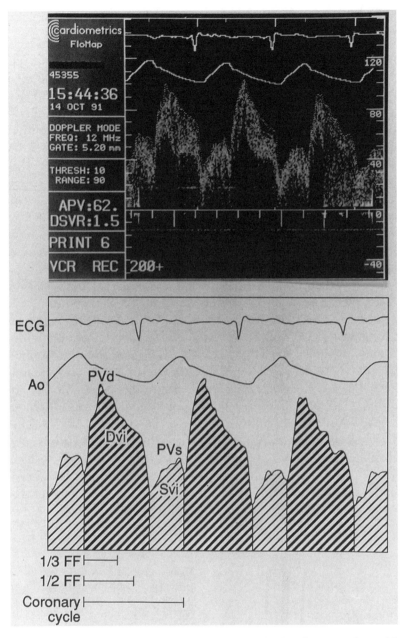

Figure 20-5 Coronary flow velocity spectra acquired with a Doppler guide-wire from a normal left anterior descending artery demonstrating smaller systolic and larger diastolic velocity components. A dotted line is visible that is continuously tracking the instantaneous peak velocity, from which the average peak velocity (APV) over the cardiac cycle is digitally generated. The schematic diagram of digitized spectral profiles below shows derivation of the diastolic velocity integral (Dvi, dark hatching), the systolic velocity integral (Svi, light hatching), and peak diastolic (PVd) and peak systolic (Pvs) velocities. Ao, aortic pressure; DSVR, diastolic-to-systolic velocity ratio. Reprinted with permission from the American College of Cardiology (Ofili EO, Kern MJ, Labovitz AJ, et al. J Am Coll Cardiol 1993, 21, 308–316).

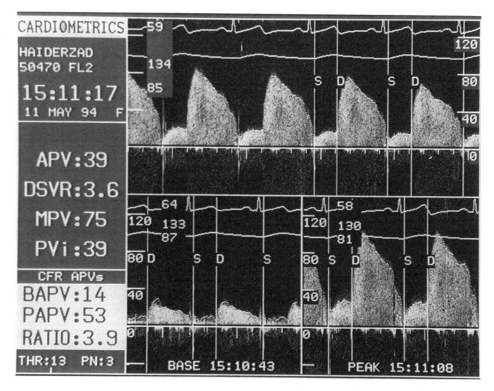

Figure 20-6 Spectral Doppler flow velocity recordings obtained using a Doppler guidewire from the normal proximal left anterior descending artery of a 45-year-old man with atypical chest pain, recorded at baseline (lower left panel) and at peak hyperemia induced by intracoronary adenosine (lower right panel); the upper panel shows the flow velocity spectra scrolling in realtime. Near the top of each panel, the ECG, arterial pressure waveform, heart rate, and systolic and diastolic BPs are simultaneously displayed. The velocity scale in centimeters per second is shown at the left or right of each panel, and continuously updated, digitally analyzed values for average peak velocity (APV), diastolic-to-systolic velocity ratio (DSVR), maximal peak velocity (MPV), peak velocity integral (PVi), and ratio of base to hyperemic APV (ratio or CFR) are shown to the far left. S and D demarcate timing of systole and diastole. Note the normal diastolic-predominant phasic flow velocity pattern and the normal CFR with a 3.9-fold increase in APV during peak hyperemia. (Reproduced with permission from Bach RG, Donohue TJ, Kern MJ. Intracoronary Doppler flow velocity measurements for the evaluation and treatment of coronary artery disease. Curr Opin Cardiol 1995;10:434–442. Copyright © by Rapid Science Publishers.)

Table 20-1   Clinical Applications of Functional Angiometry:

Intermediate (40%–70% diameter stenosis) lesion assessment
   Coronary angioplasty
   Objective data of pre-intervention distal flow impairment
   Documenting physiologic improvement after PTCA (target endpoints)
   Diagnosing inadequate or unstable PTCA result
   Managing PTCA complications
   Assessing additional lesions for multivessel PTCA
   Coronary flow reserve assessment
   Syndrome X
   Microvascular dysfunction

Potential Applications of Functional Angiometry

Functional angiometry has several clinical applications that have the potential to improve the diagnostic and therapeutic capabilities of the cardiac catheterization laboratory. These are summarized in Table 20-1. Two of these uses—the application of transstenotic flow velocity measurements to better assess coronary lesions of intermediate or indeterminate angiographic severity, and the application of poststenotic flow velocity measurements to apply physiologic criteria to percutaneous coronary intervention—represent significant advances provided specifically by the Doppler guidewire.

Physiologic Assessment of Stenosis Severity

Angiography has significant limitations for assessing the functional significance of coronary stenoses, especially with respect to stenoses falling within an intermediate severity range ($\sim$ 40%–70% diameter stenosis), where interpretation is subject to very high interobserver variability. Computer-assisted quantitative coronary angiography was developed to overcome many of the limitations of visual interpretation and incorporate algorithms to estimate the hemodynamic and flow consequences of lesions from their anatomic or geometric features. Nevertheless, quantitative angiographic techniques suffer from their own variability, and comparisons of quantitative coronary angiography–derived hemodynamic parameters and directly measured translesional hemodynamic and flow velocity variables in patients in our laboratory have demonstrated a poor correlation.

During diagnostic catheterization, or prior to intervention, the Doppler guidewire may be utilized to interrogate translesional flow dynamics to determine the physiologic significance of a coronary stenosis. This use may be particularly helpful in cases of multivessel disease or when objective evidence of regional ischemia from stress perfusion imaging or stress echocardiography is not available. Heparin (5000–10,000 units) is administered and the wire is introduced through a standard Y-connector. Flow velocity spectra are acquired in the coronary artery proximal to the stenosis (proximal enough to avoid flow acceleration due to the narrowing) and distal to the stenosis (at least 5–10 artery diameters distal to the stenosis to allow recovery of stable steady-state flow). During flow velocity measurements, maximal hyperemic flow can be generated in response to pharmacologic vasodilators such as papaverine, dipyridamole, or adenosine to assess the increase in flow velocity over basal flow and thereby derive the coronary flow reserve. In our laboratory, maximal hyperemia is most conveniently and safely induced using an intracoronary bolus injection of adenosine at doses (8–12 μg for the right and 12–24 μg for the left coronary artery) that do not induce heart block and that have an extremely rapid onset (<10 sec) and short duration of action (30–45 sec). When flow velocity data confirm a flow-limiting stenosis, PTCA may proceed without interruption, using the flowire as a guidewire. When utilized during diagnostic angiography, the finding of normal translesional flow dynamics may allow deferral of further noninvasive testing or consideration of revascularization.

By allowing interrogation of translesional and poststenotic coronary blood flow velocity, the Doppler guidewire can provide an objective assessment of the physiologic significance of coronary stenoses. Three parameters have thus far been defined that have relevance to the clinical evaluation of a particular coronary stenosis: (1) an impairment of maximal hyperemic flow expressed in the *poststenotic coronary flow reserve;* (2) an impairment of resting flow velocity across the stenosis, expressed in the translesional flow velocity *proximal-to-distal (P/D) ratio;* and (3) an impairment of the normal phasic pattern of flow velocity expressed in the poststenotic *diastolic-to-systolic velocity ratio.*

Poststenotic Coronary Flow Reserve

As a result of the autoregulatory capabilities of myocardial resistance vessels, resting coronary blood flow is kept at a fairly constant level to meet myocardial demands despite increasing degrees of epicardial obstruction (up to some critical level), but maximal hyperemic flow is increasingly impaired in relation to increasing severity for stenoses of greater than approximately 40% diameter lumen reduction. Although coronary flow reserve in the artery proximal to a severe stenosis may remain normal due to hyperemic flow to proximal branches, hyperemia in the distal artery will typically be impaired. Poststenotic coronary flow reserve thus measured with the Doppler guidewire serves as a sensitive index of lesion severity. In recent comparisons of pharmacologic stress tomographic perfusion imaging with both quantitative coronary angiography and coronary flow velocities in patients with intermediately severe coronary artery disease, the strongest correlation was found between an abnormal poststenotic coronary flow reserve by the Doppler wire (≤2.0) and the presence of reversible perfusion defects in the target perfusion zone. Both the sensitivity and specificity of flow wire–derived distal coronary flow reserve for predicting regional scintigraphic myocardial perfusion appear to be in the 85% to 95% range.

Proximal-to-Distal Velocity Ratio

An epicardial stenosis of sufficient hemodynamic severity to create significant resistance to flow in a branching coronary artery would theoretically reduce flow velocity in the poststenotic bed. Studies from our laboratory comparing translesional flow velocity parameters acquired with the flow wire and quantitative coronary angiography–derived severity indices with translesional pressure gradients during cardiac catheterization in patients with a wide range of coronary stenoses have shown that, as might be expected, absolute proximal or distal flow velocities are unable to differentiate stenosis severity. Normalization of resting poststenotic distal velocity to proximal velocity by generation of a P/D velocity ratio, however, generates a parameter that is relatively specific

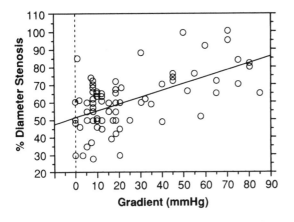

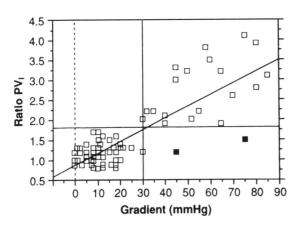

Figure 20-7 Linear regression analyses depicting relationships between translesional hemodynamics and percent diameter stenosis by (top panel) quantitative coronary angiography and (bottom panel) the ratio of P/D peak velocity integral obtained using the Doppler wire. Note the weak correlation ($r = 0.2$, $p = $ NS) between percent diameter stenosis and translesional gradient for intermediate (40%–70%) stenoses, while P/D velocity ratio of greater than 1.7 correlated highly (90%) with translesional gradients of greater than 30 mm Hg. Reprinted with permission from the American College of Cardiology (Donohue TJ, Kern MJ, Aguirre FV, et al. J Am Coll Cardiol 1993, 22, 449–458).

for critically severe lesions. Proximal-to-distal ratios at rest of greater than 1.7 are found with lesions having translesional pressure gradients of greater than 30 mm Hg, a finding that implies significant hemodynamic severity (Fig 20-7). In the subgroup of patients with intermediate stenoses, the correlation of translesional gradient and P/D ratio remains high ($r = 0.8, p < 0.001$), whereas the correlation between translesional gradient and quantitative coronary angiography–derived percent diameter stenosis is quite poor ($r = 0.2, p = NS$).

Diastolic/Systolic Velocity Ratio

As described, there is a typical phasic pattern to coronary blood flow. Due to the interaction of aortic driving pressure and intramyocardial compressive pressure, normal flow velocity spectra in the left coronary and left ventricular branches of the right coronary artery show a diastolic-predominant waveform, resulting in a normal diastolic-to-systolic velocity ratio of greater than 1.5. The phasic pattern of flow distal to an epicardial coronary narrowing depends on the relative contributions of stenotic resistance and intramyocardial resistance. In animal models, as an epicardial stenosis increases in severity to the point at which autoregulation is exhausted, viscous pressure losses across the stenosis become dominant and the distal phasic flow pattern becomes altered. Studies using Doppler flow wires during coronary angioplasty have demonstrated a reduction in diastolic-to-systolic velocity ratio distal to significant stenoses prior to intervention. In more than 50% of angiographically severe lesions studied, poststenotic phasic predominance was reversed, and the systolic velocity was higher than diastolic velocity. In response to successful PTCA, there was a return of the normal phasic pattern to distal flow velocity spectra and therefore normalization of the distal diastolic-to-systolic velocity ratio.

An example of the use of the Doppler guidewire for intermediate lesion assessment is shown in Figure 20-8. In this case, a 59-year-old man was referred to the catheterization laboratory for evaluation of chest pain after an equivocal radionuclide stress test. Angiography of the left anterior descending artery (Fig 20-8A) in left anterior oblique (LAO) projection demonstrated an eccentric proximal 80%-diameter stenosis, whereas in the right anterior oblique (RAO) view, the diameter stenosis appeared less than 50%. Figure 20-8B shows the measured translesional flow velocities (upper panels) and hemodynamics (lower panels) for this stenosis. The average peak velocity proximal to the stenosis measured 22 cm/sec and distal to the stenosis measured 26 cm/sec, yielding a P/D ratio close to 1.0. The distal spectral pattern was normal, with a diastolic-to-systolic velocity ratio of 1.7. Maximal hyperemia induced by intracoronary adenosine demonstrated a poststenotic coronary flow reserve of 2.5. These flow velocity measurements indicate this stenosis is not hemodynamically significant, a finding confirmed by the lack of any resting translesional pressure gradient.

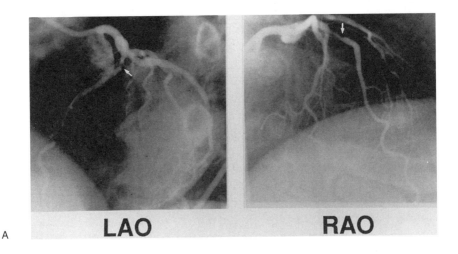

A

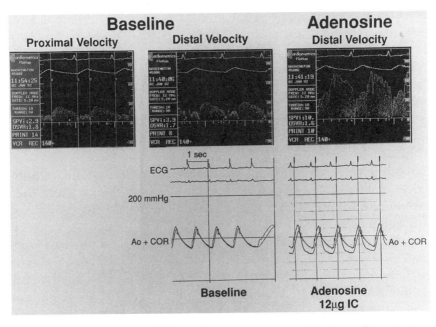

B

Figure 20-8 Translesional flow velocity assessment of intermediate steno-sis in a 59-year-old man with chest pain and equivocal radionuclide stress test, demonstrating absence of hemodynamic significance. (**A**) Cineangio-graphic frames of an eccentric stenosis in the proximal left anterior de-scending artery; LAO view shows less than 80%-diameter stenosis. In the RAO view, the diameter stenosis was less than 50%. (**B**) Flow velocity (upper panels) and translesional gradient measurements (lower panels). Proximal average peak velocity was 22 cm/sec, distal poststenotic velocity was 26 cm/sec, with a normal phasic pattern and diastolic-systolic velocity ratio (1.8). Hyperemia induced a 2.5-fold increase in poststenotic flow velocity. These findings corresponded to a translesional pressure gradient of 0 mm Hg at rest and 10 mm Hg at peak hyperemia. Ao, aorta; COR, coronary pres-sure; flow velocity scale, 0–140 cm/sec. Reprinted with permission from the American College of Cardiology (Donohue TJ, Kern MJ, Aguirre FV, et al. J Am Coll Cardiol 1993, 22, 449–458).

Limitations of Functional Angiometry for Lesion Assessment

There are recognized limitations to the use of these Doppler flow wire parameters for lesion assessment. Coronary flow reserve can be potentially affected by factors other than lesion severity, such as heart rate, BP, left ventricular hypertrophy, previous infarction, and anemia, which must be considered for correct interpretation of the data. Coronary flow velocity can be affected by all lesions within a vessel, and serial stenoses may complicate the interpretation of velocity measurements across any one site. Although an accurately measured abnormal P/D ratio alone may have high specificity for very significant stenoses (> 30 mm Hg resting gradient), this parameter can remain insensitive to functionally significant lesions with lower resting gradients. Accurate velocities proximal to the zone of acceleration may also be difficult to obtain for very proximal coronary lesions. The degree of proximal arterial branching also has a strong influence on the ability of P/D ratios to discriminate lesions, because non-branching conduits must maintain equivalent proximal and distal flow by the continuity equation. Vasoconstriction or angiographically inapparent luminal narrowing can accelerate resting flow velocity at a particular site, affecting comparisons with other sites. In proximal and mid-right coronary arteries, the P/D ratio may not be helpful in functional lesion assessment, potentially a result of the lack of significant branching typical for this portion of the right coronary artery. In addition, the diastolic-to-systolic velocity ratio of flow velocity in the proximal to mid-right coronary artery is typically less than 1.5, likely due to the lower systolic resistance in the right heart. This may limit the use of distal diastolic-to-systolic velocity ratio in discriminating lesion significance in those segments.

Although recognizing certain limits, the data provided by lesion assessment in the catheterization laboratory using the flow wire can serve as a reliable indicator of the functional significance of coronary stenoses. In patients presenting primarily for invasive evaluation, use of intracoronary flow velocity for assessment of the functional significance of coronary stenoses can provide immediate data regarding the flow-limiting characteristics of lesions and thereby aid in assessing the need for revascularization. This approach can potentially eliminate unnecessary interventional procedures and redundant noninvasive tests, as well as shorten hospital stays. Using flow wire assessment, we have encountered lesions that appear angiographically severe but are not flow limiting, lesions that are angiographically moderate but *are* flow limiting, and even lesions of equal angiographic severity in different arteries of the same patient that differ markedly in hemodynamic significance.

Doppler Flow Velocity During Coronary Interventions

Coronary intervention by angioplasty, atherectomy, or use of another catheter-based device frequently causes complex plaque disruption. It may be difficult to accurately judge the degree of residual lumen area reduction after intervention by angiography, which is relatively insensitive to intimal dissection and residual plaque burden. The Doppler guidewire provides an objective means of quantifying the functional improvement gained by a particular intervention, and can be easily integrated into the interventional procedure to provide continuous on-line assessment of the immediate physiologic consequences and the potential adequacy of intervention. Successful PTCA generally results in a significant increase in distal average peak velocity and improvement in the distal phasic flow pattern reflected in normalization of the diastolic-to-systolic velocity ratio. On guidewire pullback, the equivalence of flow velocity proximal and distal to the site of dilatation, with normalization of the proximal-to-distal mean

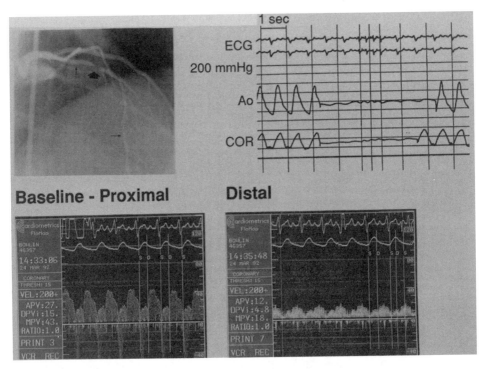

Figure 20-9   **(A)** Pre-intervention findings in a 56-year-old woman with severe unstable angina. Upper left panel shows RAO view of left coronary angiogram showing (large arrow) mid left anterior descending artery stenosis. Small arrows mark sites of proximal and distal pressure and flow recordings. Upper right panel shows translesional pressure gradient of 80 mm Hg. Lower panels show coronary flow velocity spectra recorded at proximal and distal sites using Doppler guidewire, with diminished flow velocity distal to stenosis. Abbreviations as in Figures 20-5, 20-6 and 20-8. (Reproduced with permission from Bach RG, Kern MJ, Bell C, et al. Clinical application of coronary flow velocity for stent placement during coronary angioplasty. Am Heart J 1993;125:873–877.)

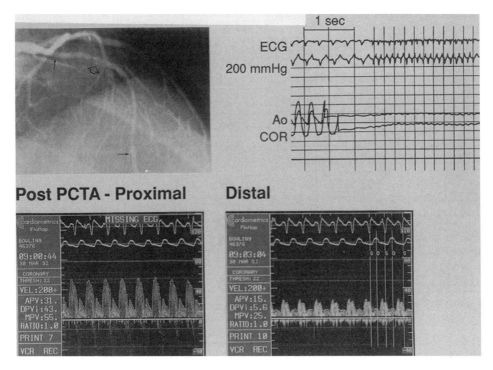

Figure 20-9 (B) Follow-up findings 6 days after PTCA with return of angina. Right anterior oblique cineangiogram (upper left), where open arrow shows site of PTCA in mid left anterior descending artery with intermediate stenosis and visible dissection. Translesional gradient (upper right) is 20 mm Hg. Coronary flow velocity spectra (lower panels) recorded proximal and distal to the site of dissection, showing diminished flow signal distal to intimal flap (P/D ratio ≥ 2), suggesting significant flow impairment by the lesion. (Reproduced with permission from Bach RG, Kern MJ, Bell C, et al. Clinical application of coronary flow velocity for stent placement during coronary angioplasty. Am Heart J 1993;125:873–877.)

velocity ratio (<1.7), can be ascertained. Failure to document sufficient improvement in distal velocity, phasic flow pattern, and P/D ratio may indicate suboptimal PTCA results and prompt further intervention. The reestablishment of normal coronary flow reserve (>2.0) is more variable in the immediate post-intervention period, although when present, may provide a strong indicator of physiologic improvement.

An example where translesional flow velocity measurements were helpful in the assessment of the flow-limiting consequences of complex coronary dissections complicating angioplasty is shown in Figures 20-9a–c. In this case, a 56-year-old woman underwent PTCA of a mid-left anterior descending artery stenosis. Initial flow velocity measurements prior to intervention (Fig 20-9a) showed findings compatible with a severe lesion, with a diminished resting

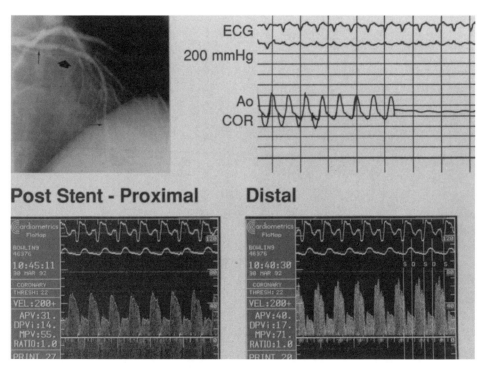

Figure 20-9   (**C**) Repeat cineangiogram (upper left), translesional gradient (upper right) and flow velocity recordings (lower panels) following stent placement in mid left anterior descending artery. Transstent pressure measurement shows no gradient. Intracoronary flow velocity spectra proximal and distal to stent show preserved distal flow signal, indicating relief of stenosis by stent. (Reproduced with permission from Bach RG, Kern MJ, Bell C, et al. Clinical application of coronary flow velocity for stent placement during coronary angioplasty. Am Heart J 1993;125:873–877.)

distal velocity (P/D ratio = 2.3) and an abnormal phasic pattern (diastolic-to-systolic velocity ratio < 1.5) associated with an 80-mm Hg translesional gradient. Following prolonged balloon dilatations, there remained a linear lucency suggestive of moderate dissection at the site, although the angiographic results appeared adequate, with brisk angiographic distal filling and 30% residual stenosis. Despite angiographic patency, repeat Doppler flow velocity measurements (Fig 20-9b) showed impaired distal flow, with a P/D ratio greater than 2.0 and reduced diastolic velocity compared with proximal spectra. The translesional gradient was 20 mm Hg. Deployment of a 2.5-mm stent at the site of dissection resulted in abolition of the gradient and complete normalization of the distal flow velocity (Fig 20-9c).

Use of the flow wire for continuous distal flow velocity monitoring during the immediate postintervention period can also allow identification of patterns of the coronary flow velocity trend over time that are unstable and associated

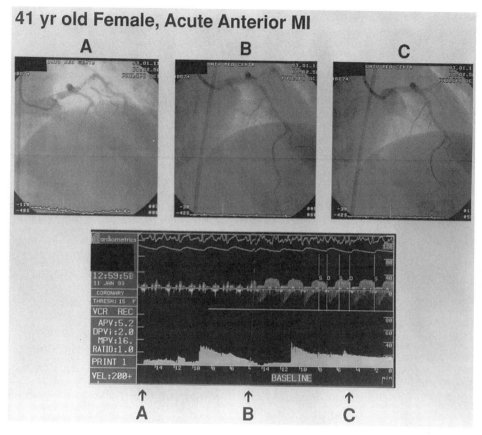

Figure 20-10 Cineangiographic frames (upper panels) of a 41-year-old woman during direct PTCA of totally occluded mid left anterior descending artery (LAD) for acute myocardial infarction (MI). Panels show (A) LAD before PTCA, (B) after first balloon dilatation, and (C) after final dilatation. The trend of average peak flow velocity (composite of continuous 15-min intervals) is shown on the lower panel and divided into phasic flow velocity spectra (upper half) and the trend plot (lower half); the velocity scale in centimeters per second is shown to the far right. Locations A, B, and C correspond to angiographic frames in the upper panel. Note initial guidewire advancement distal to occlusion detects flow velocity near zero (A); after first dilatation, hyperemia is observed, but flow velocity declines toward zero (B), predicting vessel occlusion. After final dilatation, flow velocity is stabilized (C) and vessel patency maintained. (Reproduced with permission from Kern MJ, Aguirre FV, Donohue TJ, et al. Coronary flow velocity monitoring after angioplasty associated with abrupt reocclusion. Am Heart J 1994;127:436–438).

with impending occlusion or inadequate results. These include cyclic flow variations, steadily declining average peak velocity, and abrupt cessation of flow. Figure 20-10 depicts findings from a 41-year-old woman during direct PTCA for an acute anterior myocardial infarction due to total mid-left anterior descending artery occlusion. Cineangiographic frames in the upper panels show the left anterior descending artery before PTCA (A), after the initial balloon inflation (B), and after the final inflation (C). The lower panel shows a composite trend plot covering an approximate 28-minute period during PTCA. Immediately following guidewire advancement across the occlusion into the distal vessel (point A), flow velocity near zero was recorded. After the first balloon dilatation, vessel patency was achieved and hyperemia was observed, but this was quickly followed by a declining flow velocity trend not reflected by any significant changes on angiography (point B). The declining flow predicted impending abrupt reocclusion (flow velocity falling to zero), which then responded to repeat balloon dilatation. Following the second dilatation, flow velocity stabilized for more than 10 minutes (point C), and vessel patency was maintained.

Topics of Angiometry Research

From ongoing research it appears that functional angiometry shows promise as well for other clinical applications. The flow wire can detect the velocity of collateral blood flow distal to coronary occlusions, critical stenoses, and inflated angioplasty balloons. Direct, quantitative measures of collateral blood flow in patients have not previously been possible. This application may yield exciting information previously unavailable regarding dynamic collateral physiology.

The assessment of coronary flow velocity as a quantitative means for determining the adequacy of reperfusion in patients following thrombolysis or intervention for acute myocardial infarction also represents a topic of considerable current interest. The analysis of distal flow velocity during direct or rescue intervention for acute myocardial infarction will allow correlation of quantitative measures of infarct-related artery blood flow and clinical outcome. From previous semiquantitative angiographic analyses, acute Thrombolysis in Myocardial Infarction (TIMI) flow grades in the infarct-related artery can provide prognostic data after acute myocardial infarction. The prognosis has been found to differ substantially between patients with TIMI grades 0 to 2 flow versus those with TIMI 3 flow. Preliminary studies comparing angiographic flow rate with Doppler flow velocity have demonstrated that average peak velocity is significantly lower in arteries with TIMI grades 0 to 2 flow compared with arteries with TIMI 3 flow. By examining the potential correlation between directly measured flow velocities in the infarct-related artery obtained acutely and clinical outcomes, it is possible that clinically useful physiologic and prognostic information may be derived from a quantitative analysis of coronary blood flow during myocardial infarction.

Conclusion

Functional angiometry with intracoronary translesional flow velocity measurements using the Doppler flow wire during cardiac catheterization can provide immediate data regarding the physiologic significance of coronary stenoses. This should refine the selection of cases for revascularization. Translesional and distal coronary flow velocity dynamics during procedures also provide immediate data regarding the physiologic adequacy of intervention. The analysis of coronary blood flow using the Doppler guidewire thus may overcome many of the limitations of angiography and provide a more physiologic approach to coronary diagnosis and intervention.

SELECTED READINGS

Gould KL, Kirkeeide RL, Buchi M. Coronary flow reserve as a physiologic measure of stenosis severity. J Am Coll Cardiol 1990;15:459–472.

Doucette JW, Corl D, Payne H, et al. Validation of a Doppler guidewire for intravascular measurement of coronary artery flow velocity. Circulation 1992;85:1899–1911.

Donohue TJ, Kern MJ, Aguirre FV, et al. Assessing the hemodynamic significance of coronary artery stenoses: analysis of translesional pressure–flow velocity relationships in patients. J Am Coll Cardiol 1993;22:449–458.

Kern MJ, Anderson HV, eds. A symposium: the clinical applications of the intracoronary Doppler guidewire flow velocity in patients: understanding blood flow beyond the coronary stenosis. Am J Cardiol 1993;71:1D–86D.

Segal J, Kern MJ, Scott NA, et al. Alterations of phasic coronary artery flow velocity in humans during percutaneous coronary angioplasty. J Am Coll Cardiol 1992;20:276–286.

Ofili EO, Kern MJ, Labovitz AJ, et al. Analysis of coronary blood flow velocity dynamics in angiographically normal and stenosed arteries before and after endoluminal enlargement by angioplasty. J Am Coll Cardiol 1993;21:308–316.

Uren NG, Melin JA, De Bruyne B, et al. Relation between myocardial blood flow and the severity of coronary artery stenosis. N Engl J Med 1994;330:1782–1788.

Miller DD, Donohue TJ, Younis LT, et al. Correlation of pharmacologic ^{99m}Tc-sestamibi myocardial perfusion imaging with poststenotic coronary flow reserve in patients with angiographically intermediate coronary artery stenoses. Circulation 1994;89:2150–2160.

21

CORONARY ANGIOSCOPY

Barry F. Uretsky

ULTIPLE DIAGNOSTIC MODALITIES are currently available to interrogate the coronary artery. These include contrast angiography, ultrasound, computerized tomography, magnetic resonance, Doppler flow velocity, and vascular endoscopy (angioscopy). Of these modalities only angioscopy views the artery as our eyes might see it. The importance of coronary angioscopy, particularly its value in clinical cardiology, however, is largely unknown at present. Endoscopy of other organ systems, however, has become an important diagnostic tool. One need only look to what has been accomplished with endoscopy of the gastrointestinal tract to appreciate the possibilities for its use in the coronary circulation. Endoscopic diagnosis of gastric, small intestinal, and large intestinal pathology is considered the "standard of care." Similarly, fiberoptic bronchial endoscopy (bronchoscopy) and arthroscopy are used routinely for diagnosis and treatment. More recently, videoscopic techniques have been utilized to visualize structures as part of surgical procedures performed percutaneously.

Coronary angioscopy encounters certain problems not faced in the applications noted. The most obvious is the inability to view the vessel wall in the presence of flowing blood. In addition, the structures visualized (i.e., the coronary arteries) are typically 3 to 4 mm or less. The requisite small size of the angioscope limits the complexity of the lens system. At present, there is one clinically available vascular endoscope. This chapter reviews instrumentation, technique for use, and potential clinical applications.

Instrumentation

Angioscope Catheter

The available angioscope (Fig 21-1) (ImageCath, Baxter Corp., Irvine, CA) has a single lens at its distal end. The angioscope body is composed of optical fibers (approximately 3000) that carry the image to the camera. Each fiber (2 μm in diameter) has one picture element (pixel). In general, the greater the number of pixels present, the greater the image clarity. The flexibility of optical fibers is particularly important in coronary angioscopy because the catheter must be able to negotiate bends in the coronary tree. Optical fibers are arrayed identically at the proximal and distal ends to allow the camera to produce a spatial representation of the pixels. Surrounding the 3000 receiving fibers that return the pixellated elements to the camera are 14 somewhat larger optical fibers transmitting light down the catheter into the coronary artery. The lens field of view is 50 to 55 degrees in water. As a result of this relatively limited field of view, and the inability to steer the catheter, there are occasions when the current model may not "see" intravascular pathology.[1]

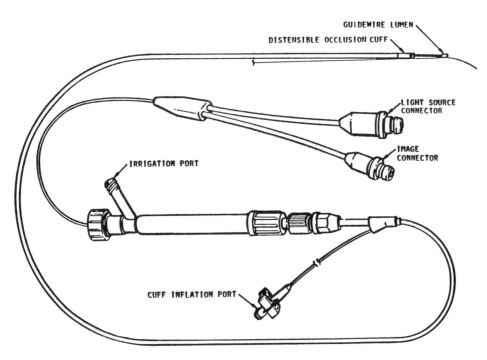

Figure 21-1 Diagram of currently used angioscope. (Courtesy of Baxter Corp., Irvine, CA.)

Guidewire Apparatus

The shaft of the angioscope is composed of the fibers as previously described. The catheter is 4.5 Fr in diameter at its largest point, which is at the catheter tip. In addition, there is a plastic sleeve of monorail design so that the catheter can be placed over a standard length (140-cm) percutaneous transluminal coronary angioplasty guidewire (0.014″) similar to a monorail angioplasty catheter. The distal end of the catheter employs a small, very compliant balloon to occlude blood flow and an irrigation system that provides infusion of warm saline or lactated Ringer's solution up to 30 ml/min. The most innovative aspect of the angioscope is the ability of the lens to travel approximately 6 cm along the guidewire while the balloon is inflated. This design provides the opportunity to visualize a long segment of the coronary artery in an over-the-wire method rather than by moving the relatively blunt tip of the angioscope itself.

External connections of the angioscope include a port for connection to the camera, a port for saline irrigation, and a port for the light source to be transmitted to the tip of the angioscope. The light source has a ratio of transmitted light from the source to light at the tip of the catheter of approximately 100:1. The light source uses a xenon arc lamp, which provides a "cold" white light.

Camera

The camera, a dedicated computerized instrument, translates the pixels to an image that can be taped on a standard VCR console and viewed on a standard television monitor. The camera utilized in the configuration of the presently available angioscope is an Optx 3000P camera (Baxter Corp., Irvine, CA), which has 300 horizontal and 300 vertical lines.

Angioscopic Technique

The current angioscope is relatively user-friendly. A complete angioscopic examination can be performed in less than 60 to 120 seconds. The catheter is prepared by calibrating the camera for colors by shining the catheter tip on a pure white surface. A 0.014″ guidewire, usually of 140 cm in length or 260 to 300 cm if an over-the-wire interventional catheter is to be performed, is inserted into the artery and distal to the lesion. The angioscopic catheter is flushed outside the patient using a power injector and is checked to ascertain that there are no leaks in the system. The connections to the light source and camera are secured and sealed in a sterile plastic bag to prevent contamination and maintain dryness of the electronic connections. The monorail system allows for insertion of the distal end without any other maneuvers except to pass it into the coronary artery. The patient is anticoagulated with 5000 to 10,000 units of heparin with an activated clotting time of greater than 300 seconds prior to catheter insertion. When the angioscope tip approaches the lesion (and distal to the left main coronary artery or the ostial right coronary artery), the highly compliant balloon is inflated and the warmed flush solution (usually lactated Ringer's) is infused up to 30 ml/min. The light source is adjusted so that image brightness level is optimized. The brightness level requires frequent modulation; as such, it is worthwhile for an assistant to be near this dial and adjust it accordingly. The angioscope is then passed to the lesion, and through the lesion on some occasions. There is not a consensus regarding the safety of passing the catheter across the lesion, but in our experience it has been complication-free. At present, still images are of limited quality because they are acquired on analog tape. As the capacity of computer memory increases, capturing and storing the images digitally will improve still-frame picture quality. Enhanced angioscopic images require analog-to-digital transfer. The tape frame chosen may be "enhanced" by accentuating borders and color differentiation. As such, these enhancements are not true reproductions of what the angioscopy sees but rather what the angioscopist thinks he sees and wants to reproduce in a static picture.

Evaluation of Coronary Lesions

Normal Vessel

The endoluminal surface of a normal vessel appears to be light gray to white, smooth, and without evidence of yellow (plaque) or red (thrombus) surface color.

Plaque

Subintimal plaquing may appear white, gray, or yellow. In addition to color, it is recognized by its bulging into the vessel separate from the guidewire. Angioscopy cannot, however, determine quantitatively the percent stenosis because optical distortion and inability to determine a reference size make quantitation not feasible at this time.

Thrombus

Thrombus (Fig 21-2) is well seen angioscopically. In fact, it is much more sensitive to the detection of thrombus than contrast angiography or intravascular ultrasound.[2-4] For large, obstructing thrombi angioscopically, an angiographic detection rate may be acceptable (50%–75%). For smaller or mural thrombi, however, the angioscope will detect such lesions whereas angiography typically will not (<30% observed angiographically). The clinical importance of

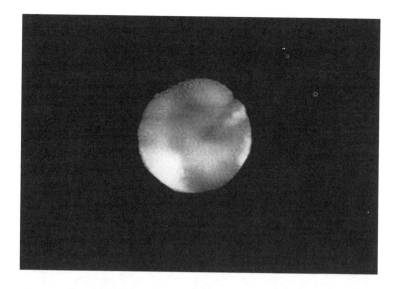

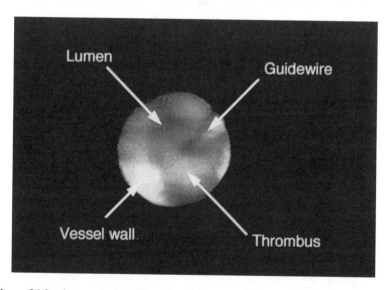

Figure 21-2   Appearance of intraluminal thrombus in unannotated and annotated photographs. Thrombus occupies the entire remaining lumen. The guidewire is at 3 o'clock. Note that the guidewire has perforated the center of the thrombus.

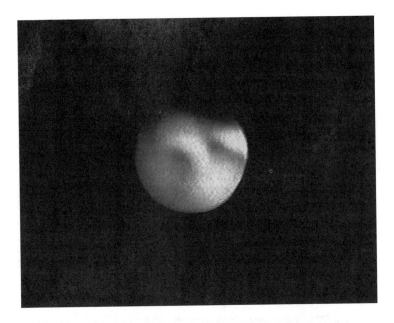

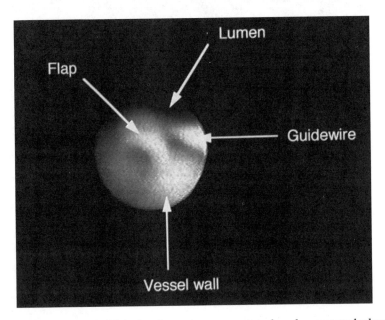

Figure 21-3   Superficial intimal tear in unannotated and annotated photographs is seen at 5 o'clock. Guidewire is at 2 o'clock.

detecting smaller thrombi is not clear at present but may represent a future strategy for improving short- and long-term interventional procedural success.

Intimal Flap

Breaks in the intima and protruding intimal flaps (Fig 21-3) are well seen angioscopically and are frequently the major element in angiographically "hazy" lesions. If, in fact, residual intimal flaps are predictive of abrupt closure, adverse short-term events, or restenosis after an interventional procedure, the angioscopy may have an important clinical use in this setting.

Collateral Blood Flow

When the vessel is occluded by means of the angioscope balloon, there are occasions when visualization is highly impaired to impossible because of retrograde filling of that arterial segment via collaterals.

Safety of Angioscopy

Angioscopic evaluation of the coronary vasculature has a good safety profile. Used correctly, it should not be associated with any deaths. There have been a few case reports of the guidewire's being entrapped by the monorail system in a knot-like structure, causing dissection and requiring emergency surgery. It should be emphasized that this instrument cannot be steered. If the operator tries to steer the wire with the angioscope in the coronary artery, the tip may become tangled, predisposing to dissection or even catheter impaction. The time of angioscopic evaluation is dictated in part by the patient's tolerance to discontinuation of antegrade coronary flow. Typically a 30- to 60-second examination can be performed before ischemia develops. The very proximal segment of the left anterior descending and circumflex arteries cannot be studied because it requires balloon occlusion of the left main artery. The learning curve for angioscopy is steep. Many centers, including our own, have had a very low (<1%) complication rate. Most adverse events are related to ischemia from prolonged occlusion of coronary flow.

Comparison with Intravascular Ultrasound

Intravascular ultrasound is a superb technique for looking at the walls of the coronary artery, (i.e., the "doughnut" itself) (see Chapter 19). Angioscopy is excellent for looking at the hole of the doughnut. Intravascular ultrasound provides information regarding the composition of plaque and the relative area of the vessel impinged upon by plaque. Angioscopy cannot evaluate these aspects of the coronary artery. On the other hand, angioscopy is particularly useful in characterizing the endoluminal surface, including the presence, quantity, and distribution of thrombus and the composition of angiographic filling defects. As such, one can envision both devices used together to interrogate a vessel. Based on angiographic studies, we have learned that certain forms of therapy are better treated by medicine, angioplasty, or surgery (see Chapter 16). Data from other interrogative techniques, such as intravascular ultrasound, Doppler ultrasound, and angioscopy, are currently in progress. Results of these studies will determine whether nonangiographic forms of vessel interrogation can either supplement or take the place of angiography as a medical decision-making test.

Lesion Nomenclature

There are several different nomenclatures for describing the findings of coronary angioscopy. These are attempts by investigators to have some common language regarding angioscopic observations. In terms of lesion description, it would be most useful to be able to quantitate the size of an intimal flap or clot. As previously noted, however, this is not feasible at present. On the other hand, one can classify it semiquantitatively based on the impingement of the residual lumen. For example, in a vessel that has a 90% angiographic or ultrasonographic lesion, the angioscope will be looking at only the 10% that is patent. That 10% in turn may be lined with large clots and a small lumen that can be seen angioscopically or an intimal plaque with no thrombus. The thrombus lesion itself may be classified by color as a red thrombus, a white thrombus, or a mixed (pink) thrombus. The white thrombus, presumed to be platelet-rich, is a particularly challenging entity. Some experienced angioscopists have not utilized this term, because they say a white thrombus cannot be discerned. Those investigators who have observed a white thrombus describe it as "cottony" or "fluffy."[3-5] The author believes he has seen a white thrombus, both alone and in association with a red thrombus.

Angioscopic Findings in Coronary Syndromes

Angioscopic findings have provided insight into the pathophysiology of coronary syndromes. Intra-operative and percutaneous angioscopy in patients with unstable angina pectoris undergoing bypass surgery has shown a high prevalence of thrombus.[5,6] It has been shown that diabetics have an even higher prevalence of thrombus-laden lesions with intimal tears, which may explain in part the finding of higher complication during interventional procedures and restenosis rates in the diabetic population.[7] In contrast, stable angina patients show a low incidence of intimal tears or thrombus. Patients with acute myocardial infarction have a very high incidence angioscopically of both red clot and intimal tears. These findings support the concept that unstable syndromes result from plaque disruption and secondary thrombus formation.

Potential Uses of Angioscopy

The absolute need for angioscopy for any clinical condition cannot be recommended unreservedly at the present time. There are, however, reasons to believe that angioscopy may be useful for the conditions described in this section.

Coronary Stenting

Coronary stenting has become a primary approach to coronary disease and may account for as much as 60% to 80% of all interventional cases in some laboratories. Intravascular ultrasound has been proposed as a method to determine apposition of the stent to the vessel wall. An alternative approach is angioscopic inspection. If stent struts are seen not to be flush with the vessel wall, one can surmise that the stent has not been adequately embedded into the vessel wall. Preliminary data in this regard have been reported, suggesting the utility of angioscopy in clinical decision making.[8]

Treatment of Unstable Angina

Unstable angina is characterized by both red and white thrombi as well as intimal flaps. It is probable that these abnormalities account in part for the relatively higher risk of adverse events in this patient group compared with patients with stable angina. Data suggest that an angioscopically present red thrombus postprocedure is predictive of acute adverse outcomes.[9]

Angiography is quite poor as compared with angioscopy in describing endoluminal morphologic abnormalities. Most treatment strategies and clinical trials to date have described angiographic parameters for prognosis and treatment strategies (see Chapter 16). Angioscopic findings may allow for a more precise treatment plan. As one example, angioscopy may define the role of therapy applied locally in patients with unstable syndromes who have an angioscopically detected thrombus. Angioscopy may aid in determining the best approach for angioscopically detected intimal dissections and/or white thrombi. Ongoing studies should help to elucidate these issues.

Prediction and Treatment of Abrupt Closure

Abrupt closure is usually an unpredictable event. It may be possible, however, to determine a "risk score" based on postprocedure angioscopy to predict the highest risk group for closure. We have found that patients who developed abrupt closure postangioplasty tended to have more angioscopically detected intimal disruption and mural thrombi than patients who did not develop abrupt closure.

Evaluation of an Intravascular Filling Defect

Angiography is poor in determining the contents of intravascular filling defects.[2–4] Because the treatments of thrombus, intimal dissections, and protruding plaque are different, angioscopy is able to identify the composition of the filling defects and thus guide therapeutic decisions.

Interventional Procedural Success

Interventional procedural success at present is defined using angiographic endpoints. Ultrasound studies have demonstrated that after angiographic procedural "success" with debulking devices such as directional or rotational atherectomy, a significant quantity of plaque remains. Likewise, it has been found angioscopically that with angiographic "success," postprocedure thrombi and moderate-to-large intimal flaps frequently remain.[2,3] Because it is the size of the hole of the doughnut that is important for procedural success, direct visualization of the vessel after angiographic success may provide information to determine whether further intervention is required to enlarge the lumen by stenting or eliminating tissue (intimal tears or protruding plaque) or clot within the hole.

Evaluation of Saphenous Vein Grafts

Angioscopy is ideal for studying saphenous vein grafts. The large size of the grafts allows for easy passage of the angioscope. If a therapeutic procedure is contemplated, angioscopy can define the nature of the lesion. The "cottage cheese" lesion that has been described in old degenerated vein grafts is very friable and prone to embolization. Old grafts also may contain friable clots, also prone to embolize. On the other hand, there are some vein graft lesions that may have only fibrotic lesions. Angioscopy may be useful in deciding on the therapeutic approach and response to therapy.

Conclusion

Angioscopy is a promising technique. As we learn more about the predictive nature of angioscopic findings, we may use this technique as a guide to therapy.[9] One can envision its use alongside a therapeutic modality, such that rather than depending on x-ray shadows, we will be able to directly see the lesion and intervene, utilizing angioscopy to optimize the result.

SELECTED READINGS

1. Uretsky BF, Denys BG, Ragosta M, Counihan P. Accuracy of angioscopy in diagnosing endoluminal lesions. Eur Heart J 1994;15:433.
2. Ramee S, White CJ, Collins TJ, et al. Percutaneous angioscopy during coronary angioplasty using a steerable microangioscope. J Am Coll Cardiol 1991;17:100–105.
3. Uretsky BF, Denys BG, Counihan PC, Ragosta M. Angioscopic evaluation of incompletely obstructing coronary intra-luminal filling defects: comparison to angiography. Cathet Cardiovasc Diagn 1994;33:323–329.
4. den Heijer P. Coronary angioscopy. The Hague, Netherlands: Drukkerij Opmeer, 1994.
5. Mizuno K, Satomura K, Miyamoto A, et al. Angioscopic evaluation of coronary artery thrombi in acute coronary syndromes. N Engl J Med 1992;326:287–291.
6. Sherman CT, Litvack F, Grundfest W et al. Coronary angioscopy in patients with unstable angina pectoris. N Engl J Med 1986;315:913–919.
7. Silva JA, Escobar A, Collin TJ, et al. Unstable angina: a comparison of angioscopic findings between diabetic and nondiabetic patients. Circulation 1995;92:1731–1736.
8. Teirstein PS, Schatz RA, Wong SC, Rocha-Singh KJ. Coronary stenting with angioscopic guidance. Am J Cardiol 1995;75:344–347.
9. Feld, Gania M, Carell WK, et al. Comparison of angioscopy, intravascular ultrasound imaging, and quantitative coronary angiography in predicting clinical outcome after coronary intervention in high risk patients. J Am Coll Cardiol 1996;28:97–105.

IV

THERAPEUTIC
INTERVENTIONS

22

INTRA-AORTIC BALLOON PUMP COUNTERPULSATION

Michael Ragosta

Concepts and Physiology

THE INTRA-AORTIC BALLOON pump (IABP) consists of a catheter with a long, cylindrical balloon with a volume of between 30 and 50 ml that is placed in the descending thoracic aorta and timed to inflate during diastole and deflate during systole. By inflating during diastole, the balloon pump displaces aortic blood and increases early diastolic pressure within the aorta. This is known as *diastolic augmentation* and is responsible for the increased perfusion pressure afforded by the device. The balloon deflates rapidly during end-diastole and the isovolumic phase of early systole, creating a potential space of 30 to 50 ml within the aorta, thereby lowering the impedance of the aorta and reducing end-diastolic pressure. The left ventricle pumps against a lower pressure (afterload), reducing the work of the left ventricle and lowering myocardial oxygen consumption. Forward flow and cardiac output are improved and a lower oxygen demand reduces myocardial ischemia. These are the principal beneficial hemodynamic effects of aortic balloon counterpulsation: aortic diastolic pressure augmentation and systolic afterload reduction and resulting in improved left ventricular performance and reduced myocardial oxygen demand.

The IABP is not a cardiopulmonary bypass device. Because the device is triggered by the ECG and works predominantly by reducing afterload and augmenting diastolic pressure, the beneficial effect of the IABP depends on the patient's intrinsic rhythm and cardiac output. The IABP will not work in a patient with asystole or ventricular fibrillation, and its effectiveness is reduced in patients with arrhythmia. Patients with massive pump failure may not be very responsive to this maneuver.

Effect on Systemic Hemodynamics and Coronary Blood Flow

The intra-aortic balloon results in numerous beneficial systemic hemodynamic effects in patients with cardiogenic shock, ischemic syndromes, and left heart failure. Left ventricular afterload and preload are reduced. Aortic counterpulsation will decrease aortic systolic pressure by 10% to 20% due to the reduction in afterload. Pulmonary capillary wedge pressure (PCWP) (i.e., left ventricular preload) will decrease approximately 20%, reflecting decreases in left ventricular end-diastolic pressure and left atrial pressure secondary to afterload reduction. Diastolic augmentation will enhance diastolic BP 30% to 90% above baseline. Mean arterial BP will subsequently increase 30% to 40%. Cardiac output and stroke volume generally increase by 20%, and heart rates either are unaffected or may decrease slightly as a consequence of hemodynamic improvement. Systemic vascular resistance usually drops, although this response is variable. Parameters of global left ventricular function generally improve on the balloon pump. In patients with cardiogenic shock and acute myocardial infarction, left ventricular end-diastolic volume decreases with a proportionally greater reduction in left ventricular end-systolic volume, resulting in increased ejection fraction. The improvement in indices of global ventricular function are not due to an improvement in myocardial contractility but instead reflect the sensitivity of these indices to changes in afterload.

The effect of aortic counterpulsation on coronary blood flow varies depending on the underlying hemodynamics, degree of coronary arterial narrowing, and the method by which blood flow is estimated. In experimental models, normotensive dogs without flow-limiting lesions in the coronary artery show no change in coronary blood flow during counterpulsation, whereas animals with hypotension and flow-limiting coronary stenoses show an increased coronary blood flow. Early studies in humans using the thermodilution method to measure global coronary blood flow showed conflicting results, with some studies demonstrating improved coronary blood flow and others showing no change with aortic counterpulsation. The recent availability of the intracoronary Doppler flow wire has clarified the effect of aortic counterpulsation on coronary blood flow. In human subjects, aortic counterpulsation increases coronary blood flow velocity in the proximal prestenotic segment of the coronary artery and in the distal artery only if there is no significant stenosis present (Fig 22-1). When a significant stenosis is present, coronary blood flow velocity in the distal artery does not increase with the IABP. These studies suggest that the dramatic relief of ischemia afforded by the IABP in patients with critical coronary stenoses is due to the beneficial effects on afterload and preload, which decrease myocardial oxygen demand, rather than via a direct increase in coronary blood flow.

The effect of the IABP on human collateral flow is not well characterized. It is speculated that aortic counterpulsation improves collateral flow. Evidence for this phenomenon in humans with coronary artery disease is lacking and con-

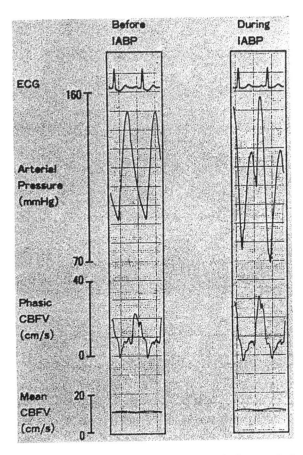

Figure 22-1   Intracoronary Doppler flow velocity before and during intra-aortic balloon counterpulsation in a patient who underwent successful angioplasty, demonstrating an increase in phasic coronary blood flow velocity (CBFV). (Reproduced with permission from Ishihara M, Sato T, Tateishi H, et al. Effects of intra-aortic balloon pumping on coronary hemodynamics after coronary angioplasty in patients with acute myocardial infarction. Am Heart J 1992;124:1133–1138.)

sists predominantly of case reports and clinical anecdotes. One study found augmentation of collateral flow as assessed by Doppler flow wire (seen as reversal of flow velocity) in one patient but no augmentation in two additional patients studied, and another investigator found no augmentation of diastolic pressure across a stenosis with aortic counterpulsation during coronary occlusion during angioplasty in three patients. Whether collateral flow is improved by aortic counterpulsation remains speculative until further studies are performed using better techniques to study collateral flow, such as myocardial contrast echocardiography.

Indications and Contraindications

Originally designed for patients with shock in the setting of an acute infarction, the IABP is now used for many other indications (Table 22-1). The most common indications are for the treatment of patients with cardiogenic shock and for the treatment of unstable angina refractory to medical therapy in patients awaiting revascularization.

The acute hemodynamic effects of the IABP are impressive and result in clinical stability in the majority of patients with cardiogenic shock from acute infarction. Despite these beneficial effects on hemodynamics, the IABP has not favorably affected the high in-hospital and long-term mortality, because the IABP cannot reverse extensive myocardial damage, an important determinant of long-term survival. Aggressive reperfusion therapy appears to favorably impact on the mortality of cardiogenic shock complicating infarction, and the IABP is a highly effective method of stabilizing the patient's hemodynamics,

Table 22-1   Indications for Intra-aortic Balloon Pump

Cardiogenic shock
Unstable angina refractory to medical therapy
Prior to coronary bypass surgery in high-risk patients
Mechanical complication of acute infarction (MR, VSD)
Severe MR
Decompensated aortic stenosis
Adjunct to PTCA in high-risk patients
Refractory ventricular tachycardia
Threatened closure after dissection from PTCA
Adjunct to thrombolysis or PTCA in acute MI to maintain vessel patency
Refractory congestive heart failure
Prophylaxis prior to noncardiac surgery in selected patients with CAD
"Bridge" to cardiac transplant

Abbreviations: MR, mitral regurgitation; VSD, ventricular septal defect; PTCA, percutaneous transluminal coronary angioplasty; MI, myocardial infarction; CAD, coronary artery disease.

thereby allowing survival until coronary revascularization can be accomplished. The balloon pump is very effective at alleviating ischemia in patients with unstable angina refractory to medical therapy, and has been demonstrated to decrease the risk of emergency coronary bypass surgery in this setting. Although the IABP results in symptomatic improvement in patients with medically refractory unstable angina, it does not appear to modify infarct size or alter morbidity or mortality when initiated as primary therapy for acute myocardial infarction.

The IABP is useful to stabilize patients with poor ventricular function or tenuous hemodynamics pre- and postoperatively for coronary bypass surgery. It can be life-saving in patients with mechanical complications of acute myocardial infarction, such as acute mitral regurgitation or ventricular septal rupture, and has been used with some success in patients with acutely decompensated critical aortic stenosis, presumably due to its effect on increasing coronary perfusion. The IABP has performed favorably in the support of patients undergoing "high-risk" angioplasty, defined as patients with either severe ventricular dysfunction (ejection fraction < 30%), a single remaining arterial conduit requiring angioplasty, angioplasty of an unprotected left main stem, or multivessel angioplasty complicated by hypotension. Other less common indications include the treatment of refractory ventricular tachycardia, treatment of recurrent acute closure after balloon angioplasty, as an adjunct to prevent reocclusion following mechanical or pharmacologic reperfusion in acute myocardial infarction, and as a relatively long-term "bridge" in patients with severe left ventricular dysfunction awaiting cardiac transplantation. The prophylactic use of the IABP in patients with extensive coronary artery disease prior to major noncardiac surgery appears beneficial in those with a high preoperative risk in whom revascularization is not an option either because of inoperable coronary disease, because of a severe co-existing condition such as advanced malignancy, or because the noncardiac surgery is emergent.

Contraindications (Table 22-2) include significant aortic insufficiency, aortic dissection and aortic aneurysm, sepsis, and the presence of iliac or femoral artery obstructive vascular disease. Because the IABP decreases left ventricular end-diastolic pressure, resulting in decreased left atrial pressure, the IABP has been reported to cause significant right-to-left shunting, leading to clinical in-

Table 22-2   Contraindications for Intra-Aortic Balloon Pump

Significant aortic insufficiency
Aortic aneurysm or dissection
Sepsis
Peripheral vascular disease
Significant arteriovenous shunt (i.e., patent ductus arteriosus)
Atrial septal defect or patent foramen ovale and elevated right atrial pressure
Severe coagulopathy
No clear surgical endpoint (revascularization or transplant)

stability in a patient with a patent foramen ovale and elevated right atrial pressure secondary to right ventricular infarction. Use of the IABP in patients known to be at increased risk for complications, such as in women or in patients with small body habitus, diabetes mellitus, and peripheral vascular disease, requires careful judgment of the risk-to-benefit ratio. Although prior peripheral vascular surgery in the femorals, iliacs, or aorta may preclude placement of a percutaneous IABP, the device has been successfully inserted surgically in patients with Dacron aortofemoral grafts. The IABP has an acceptable complication rate and is not contraindicated in the very elderly or in patients who received thrombolysis. The IABP should be inserted only in those patients with a clear treatment plan. This is particularly important in patients with unstable angina and no clear surgical endpoint and in those with refractory heart failure who are not suitable for transplantation.

Equipment

Aortic counterpulsation is performed by using a catheter with a polyurethane balloon and a pumping device (console) that synchronizes inflation and deflation of the balloon. Helium is used as the inflation gas because of its low viscosity, allowing smaller catheter size and rapid inflation and deflation. Manufacturers with devices approved for use in the United States include Datascope (Paramus, NJ), St. Jude Medical, Kontron (Everett, MA), and Mansfield (Mansfield, MA). Each manufacturer produces similar catheters and consoles (Figs 22-2 and 22-3). Adult catheter sizes range from 8.5 Fr (single-lumen catheter) to 10.5 Fr (double-lumen catheter), and balloon volume varies between 30 and 50 ml. In the United States, most physicians use double-lumen balloon catheters so that they can use the wire-guided percutaneous insertion technique (see next section) and can monitor central aortic pressure to assist in timing. Currently, 9.5-Fr catheters with 40-ml balloons are the most popular, with 30-ml balloons reserved for persons with small stature and 50-ml balloons for those with large stature.

Insertion, Proper Use, and Removal

Percutaneous Insertion Techniques

Before 1980, all IABPs were inserted surgically using a Dacron graft anastomosed to the common femoral artery and were removed by primary closure. The development of a double-lumen catheter led to the wire-guided percutaneous approach in the early 1980s. The success rate is similar to surgically inserted pumps (>90%), but the IABP technique is faster and easier and has essentially replaced the surgical technique.

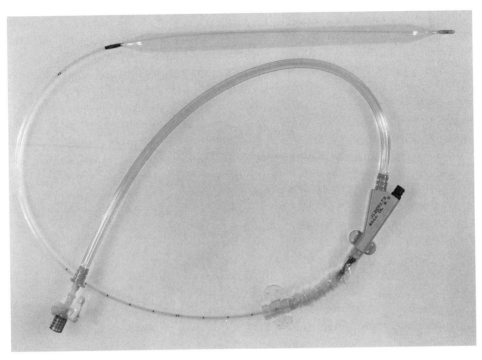

Figure 22-2   An IABP catheter. (Courtesy of Datascope Inc., Paramus, NJ.)

Percutaneous insertion is accomplished from the femoral artery. The skin overlying both femoral arteries is shaved, sterilized with an iodine solution, and draped with sterile linen. Adequate local anesthesia is important for patient comfort during insertion of the large sheath and requires a minimum of 20 ml of 1% lidocaine infiltrated into the skin and around the artery. After local anesthesia is achieved, a 5-mm skin incision is created, and the subcutaneous tissue is spread with the tips of a needle-nosed forcep. Arterial access is obtained using the Seldinger technique (described in Chapter 4) with a J-tipped guidewire (note that the standard wire used for diagnostic catheterization is 0.035″– 0.038″; the central lumen of most IABP catheters requires a 0.030″ or 0.032″ guidewire). The guidewire is advanced through the iliac artery to the descending aorta and should pass without resistance. Assessment of iliac tortuosity is important and can be accomplished by observing the course of the guidewire through these vessels by fluoroscopy. If there is resistance to the passage of the J-tipped guidewire, it may be necessary to use the opposite artery. If resistance is encountered from the contralateral side, iliac and aortic angiography should be performed by using a small (5- or 6-Fr) sheath or dilator and hand injections of contrast. Tortuous iliacs may require a long arterial sheath to allow successful insertion. Obstructive vascular disease in the aorta or iliacs precludes percutaneous balloon placement and necessitates surgical implantation in the axillary artery or thoracic aorta.

Assuming the J-tipped guidewire advances smoothly through the iliacs and aorta, the Seldinger needle is removed while pressure is applied to the femoral artery to prevent bleeding and hematoma formation. An 8-Fr dilator is inserted over the guidewire and advanced into the femoral vessels to create a smooth track for the insertion of the larger sheath. The dilator is removed, gentle pressure is applied to the artery, and the large-bore (usually 9.5-Fr) sheath along with its dilator is positioned in the femoral artery. When the sheath is in place, the dilator is removed, taking care to maintain the guidewire in its position high in the thoracic aorta. Some sheaths bleed around the guidewire; hemostatic sheaths are recommended because they prevent blood loss while the balloon pump is advanced on the guidewire to the sheath. If a nonhemostatic sheath is used, pinching of the sheath below its diaphragm will stop back-bleeding until the balloon catheter reaches the sheath. The IABP catheter is then advanced over the guidewire under fluoroscopic guidance so that the radio-

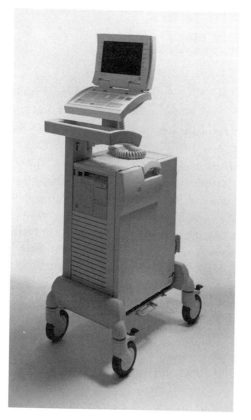

Figure 22-3   An IABP console. (Courtesy of Datascope Inc., Paramus, NJ.)

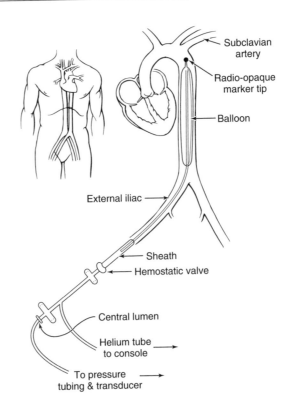

Figure 22-4 Proper position of the IABP catheter in the body.

opaque marker tip lies below the origin of the left subclavian artery, which can be identified radiographically as the level of the carina or left mainstem bronchus (Fig 22-4). With the IABP catheter in this final position, the guidewire is removed and the central lumen is aspirated, flushed with heparinized saline, and connected to a pressure transducer. Insertion of sheathless balloon catheters is accomplished in a similar manner, except that the skin and subcutaneous tissue are first dilated with a 7-Fr dilator and the balloon catheter is advanced over the guidewire without placing a sheath in the femoral artery. Occasionally, bleeding around the catheter may occur when using a sheathless insertion technique; some clinicians backload a short sheath on the catheter prior to insertion, and if significant oozing around the catheter site occurs, the sheath is slipped over the catheter into the femoral artery to control bleeding.

Prior to initiation of counterpulsation, the balloon is filled with helium gas. As the balloon fills, fluoroscopy of the balloon should be performed to be sure the balloon is unwrapping fully and that there are no kinks or obstructions to filling. To prevent thrombus and thromboembolism, a heparin bolus of 5000 units followed by an infusion of 800 to 1200 units/hr to prolong the partial thromboplastin time approximately two times control. The sheath and balloon catheter are sutured securely to the skin to avoid kinking, and a sterile dressing is applied. Prophylactic antibiotics are administered by some clinicians; their routine use is not recommended unless a breach in sterile technique occurred during insertion.

After the IABP is inserted and counterpulsation initiated, the patient must remain on strict bed rest with no hip flexion beyond 10 or 20 degrees. Analgesics prescribed at regular intervals are effective in alleviating incisional discomfort and back pain. It is important to observe the patient carefully for any potential complications, with special attention given to the assessment of limb perfusion and the status of distal arterial pulses in both extremities. The insertion site must be observed for bleeding, hematoma formation, and signs of local infection. Obtaining frequent vital signs is important for the detection of occult infection or bleeding, and periodic monitoring of hematocrit, WBC count, and platelet count should be performed. Any complaint of abdominal, back, flank, or extremity pain must be taken seriously and carefully assessed. Nurses should not attempt to routinely draw blood samples from the central lumen of the balloon catheter. If the arterial waveforms appear "damped," a thrombus may have formed within the lumen. If aspiration of the central lumen is not possible, the central lumen should be capped and pressure monitoring discontinued from this site; the temptation to flush a catheter that does not aspirate must be resisted.

Timing and Proper Use of the Intra-Aortic Balloon Pump

Effective counterpulsation is critically dependent on proper timing of inflation and deflation. The electrocardiographic impulses are used to establish timing after they are correlated with aortic valve opening and closing on the central aortic pressure tracing. The arterial waveforms generated from the catheter's central lumen are used to confirm that timing of inflation and deflation is associated with the hemodynamic effects desired. Fine tuning of inflation and deflation is based on these central aortic waveforms. Use of a radial artery catheter is less desirable because of the delay seen in the peripheral arteries.

To establish appropriate timing, a 1:2 or 1:3 counterpulsation sequence is used with the pump volume set at 40 ml. Inflation should occur immediately after aortic valve closure and be timed to coincide with the dicrotic notch on the central aortic waveform. Deflation should occur just prior to aortic valve opening and left ventricular ejection during the isovolumic phase of early systole (usually coinciding with the R wave on the ECG). Figure 22-5 demonstrates the characteristic central aortic waveforms seen with the proper timing of counterpulsation. Inflation begins on the dicrotic notch and results in a rise in aortic diastolic pressure known as the augmentation wave (a), which should be greater than aortic systolic pressure (b). With deflation at end-diastole, aortic diastolic pressure drops sharply with the aortic end-diastolic pressure (c), typically 10 to 15 mm Hg lower than the aortic end-diastolic pressure of a nonaugmented beat (d).

Figure 22-5 Proper timing of inflation and deflation. Counterpulsation is set at 1:2, indicating that the inflation and deflation sequence occurs with every other beat. a, augmentation wave; b, aortic systolic pressure with counterpulsation; c, aortic end-diastolic pressure of the augmented beat; d, aortic end-diastolic pressure of the nonaugmented beat. See text for details.

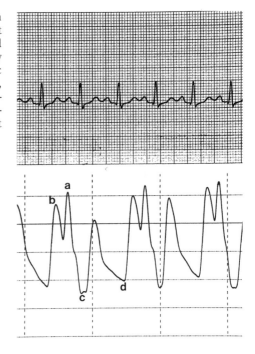

Examples of incorrect timing as seen in Figure 22-6. *Early inflation* (Fig 22-6A) is undesirable because it occurs when the aortic valve is still open and results in early closure of the aortic valve with impairment of ventricular emptying and a subsequent drop in stroke volume and cardiac output. Aortic regurgitation also may occur, which will increase the work of the heart, thereby increasing myocardial oxygen demand. Early inflation appears as a superimposition of the augmentation wave on the systolic wave. It is corrected by moving inflation to the right until the dicrotic notch is visible and then backing it up slightly so that inflation coincides precisely with the dicrotic notch. *Late inflation* (Fig 22-6B) results in inefficient counterpulsation with attenuated augmentation. It is characterized by the obvious presence of the dicrotic notch and a suboptimal augmentation wave. *Early deflation* (Fig 22-6C) produces minimal beneficial effect because of the short duration of diastolic augmentation. The balloon has already deflated well before the isovolumic phase of systole, thereby limiting the afterload reducing effect of aortic counterpulsation. A characteristic broad, U-shaped deflection is seen. If deflation continues after the isovolumic phase of systole, ventricular ejection may begin against an incompletely deflated balloon, resulting in increased rather than decreased afterload (*late deflation*). Obvious detrimental effects include increased myocardial oxygen demand, decreased stroke volume, and diminished cardiac output. The pressure waveform seen in late deflation is characterized by a higher aortic end-diastolic pressure than that of a non-augmented beat (Fig 22-6D).

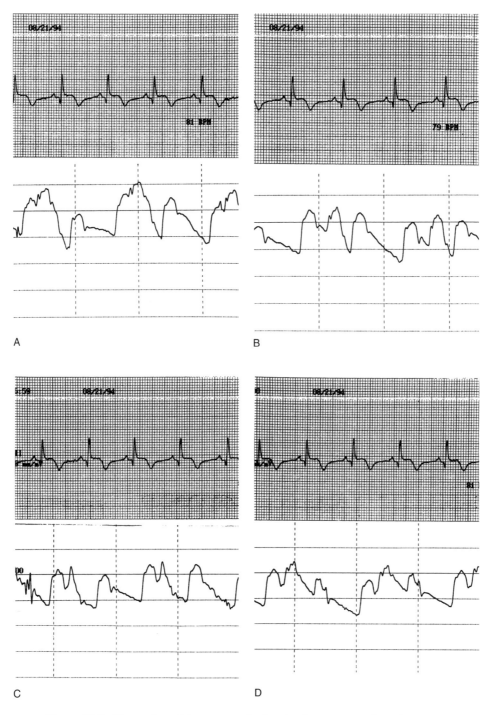

Figure 22-6 Examples of improper timing in the same patient (counter-pulsation at 1:2): **(A)** Early inflation, **(B)** late inflation, **(C)** early deflation, **(D)** late deflation.

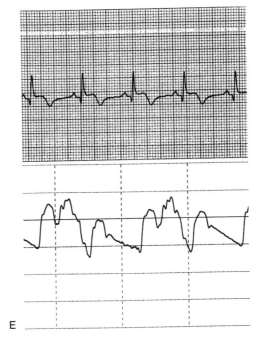

Figure 22-6 (E) Proper timing. See text for details.

Arrhythmias interfere with proper timing of the IABP. Tachycardia shortens diastole, and so deflation should be adjusted to occur earlier. With rates greater than 120 bpm, current balloon pumps cannot fill and empty fast enough. Optimal hemodynamics may be obtained by switching to 1:2 counterpulsation. Marked arrhythmias, as seen in atrial fibrillation, multifocal atrial tachycardia, and frequent ventricular ectopy, result in very inefficient augmentation, limiting the balloon pump's usefulness. Future advances in IABP technology include the development of closed-loop systems, which time inflation and deflation on a beat-by-beat basis, thereby increasing the effectiveness of balloon counterpulsation in patients with marked arrhythmias.

Weaning from Counterpulsation and Removal of the Balloon Pump

Determination of a patient's suitability for weaning from counterpulsation depends on the indication for counterpulsation. In general, patients who underwent placement of the IABP for medically refractory angina can be weaned from counterpulsation rather quickly (as soon as 1–2 hr) once successful revascularization has been accomplished by either coronary bypass surgery or angioplasty. Patients with balloon pumps inserted for cardiogenic shock or refractory heart failure, however, should demonstrate hemodynamic stability before weaning is attempted. Objective evidence of hemodynamic stability in patients with shock or heart failure requires a stable arterial BP, adequate cardiac output, and lack of pulmonary congestion or volume overload. Suggested parameters to help assess the appropriate time for weaning include a mean arterial BP greater than 70 mm Hg, a systolic arterial pressure or augmented diastolic pressure in excess of 90 mm Hg, a cardiac index above 2.2 liters/min/m^2, and a PCWP less than 18 to 20 mm Hg. Achievement of these parameters in a patient with profound pump failure often requires simultaneous use of inotropic or pressor support.

Weaning is initiated by decreasing counterpulsation from 1:1 to 1:2. The patient is closely watched for signs of decompensation. With continued hemodynamic stability, counterpulsation can be further decreased to 1:3 or 1:4. Removal of the IABP can be considered if the patient's clinical condition remains stable with 1:3 or 1:4 counterpulsation. An alternative method of weaning is to maintain 1:1 counterpulsation but gradually decrease the balloon volume during weaning until there is little or no circulatory assistance. Successful weaning can be accomplished using either technique.

When the patient's status allows removal of the pump, anticoagulation is discontinued and the balloon pump is placed on infrequent pumping (1:3, 1:4, 1:8) to prevent clots from forming on the deflated balloon. When the activated clotting time is less than 150 seconds, the pump can be removed. Premedication with 2 to 4 mg of intravenous (IV) morphine sulfate and infiltration of the femoral artery site with 20 ml of 1% lidocaine are recommended prior to balloon pump removal to prevent discomfort and to reduce the incidence of a vagal reaction. Because the removal of a large-bore sheath coupled with compression of the femoral artery can result in stimulation of vagal afferents and a profound vagal reaction leading to hypotension and bradycardia, the patient's rhythm and BP must be monitored. A well-functioning IV line should be present and atropine readily available. The balloon pump is turned off and suction is applied to the balloon lumen of the catheter with a syringe in order to collapse the balloon. Once a balloon has been inflated, it retains a high profile and can no longer pass through the sheath. Therefore, the balloon catheter is withdrawn to the sheath, and then the catheter and sheath are removed from the body as one unit. Clots may form on the balloon catheter and may be dragged to the puncture site during removal of the catheter and sheath. Therefore, the puncture site must be allowed to bleed freely for 1 to 2 seconds while pressure is applied both proximal to and then distal to the insertion site to help expel any thrombus that may have been inadvertently carried to the site during catheter removal. This method of removal is very important to prevent distal embolization of clot. The arterial puncture site is compressed for 30 to 60 minutes until hemostasis is achieved, with careful assessment of the distal pulses made during the compression. A sterile dressing is applied and the patient kept at strict bed rest for at least 12 hours after the sheath is removed. The puncture site and distal pulses should be assessed frequently (every 15 min for the first hour, once per hour for 2 hours, then every 4 hours).

Complications

The IABP is associated with a fairly high complication rate, and all physicians who utilize this device must be aware of all possible complications as well as their management. The overall complication rates vary from 8% to 45% depending on the era, technique, and equipment used as well as the definition of a complication by the reporting author. In the modern era, utilizing 9.5-Fr catheters and the wire-guided percutaneous approach, the expected complication rate is in the 10% to 20% range. The newer, sheathless methodology may result in even lower complication rates.

Table 22-3 lists the wide range of complications reported in the literature. Deaths attributable to the IABP are rare (<0.5%). Unsuccessful insertions are seen in 5% to 6% of attempts. By far the most commonly observed complications are vascular in nature, accounting for between 80% and 90% of all IABP-related complications. Vascular complications include local bleeding, retroperitoneal bleeding, hematoma, vessel perforation, pseudoaneurysm formation, and acute arterial insufficiency in the affected limb. Acute arterial insufficiency is potentially limb threatening, and the manifestations vary along a spectrum from asymptomatic loss of distal arterial pulses to gangrene. Symptoms include pain in the foot or leg, paresthesias, and the loss of motor or sensory function. Development of ischemic ulcers or gangrene may be seen in patients with prolonged use of the IABP. Physical examination of a patient with limb ischemia may reveal diminished or absent pulses, coolness of the extremity, pallor, and possibly swelling or edema.

There are several mechanisms by which a patient with an IABP may develop limb ischemia, the most common of which is from mechanical obstruction of the femoral artery due to the large size of the arterial sheath and balloon catheter. This mechanism is especially operative in female patients, patients with peripheral vascular disease, and patients with small stature because of the smaller size of the arterial lumen. Other mechanisms include thrombosis, embolism, and the creation of an intimal flap during insertion of the device. Rarely, aortic dissection or aortic perforation may manifest as limb ischemia because of an occlusive aortic intimal flap in the case of aortic dissection or because of the development of a retroperitoneal hematoma and extrinsic arterial compression in the case of aortic or iliac perforation. In general, removal of the balloon pump will restore circulation to the threatened limb in about half of patients with acute limb ischemia. The remaining patients may require a surgical procedure in addition to removal of the balloon pump, such as thrombectomy or embolectomy, vascular repair or grafting, or, more rarely, amputation. In the rare patient who develops limb-threatening ischemia who will not tolerate removal of the balloon pump, surgical bypass, such as a femorofemoral bypass graft, may be required to maintain limb viability.

Table 22-3 Complications of Intra-aortic Balloon Pump

I. Relatively common complications
  A. Vascular complications
    1. Local bleeding
    2. Retroperitoneal bleeding
    3. Hematoma
    4. Vessel perforation
    5. Pseudoaneurysm
    6. Arterial insufficiency
      a. Asymptomatic loss of pulses
      b. Paresthesias
      c. Leg pain
      d. Motor deficit
      e. Ulcer or gangrene
    7. Aortic dissection
  B. Infectious
    1. Local wound infection
    2. Bacteremia (with/without sepsis)
II. Rare complications
    1. Persistent lymph drainage or lymph edema
    2. Foot drop
    3. Femoral cutaneous nerve damage (dysesthesia syndrome)
    4. Cerebrovascular accident
    5. Compartment syndrome
    6. Hemolysis
    7. Thrombocytopenia
    8. Helium embolism
    9. Vascular entrapment of balloon
    10. Spinal cord necrosis and paraplegia
    11. Mesenteric infarction
    12. Renal or splenic infarction

Other complications are less common and are observed in less than 5% to 10% of insertions. These include local wound infection and sepsis, persistent lymph drainage, foot drop, femoral cutaneous nerve damage (dysesthesia syndrome), cerebrovascular accident, and compartment syndrome from prolonged limb ischemia. Thrombocytopenia and hemolysis have been reported in the early literature. Rupture of the balloon may result in helium embolism, causing neurologic syndromes, or may result in bleeding and thrombosis within the balloon lumen, causing entrapment of the balloon while attempting to remove it. Spinal cord necrosis and paraplegia, mesenteric infarction, and renal or splenic infarction have also been described and are due to embolism (either atheromatous or thrombotic) to arterial branches of the aorta.

There is no difference in overall complication rate between the percutaneous wire-guided insertion technique and the open surgical insertion technique. Slight differences in individual complications are seen between these two insertion techniques, with a greater incidence of local infection and bleeding in the surgically inserted group and a higher incidence of local vascular complications in patients with percutaneous insertions. Percutaneous insertions are faster to insert, with a more rapid time to onset of counterpulsation.

Clinical factors responsible for increasing the risk of the IABP have been studied extensively. There is near-uniform agreement that female gender, diabetes, obesity, and the presence of peripheral vascular disease are associated with greater risk for vascular complications. Age, method of insertion, adequacy of anticoagulation, balloon size, and duration of insertion do not appear to be associated with a greater risk of vascular complications. Prolonged insertion (longer than 5 days) is fairly well tolerated, with sustained beneficial hemodynamic effects and no greater risk of vascular complication. There is, however, an increased risk of infection in patients with prolonged IABP use.

Specific Problems and Issues Related to the Use of the Intra-aortic Balloon Pump

Asymptomatic Loss of Pulses

The most common complication of the IABP is the asymptomatic loss of distal pulses. In most cases, this is due simply to mechanical obstruction of the lumen from the large-bore sheath and catheter. The distal pulses should be assessed by Doppler, and, if pulses are not obtainable, careful assessment of the neurologic and perfusion status of the extremity should be performed. The balloon pump will most likely need to be removed, because this is a potentially limb-threatening complication. Once the balloon is removed, the pulses return in about 50% of cases and require no further evaluation. Failure of distal pulses to return after removal of the balloon pump must be evaluated and treated promptly by a vascular surgeon.

Blood in the Helium Tube Connecting the Catheter to the Console

When blood is seen in the clear plastic tube that shuttles helium gas from the console to the balloon catheter, this indicates a tear in the membrane of the balloon. Helium may leak and the balloon pump may fail to augment properly. In some cases, however, the balloon pump continues to augment properly and no alarms sound. Whenever blood is seen in the tube connecting the IABP catheter to the console, the balloon must be removed immediately. Catheter entrapment, requiring surgical removal of the catheter, has been noted due to the presence of desiccated thrombi ("gravel") forming within the balloon, preventing proper deflation and obviating percutaneous removal.

Tachycardia

Heart rates greater than 120 bpm often do not allow proper timing and result in ineffective counterpulsation. If the patient's tachycardia cannot be slowed, switching to 1:2 counterpulsation and timing deflation to occur earlier in the cardiac cycle (because of shortened diastole) may be useful. Use of the device in patients with marked arrhythmia, such as rapid atrial fibrillation and frequent ventricular ectopy, is of limited effectiveness.

Prolonged Use of the Intra-aortic Balloon Pump

Prolonged use (>5 days) of the IABP may be necessary in patients with severe ventricular dysfunction who are awaiting cardiac transplantation. The beneficial hemodynamic effects of counterpulsation continue, and the vascular complication rate is not increased; the risk of infection may be increased with prolonged use. It is the experience of many transplant centers to routinely change the IABP every 7 to 10 days in balloon-dependent patients who are awaiting cardiac transplantation. If infection develops, it is necessary to provide broad-spectrum coverage, because both typical skin pathogens and hospital-acquired, gram-negative bacteria have been cultured from blood and catheter tips.

If prolonged use of the IABP is anticipated, patient comfort can be improved by surgical insertion of the balloon via a Dacron tube graft sewn to the iliac artery. This allows the patient to sit upright and ambulate.

Cardiac Catheterization with Intra-aortic Balloon Pump in Place

Left heart catheterization is sometimes necessary in patients in whom the IABP is already in place. This can safely be performed by transiently turning off the balloon pump during all catheter exchanges in order to prevent the diagnostic catheter tip from tearing the balloon.

Other Percutaneous Cardiopulmonary Bypass Systems

The IABP is by far the most popular circulatory assist device because of its ease of insertion, wide familiarity, and acceptable complication rate. More technically complicated percutaneous assist devices have been developed that are able to provide better circulatory assistance independent of the patient's underlying rhythm and cardiac output. A full discussion of these and other circulatory assist devices is beyond the scope of this chapter and are described only briefly.

The Bard percutaneous cardiopulmonary support (CPS) system (Bard, Inc., Murray Hill, NJ) is accomplished using large-bore (18- to 20-Fr) catheters inserted in the femoral artery and vein using the Seldinger technique and pro-gressive dilatation. The venous catheter is advanced to the right atrium, and the arterial catheter is placed in the aorta. A centrifugal pump aspirates blood from the right atrium to a membrane oxygenator system and pumps oxygenated blood into the aorta at a rate of 4 to 6 liters/min.

This technique has been used prior to and as a stand-by assist device for an-gioplasty in high-risk patients and has been used in patients with shock and re-fractory cardiopulmonary arrest. Insertion of the large cannulae is technically challenging, is associated with a vascular complication rate in the 40% range, and has a much greater expense than the IABP. For these reasons, this tech-nique has not gained widespread acceptance.

Another percutaneous left ventricular assist device currently under refine-ment is the Hemopump (Nimbus, Johnson and Johnson, New Brunswick, NJ). This is not a cardiopulmonary bypass unit; rather, this device assists the left ven-tricle directly. Although it is not dependent on the patient's underlying cardiac rhythm, this device does depend on adequate pulmonary venous return. The device consists of a 21-Fr catheter with a rotating turbine (the Archimedes screw principle) placed across the aortic valve and into the left ventricle via an anastomosed tube graft from the femoral artery. Blood is pumped in a non-pulsatile fashion continuously throughout the cardiac cycle at a flow rate of 3 to 4 liters/min. Smaller devices suitable for percutaneous placement are under development.

SELECTED READINGS

Alcan KE, Stertzer SH, Wallsh E, et al. Comparison of wire-guided percutaneous insertion and conventional surgical insertion of intra-aortic balloon pumps in 151 patients. Am J Med 1983;75:24–28.

Alderman JD, Babliani GI, McCabe CH, et al. Incidence and management of limb ischemia with percutaneous wire-guided intra-aortic balloon catheters. J Am Coll Cardiol 1987;9:524–530.

Bengston JR, Kaplan AJ, Pieper KS, et al. Prognosis in cardiogenic shock after acute myocardial infarction in the interventional era. J Am Coll Cardiol 1992;20:1482–1489.

Busch HM, Cogbill TH, Gundersen AE. Splenic infarction: complication of intra-aortic balloon counterpulsation. Am Heart J 1985;109:383–385.

Cowell RPW, Paul VE, Ilsley CDJ. The use of intra-aortic balloon counterpulsation in malignant ventricular arrhythmias. Int J Cardiol 1993;39:219–221.

DeWood MA, Notske RN, Hensley GR, et al. Intra-aortic balloon counterpulsation with and without reperfusion for myocardial infarction shock. Circulation 1980;61:1105–1112.

Eltchaninoff H, Dimas AP, Whitlow PL. Complications associated with percutaneous placement and use of intra-aortic balloon counterpulsation. Am J Cardiol 1993;71:328–332.

Flaherty JT, Becker LC, Weiss JL, et al. Results of a randomized prospective trial of intra-aortic balloon counterpulsation and intravenous nitroglycerin in patients with acute myocardial infarction. J Am Coll Cardiol 1985;6:434–446.

Flynn MS, Kern MJ, Donohue TJ, et al. Alterations of coronary collateral blood flow velocity during intra-aortic balloon pumping. Am J Cardiol 1993;71:1451–1455.

Folland ED, Kemper AJ, Khuri SF, et al. Intra-aortic balloon counterpulsation as a temporary support measure in decompensated critical aortic stenosis. J Am Coll Cardiol 1985;5:711–716.

Frederiksen JW, Smith J, Brown P, Zinetti C. Arterial helium embolism from a ruptured intra-aortic balloon. Ann Thorac Surg 1988;46:690–692.

Freed PS, Wasfie T, Zado B, Kantrowitz A. Intra-aortic balloon pumping for prolonged circulatory support. Am J Cardiol 1988;61:554–557.

Fuchs RM, Brin KP, Brinker JA, et al. Augmentation of regional coronary blood flow by intra-aortic balloon counterpulsation in patients with unstable angina. Circulation 1983;68:117–123.

Funk M, Gleason J, Foell D. Lower limb ischemia related to use of the intra-aortic balloon pump. Heart Lung 1989;18:542–552.

Georgeson S, Coombs AT, Eckman MH. Prophylactic use of the intra-aortic balloon pump in high-risk cardiac patients undergoing noncardiac surgery: a decision analytic review. Am J Med 1992;92:665–678.

Gold HK, Leinbach RC, Sanders CA, et al. Intra-aortic balloon pumping for control of recurrent myocardial ischemia. Circulation 1973;47:1197–1203.

Goldberg MJ, Rubenfire M, Kantrowitz A, et al. Intra-aortic balloon pump insertion: a randomized study comparing percutaneous and surgical techniques. J Am Coll Cardiol 1987;9:515–523.

Gottlieb SO, Brinker JA, Borkon M, et al. Identification of patients at high risk for complications of intra-aortic balloon counterpulsation: A multivariate risk factor analysis. Am J Cardiol 1984;53:1153–1139.

Gurbel PA, Anderson RD, MacCord CS, et al. Arterial diastolic pressure augmentation by intra-aortic balloon counterpulsation enhances the onset of coronary artery reperfusion by thrombolytic therapy. Circulation 1994;89:361–365.

Hasan RIR, Deiranyia AK, Yonan NA. Effect of intra-aortic balloon counter-pulsation on right-left shunt following right ventricular infarction. Int J Cardiol 1991;439–442.

Horowitz MD, Otero M, deMarchena EJ, et al. Intra-aortic balloon entrapment. Ann Thorac Surg 1993;56:368–370.

Ishihara M, Sato H, Tateishi H, et al. Intra-aortic balloon pumping as the postangioplasty strategy in acute myocardial infarction. Am Heart J 1991;121:385–389.

Ishihara M, Sato H, Tateishi H, et al. Effects of intra-aortic balloon pumping on coronary hemodynamics after coronary angioplasty in patients with acute myocardial infarction. Am Heart J 1992;124:1133–1138.

Kahn JK, Rutherford BD, McConahay DR, et al. Supported "high risk" coronary angioplasty using intra-aortic balloon pump counterpulsation. J Am Coll Cardiol 1990; 15:1151–1155.

Kantrowitz A, Tjonneland S, Freed PS, et al. Initial clinical experience with intra-aortic balloon pumping in cardiogenic shock. JAMA 1968;203:135–140.

Kantrowitz A, Wasfie T, Freed PS, et al. Intra-aortic balloon pumping 1967 through 1982: analysis of complications in 733 patients. Am J Cardiol 1986;57:976–983.

Katz ES, Tunick PA, Kronzon I. Observations of coronary flow augmentation and balloon function during intra-aortic balloon counterpulsation using transesophageal echocardiography. Am J Cardiol 1992;69:1635–1639.

Kern MJ, Aguirre F, Bach R, et al. Augmentation of coronary blood flow by intra-aortic balloon pumping in patients after coronary angioplasty. Circulation 1993;87: 500–511.

Kern MJ, Aguirre FV, Tatineni S, et al. Enhanced coronary blood flow velocity during intra-aortic balloon counterpulsation in critically ill patients. J Am Coll Cardiol 1993; 21:359–368.

Kvilekval KHV, Mason RA, Newton GB, et al. Complications of percutaneous intra-aortic balloon pump use in patients with peripheral vascular disease. Arch Surg 1991;126: 621–623.

Langou RA, Geha AS, Hammond GL, Cohen LS. Surgical approach for patients with unstable angina pectoris: role of the response to initial medical therapy and intra-aortic balloon pumping in perioperative complications after aortocoronary bypass grafting. Am J Cardiol 1978;42:629–633.

Lazar JM, Ziady GM, Dummer SJ, et al. Outcome and complications of prolonged intra-aortic balloon counterpulsation in cardiac patients. Am J Cardiol 1992;69:955–958.

Leung WH. Coronary and circulatory support strategies for percutaneous transluminal coronary angioplasty and high-risk patients. Am Heart J 1993;125:1727–1738.

MacDonald JG, Hill JA, Feldman RL. Failure of intra-aortic balloon counter-pulsation to augment distal coronary perfusion pressure during percutaneous transluminal coronary angioplasty. Am J Cardiol 1987;59:359–361.

MacKenzie DJ, Wagner WH, Kulber DA, et al. Vascular complications of the intra-aortic balloon pump. Am J Surg 1992;164:517–521.

McBride LR, Miller LW, Naunheim KS, Pennington DG. Axillary artery insertion of an intra-aortic balloon pump. Ann Thorac Surg 1989;48:874–875.

Miller JS, Dodson TF, Salam AA, Smith RB. Vascular complications following intra-aortic balloon pump insertion. Am Surg 1992;58:232–238.

Moulopoulos SD, Topaz S, Kolff WJ. Diastolic balloon pumping (with carbon dioxide) in the aorta: a mechanical assistance to the failing circulation. Am Heart J 1962; 63:669–675.

Mueller H, Ayres SM, Conklin EF, et al. The effects of intra-aortic counterpulsation on cardiac performance and metabolism in shock associated with acute myocardial infarction. J Clin Invest 1971;50:1885–1900.

Nash IS, Lorell BH, Fishman RF, et al. A new technique for sheathless percutaneous intra-aortic balloon catheter insertion. Cathet Cardiovasc Diagn 1991;23:57–60.

Ohman EM, Califf RM, George BS, et al. The use of intra-aortic balloon pumping as an adjunct to reperfusion therapy in acute myocardial infarction. Am Heart J 1991; 121:895–901.

Ohman EM, George BS, White CJ, et al, for the Randomized IABP Study Group. Use of aortic counterpulsation to improve sustained coronary artery patency during acute myocardial infarction. Results of a randomized trial. Circulation 1994;90:792–799.

O'Rourke MF, Norris RM, Campbell TJ, et al. Randomized controlled trial of intra-aortic balloon counterpulsation in early myocardial infarction with acute heart failure. Am J Cardiol 1981;47:815–820.

Powell WF, Dagget WM, Magro AE, et al. Effects of intra-aortic balloon counterpulsation on cardiac performance, oxygen consumption, and coronary blood flow in dogs. Circ Res 1970;26:753–764.

Riggle KP, Oddi MA. Spinal cord necrosis and paraplegia as complications of the intra-aortic balloon. Crit Care Med 1989;17:475–476.

Schecter D, Murali S, Uretsky BF, et al. Vascular entrapment of intra-aortic balloon after short-term balloon counterpulsation. Cathet Cardiovasc Diagn 1991;22:174–176.

Scheidt S, Wilner G, Mueller H, et al. Intra-aortic balloon counterpulsation in cardiogenic shock. Report of a cooperative clinical trial. N Engl J Med 1973;288:979–984.

Shahian DM, Jewell ER. Intra-aortic balloon pump placement through Dacron aorto-femoral grafts. J Vasc Surg 1988;7:795–797.

Shahian DM, Neptune WB, Ellis FH, Maggs PR. Intra-aortic balloon pump morbidity: a comparative analysis of risk factors between percutaneous and surgical techniques. Ann Thorac Surg 1983;36:644–651.

Sisto DA, Hoffman DM, Fernandes S, Frater RWM. Is use of the intra-aortic balloon pump in octogenarians justified? Ann Thorac Surg 1992;54:507–511.

Suneja R, Hodgson JM. Use of intra-aortic balloon counterpulsation for treatment of recurrent acute closure after coronary angioplasty. Am Heart J 1993;125:530–532.

Tatar H, Cicek S, Demirkilic U, et al. Vascular complications of intra-aortic balloon pumping: unsheathed versus sheath insertion. Ann Thorac Surg 1993;55:1518–1521.

Vignola PA, Swaye PS, Gosselin AJ. Guidelines for effective and safe percutaneous intra-aortic balloon pump insertion and removal. Am J Cardiol 1981;48:660–664.

Wasfie T, Freed PS, Rubenfire M, et al. Risks associated with intra-aortic balloon pumping in patients with and without diabetes mellitus. Am J Cardiol 1988;61:558–562.

Weiss AT, Engel S, Gotsman CJ, et al. Regional and global left ventricular function during intra-aortic balloon counterpulsation in patients with acute myocardial infarction. Am Heart J 1984;108:249–254.

Willerson JT, Curry GC, Watson JT, et al. Intra-aortic balloon counterpulsation in patients with cardiogenic shock, medically refractory left ventricular failure and/or recurrent ventricular tachycardia. Am J Med 1975;58:183–191.

Williams DO, Korr KS, Gewirtz H, Most AS. The effect of intra-aortic balloon counterpulsation on regional myocardial blood flow and oxygen consumption in the presence of coronary artery stenosis in patients with unstable angina. Circulation 1982;66:593–597.

23

RETRIEVAL OF FOREIGN BODIES

Ronald E. Vlietstra

FOREIGN BODIES IN the circulatory system are usually of medical origin (i.e., iatrogenic). They include fragments of infusion and diagnostic catheters, sheaths, and guidewires. These are the medical equivalent of the debris left in the outer atmosphere by space program explorers. In the past, recovery of intravascular foreign bodies was possible only by surgery, but today percutaneous techniques are increasingly used.

The retrieval of foreign bodies poses special challenges. Capturing, detaching, and extracting procedures must be accomplished without vascular tearing, embolism, and hemorrhage. These difficulties are often compounded by problems in finding the foreign object and precisely locating its position.

Each of these unusual cases is unique and requires individual planning. There should be preprocedural discussion of the issues involved, not only with the patient but also with colleagues. Surgical back-up should be considered. Operators need to be sensitive to the issue that some of the steps involved in foreign body extraction may require catheters being used for nonapproved indications.

Fortunately, the problem of foreign body extraction is not a frequent one. It is often not addressed in cardiac laboratory textbooks, and even in large catheterization laboratories some months may pass without having to deal with this problem. The infrequency of the issue can be partly attributed to the resilience of modern catheter materials. Even more important, however, it is the careful attention paid to preventing damage to intravascular equipment. Most intravascular foreign bodies are avoidable.

Avoiding Foreign Bodies

A number of steps can be taken to avoid foreign bodies, being introduced into the vascular system.

1. Use equipment only as it was intended to be used. Attempted modification of its shape or application may lead to breakage.

2. Limit twisting of catheters, and ensure that the distal end is free (i.e., not trapped). Excessive manipulation of catheters may produce knotting; any manipulations, other than flotation, should be performed with fluoroscopic guidance.

3. Secure the extravascular (free) end of any wire or catheter that could migrate into the body. For chronic implants (e.g., pacemaker leads), nonabsorbable suture should be used.[1]

4. Do not advance needles over catheters or wires. The sharp cutting edge of the needle may shear off the end. Specially designed dilators are available for passage over catheters and wires.

5. Maintain sterile technique so that chronically implanted equipment will not become infected and require removal.

6. Obtain full training in the use of new devices to minimize their higher potential for problems.

Types of Foreign Bodies

As mentioned, most intravascular foreign bodies are of iatrogenic origin. They include fragments of intravascular infusion catheters, pacemaker leads and fragments thereof, pieces of sheaths and guidewires, misplaced stents, other coronary device components, and components of heart valves and other prostheses.[2,3] Malfunctioning catheter systems may also be a problem (e.g., a balloon catheter that has not deflated). They may also include knotted or kinked catheters or occlusive balloons that have dislodged from their intended positions. Occasionally, noniatrogenic foreign bodies may be encountered; examples are bullets, lead shot, and fragments of needles used for administering illicit drugs.[4,5]

Foreign bodies may be located at any site in the circulation. In the absence of a right-left communication, those on the venous side carry a lower embolic risk, but they are quite susceptible to infection and thrombus formation. On the arterial side, foreign bodies may cause arterial obstruction and infarction either by themselves or when they serve as a nidus for thrombosis and/or embolism.

An important distinction is whether the object is radiopaque. This will determine how well fluoroscopic x-ray can be used for localization.[6]

When to Retrieve

Not every foreign body must be extracted. A careful assessment should be made, weighing removal risks against the risks of leaving the foreign body in situ.

Foreign bodies pose risks mainly from infection and thrombosis. The risk of the former is relatively small, but once it occurs, removal of the foreign body is almost mandatory. Typically, this is most commonly an issue with chronic pacemaker leads, from which retained infected lead fragments may cause recurrent bacteremia.[7,8]

Thrombosis poses particular hazards for the arterial circulation wherein occlusion or embolism may be produced. Guidewire fragments lodged in a coronary artery (or one of its branches) may lead to myocardial infarction. They also may lead to cerebral embolism if part of a guidewire fragment lies free in the aorta. A small, noninfected, firmly attached foreign body in the venous circulation or in an already occluded artery may not need removal.

There is also significant potential for patient concern, even when foreign bodies have relatively low intrinsic risk (e.g., an infusion catheter fragment lodged in a pulmonary artery branch). At times, this patient concern may be the most important factor leading to foreign body retrieval.

On the other hand, there are risks to foreign body removal. These include vascular tearing at or near the site where the foreign body is lodged or attached. It may lead to significant hematoma or even hemopericardium. There also may be vascular injury during the extraction process, especially if the foreign body is bulky or knotted. Surgical stand-by or intervention is sometimes needed to effect a safe extraction. Chordal entanglement may cause permanent valvular insufficiency, especially in the case of the tricuspid valve. Arrhythmias may occur when strenuous effort is applied to incarcerated pacemaker leads. Embolism of foreign body fragments also may occur.

The devices used for extraction carry potential risk. The stiffness of extraction or snare catheters may cause cardiac perforation. Normally functioning pacemaker leads may be dislodged by extraction efforts.

Localization of the Foreign Body

Successful retrieval is dependent on precise localization of the foreign body. Adequate localization in turn depends on high-quality x-ray fluoroscopy and precise knowledge of vascular anatomy.

For large radiopaque foreign bodies (e.g., pacemaker leads), single-plane x-ray fluoroscopy may be sufficient. In locating more peripheral objects, however, such as those located in pulmonary artery branches, biplane fluoroscopy may be particularly useful. Contrast dye injection may be needed to better define the location of objects in the coronary arteries and any site of entrapment.

Ultrasound imaging may reveal information unappreciated by fluoroscopy. For example, infected pacemaker leads may be covered with a thrombus. This infected mass may embolize during lead extraction. Such a clot is not visible on x-ray fluoroscopy but usually can be seen easily with two-dimensional echocardigraphy. Intravascular ultrasound has been used to detect small objects that are not visible by other means.[2] Instances in which computed tomography has proven especially useful have also been described (e.g., in locating embolized metallic valve leaflets).[3]

There is obvious advantage to having all intravascular products radiopaque. This is of help not only for retrieval, but also for determining proper location for normal operation. Central infusion lines and Swan-Ganz catheters have incorporated this feature. Initial coronary stents have been manufactured from stainless steel, which is not radiopaque. However, these are now being replaced by radiopaque tantalum and nitinol.

Tools

A wide variety of tools may be useful in percutaneous foreign body extraction (Table 23-1). Some of these tools are part of the usual diagnostic catheterization selection, while others are specially designed for foreign body extraction.

In the former category stiffer core guidewires may be used to help unkink catheters. A balloon catheter may be inflated inside an escaped stent to allow its recovery. Myocardial biopsy forceps may be the method of grabbing a small foreign body or a pacing lead.[9,10] A pigtail catheter may be used to coil up an escaped wire.

A variety of specially designed tools also are available. Those intended for removing thrombus from the circulation (e.g., the pulmonary extraction catheter) are not discussed in this chapter.[11]

Table 23-1   Retrieval Tools

General catheters
Preformed diagnostic catheters
Stiffer core guidewires
Balloon catheters
Biopsy forceps
Special devices
Dotter retriever
Snare loops
Retrieval forceps
Lead extractors

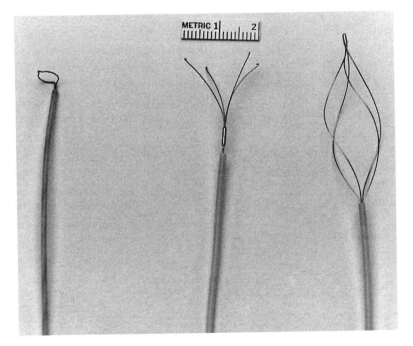

Figure 23-1   Three types of retrieval device. (Left) Snare, (middle) biliary forceps, and (right) Dotter retriever. (Courtesy of Dr. K.N. Garrett.)

Dotter Retriever

The Dotter retriever uses an inner wire cage, or basket, and an outer sheath to trap fragments for extraction (Fig 23-1, right). Commercially made devices come in a variety of sizes.

The item to be secured is approached, usually from the femoral vein or artery (whichever is appropriate). First, the sheath is inserted over a guidewire, and the basket snare is subsequently inserted. Once a free component of the foreign body can be positioned within the basket, the sheath is advanced so that the two components are locked together (see Fig 23-8c). This traps the foreign body and allows for extraction.[12]

Snare Catheter

A variety of wire loops are available that allow foreign bodies to be snared and withdrawn into a catheter sheath (Fig 23-1, left). Some of these are made in small sizes, down to 2 mm, allowing for their passage within small arteries, including the coronary arteries (e.g., Microvena, Minneapolis, MN). Usually, the retrieved foreign body must be doubled over to be withdrawn into the guide catheter, but for wires that cannot be doubled over, a snare-and-capture technique has been described.[13] The wire fragment is trapped in the snare and guided into the distal end of another catheter (Fig 23-2).

Retrieval Forceps

A small (3-Fr) retrieval forceps is now available (Fig 23-3) that allows access to peripheral artery branches and possibly even coronary arteries.[14] This may be especially useful for guidewire fragment and stent retrieval. This device, which has a distal flexible spring coil tip to minimize vascular trauma, can be positioned through a large-lumen guide catheter. Once the foreign body is grasped, it can be withdrawn via the guide catheter. Other devices primarily designed for use within other anatomic sites (e.g., biliary forceps) may be employed for vascular purposes (see Fig 23-1, middle).

Lead Extractors

At least two different systems have been developed specifically for extracting chronic pacemaker leads that are firmly attached to the heart's endocardium. In the United States, the largest experience has been with the Cook system (Cook Pacemaker Corporation, Leechburg, PA). This system uses a set of locking stylets and dilator sheath via the subclavian or cephalic vein, or tip-deflecting wire guides, Dotter baskets, and sheaths with a transfemoral approach

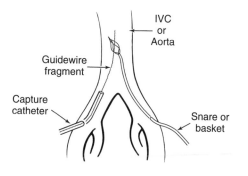

Figure 23-2 Snare-and-capture technique for extracting guidewire fragments that resists doubling over. IVC, inferior vena cava.

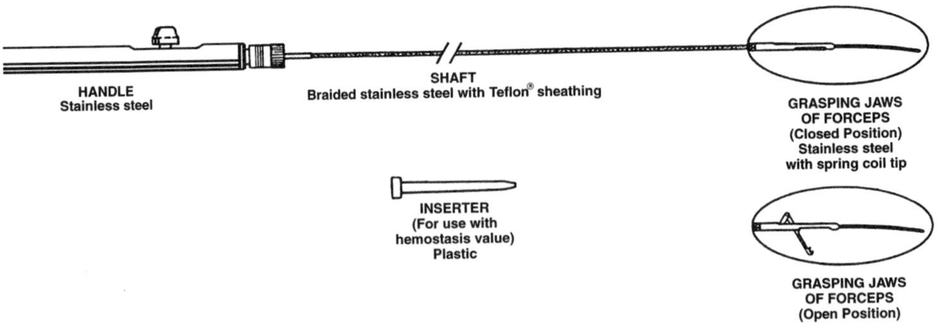

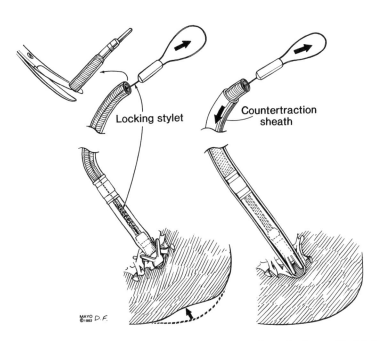

HANDLE
Stainless steel

SHAFT
Braided stainless steel with Teflon® sheathing

**GRASPING JAWS
OF FORCEPS**
(Closed Position)
Stainless steel
with spring coil tip

INSERTER
(For use with
hemostasis value)
Plastic

**GRASPING JAWS
OF FORCEPS**
(Open Position)

Figure 23-3   Vascular retrieval forceps. The distal spring coil tip prevents inadvertent engagement of the vascular wall. (Courtesy of Cook Inc, Bloomington, IN.)

Locking stylet

Countertraction
sheath

Figure 23-4   Locking stylet/countertraction sheath technique. (Left) The connector pin is transected and the locking stylet advanced to the lead tip. Traction is applied via the stylet. (Right) If the lead cannot be dislodged by traction on the stylet alone, countertraction sheath(s) may be used. Traction is then applied to the stylet while countertraction prevents invagination of the endocardial surface. (Courtesy of Dr. D.L. Hayes, Mayo Clinic.)

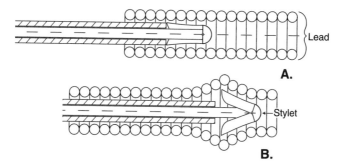

Figure 23-5 **(A)** The VascoMed extraction stylet is threaded fully through the pacemaker lead. **(B)** The stylet tip is opened so that it tightly engages the distal inner lead coils. Traction on the stylet will then be transmitted to the lead tip.

(Fig 23-4). The principle of this device is that an appropriately sized locking stylet is advanced through the inner lumen of the pacemaker electrode. The locking stylet has an expandable coil at its tip. Using counterclockwise rotation, this coil becomes entwined with the inner coil of the electrode near its distal tip. Traction is then applied to the locking stylet, and frequently this alone allows lead removal. If not, external dilator sheaths can be passed over the pacemaker electrode and used to apply countertraction to the tip of the electrode where it is firmly attached to the endocardium.

An alternative extraction stylet has been developed in Germany (VascoMed, Weil am Rhein, Germany). It has been tested less extensively than the Cook device and is not yet marketed in the United States (Fig 23-5).[15]

Specific Situations

An approach can be described for handling the problems most likely to be encountered. It must be remembered that each case is unique, and that experienced opinion should be sought, often including surgical back-up.

Knotted or Kinked Catheter

The incidence of this problem increases with vigorous catheter manipulation and is more frequent with thin-walled catheters. If a kink occurs, there should be an effort to move the kinked portion of the catheter into a large-lumen vessel, such as the inferior vena cava or aorta. An attempt should be made to catch the tip of the catheter on a side branch or with a snare and, if possible, to pass a guidewire through the lumen.

If an actual true knot has been formed, it may be necessary to introduce a catheter (e.g., a sidewinder catheter) through another vessel to help disentangle the knot (Fig 23-6). More often, there is an apparent knot that has

Figure 23-6   Use of a sidewinder catheter to disentangle a knot. IVC, inferior vena cava.

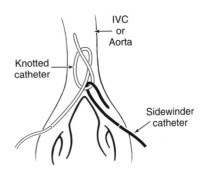

formed due to coiling of the catheter. This can usually be untwisted by judicious reverse rotation. Forcible extraction should be avoided because of the risks for vascular trauma. Surgical extraction may be required if none of these approaches is successful.

Catheter Fragment in the Right Heart

Such a fragment is usually lying free and relatively unembedded in heart muscle. It may be difficult to visualize, thus attempts at extraction should be undertaken in the highest quality fluoroscopy suite. Usually, a snare or Dotter-type retriever is the best device to use, and the best approach is usually from either the right femoral or the internal jugular vein. The catheter fragment may be doubled over and drawn into the Dotter or snare retriever sheath. Usually, it is best to withdraw the whole device as a single unit from the venous entry site.

Retained Pacemaker Lead

Removal of a retained pacemaker lead is usually performed when dealing with an infected or embolized lead. Uncommonly, the presence of multiple leads may indicate the removal of one or more to minimize the risk of subclavian vein thrombosis.

A number of approaches have been used to remove retained pacemaker leads. If the lead has been in only a short time, simple traction may be sufficient (Fig 23-7). A stylet may help stiffen the lead, and any screw device may need loosening.

With more long-term leads, simple traction may not be sufficient.[16] This is especially true of the more elastic polyurethane materials, compared with the stiffer silicone material. The lead may be trapped from below using a pigtail catheter and/or a Dotter basket (Fig 23-8a). It may then be withdrawn via the femoral vein (Fig 23-8b, c). This approach can be successful in as many as three-fourths of incarcerated leads.[17]

A second approach uses the Cook extraction system and is sometimes called the Byrd method.[18] A specifically designed stylet is passed to secure the lead for

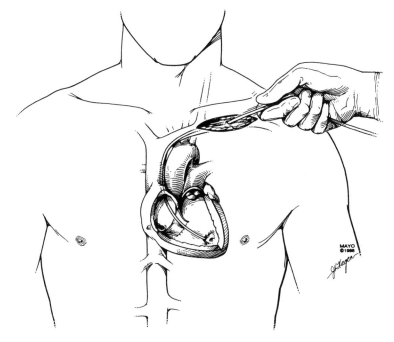

Figure 23-7 Simple traction on the lead allows extraction of most recent implants and some long-term silicone leads. Any active fixation mechanism (e.g., a screw) must be disengaged.

better traction (see Fig 23-4). A countertraction catheter, or catheters, can be advanced over the lead to free adhesions and may be used coming from either the subclavian or the femoral vein. In experienced hands, this approach can be highly successful and safe.[19]

The Telectronics Accufix atrial J-lead (Englewood, CO) presents unique challenges for extraction.[20] Over time, the J-shaped stiffening wire incorporated into the lead's outer insulation has been known to fracture in at least 10% to 20% of implants. When a fractured end extrudes through the lead insulation, it may cause cardiac laceration and tamponade. The stiff extruded J-wire also poses unique problems for extraction. Atrial and superior vena caval tears can be readily produced. Consultation with a lead-extraction expert and/or Telectronics is recommended.

Fragment of Guidewire in Coronary Artery

The growing use of coronary interventional procedures has led to a number of device problems. It is estimated that approximately 1 in 1000 of these procedures will be complicated by a foreign body's being deposited within the circulation.[21] Most commonly, this will be a piece of flimsy guidewire left within a coronary artery or one of its branches. This may be related to overmanipulation

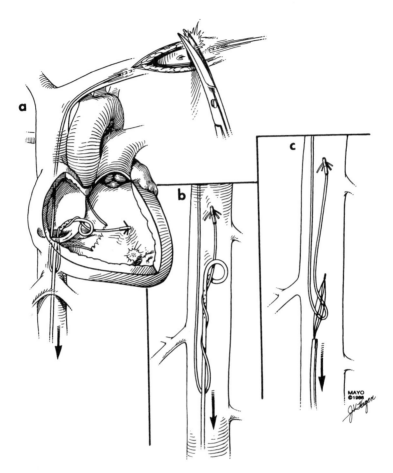

Figure 23-8 Using a femoral venous approach, a pigtail catheter can be used to (**a**) entwine the lead and (**b**) withdraw it into the inferior vena cava. Redundant lead outside the subclavian vein can be transected. (**c**) The lead, now free, can be captured and withdrawn through the femoral vein using a Dotter retriever.

of a trapped guidewire tip during balloon angioplasty, or it may be a cut-off fragment damaged during atherectomy. Tortuous and calcified vessels are especially at risk for this kind of problem.

An important decision is whether such a foreign body should be retrieved at all. If it lies completely within an occluded coronary artery or if it can be stented, there may be little risk in leaving it. If it extends out into the aorta or if it lies within a patent coronary artery, however, there is a risk of thrombotic occlusion or distal fragmentation or clot embolism.[21] Generally, such fragments should be removed percutaneously or by open-heart surgery (if percutaneous extraction is not feasible).

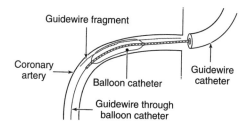

Figure 23-9 A balloon catheter may be inflated to trap a nonimpacted guidewire fragment. Gentle traction may then be used to withdraw the fragment into the guide catheter.

A variety of methods have been employed. If possible, an active grabbing device would seem best (e.g., a snare or basket retriever). This will be easiest if the proximal guidewire extends out into the aorta.[22]

For fragments lying within the coronary artery, a balloon catheter may be inflated to trap the fragment (Fig 23-9) and deliver it back into the guide catheter.[21] Two guidewires may be used to make a coil and so trap the fragment.[23] Finally, for a proximal fragment in a large coronary artery, small-caliber retrieval forceps could be used. None of these methods has been used with great frequency, however, and each should be adapted to best meet the unique characteristics of the problem at hand.

Misplaced coronary stents are likely to be seen increasingly, because they occur in about 1% of stent procedures. Fortunately, they are often innocuous. Snares, forceps, and baskets have been used for successful retrieval.[24] At times, inflating a balloon catheter in or beyond the stent may help in its retrieval.[25] Improved retrieval devices are in the developmental phase.

SELECTED READINGS

1. Trigano JA, Batson R, Lauribe P, et al. Intrapulmonary artery coiling of a permanent pacing lead. Clin Cardiol 1994;17:451–452.
2. Miller SF, McCowan TC, Eidt JF, et al. Embolization of a prosthetic mitral valve leaflet: localization with intravascular US. J Vasc Interv Radiol 1991;2:375–378.
3. Tsui BC, Kinley CE, Miller RM. Optimal imaging techniques for locating leaflets after escape from prosthetic heart valves. Can Assoc Radiol J 1994;45:93–96.
4. Abad J, Merino MJ, Alted E. Case report: wandering intravascular bullet with aortic pseudoaneurysm. Clin Radiol 1993;47:355–356.
5. Kulaylat MN, Barakat N, Stephan RN, Gutierrez I. Embolization of illicit needle fragments. J Emerg Med 1993;11:403–408.
6. McIvor ME, Kaufman SL, Satre R, et al. Search and retrieval of a radiolucent foreign object. Cathet Cardiovasc Diagn 1989;16:19–23.
7. Choo MH, Holmes DR Jr, Gersh BJ, et al. Permanent pacemaker infections: characterization and management. Am J Cardiol 1981;48:559–564.
8. Brodman R, Frame R, Andrews C, Furman S. Removal of infected transvenous leads requiring cardiopulmonary bypass or inflow occlusion. J Thorac Cardiovasc Surg 1992;103:649–654.
9. Kratz JM, Leman R, Gillette PC. Forceps extraction of permanent pacing leads. Ann Thorac Surg 1990;49:676–677.
10. Hartzler GO. Percutaneous transvenous removal of a bullet embolus to the right ventricle. J Thorac Cardiovasc Surg 1980;80:153–154.
11. Greenfield LJ. Catheter pulmonary embolectomy. Chest 1991;100:593–594.
12. Dotter CT, Rösch J, Bilbao MK. Transluminal extraction of catheter and guide fragments from the heart and great vessels; 29 collected cases. Am J Roentgenol 1971;111:467–472.
13. Park JH, Yoon DY, Han JK, et al. Retrieval of intravascular foreign bodies with the snare and catheter capture technique. J Vasc Interv Radiol 1992;3:581–582.
14. Selby JB, Tegtmeyer CJ, Bittner GM. Experience with new retrieval forceps for foreign body retrieval in the vascular, urinary, and biliary systems. Radiology 1990;176:535–538.
15. Alt E, Theres H, Busch U, et al. Removal of three infected pacemaker leads by means of a new extraction stylet: a case report. Herzschr Elektrophys 1991;2:29–34.
16. Madigan NP, Curtis JJ, Sanfelippo JF, et al. Difficulty of extraction of chronically implanted tined ventricular endocardial leads. J Am Coll Cardiol 1984;3:724–731.
17. Espinosa RE, Hayes DL, Vlietstra RE, et al. The Dotter retriever and pigtail catheter: efficacy in extraction of chronic transvenous pacemaker leads. PACE 1993;16:2337–2342.
18. Byrd CL, Schwartz SJ, Hedin NB. Intravascular techniques for extraction of permanent pacemaker leads. J Thorac Cardiovasc Surg 1991;101:989–997.
19. Colavita PG, Zimmern SH, Gallagher JJ, et al. Intravascular extraction of chronic pacemaker leads: efficacy and follow-up. PACE 1993;16:2333–2336.
20. Lloyd M, Hayes D, Holmes DR. Atrial "J" pacing lead retention wire fracture: radiographic assessment, incidence of fracture, and clinical management. PACE 1995;18:958–964.
21. Hartzler GO, Rutherford BD, McConahay DR. Retained percutaneous transluminal coronary angioplasty equipment components and their management. Am J Cardiol 1987;60:1260–1264.
22. Steele PM, Holmes DR Jr, Mankin HT, et al. Intravascular retrieval of broken guide wire from the ascending aorta after percutaneous transluminal coronary angioplasty. Cathet Cardiovasc Diagn 1985;11:623–626.
23. Gurley JC, Booth DC, Hixson C, Smith MD. Removal of retained intracoronary percutaneous transluminal coronary angioplasty equipment by a percutaneous twin guidewire method. Cathet Cardiovasc Diagn 1990;19:251–256.

24. Foster-Smith KW, Garratt KN, Higano ST, Holmes DR Jr. Retrieval techniques for managing flexible intracoronary stent misplacement. Cathet Cardiovasc Diagn 1993;30:63–68.
25. Rozenman Y, Burstein M, Hasin Y, Gotsman MS. Retrieval of occluding unexpanded Palmaz-Schatz stent from a saphenous aorto-coronary vein graft. Cathet Cardiovasc Diagn 1995;34:159–161.

24

TEMPORARY PACING

Stephen Keim

CATHETERIZATION AND ELECTROPHYSIOLOGY laboratories have been increasingly utilized for a variety of interventional electrophysiologic procedures, including the implantation of permanent pacemakers and defibrillators. This chapter is limited to the techniques and procedures of cardiac pacing performed by the cardiac angiographer. A variety of modalities are available to the cardiologist to temporarily treat the patient with transient life-threatening arrhythmias in the catheterization laboratory or as an adjunct to the physiologic assessment of cardiovascular dysfunction. The indications for temporary and permanent pacing have been well delineated in policy statements.[1] This chapter discusses temporary pacing from the catheterization laboratory perspective.

Indications for Temporary Pacing

Because the patient is undergoing either a diagnostic or interventional procedure, the acuity is usually higher and the tolerances for hemodynamic instability narrower than for a patient not undergoing any of these procedures. The invasive cardiologist must be aware of the broader indications of temporary pacing as it applies to the overall clinical situation outside of the laboratory (Table 24-1).

Table 24-1   Indications for Pacing in the Catheterization Laboratory

Bradycardia
  Sinus node dysfunction
  Medically unresponsive hypervagatonia
  Second degree AV block: type 1 or type 2
  Third-degree AV block
Prophylactic
  Preexisting bundle branch block with contralateral heart catheterization or biopsy
  Coronary intervention of right or dominant coronary artery
  Cardioversion in suspected sick sinus syndrome
Physiologic assessment
  Determination of myocardial ischemic threshold
  Severity of moderate stenotic AV valves
  Optimal AV delay in dilated or hypertrophic cardiomyopathy and acute ischemic syndromes
Antitachycardia pacing
  Termination of atrial flutter
  Termination of ventricular tachycardia

Sinus Bradycardia

Hemodynamically significant bradycardia that is unresponsive to pharmacologic maneuvers, such as atropine, and that is expected to recur is the predominant indication for pacing in the catheterization laboratory.[2] The intrinsic heart rate is physiologically determined by the sinus node or a subsidiary supraventricular pacemaking focus. Sinus arrest is common with intracoronary injection, particularly with ionic contrast agents, but is significant in less than 0.3%.[2] Significant sinus bradycardia during intracoronary injection usually responds to having the patient cough several times. This maintains enough cardiac output to clear the coronary bed of contrast. In patients who cannot tolerate repeated, short episodes of bradycardia, pacing may be required. Bradycardia secondary to induced hypervagatonia during initial vascular access is probably one of the most common causes of sinus bradycardia in the catheterization laboratory. This event is usually managed with fluids, oxygen supplementation, and atropine. Patients with severe coronary artery disease or critical aortic stenosis may not tolerate even a short period of hypotension and may require pacing if a vasovagal reaction is anticipated. Supraventricular pacing foci are sensitive to autonomic tone and generally are responsive to atropine or low-dose catecholamines. It is important to recall that the so-called vasovagal reaction has both a cardioinhibitory (bradycardic) and a vasodepressor (vasodilator) effect. Pacing will correct the bradycardia, but the increase in heart rate may not be able to support cardiac output if vasodilation is significant. Chronic and transient dysfunction of the sinus node can occur with ischemia arising from the sinus node artery. During occlusion of the artery, for example, during angioplasty of the proximal right coronary artery, sinus arrest, and bradycardia may occur. Bradycardia may be profound, and unless there is atrioventricular (AV) nodal ischemia, a junctional escape takes over.

Atrioventricular Block

Atrioventricular block is a more ominous finding in the laboratory, because the ventricular escape is less reliable and less likely to be at a rate that will support adequate cardiac output. In the ischemic setting, AV nodal block may be atropine-resistant, so the precise determination of the level of block—intranodal versus infranodal—is less relevant to whether temporary pacing is indicated. The operator must decide whether the AV block will persist or recur and be profound enough to compromise the patient in the periprocedural period. If the patient is experiencing an acute ischemic attack and has heart block at any level, it is prudent to place a temporary pacemaker for the procedure. Indications for temporary pacing in the coronary care unit during an acute myocardial infarction are well recognized and deal with the probability of the development of complete AV block and profound bradycardia. In the catheterization laboratory, especially if intervention is planned, even transient bradycardia may compromise the procedure, and pacing should be utilized if AV block is present.

Prophylactic Pacing

Prophylactic placement of a transvenous temporary pacemaker is controversial and depends on the laboratory's ability to deal quickly with a sudden emergency and their experience with transcutaneous pacing. Venous access and having the equipment available may be sufficient for some laboratories. Other laboratories, experienced and proficient in transcutaneous pacing, may feel that no special precautions are necessary. It has been traditionally suggested that a temporary pacemaker be placed prophylactically during right heart catheterization for patients with left bundle branch block, because traumatic right bundle branch block occurs in approximately 5% of cases with right heart catheter placement.[2-4] Pulmonary artery catheters are now available that have intrinsic pacing electrodes that obviate much of the concern.[5] Traumatic left bundle branch block occurs in less than 1% of left heart catheterizations; as such, most operators do not routinely place a temporary pacemaker for left heart catheterization, but this depends on the practices of the laboratory.[2,6] Although temporary pacemakers are not routinely placed for angioplasty procedures, bradycardia is certainly more common with some of the newer techniques (atherectomy), and consideration of patient stability and length of procedure must be taken into account when deciding to forego placement of a temporary pacing catheter. Finally, for a patient with known sick sinus syndrome or on medications that produce negative chronotropic effects, placement of a temporary pacing catheter during catheterization may be prudent, because postcardioversion bradycardia (after atrial fibrillation) is common.

Physiologic Assessment

Rapid cardiac pacing may be required to assess a variety of hemodynamic problems. Rapid atrial pacing may be an adjunct to induce ischemia in patients with moderate epicardial coronary disease.[7] Lactate metabolism and release of ischemic metabolites (adenosine) may be determined with concomitant coronary sinus sampling as a method of determining the significance of moderate coronary stenosis.[8,9] Mitral stenosis may be demonstrated to be significantly more deleterious with exercise or in patients unable to exercise with rapid atrial pacing. Arterioventricular sequential pacing at variable rates and AV intervals may be used to optimize the timing of atrial and ventricular systole and improve hemodynamics in patients with advanced heart failure or hypertrophic cardiomyopathy.[10,11] In the setting of acute right ventricular failure, AV sequential pacing may be utilized to improve left ventricular filling and cardiac output.

Antitachycardia Pacing

The angiographer is occasionally confronted with unstable tachycardias, which preferably are treated without countershock.[2] Most supraventricular and ventricular tachycardias may be definitively treated with DC cardioversion, but this usually requires sedation. The majority of hemodynamically tolerated atrial or ventricular tachycardias may be successfully terminated with pacing. In the setting of polymorphic ventricular tachycardia associated with long QTc and pauses (torsades de pointe), the angiographer may be asked to place a temporary pacemaker to suppress the tachycardia.

Methods of Pacing

There are basically four methods of pacing the heart in the catheterization laboratory: transcutaneous, transesophageal, transvenous, and transthoracic. Each has its advantages in the acute establishment of a stable heart rate, patient tolerability, complications, and stability after leaving the catheterization laboratory.

Transcutaneous Pacing

Transcutaneous external pacing utilizes large gel adhesive electrodes placed on the thorax either in an anterior-posterior location or in a more classical sternum-apex position.[12] The large surface area and long pulse width allow for enough current to pass through the chest wall muscles to activate the excitable myocardium (20–149 mA). This is the safest modality of pacing, and pacing may be initiated within a minute of identification of a problem. Many of the newer defibrillation systems have concomitant external pacing capabilities. The major disadvantage is the variable capture rate. Ischemic myocardium, acidemia, electrolyte abnormalities, pericardial effusions, and mechanically ventilated patients, all common to the catheterization laboratory, contribute to an unpredictable capture rate of between 52% and 93%.[13] At higher pacing currents, chest wall stimulation invariably occurs, requiring patient sedation.[14] It is frequently difficult to verify capture of myocardium with monitors because of the large depolarization artifact, and verification of a generated pulse with each pacing artifact is requisite. Only recently have radiopaque patches been developed, allowing angiography to be performed with the patches in place.

Transesophageal Pacing

Transesophageal pacing utilizes a specialized pill electrode or catheter passed through the nares and positioned in the esophagus behind the left atrium.[15] In addition, a special pulse generator capable of delivering a wide impulse—10 to 15 milliseconds up to 50 mA—is required. This technique requires experience and special equipment. It also requires a high level of patient cooperation and stability, because the electrode is passed approximately 20 to 40 cm into the esophagus behind the left atrium. Atrial capture is usually accomplished in about 85% of cases. Because of the highly complex lead placement and the lack of ventricular capture, it has virtually no use in pacing for heart block. It has been used to terminate atrial or AV reentrant tachycardias, with a success rate of about 90%, and for some limited electrophysiologic studies.[16,17] Because no venous access is required, it is more popular as an outpatient and pediatric technique than as a procedure in the catheterization laboratory.

Transvenous Pacing

Transvenous pacing is clearly the technique of choice for almost all catheterization laboratory procedures. It is generally regarded as the most technically demanding, but it is clearly the most familiar for the invasive cardiologist. In the laboratory, venous access is either present or easily obtained in order to respond emergently. Transcatheter pacing is the most reliable method of pacing, allowing the atria, ventricle, or both to be consistently paced.

Venous access may be accomplished in several ways, and the short- and long-term goals of pacing should be considered. The safest, quickest, and easiest access in the laboratory is usually from the femoral vein. If pacing is known to be needed for the procedure and inferior venous access is not possible (e.g., inferior vena caval obstruction), the brachial, subclavian, or internal jugular approaches are available. After leaving the laboratory, patient tolerability is highest with the subclavian approach and lowest with the femoral approach. The subclavian approach has the highest incidence of acute complications (1%–3%). For longer periods, the femoral approach has the highest incidence of infection, phlebitis, and lead dislodgment, so it is not ideal for pacing outside of the laboratory for more than 24 hours.[18,19]

Placement of the venous pacing catheter begins with the same approach described in Chapter 4. A venous sheath with a lock-down diaphragm is probably best used in most circumstances. Fluoroscopy is always available in the laboratory, so blind approaches are not necessary. Temporary pacing catheters are usually woven Dacron or plastic and are available in a variety of curves and flexibilities (Fig 24-1). Balloon-tipped flow-directed catheters may still be useful, even when fluoroscopy is available. Placement of the tip of the catheter should be within the right ventricular apex. If an inferior approach is used, the catheter is advanced to the tricuspid valve. On entering the right atrium, the lead should be torqued counterclockwise to direct the tip anteriorly through the valve and into the ventricle. After crossing the valve and entering well into the right ventricle, the catheter should be turned clockwise, directing the tip against the septum. The most common error is crossing the tricuspid valve too inferiorly and applying clockwise rotation too early. This allows the tip to be

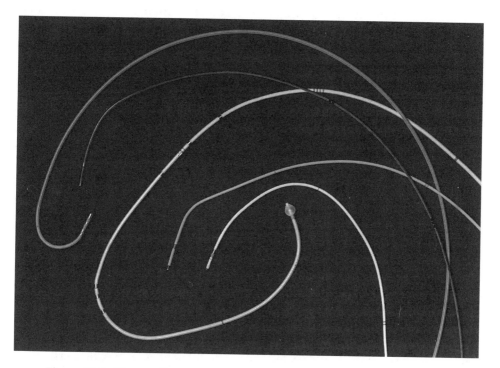

Figure 24-1 Types of temporary pacing catheters. (From left to right) 6-Fr steerable quadripolar; 5-Fr standard straight; 7-Fr balloon tip pressure monitoring with ventricular pacing (distal electrode pair) and atrial pacing (proximal three metal rings) for AV sequential pacing; 5-Fr angled or curved bipolar catheter; and 5-Fr balloon tip (deflated) flow-directed pacing.

caught on the moderator band and right ventricular trabeculations. If this occurs, the operator should withdraw the tip and enter through the valve from a more cephalad and anterior direction. The lead will take a gentle arc through the tricuspid valve and be pointed inferiorly. There should be a minimal amount of lead movement with systole. Catheter movement should be tested by the patient deep-breathing and coughing. For a short procedure, some operators prefer to use an angled catheter and place it in the right ventricular outflow or inflow tract. This is not a stable position if the patient leaves the laboratory with the catheter in place.

Placement of the catheter from the superior approach is similar in technique. The tip is advanced to the tricuspid valve and turned either clockwise or counterclockwise to direct the tip anteriorly. Sometimes the catheter is too straight and cannot be directed anteriorly. One may either use a flow-directed balloon-tipped catheter at this point or attempt to catch the tip in the hepatic vein. Gentle pressure is applied and the catheter torqued, allowing the middle portion to prolapse across the valve into the right ventricle. The catheter is then pulled back, and counterclockwise rotation is applied as the tip is freed up. This will generally place the tip of the catheter in the inflow tract directed posteriorly toward the outflow tract. The catheter is then advanced with clockwise rotation, directing it anteriorly away from the septum. The final advancement requires counterclockwise rotation. This will cause the tip to edge down the septum to the apex. A common mistake is to leave the tip superiorly with the tip pointing up or horizontally. Stable position is with the tip deflected inferiorly and again with minimal movement in systole.

Stable temporary atrial leads require a good bit of experience and are best placed with fluoroscopic assistance. The right atrium is the easiest chamber to reach and pace quickly, but stable pacing position is usually found within the atrial appendage. Temporary tined atrial leads are not widely available, and so one must rely on placement within the atrial appendage. This is best achieved when the catheter has a J-tipped deflection for the superior approach or a Cournand-type curve for the femoral approach. Steerable electrophysiologic recording and pacing catheters are particularly useful if the atrial appendage is not present and an alternative right atrial site is needed. The atrial appendage is directed anteriorly above the tricuspid annulus. Its motion, however, is horizontal in anteroposterior fluoroscopy. Multiple planes are frequently helpful in verifying stable location. Again, movement with coughing and deep breathing should be tested. The coronary sinus in its proximal portion courses along the left atrium, and atrial pacing may be performed. More distally, the coronary sinus crosses over the left ventricle, and ventricular pacing may be performed. The threshold in the coronary sinus is frequently high, but in many patients it may be a more stable location than the atrial appendage. The pacing threshold difference between atrial and ventricular pacing may be so narrow that atrial capture and ventricular capture occur simultaneously, thus losing the advantage of AV synchrony.

Once a catheter is in stable position, threshold testing should be performed. Temporary pacing leads are constructed so that the distal electrode is universally used as the cathode (− for negative terminal) and the ring is used as the anode (+ for positive terminal). The pacing catheter is attached through a connecting cable to a temporary pacemaker. Most temporary pacemakers are constant current devices with a fixed pulse width of 0.5 milliseconds (Fig 24-2). Pacing is usually started at 10 to 15 beats faster than the intrinsic rate with a 5-mA output. If asystole or extreme bradycardia is present, the pacing is performed at 70 beats per minute (bpm). If capture is not present at this output, repositioning should be performed. Once capture is demonstrated at 5 mA, the current is slowly decreased and the monitor is observed for loss of capture. The threshold is defined as the lowest capturing current. Pacing thresholds should

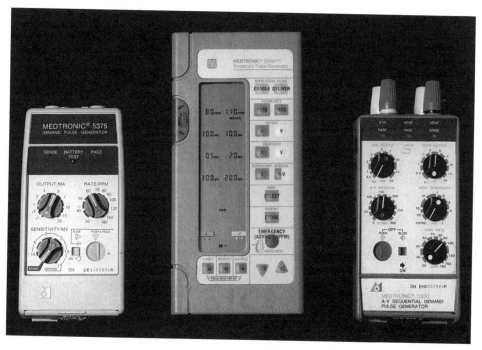

Figure 24-2 Types of temporary pacemakers. At the left is the standard single-chamber demand pacemaker with controls for current strength, rate, and sensitivity settings. In the middle is a fully programmable AV sequential pacemaker that is able to pace in most common modes at variable rates and AV intervals. At the right is the standard dual-chamber pacemaker. The mode is not programmable and operates as a DVI pacemaker. Only the ventricular rate is sensed while pacing is performed in the ventricle and atrium. There is a wide range of programmable AV delays.

be less than 1 mA. Pacing is then set at two- or threefold the threshold to ensure a safety margin. Pacing at higher current strengths poses a risk of induction of ventricular fibrillation, especially in the ischemic myocardium.[20]

Sensing thresholds are tested by setting the pacing rate at 10 to 20 bpm less than the intrinsic rate. The pacemaker is set at the most sensitive setting and gradually decreased until asynchronous pacing is identified. A 50% margin of safety is then set.

After adequate pacing and sensing thresholds are determined, the pacing catheters and the connections are secured. If dual-chamber pacing is being performed, the AV interval will need to be programmed. A default of 150 milliseconds is frequently used, but the optimal AV delay may be longer if the intrinsic QRS needs to be monitored, or less if ventricular compliance is low.

The most serious complications from transvenous pacing are from vascular or myocardial damage. The subclavian and jugular approaches may be additionally complicated by a pneumothorax. The laboratory needs to be prepared to deal with these complications by having chest tube and pericardiocentesis trays available. Cardiac perforation has been reported to be as high as 20% in long-term temporary pacing.[21] The incidence of this complication is probably lower now with the development of small, more flexible catheters. In a patient who requires temporary, prolonged, and intense anticoagulation, cardiac perforation should be diligently anticipated. The most frequent finding is inappropriate pacing with loss of sensing and an increase in the pacing thresholds. Fluoroscopy will help define if the catheter has been pulled back or advanced through the epicardium. Cardiac perforation is usually associated with chest pain in the conscious patient.

Transthoracic Pacing

Transthoracic pacing has little utilization in the catheterization laboratory with the availability of fluoroscopy. Although access is quickly achieved, the great potential for pericardial hemorrhage, tamponade, pneumothorax, and lead instability makes it an unattractive choice of pacing. A variety of kits are available, however. The right ventricle is entered by using a left parasternal approach as in pericardiocentesis. A bipolar wire lead is advanced as far as possible through the needle. The needle is withdrawn, and the wire is connected to the pacemaker. The anodal ring is ideally placed on the epicardial surface, but any subcutaneous position is adequate. If capture is not possible, the wire is manipulated and gradually withdrawn until capture occurs or the wire is pulled out of the chest.

Alternative Pacing

The mechanical pacing option is frequently overlooked by the inexperienced angiographer. A precordial thump can generate enough myocardial depolarization to cause ventricular contraction. It need not be hard, but sequential precordial thumps are obviously distressing to the patient. The previously mentioned coughing maneuver can generate extrathoracic pressures adequate to maintain consciousness for 30 to 60 seconds. Frequently overlooked options available to the angiographer for short-term emergent heart rate support include direct mechanical stimulation of the heart. When heart block and asystole occur during the crossing of the aortic valve, the first impulse is to withdraw the catheter. By jiggling the catheter against the left ventricular myocardium, ventricular ectopic beats at a sufficient rate may be induced for a period long enough to establish a more stable pacing arrangement. If the catheter is withdrawn, recrossing the aortic valve during asystole may not be possible. The guidewire may be advanced through the end-hole catheter and be used as a unipolar catheter with a skin electrode similar to the transthoracic pacing concept. This is frequently associated with high pacing thresholds but can be more stable than catheter manipulation. Epicardial unipolar pacing may be performed through the coronary artery with an angioplasty guidewire in a similar fashion.

Antitachycardia Pacing

Several tachycardia rhythms of either automatic or reentrant mechanism may be terminated by rapid pacing. Generally, this involves pacing the chamber in which the reentrant circuit exists. For atrial tachycardias, atrial flutter, or AV nodal reentrant tachycardia, rapid atrial pacing is extremely effective at termination. If ventricular tachycardia is stable enough to place a pacing catheter, pace termination is the preferred method of termination.

Regardless of the type of tachycardia, overdrive pacing is usually initiated at 10 to 20 bpm faster than the tachycardia. For some rhythms, this may require pacing at very fast rates (e.g., 300 bpm). If possible, a quadripolar catheter, which allows both pacing and recording of intracardiac signals, is helpful. It can be difficult to be sure of myocardial capture with some of the rapid atrial beats from surface tracings (Fig 24-3). Pacing is continued until capture is achieved for 4 to 6 beats. Then, pacing is abruptly turned off, and assessment of efficacy is made. If the tachycardia continues, pacing can be extended in duration or increased in rate. The major complication of this technique is the acceleration of the rhythm to an unstable faster tachycardia or fibrillation. Therefore, cardiac defibrillation needs to be available immediately when overdrive termination is being performed. Pacing cardioversion has the advantage over DC cardioversion because sedation is not required and because posttachycardia pauses can be treated immediately with physiologic pacing.

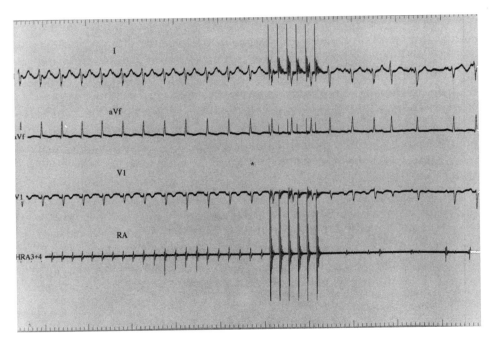

Figure 24-3 Pace termination of atrial flutter with 2:1 AV block. Shown are surface lead I, aVf, and V1, along with an intracardiac recording from a quadripolar pacing catheter in the right atrium (RA). Six pacing impulses are seen, delivered at a rate 10 bpm faster than the atrial rate (asterisk). Note how atrial activity is difficult to discern from the surface tracings, especially during atrial burst pacing. Intracardiac tracings aid in the determination of the proper pacing rate, and myocardial capture is more easily identified.

SELECTED READINGS

1. Dreifus LS, Fisch C, Griffin JC, et al. Guidelines for implantation of cardiac pacemakers and antiarrhythmia devices. A report of the American College of Cardiology/American Heart Association Task Force on assessment of diagnostic and therapeutic procedures. J Am Coll Cardiol 1991;18:1–13.

2. Braunwald E, Swan HJC, eds. Cooperative study on cardiac catheterization. Circulation 1968;1(suppl III):1.

3. Sprung CL, Elser B, Schein RMH, et al. Risks of right bundle branch block and complete heart block during pulmonary artery catheterization. Crit Care Med 1989; 17:1–3.

4. Morris D, Mulvihill D, Lew WYW, et al. Risk of developing complete heart block during bedside pulmonary artery catheterization in patients with left bundle branch block. Arch Intern Med 1987;14:2005–2010.

5. Trankina MF, White RD. Perioperative cardiac pacing using an atrioventricular pacing pulmonary artery catheter. J Cardiothorac Anesth 1989;3:154–162.

6. Harvey JR, Wyman RM, McKay RG, Baim DS. Use of balloon flotation catheters for prophylactic temporary pacing during diagnostic and therapeutic catheterization procedures. Am J Cardiol 1988;62:941–944.

7. Sowton GE, Balcon R, Cross D, Frick MH. Measurement of the angina threshold using atrial pacing. Cardiovasc Res 1967;1:301–307.

8. Parker JO, Chiong MA, West RO, Case RB. Sequential alterations in myocardial lactate metabolism, S-T segments, and left ventricular function during angina induced by atrial pacing. Circulation 1969;40:113–131.

9. Rios JC, Herwitz LE. Electrocardiographic responses to atrial pacing and multistage treadmill testing. Correlation with coronary anatomy. Am J Cardiol 1974;34: 661–666.

10. Fananapazir L, Cannon RO III, Tripodi D, et al. Impact of dual-chamber permanent pacings in patients with obstructive hypertrophic cardiomyopathy with symptoms refractory to verapamil and B-adrenergic blocker therapy. Circulation 1992;85: 2149–2161.

11. Brecker SJD, Xiao HB, Sparrow J, et al. Effects of dual chamber pacing with short atrioventricular delay in dilated cardiomyopathy. Lancet 1992;340:1308–1312.

12. Zoll PM. Noninvasive cardiac stimulation revisited. PACE 1990;13:2014–2016.

13. Zoll PM, Zoll RH, Falk RH, et al. External noninvasive temporary cardiac pacing: clinical trials. Circulation 1985;71:937–944.

14. Klein LS, Miles WM, Heger JJ, et al. Transcutaneous pacing: patient tolerance, strength interval relations, and feasibility for programmed electrical stimulation. Am J Cardiol 1988;62:1126–1129.

15. Gallagher JJ, Smith WM, Kerr CR, et al. Esophageal pacing: a diagnostic and therapeutic tool. Circulation 1982;65:336–341.

16. Guarnerio M, Furlanello, Del Greco M, et al. Transesophageal atrial pacing: a first choice technique in atrial flutter therapy. Am Heart J 1989;117:1241–1252.

17. Benson DW JR, Dunnigan A, Sterba R, Benditt D. Atrial pacing from the esophagus in the diagnosis and management of tachycardia: role of transesophageal pacing. Pediatrics 1983;102:40–46.

18. Hynes JK, Holmes DR, Harrison CE. Five year experience with temporary pacemaker therapy in the coronary care unit. Mayo Clinic Proc 1983;58:122–126.

19. Nolewajka AJ, Goddard MD, Brown TC. Temporary transvenous pacing and femoral vein thrombosis. Circulation 1980;62:646–650.

20. Merx W, Han J, Yoon M. Effects of unipolar cathodal and bipolar stimulation of vulnerability of ischemic ventricles to fibrillation. Am J Cardiol 1975;35:37–41.

21. Silver MD, Goldschlager N. Temporary transvenous pacing in the critical care setting. Chest 1988; 93:607–613.

APPENDIX

CONVERSION FACTORS
AND NORMAL VALUES FOR
COMMONLY USED VARIABLES

I. Conversion factors

millimeter (mm)	= 0.001 m	=	0.039 inches	= 0.33 Fr
micron (μ)	= 0.001 mm			
millimeters of mercury (mm Hg)	= 13.6 mm H_2O	=	1337.7 dynes cm^{-2}	
atmosphere (atm)	= 760 mm Hg	=	14.6 lb/sq in	
French (Fr)	= 0.33 mm	=	0.013 inches	

II. Normal values of pressure, flow, and resistance

A. Normal values of cardiac pressures

	Systolic	Diastolic	a wave	v wave	Early DP	End DP	Mean
RA			2–10	2–10			0–8
RV	15–30				0–2	0–8	
PA	15–30	5–15					10–15
LA(PCW)			4–16	4–16			2–12
LV	100–140				0–4	4–12	
Ao	100–140	60–86					70–100

Abbreviations: Ao, aortic; DP, diastolic pressure; LA, left atrial; LV, left ventricular; PA, pulmonary arterial; PCW, pulmonary capillary wedge; RA, right atrial; RV, right ventricular.

B. Normal values for cardiac flow

	Range
Cardiac output (liters/min)	5.2–7.4
Cardiac index (liters/min/m²)	2.5–4.2
Stroke volume (ml/beat)	70–94
Stroke index (ml/beat/m²)	30–65
Ateriovenous oxygen difference (O_2 vols %)	4.0–5.5
Oxygen consumption index (liters O_2/min/m²)	110–140

C. Resistances (dynes-sec-cm^{-5})

	Range
Systemic	900–1500
Pulmonary vascular (arteriolar)	50–150
Total pulmonary	100–300

III. Other cardiac variables

	Range
LV ejection fraction (%)	50–80
LV diastolic volume index (ml/m^2)*	50–90
LV systolic volume index (ml/m^2)*	20–40
Heart rate	60–100

Normal values are based on a review of the medical literature.

*Each catheterization laboratory should determine its normal values for this parameter. (Normal values are based on biplane area-length or Simpson's rule calculation.)

We have attempted to determine the conversion factor for "gauge," as in "18-gauge needle." In fact, there is no constant. Each gauge needle is different in size and described in standardized tables.

INDEX